Target Organ Toxicology Series

Toxicology of the Kidney

Second Edition

Target Organ Toxicology Series

Series Editors
A. Wallace Hayes, John A. Thomas, and Donald E. Gardner

Toxicology of the Kidney, Second Edition
Jerry B. Hook and Robin S. Goldstein, editors, 576 pp., 1993

Cardiovascular Toxicology, Second Edition
Daniel Acosta, Jr., editor, 576 pp., 1992

Ophthalmic Toxicology
George C. Y. Chiou, editor, 352 pp., 1992

Neurotoxicology
Hugh A. Tilson and Clifford L. Mitchell, editors, 416 pp., 1992

Toxicology of the Lung
Donald E. Gardner, James D. Crapo, and Edward J. Massaro, editors, 540 pp., 1988

Endocrine Toxicology
John A. Thomas, Kenneth S. Korach, and John A. McLachlan, editors, 414 pp., 1985

Immunotoxicology and Immunopharmacology
Jack H. Dean, Michael I. Luster, Albert E. Munson, and Harry Amos, editors, 528 pp., 1985

*__Reproductive Toxicology__
Robert L. Dixon, editor, 368 pp., 1985

Toxicology of the Blood and Bone Marrow
Richard D. Irons, editor, 192 pp., 1985

Toxicology of the Eye, Ear, and Other Special Senses
A. Wallace Hayes, editor, 264 pp., 1985

*__Toxicology of the Immune System__
Jack H. Dean and Albert E. Munson, editors, 528 pp., 1985

Cutaneous Toxicity
Victor A. Drill and Paul Lazar, editors, 288 pp., 1984

Intestinal Toxicology
Carol M. Schiller, editor, 252 pp., 1984

Cardiovascular Toxicology
Ethard W. Van Stee, editor, 400 pp., 1982

---

*Out of print.

Target Organ Toxicology Series

Toxicology of the Kidney

Second Edition

Editors

Jerry B. Hook, Ph.D.
Senior Vice President and Director,
Development
Research and Development
SmithKline Beecham Pharmaceuticals
King of Prussia, Pennsylvania

Robin S. Goldstein, Ph.D.
Assistant Director, Biochemical Toxicology
Research and Development
SmithKline Beecham Pharmaceuticals
King of Prussia, Pennsylvania

Raven Press New York

Raven Press, Ltd., 1185 Avenue of the Americas, New York, New York 10036

Made in the United States of America

Library of Congress Cataloging-in-Publication Data

Toxicology of the kidney / editors, Jerry B. Hook, Robin S. Goldstein.
—2nd ed.
p. cm.
Includes bibliographical references and index.
ISBN 0-88167-885-6
1. Nephrotoxicology. I. Hook, Jerry B. II. Goldstein, Robin S.
[DNLM: 1. Kidney—drug effects. 2. Kidney Diseases—chemically induced. 3. Kidney Function Tests. WJ 300 T755]
RC918.N45T68 1992
616.6′1—dc20
DNLM/DLC
for Library of Congress 92-49644
CIP

The material contained in this volume was submitted as previously unpublished material, except in the instances in which some of the illustrative material was derived.

Great care has been taken to maintain the accuracy of the information contained in the volume. However, neither Raven Press nor the editors can be held responsible for errors or for any consequences arising from the use of the information contained herein.

9 8 7 6 5 4 3 2 1

Contents

Contributing Authors

Mauro Abbate, M.D. *Mario Negri Institute for Pharmacological Research, Via Gavazzeni 11, 24100 Bergamo, Italy*

George L. Bakris, M.D., F.A.C.P. *Renal Division, University of Texas, Health Science Center, 7703 Floyd-Curl Drive, San Antonio, Texas 78284-7882*

William M. Bennett, M.D. *Division of Nephrology and Hypertension, Department of Medicine, Oregon Health Sciences University, 3181 SW Sam Jackson Park Road, Portland, Oregon 97201-3098*

William O. Berndt, Ph.D. *Department of Pharmacology, College of Medicine, University of Nebraska Medical Center, 600 South 42nd Street, Omaha, Nebraska 68198-6810*

Richard F. Borch, M.D., Ph.D. *Department of Pharmacology, University of Rochester Medical Center, School of Medicine and Dentistry, 601 Elmwood Avenue, Rochester, New York 14642*

Mayer Brezis, M.D. *Department of Medicine, Hadassah University Hospital, Mount Scopus, Jerusalem, Israel*

E. A. Conner, Ph.D *Program in Toxicology, University of Maryland, 660 West Redwood Street, Baltimore, Maryland 21201-1596*

Daniel R. Dietrich, Ph.D. *Institute of Toxicology, Swiss Federal Institute of Technology and University of Zurich, CH-8603 Schwerzenbach, Switzerland*

Geoffrey G. Duggin, M.D., F.R.A.C.P. *Toxicology Unit, Royal Prince Alfred Hospital, Missenden Road, Camperdown NSW. 2050, Australia*

Adnan A. Elfarra, Ph.D. *Department of Comparative Biosciences, University of Wisconsin, School of Veterinary Medicine, 2015 Linden Drive West, Madison, Wisconsin 53706*

Franklin H. Epstein, M.D. *Department of Medicine, Beth Israel Hospital, and the Harvard Center for the Study of Kidney Diseases, Harvard Medical School, 25 Shattuck Street, Boston, Massachusetts 02215*

Ernest C. Foulkes, Ph.D. *Department of Environmental Health, University of Cincinnati College of Medicine, 3223 Eden Avenue, Cincinnati, Ohio 45267-0056*

B. A. Fowler, Ph.D. *Program in Toxicology, University of Maryland, 660 West Redwood Street, Baltimore, Maryland 21201-1596*

Robin S. Goldstein, Ph.D. *Department of Toxicology, SmithKline Beecham Pharmaceuticals, 709 Swedeland Road, King of Prussia, Pennsylvania 19406*

Lewis B. Kinter, Ph.D. *Departments of Investigative Toxicology and Experimental Pathology, SmithKline Beecham Pharmaceuticals, 709 Swedeland Road, King of Prussia, Pennsylvania 19406*

Serrine S. Lau, Ph.D. *Division of Pharmacology and Toxicology, College of Pharmacy, The University of Texas at Austin, Room 5.112, Austin, Texas 78712*

Lois D. Lehman-McKeeman, Ph.D. *Human and Environmental Safety Division, Miami Valley Laboratories, Procter and Gamble Company, P.O. Box 398707, Cincinnati, Ohio 45239-8707*

Daniela Macconi, Ph.D. *Mario Negri Institute for Pharmacological Research, Via Gavazzeni, 11, 24100 Bergamo, Italy*

Terrence J. Monks, Ph.D. *Division of Pharmacology and Toxicology, College of Pharmacy, The University of Texas at Austin, Room 5.112, Austin, Texas 78712*

Steen Olsen, M.D., Ph.D. *University Institute of Pathology, Aarhus Kommunehospital, DK-8000 Aarhus C, Denmark*

George A. Porter, M.D., F.A.C.P. *Division of Nephrology and Hypertension, Department of Medicine, Oregon Health Sciences University, 3181 SW Sam Jackson Park Road, Portland, Oregon 97201-3098*

Lorraine C. Racusen, M.D. *Department of Pathology, The Johns Hopkins University School of Medicine, 725 North Wolfe Street, Baltimore, Maryland 21205*

Giuseppe Remuzzi, M.D. *Mario Negri Institute for Pharmacological Research, Via Gavazzeni, 11, 24100 Bergamo, Italy, and Division of Nephrology, Ospedali Rianiti di Bergamo, 24100 Bergamo, Italy*

Brian G. Short, D.V.M., Ph.D. *Departments of Investigative Toxicology and Experimental Pathology, SmithKline Beecham Pharmaceuticals, 709 Swedeland Road, King of Prussia, Pennsylvania 19406*

Kim Solez, M.D., F.R.C.P.C. *Department of Pathology, The University of Alberta, Room 53402, Walter Mackenzie Health Sciences Center, 8440 112 Street, Edmonton, Alberta, Canada T6G 2R7*

James A. Swenberg, D.V.M., Ph.D. *Departments of Environmental Sciences and Engineering and Pathology, University of North Carolina, Chapel Hill, North Carolina 27599–7095*

Bruce M. Tune, M.D. *Laboratory of Renal Pharmacology, Division of Nephrology, Department of Pediatrics, Stanford University School of Medicine, 300 Pasteur Drive, Stanford, California 94305-5119*

Jan J. Weening, M.D. *Department of Pathology, University of Amsterdam, Academic Medical Center, Meibergdreef 9, 1105 AZ Amsterdam, The Netherlands*

Preface

The kidney plays a vital role in certain endocrine functions. Abnormalities caused by toxic chemicals or other interventions can have profound effects on these functions and, consequently, on total body function. Nevertheless, the predominant "work" of the kidney is reabsorption of filtered nutrients, salts, and water in appropriate proportions to maintain fluid and electrolyte balance in the body. As a result, the two human kidneys filter upwards of 180 liters a day, reabsorbing between 98 and 99 percent and eliminating the remainder as waste material in water. These multiple reabsorptive functions are highly energy dependent and, as such, are vulnerable to chemically-induced injury. Fortunately, the kidneys have considerable reserve and can repair a significant amount of damage. But when injury is massive and acute, or chronic in nature, to the degree that regenerative capacity is overwhelmed, the consequences to the total organism are profound.

The dynamic nature of kidney function is inextricably linked to its highly complicated structure. At every level of complexity, ranging from the clear demarcation of cortex and medulla, endothelial-rich blood vessels and epithelial tubules, proximal and distal tubules, S1, S2, and S3 cell types of the proximal tubule to mitochondria and endoplasmic reticulum, kidney structure and its attendant biochemistry support very specific functions. From an understanding of the specificity of anatomy, biochemistry, and physiology comes an understanding of site-selective toxicity and its relationship to total organ and body function.

Fortunately for the toxicologist, there are many correlations between nephrotoxicity seen in animals and in humans. In several cases, conditions previously thought to be renal disease in humans upon close examination have been shown to reflect chemically-induced injury. A major theme of this edition is the correlation between renal injury in humans and animals and how knowledge from one species can be transferred to another, thus supporting the use of animal models to understand the mechanisms and potential risks of chemical exposure to humans.

This edition is focused initially on an understanding of the correlation between anatomy, biochemistry, and physiology of the kidney and how this is related to normal renal functions, and how we assess those functions. From there we develop the concepts of clinical nephrotoxicity and renal failure in humans and how animal models can be used to understand the mechanisms of human renal disease. Further emphasis is placed on the correlation between biochemical heterogeneity within the kidney and site-specific nephrotoxicity, followed by mechanistic definitions of specific classes of nephrotoxicants ranging from human drugs and diagnostic agents to a variety of toxicants found in the environment. Last, we include a major chapter on the mechanisms of renal carcinogenesis.

It is our intention that this edition will serve as an introduction for some, a review for others, and a text for many. But, most important, we hope it serves as a stimulus for all to continue in this important work of understanding the mechanisms of chemically-induced injury to the kidney.

Jerry B. Hook
Robin S. Goldstein

Acknowledgments

The editors are indebted to each of the contributors for providing outstanding chapters. We also wish to express our sincere gratitude to Marie Iacovelli for her invaluable assistance and administrative support in this endeavor.

Target Organ Toxicology Series

Toxicology of the Kidney

Second Edition

Toxicology of the Kidney, Second Edition,
edited by Jerry B. Hook and Robin S. Goldstein.
Raven Press, Ltd., New York © 1993.

1

Anatomy and Physiology of the Kidney

A Brief Review

Lewis B. Kinter and Brian G. Short

Departments of Investigative Toxicology and Experimental Pathology, SmithKline Beecham Pharmaceuticals, King of Prussia, Pennsylvania 19406

Over a century ago the French physician and physiologist Claude Bernard noted that higher animals "have really two environments: an external environment (milieu exterieur) in which the organism is situated, and an internal environment (milieu interieur) in which the tissue elements live" (1). Bernard recognized that although the external environment was variable and beyond the control of vital mechanisms, "all the vital mechanisms, however varied they may be, have only one object, that of preserving constant the conditions of life in the internal environment." During the past 50 years our knowledge of the pivotal role of the kidneys in the regulation of the volume and composition of Bernard's "milieu interieur" has increased to include molecular descriptions of mechanisms involved, and during the past 25 years, coincident with elucidation of the mechanisms of renal functions, an increasingly detailed understanding and appreciation of the mechanisms of chemical-induced renal toxicity has emerged.

The unusual susceptibility of the mammalian kidney to the adverse effects of toxicants can be attributed in large measure to the anatomic, physiological, and biochemical features of the kidney. The disproportionately large blood flow to the kidneys, which both supports the high rate of glomerular filtration and sustains the high rate of renal metabolism, results in greater exposure of the kidneys to blood-borne chemicals. During the process of solute and water reabsorption along the nephron, the tubular fluid becomes enriched in those chemicals that remain in the urine, thus exposing the cells of the nephron to potentially high concentrations of toxicants. Chemicals with low aqueous solubilities may precipitate or crystallize in the tubular fluid of the distal nephron and obstruct the nephron and/or destroy the integrity of the tubular epithelium. Chemicals may contribute both directly and indirectly to calculus formation in the renal pelvis and urinary bladder. Chemicals that are substrates for one of the organic solute transport systems may accumulate within and damage the cells of the proximal tubule. Intrinsic metabolism of nontoxic chemicals can produce toxic metabolites within the kidneys. Finally, chemicals may directly or indirectly interrupt one or more essential cellular functions resulting in damage to kidney structures and functions. This chapter summarizes current concepts of renal morphology and physiology that underpin the discussions of renal toxicology that follow in subsequent chapters. The reader is referred to several excellent modern texts for more comprehensive discussions of the topics presented in this chapter.

The kidneys are paired, bean-shaped organs that lie next to the spine in the retroperitoneal cavity. The kidneys consist of 10^4 to 10^6 or more nephrons (depending upon species), each nephron contacting the renal blood flow at its proximal end (the glomerulus), and each coalescing at its distal end with other nephrons before terminating at the tip of the renal papilla in the renal pelvis. The glomerular filtrate, an ultrafiltrate of plasma that leaves the cardiovascular compartment and enters the nephrons, represents ~20% of the normal renal plasma flow and, hence, 2% to 3% of the normal cardiac output. The final urine excreted by the kidneys is generally $< 1\%$ of the original glomerular filtrate and contains the excess solutes, wastes, and unreabsorbed toxicants concentrated within its volume. Greater than 99% of the glomerular filtrate is reabsorbed by the nephrons and returned to the circulation each day. This seemingly inefficient process of mass filtration and reabsorption is the basis of a continuous iterative process by which the kidneys excrete, over a period of hours to days, exactly the balance between water and solute intake and metabolic, fecal, and insensitive water and solute losses so as to maintain the volume and composition of the extracellular fluid constant at fixed set-points.

The kidneys regulate both the volume and composition of the extracellular fluid by regulating the renal excretion of its solutes and water. The physiological significance of renal regulation of the extracellular fluid is illustrated in Guyton's (2) description of the critical dependence of arterial blood pressure upon renal solute excretion (the renal function curve). The relationship is a basis for understanding the central role of the kidneys in the regulation of blood pressure.

In addition to their principal functions as osmoregulatory organs and their participation in the regulation of arterial pressure, the kidneys produce erythropoietin, a hormone regulating the production of erythrocytes (3). The kidneys hydroxylate 25-OH-cholecalciferol at either the 1α or 24 position to form two vitamin D metabolites with different potencies to promote bone resorption and calcium and phosphorus absorption from the gut (4). The kidneys release renin into the circulation and regulate the activity of the peripheral renin-angiotensin-aldosterone system (5). The kidneys regulate acid-base balance (6). Finally, the kidneys produce many autocoids and cytokines, which act to modify renal biochemical pathways and functions (7). These functions may be impacted indirectly as a result of chemical-induced nephrotoxicity.

ANATOMY OF THE MAMMALIAN KIDNEY

Structural Organization

The simple unipapillary kidney is found in the majority of small mammals such as the rat and rabbit. The crest kidney is found in moderate-sized mammals such as the cat, dog, and sheep. A multipapillary kidney is present in humans and pigs. The renal cortex of the unipapillary and crest kidney surrounds the pyramid-shaped renal medulla. The papilla, the bottom portion of the medulla, projects into the renal pelvis. The relationship between kidney size and number of papillae is shown in Table 1. The renal pelvis represents the expanded upper extension of the ureter.

The cortical parenchyma is divided into the cortical labyrinth and medullary rays (Fig. 1). Despite their name, the medullary rays are actually a part of the cortex. The medulla is divided into the outer and inner medulla. The outer medulla in the rat, but not in the dog, is subdivided into the outer and inner stripes (OSOM and ISOM), and the junction between these two zones is often erroneously referred to as the corticomedullary junction. The innermost part of the inner medulla forms the papilla.

Nephron Topography

Cortex

The cortical labyrinth contains the interlobular vessels, glomeruli, proximal and distal convoluted tubules, connecting tubules, initial collecting tubules, and rich capillary networks (Fig. 2). The medullary rays contain the proximal and distal straight tubules and collecting ducts. Generally the straight tubules of superficial nephrons are more centrally located within the medullary rays, whereas those of juxtamedullary nephrons occupy a more peripheral position.

Outer Medulla

The outer stripe contains the terminal segments of the proximal straight tubules, the ascending limbs, and the collecting ducts. This region is further characterized by

TABLE 1. *Relationship between kidney size and the number of papillae/kidney*[a]

Parameter	Gerbil	Rat	Rabbit	Sheep	Pig	Cow
Kidney weight (g)	0.3	1	9	45	130	400
No. of papillae	1	1	1	5	7	15

[a]The table documents average individual kidney weights and the average number of papillae (renalomedullary pyramids) per kidney. (C. Sarmousakis, unpublished data.)

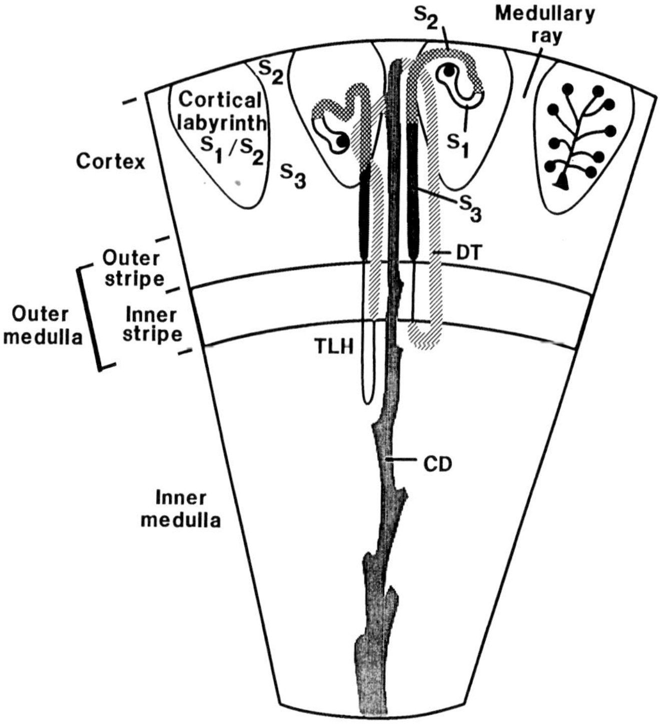

FIG. 1. Schematic diagram of the kidney illustrating topographical location of nephrons and collecting duct within various regions of the rat kidney. Note the location of S_1 and early S_2 segments within the cortical labyrinth, the late S_2 segments within the tips of the medullary rays, and the S_3 segments within the base of the medullary rays and outer stripe of the outer medulla. TLH, thin limb of Henle; DT, distal tubule; CD, collecting duct (69).

the absence of the thin limbs of Henle. The inner stripe contains thin descending limbs, thick ascending limbs, and collecting ducts. There are no straight segments of the proximal tubule in the inner stripe. Vascular bundles, which are cone-shaped aggregations of descending and ascending vasa recta, develop in the outer stripe, but are more prominent in the inner stripe. The descending limbs of short loops descend within vascular bundles in animals with a high urine concentrating ability, such as the rat. Significant countercurrent exchange processes occur between ascending vasa recta and the thin descending limbs of short loops.

Inner Medulla

Species with a high urine concentrating ability have a prominent inner medulla. The inner medulla contains thin descending and ascending limbs of long loops and collecting ducts and is characterized by the absence of thick ascending limbs.

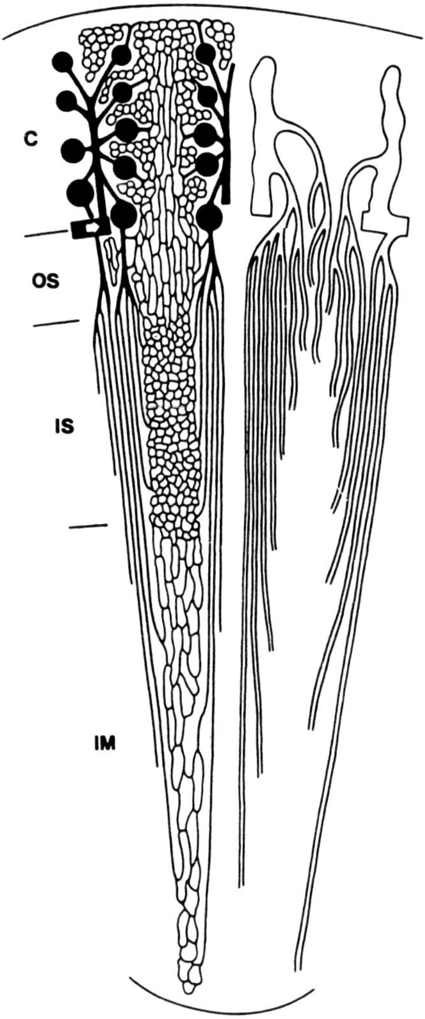

FIG. 2. Schematic diagram of the microvasculature of the rat kidney. The left side shows the arterial vessels and capillaries. An arcuate artery (*arrow*) gives rise to an interlobular artery, from which afferent arterioles originate to supply the glomeruli. The vasa efferentia of the juxtamedullary glomeruli descend into the medulla and divide into the descending vasa recta, which, together with ascending vasa recta, form the vascular bundles of the renal medulla. At intervals, descending vasa recta leave the bundles to feed the adjacent capillaries. The right side shows the venous vessels. The interlobular veins start in the superficial cortex. In the inner cortex, they, together with the arcuate veins, receive the ascending vasa recta from the medulla. The vasa recta ascending from the inner medulla all traverse the inner stripe within the vascular bundles, whereas most of the vasa recta from the inner stripe ascend outside the bundles. Both of these types of ascending vasa recta traverse the outer stripe as wide, tortuous channels. C, cortex; OS, outer stripe; IS, inner stripe; IM, inner medulla (8).

Renal Vasculature

Within the renal sinus, the single renal artery divides into several interlobar arteries, which enter the renal tissue at the border between the cortex and medulla. Interlobular arteries branch from the arcuate arteries and ascend into the cortex. As the interlobular arteries ascend, they give rise to the afferent arterioles that supply the glomerular capillaries of the renal corpuscle. The glomerular capillaries converge to form the efferent arteriole, which exits from the renal corpuscle. The efferent arterioles of midcortical and superficial renal corpuscles give rise to a highly complex and tortuous peritubular capillary network associated with the cortical convoluted proximal and distal tubules. In contrast, the efferent arterioles draining juxtamedullary renal corpuscles form the descending vasa recta, which descend into the medulla, giving rise to capillaries at various levels. The blood flow to the medulla is much less in volume and is slower than that in the cortex. The cells in the medulla depend on glycolysis to supply energy because oxygen tension is lower in the medulla than the cortex. The juxtaposition of the arterial and venous limbs of the vasa recta creates a countercurrent exchange system that permits rapid equilibration of incoming and outgoing plasma with the increasing axial hypertonicity of the medullary interstitium. This arrangement of capillary loops acts to stabilize the renal concentrating mechanism while returning excess solutes reabsorbed from the segments of Henle's loop and the collecting ducts to the circulation. The ascending vasa recta are the draining vessels of the renal medulla. The descending and ascending vasa recta of the medulla form vascular bundles, which are located beneath the cortical labyrinth. The interbundle regions are located beneath the cortical medullary rays (8,9). The renal veins (interlobular veins, arcuate veins) accompany the corresponding arteries.

The glomerular and postglomerular capillaries of the kidney represent a portal system. The principal resistance vessels are the afferent and efferent arterioles that regulate the inflow and outflow of blood from the glomerular capillary. Regulation of the vascular tone of these arterioles ensures that hydrostatic pressure is relatively constant along the glomerular capillary. Several lines of evidence suggest that the afferent and efferent arterioles are separately regulated. Studies of isolated perfused glomerular arterioles have shown differential responsiveness to many constrictor substances, including catecholamines, peptides (vasopressin, angiotensin), and arachidonic acid metabolites (10,11). Interestingly, both arterioles show similar responsiveness to dopamine and DA_1 agonists, suggesting that the heterogeneity of responsiveness to some constrictors may be of physiological significance (12). Endothelin, another vasoconstrictor peptide, is present along the endothelium of the small and medium-sized blood vessels in all regions of the kidney (13). However, the renal vasoconstrictor effect of endothelin is sustained for several hours, leading most investigators to consider a pathophysiological role, rather than a physiological regulatory role, of the peptide likely (14). Studies of Barajas (15) have shown that both arterioles are innervated; however, whether they are differentially controlled is not known.

Relatively little is known about the physiology of the postglomerular vasculature. In the peritubular capillary network the hydrostatic pressure is $\leq$15% of renal artery pressure and the transcapillary oncotic pressure difference exceeds the prevailing hydraulic pressure difference, thereby favoring fluid absorption into these capillaries (16). It is generally assumed that the postglomerular capillary beds perfuse the proximal and distal convoluted tubules of the parent nephron. This is incorrect. Cortical vascular-tubular relationships have been best described in the dog and human kidneys (17,18). These studies show that except for those convoluted tubule segments in the subcapsular cortex, the efferent peritubular capillary network and the nephron arising from each glomerulus are dissociated. In addition, even though many superficial proximal and distal convoluted tubules are perfused at least in part by peritubular capillaries arising from the parent glomerulus of the same nephron, the loops of Henle of those nephrons, descending into the medullary ray, are perfused successively by blood emerging from many midcortical glomeruli through efferent arterioles that extend into the ray. Nephrons originating from midcortical glomeruli have proximal and distal convoluted tubule segments lying close to the interlobular axis in the region above the glomerulus of origin. This region is perfused by capillaries arising from efferents of more superficial glomeruli. The loops of Henle of midcortical glomeruli are exposed to blood from efferent arterioles of many deeper glomeruli. In the inner cortex, many nephrons arise from glomeruli that have efferent vessels that supply the medulla. The convoluted segments of these nephrons lie above the glomeruli, sometimes within the complex network next to the interlobar axis and sometimes in regions perfused by capillaries of other inner cortical glomeruli. Hence, the organization of cortical tubule segments and their vasculature form a complex continuum along the interlobular axis.

Because of the high percentage of the cardiac output delivered to the kidneys, renal vasculature receives high exposures to circulating toxicants. The polyene antibiotic amphotericin B produces renal vasoconstriction that is maximal during infusion of the drug and is characterized by decreases in renal blood flow and glomerular filtration rate and an increase in renal vascular resistance. The acute toxic effects of amphotericin B on renal hemodynamics may represent a direct effect of the drug on the renal vasculature coupled with a secondary effect on the renal autoregulatory response (19). The frank nephrotoxicity that occurs in response to heavy metal exposures is also likely due, in part, to ischemia secondary to renal vasoconstriction (20). Cyclosporine-induced glomerular dysfunction may involve up-regulation of glomerular endothelin receptors (21).

Nephrons and Collecting Duct Systems

The specific structural units of the kidneys are the nephrons. In the rat, each kidney contains 25,000 to 35,000 nephrons (22). The nephron consists of a renal corpuscle connected to an elongated tubule component composed of the proximal tubule, thin limb of Henle, and the distal tubule. Proximal tubules are composed of a convoluted part in the cortical labyrinth and straight part in the medullary ray and the OSOM (the pars recta, Fig. 1). Precisely at the junction between the OSOM and the ISOM, the proximal tubule abruptly narrows down, becomes thin-walled, and undergoes a radical change in its structure to become the thin limb of Henle. The length of the thin limb of Henle varies among nephrons, and the ascent of thin limbs is limited to a specific subpopulation of nephrons. Distal tubules connect to thin limbs, and are composed of the thick ascending limb; the macula densa, which is part of the juxtaglomerular apparatus; and the distal convoluted tubule. The thick ascending limb arises in the ISOM, enters the cortical medullary rays, and eventually intertwines with its own glomerulus to continue as the macula densa. The macula densa comes into contact with the extraglomerular mesangium and afferent and efferent arterioles. Thereafter, the nephron continues as the distal convoluted tubule, which courses randomly throughout the cortical labyrinth, sometimes in contact with the proximal tubule of the same nephron, and sometimes in contact with the proximal tubules of other nephrons. The collecting ducts are formed in the renal cortex by the joining of distal convoluted tubules of several nephrons via connecting tubules. The collecting ducts descend within the medullary rays, traverse the outer medulla, then fuse successively in the inner medulla. The collecting duct system is not strictly considered to be a part of the nephron, since it is derived from the uretic bud. However, for ease of understanding, the term *nephron* in this chapter means the nephron as well as the entire collecting duct.

Nephron Heterogeneity

Based on the location of the renal corpuscles within the cortex, three types of nephrons are distinguished: superficial, midcortical, and juxtamedullary (23). According to the lengths of the loops of Henle, two types of nephrons are distinguished: short- and long-looped nephrons. Short loops turn back in the outer medulla, near the junction of the inner medulla in the rat. Although short loops descend as thin limbs, they continue into the thick ascending limbs near the hairpin turn. The long loops turn back at successive levels of the inner medulla; only a few reach the tip of the papilla. Long loops have a long descending thin limb extending into the inner medulla and a long ascending thin limb that continues into the thick ascending limb at the border between the inner and outer medulla. The long loops generally belong to the deeper renal corpuscles and the short loops to the more superficially situated corpuscles. Most species have short and long loops; an exception is the dog, which is known to have only long loops. Correlations between the ratio of short and long loops and renal functions (e.g., renal concentrating ability) are not obvious. For example, species with high urine concentrating ability, such as the rat, have greater numbers of short loops than long loops (22).

However, even the designation of superficial, midcortical, and juxtamedullary nephrons vastly understates the true complexity of nephron heterogeneity. In 70 nephrons from a series of human kidneys in which both the glomerulus and the tip of the loop of Henle could be identified, Beeuwkes (personal communication) noted a nearly linear relationship between depth of the glomerulus within the cortex and the depth at which the loop of Henle turned within the medulla (Fig. 3). Beeuwkes also noted a number of loops that actually turned within the cortex and stated that these "cortical loops" tended to originate from the most superficial cortical glomeruli. Conversely, loops that turned most deeply within the papilla tended to originate from juxtamedullary glomeruli.

Hence, the heterogeneity of nephron organization, like the heterogeneity of renal vasculature organization within the kidney, is also most accurately described as a

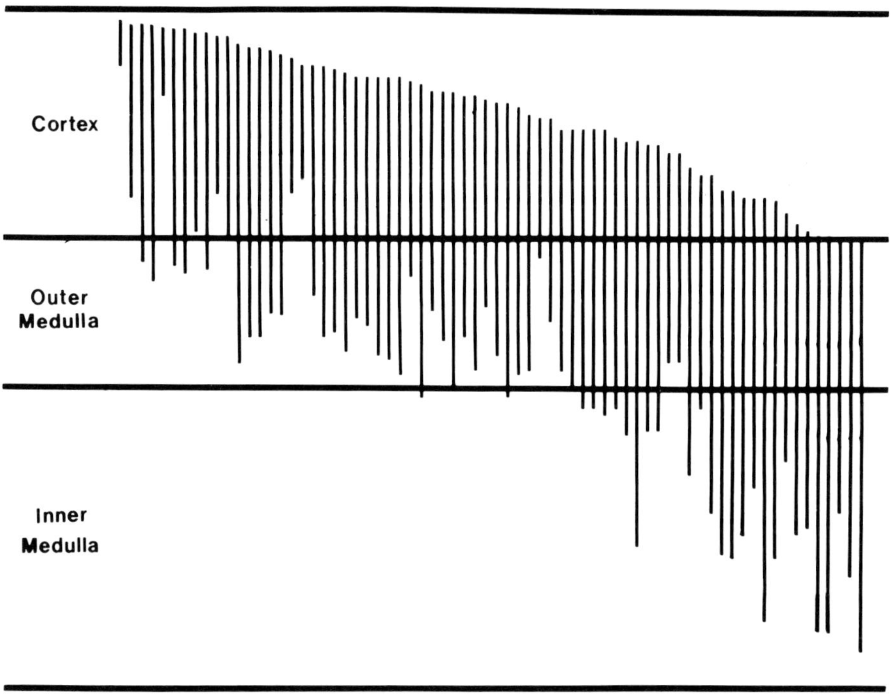

FIG. 3. The positions of the glomeruli and the turning points of their respective loops of Henle for 70 *in situ*–perfused nephrons from a series of human kidneys in which perfusion was sufficient to identify both structures (70).

continuum related to the relative positions of the glomeruli along the interlobular axis. The complementary heterogeneities of the nephrons and their associated vasculature may provide the anatomical basis for observations of shifts in the distribution of cortical blood flow, and suggest that nephrons and/or nephron segments may actually be "recruited" in a complex fashion in response to physiological stimuli (24). The complexity of vascular-tubular relationships in the renal cortex may account for the kidney's resilience to some toxicants while also accounting for the profound disruptions in cortical functions that accompany relatively subtle changes in cortical histology.

STRUCTURE AND FUNCTION OF THE GLOMERULUS

Renal Corpuscle

The renal corpuscle consists of a tuft of specialized capillaries attached to the mesangium, both of which are enclosed in the pouch-like blind extension of the tubule (Fig. 4). Capillaries are covered by epithelial cells, forming the visceral layer of Bowman's capsule (Fig. 5). A central region of mesangial cells is surrounded by mesangial matrix material. A reflection of squamous epithelial cells at the vascular pole, where afferent and efferent arteries enter and exit, becomes the parietal cell layer of Bowman's capsule. Between the two epithelial layers is a narrow cavity called Bowman's space. Although the term *glomerulus* refers to the tuft portion of the renal corpuscle, this term will be used throughout this chapter instead of renal corpuscle to refer to that portion of the nephron composed of the glomerular tuft and Bowman's capsule. The diameter of the glomerulus is approximately 120 μm in the rat (25). Juxtaglomerular renal corpuscles can exceed the diameter of midcortical and superficial nephrons by up to 50%. The filtration barrier between the blood and the urinary space is composed by fenestrated endothelium, the peripheral glomeru-

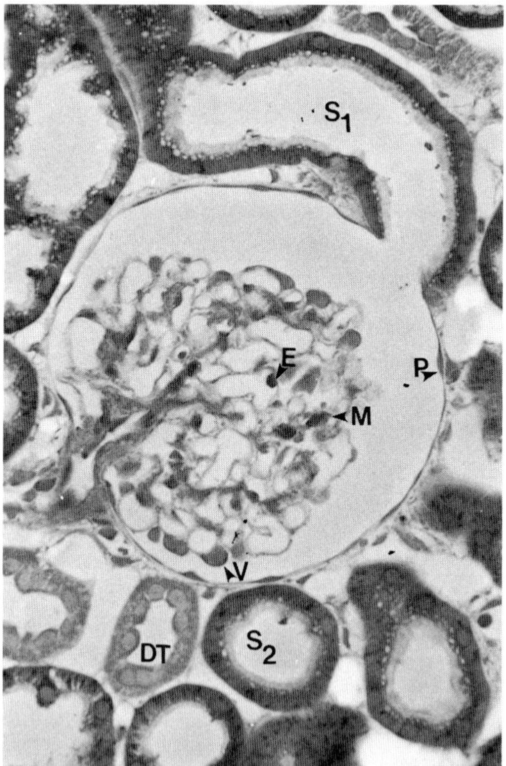

FIG. 4. Photomicrograph of a normal rat glomerulus demonstrating a visceral epithelial cell (V), mesangial cell (M), endothelial cell (E), and parietal epithelial cell (P). S_1 proximal tubules have a taller brush border and numerous apical vacuoles compared to S_2 proximal tubules. Note the distal convoluted tubule (DT). (Glycol methacrylate, $\times 510$.)

lar basement membrane (GBM), and the slit pores between the foot processes of the visceral epithelial cells, or podocytes.

Endothelial Cells

Spread along the thick GBM facing the capillary lumen, endothelial cells are large flat cells with characteristic round fenestrae and a lack of micropinocytotic vesicles (Figs. 6 and 7). Thin diaphragms extend across these fenestrae, but do not pose a significant barrier to the passage of macromolecules. Fenestrated regions of the endothelium represent approximately 54% of the total surface area, whereas nonfenestrated ridge-like structures are found near the cell borders. The surface of the endothelial cells is negatively charged by polyanionic surface glycoproteins. Podocalyxin, the principal sialoprotein of glomerular endothelial and epithelial

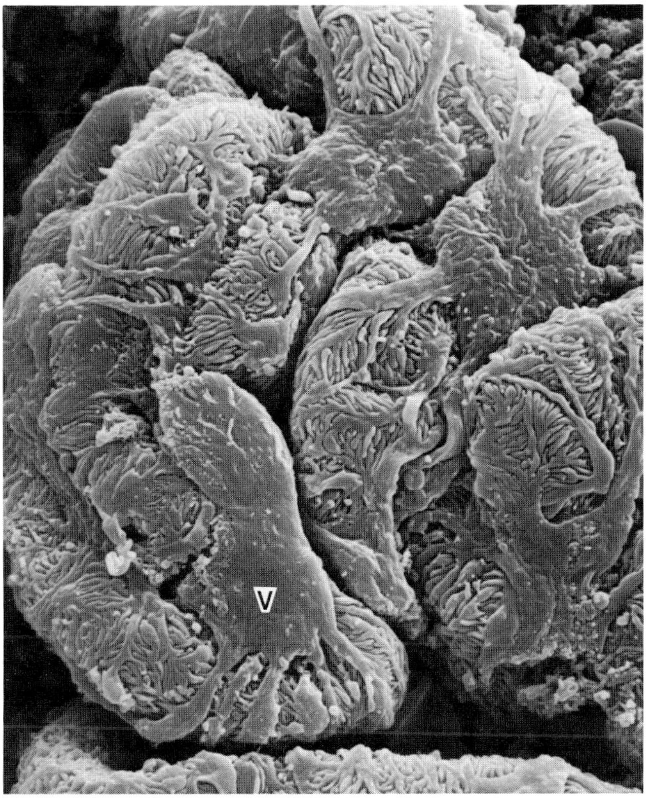

FIG. 5. Scanning electron micrograph of a normal monkey glomerulus. Visceral epithelial cells (V) wrap around individual capillary loops, extending multiple processes outward. (×3,120.)

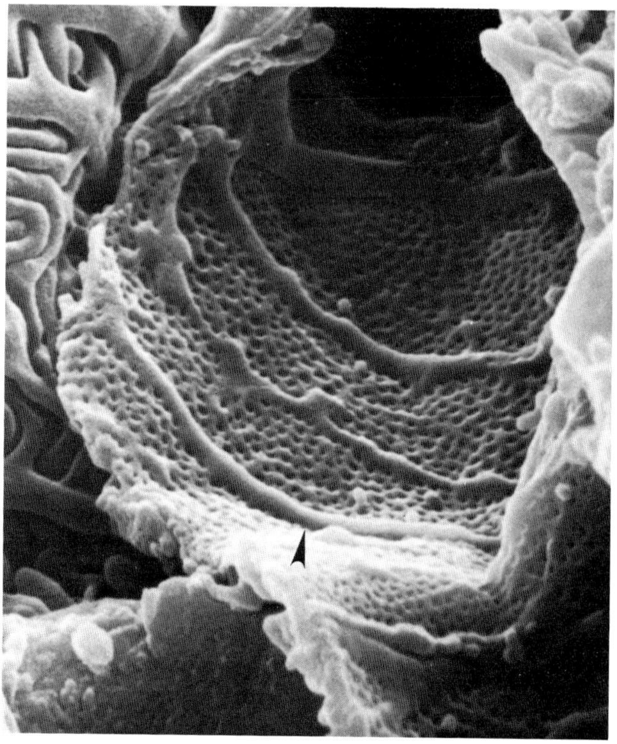

FIG. 6. Scanning electron micrograph illustrating the endothelial surface of a glomerular capillary from a normal monkey. The nonfenestrated ridge (*arrowhead*) separates the fenestrae or epithelial pores (*arrows*). (×19,500.)

cells, imparts the negative charge (26). Glomerular endothelial cells form the initial barrier keeping the cellular constituents of the blood and the platelets within the glomerular vasculature while permitting dissolved solutes to be filtered into Bowman's space. The glomerular endothelial cells contribute to the charge-selective properties of the glomerular capillary wall, tending to favor filtration of neutral and positively charged molecules, while retarding the filtration of negatively charged molecules.

Mesangial Cells

Mesangial cells with the surrounding matrix compose the mesangium, which is separated from the capillary lumen by the endothelium (Fig. 7). Mesangial cells are irregularly shaped cells with elongated cytoplasmic processes in which filaments of contractile proteins (actin and myosin) are found, suggesting their origin from muscle cells. The mesangial matrix contains glycosaminoglycans, fibronectin, and laminin.

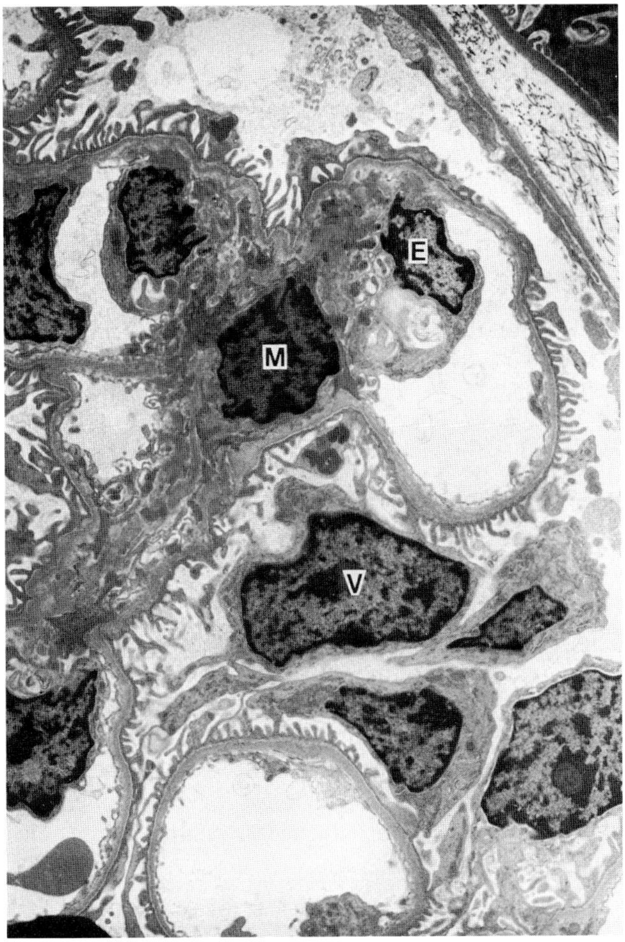

FIG. 7. Transmission electron micrograph illustrating a portion of the glomerulus from the normal monkey. Note the relationship between visceral epithelial cells (V), mesangial cells (M), and endothelial cells (E). (×4,176.)

The glomerular mesangial cells are specialized pericytes that contribute structural support and contractile and phagocytic properties. Glomerular mesangial cells possess many of the functional properties of smooth muscle cells. These cells contain surface receptors for a large number of catecholamines, peptides, and other vasoactive substances (prostaglandins, leukotrienes, platelet activating factor) and contract or relax *in vitro* in response to these agents (27). However, the role of mesangial tone in the control of glomerular hemodynamics *in vivo* is not known. Glomerular mesangial cells also produce prostaglandins, and in response to cytokines such as platelet-derived growth factor and tumor necrosis factor, produce interleukin-1, and epithelial growth factor, all of which may affect mesangial cell function and proliferation, and modulate glomerular injury in kidney disease (28). Phagocytic activities are shared by both the mesangial cells and bone marrow–derived monocyte-macrophages also residing in the mesangium.

Epithelial Cells

Visceral epithelial cells, also known as podocytes, have large cell bodies and long cytoplasmic ramifications, the primary processes, which divide into foot processes and come into direct contact with the lamina rara externa of the glomerular basement membrane (Figs. 5 and 7). Adjacent foot processes are derived from different podocytes. Podocytes contain well-developed Golgi complexes, prominent lysosomes, and large numbers of microtubules and microfilaments. Actin and myosin filaments have also been observed in podocytes. Filtration slits are spaces between foot processes, which are bridged by a thin, zipper-like diaphragm called the filtration slit membrane. The role of this structure in the determination of the permselectivity of the filtration barrier is controversial. A negatively charged surface coat rich in sialic acid covers the foot processes. Immunohistochemical studies have revealed the presence of podocalyxin on the urinary, but not the basal, surface of the podocytes. Negatively charged sites on these cells are important for the maintenance of normal structure and function of the filtration barrier. Foot process fusion, a replacement of pedicels by a continuous cytoplasmic band along the lamina rara externa, is associated with proteinuria. Podocytes are often observed with endocytic inclusions and are thought to play a role in reabsorbing proteins from the glomerular filtrate. Podocytes are also thought to contribute to the maintenance of the glomerular basement membrane.

Glomerular Basement Membrane

The glomerular basement membrane is composed of a central dense layer, the lamina densa, and two thinner, electron-lucent layers, the lamina rara externa and the lamina rara interna (Fig. 8). The thickness of the capillary basement membrane of the rat glomerulus is 132 nm (26). The glomerular basement membrane is composed of type IV and type V collagen, laminin, fibronectin, entactin, and nidogen. The glomerular basement membrane also possesses fixed negatively charged sites that influence the filtration of macromolecules. The anionic sites are rich in glycosaminoglycans, particularly heparan sulfate. The glomerular basement membrane, especially the lamina densa, is chiefly responsible for the permselective properties of the glomerulus, allowing passage of small molecules but restricting the passage of molecules the size of, or larger than, albumin.

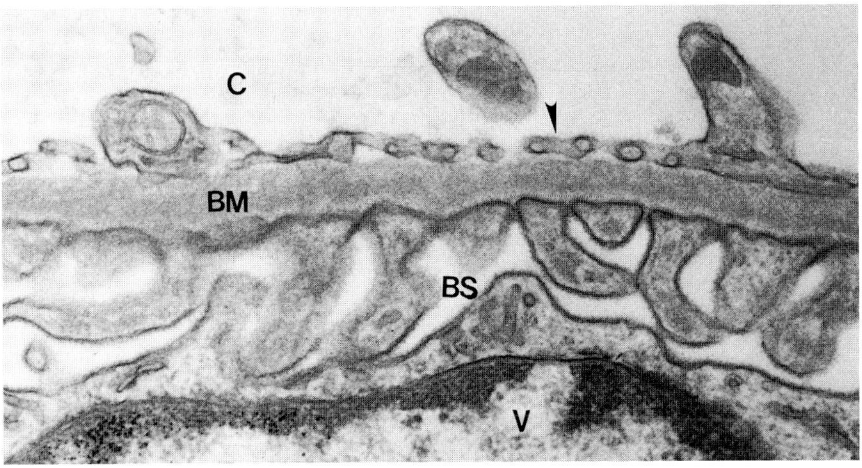

FIG. 8. Transmission electron micrograph illustrating a portion of the glomerular basement membrane from a normal monkey. The endothelial fenestrations are covered by a thin diaphragm (*arrowhead*). Capillary lumen (C), glomerular basement membrane (BM), Bowman's space (BS), and visceral epithelial cell (V) are shown. (×32,550.)

Glomerular Filtration

Glomerular filtration occurs within the renal corpuscle and refers to the process of ultrafiltration of plasma under pressure through the permselective glomerular capillary endothelium. The process of glomerular filtration separates the plasma water and its nonprotein solutes (crystalloids), which enter the most proximal end of the nephron (Bowman's space), from the blood cells and protein macromolecules (colloids) that normally remain in the vascular compartment. The same Starling forces that determine fluid movement along systemic capillaries drive ultrafiltration along glomerular capillaries (Fig. 9). Additional properties of individual solutes that contribute to their relative "filterability" by the glomerulus include molecular size, shape, flexibility and deformability, and charge. The limits of glomerular capillary permeability are suggested by the fact that hemoglobin (65 Å diameter) and smaller proteins such as albumin (36 by 150 Å) are not freely filtered but do get through the membrane in small amounts. Hence, the glomerular capillary behaves as if it were a filtering membrane containing aqueous "pores" with a diameter of 75 to 100 Å (29). In addition, the presence of fixed negatively charged glycoproteins on the surfaces of the components of the glomerular capillary wall favor the filtration of neutral and positively charged solutes, compared to negatively charged solutes of the same effective molecular radius (27).

The high rates of glomerular filtration result in large exposures of all the glomerular structures to toxicants. The aminonucleoside puromycin produces loss of organization of the normally slender, interdigitating glomerular epithelial cell foot processes, replacing them instead with nearly continuous sheets of epithelial cytoplasm,

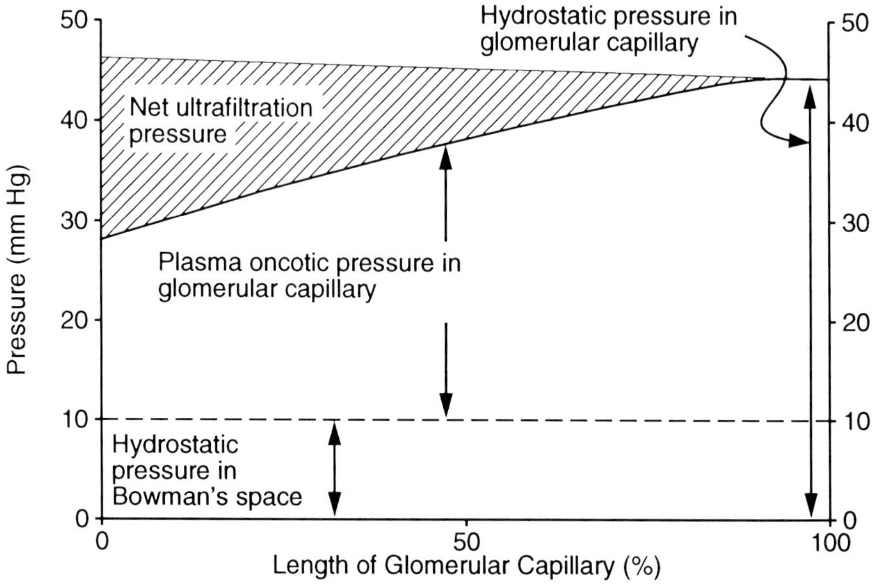

Balance of Mean Values	
Hydrostatic pressure in glomerular capillary	45 mm Hg
Hydrostatic pressure in Bowman's space	10
Plasma oncotic pressure in glomerular capillary	27
Oncotic pressure of fluid in Bowman's space	0*
Net ultrafiltration pressure	8 mm Hg

FIG. 9. Distribution of Starling forces along the glomerular capillary. Hydrostatic pressure (P_c) is shown on the *vertical axes*, distance along the glomerular capillary (as a percent of total length) is shown along the *horizontal axis*. P_c is virtually constant within the renal corpuscle. The *horizontal dashed line* depicts the hydrostatic pressure in Bowman's space. This pressure is constant as a function of capillary length because the capillary is suspended within the renal corpuscle. The *curve* separating the *hatched* and *open* areas depicts the increasing oncotic pressure within the glomerular capillary (π_p) with increasing distance along the capillary. The increase in π_p is a reflection of the loss of plasma ultrafiltrate from the vascular compartment into Bowman's space (*, the oncotic pressure of the fluid in Bowman's space is negligible as the ultrafiltrate and contains virtually no protein). The *hatched* area depicts the decreasing net ultrafiltration pressure as a function with increasing distance along the capillary. The relationship implies that net ultrafiltration is most rapid along the initial length of the glomerular capillary and may not occur at all along the more distal portions. In contrast to systemic capillary beds, net reabsorption of the fluid in Bowman's space into the glomerular capillary (i.e., a negative net ultrafiltration pressure) is not thought to occur in the renal corpuscle (29).

giving rise to the term *foot process fusion* (26). Aminoglycoside antibiotics also produce changes in glomerular ultrastructure and decreased the glomerular capillary ultrafiltration coefficient (20). These drugs can neutralize the fixed anionic changes on the glomerular endothelium and reduce or eliminate the charge-selective properties of the ultrafiltration barrier, in a fashion similar to that described in nephrotoxic serum nephritis. Glomerular structures are also susceptible to immunologic injury, which may occur as a primary or secondary action of the toxicant (20).

Juxtaglomerular Apparatus

The juxtaglomerular apparatus (JGA) is a structural complex located at the hilus of the renal glomerulus where a modified portion of the ascending thick limb, the macula densa, enters into intimate contact with the vascular pole of the same nephron. The vascular component of the JGA includes the afferent and efferent arterioles of the glomerulus. The vascular component also includes the juxtaglomerular granular cells and the extraglomerular mesangium, a roughly triangular-shaped region between the arterioles. The JGA is innervated by sympathetic nerve fibers.

Juxtaglomerular granular (JG) cells cannot be identified in routine paraffin sections stained with hematoxylin and eosin, but they are easily demonstrated with immunocytochemical methods. Ultrastructurally, these cells contain myofilaments and membrane-bound granules of different sizes and shapes that exhibit periodicity. JG cells are immunoreactive to renin. Recent immunocytochemical studies suggest that angiotensin II coexists in the same granules (25).

The extraglomerular mesangium is also called the lacis, or the cells of Goormaghtigh (25). The extraglomerular mesangium is continuous with the intraglomerular mesangium, and it is composed of cells that are similar in ultrastructure to mesangial cells. Gap junctions are commonly observed between the various cells of the juxtaglomerular apparatus, as well as between extraglomerular and intraglomerular mesangial cells, suggesting that the extraglomerular mesangium may serve as a functional link between the macula densa and the glomerular arterioles and mesangium.

In the JGA, the region of the thick ascending limb is called the macula densa because the nuclei are close together, appearing as a condensation of nuclei near the vascular pole. Mitochondria are few in number and more randomly distributed, as compared to the contiguous thick ascending limb. The basement membrane is fused with the basement membrane of surrounding granular cells. The macula densa contains a lower level of sodium-potassium–adenosine triphosphatase (Na-K– ATPase) activity and Tamm-Horsfall protein than the remaining thick ascending limb. The lower Tamm-Horsfall protein content suggests that this may be a water-permeable window in the relatively water-impermeable thick ascending limb of Henle.

The physiological significance of the juxtaglomerular apparatus is that it contains the structures that produce and release renin into the circulation, and perhaps also into the renal cortical interstitium. There are two proposed mechanisms regulating renin release: the macula densa mechanism and the stretch mechanism. The macula densa mechanism postulates that changes in the sodium or chloride concentrations in the early distal tubule, at the level of the macula densa, can control the intrarenal release of renin. According to the stretch receptor mechanism, alterations in the volume and stretch of the afferent arteriole regulate renin release (25). Recent studies using an isolated glomerular/JGA preparation have shown that physiological changes in NaCl concentration, and not NaCl delivery or tubule fluid flow rate at the macula densa, are associated with the largest changes in renin secretion from the adjacent juxtaglomerular granular cells (30).

Glomerular Autoregulation and Tubuloglomerular Feedback

Autoregulation refers to the kidney's ability to maintain renal blood flow and glomerular filtration rate constant over a wide range of renal perfusion pressures (31). Autoregulation of blood flow is known in virtually all tissues and is thought to be at least in part an intrinsic myogenic response regulated by local metabolic factors. Changes in renal vascular resistance that lead to consistency of renal blood flow and glomerular filtration have been recorded for denervated and isolated kidney preparations (31,32), suggesting that neither neural nor endocrine factors are required. Autoregulatory phenomena are observed in isolated perfused afferent and efferent arterioles. Autoregulation of glomerular filtration appears to be a consequence of the autoregulation of glomerular plasma flow and glomerular capillary pressure (33). Autoregulatory perfusion pressure ranges are reset upward in hypertension (34).

Although less is known about the autoregulatory capacity of the inner cortical and medullary microcirculations, the available data suggest that autoregulation in these zones is also relatively efficient (16). Local myogenic and metabolic mechanisms have been proposed for renal autoregulation but conclusive evidence for either of these mechanisms is still elusive (35). It has also been proposed that adjustments in renal vascular resistance in response to alterations in renal perfusion pressure are mediated by a tubuloglomerular feedback loop. The specialized cells of the macula densa located between the end of the thick ascending limb of Henle and the early distal convoluted tubule are found at the junction of the afferent arteriole, the glomerulus, and the efferent arteriole of the same nephron and form the juxtaglomerular apparatus (see above). This anatomical arrangement has widely been speculated to be a feedback system whereby stimuli received at the macula densa are transmitted to the arterioles of the same nephron to alter glomerular filtration rate and/or renin release. Many studies have now shown that changes in the composition of the fluid flowing past the macula densa elicit rapid changes in glomerular filtration of the same nephron (36). Increases in the delivery of fluid out of the proximal tubule result in decreases in filtration rate of the same nephron. Although it is possible that a common transduction pathway for tubuloglomerular feedback and renin release exists at the macula densa, whether or not changes in local concentrations of angiotensin II mediate tubuloglomerular feedback vasoconstriction of glomerular arterioles or mesangium is not known (16,37).

The effects of toxicants on the juxtaglomerular apparatus, renal autoregulation, and tubuloglomerular feedback are poorly described. Chronic administration of drugs that inhibit the production or activity of angiotensin II (angiotensin II converting enzyme inhibitors and angiotensin II receptor antagonists) produce hyperplasia of the juxtaglomerular granular cells, probably by interrupting negative feedback inhibition of renin production/release by angiotensin II. Drugs that block the activity of the renin-angiotensin-aldosterone system displace the renal function curve to the left, toward lower arterial pressure for the same level of renal solute excretion (2). The mechanism of this effect is unknown but could include renal autoregulatory and tubuloglomerular feedback mechanisms. It has also been suggested that tubuloglomerular feedback mediates amphotericin B–induced vasoconstriction (38).

STRUCTURE AND FUNCTION OF THE RENAL TUBULES AND INTERSTITIUM

Proximal Tubule

The proximal tubule is the most common site of nephrotoxicity and renal carcinogenesis. In several animals, including the rat, the rabbit, the mouse, and the rhesus monkey, three morphologically distinct segments, S_1, S_2, and S_3 (or P_1, P_2, and P_3), can be distinguished to comprise the pars convoluta and pars recta of the proximal tubule (Fig. 1). The structural features that distinguish the three segments of the proximal tubule in the rat have been described in detail by Maunsbach (39,40). The S_1 segment comprises the initial portion of the proximal convoluted tubule (Fig. 10). Epithelial cells of the S_1 segment possess a tall brush border and a well-developed vacuolar lysosomal system (Fig. 11). The basolateral membrane is extensively interdigitated, and many long mitochondria fill the basal portion of the cell, an arrangement that is characteristic of epithelia involved in active transport. The S_2 segment comprises the end of the convoluted segment and the initial portions of the straight segments in the medullary ray (Fig. 10). Epithelial cells of the S_2 segment are not as tall as those of the S_1, and possess a shorter brush border and fewer apical vacuoles and mitochondria than the S_1 cells. The number and size of lysosomes vary between species and between males and females. Lysosomes in the male rat are characteristically numerous and large in the S_2 epithelial cells (Figs. 10 and 12). α_{2u}-Globulin, a low molecular weight protein synthesized by the liver, is the major component of these protein droplets in male rats (Fig. 13) (41). The S_3 segment comprises the distal portion of straight segments of the medullary ray, which extend to the junction of the outer and inner stripe of the outer medulla (Fig. 13). The length of the brush border of the S_3 segment is tall and dense in the rat, but much shorter in the rabbit and intermediate in the human. The S_3 cells have rare apical vacuoles, and fewer and smaller lysosomes and mitochondria than the S_1 and S_2 cells. Peroxisomes are quite prominent in the S_3 cells (Fig. 13). Lateral cell processes and invaginations are absent.

The transitions between cell types are gradual. Distinguishing features of the three cell types are best observed by electron microscopy, but segment identification by light microscopy can be conducted with perfusion, rather than immersion

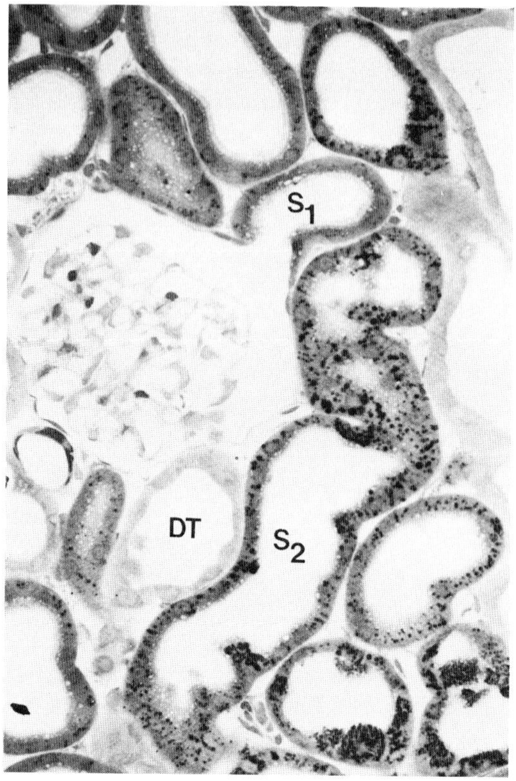

FIG. 10. Light micrograph of kidney from a male rat. Epithelial cells of the S_1 segment in the initial portion of the proximal tubule have a tall brush border. Epithelial cells of the S_2 segment have a shorter brush border and the cytoplasm in this young rat is filled with various amounts of small, round to angular protein droplets. These droplets are usually undetectable with H&E stain, but are apparent with Lee's methylene blue basic fuchsin stain. (Glycol Methocrylate, ×280.)

fixed tissue. For light microscopic identification of segments, best results are achieved with sections 2 to 3 μm thick, stained with Lee's methylene blue basic fuchsin (Fig. 10).

In the dog, four specific morphological regions have been defined, with an extremely large number of lipid droplets in the late proximal tubule (42). Many ultrastructural features of the dog kidney more closely resemble those seen in the human kidney than those in the rat. Since species variations occur, physiological differences among the species should be anticipated (43).

Histochemical studies of the proximal tubule have been useful in identifying the structural and functional heterogeneity of this important region of the nephron (44). The brush border stains with the periodic acid-Schiff (PAS) technique. Enzyme histochemical markers for the plasma membrane of the brush border include alkaline phosphatase, γ-glutamyl transpeptidase, and Na-K–ATPase. Lysosomes are

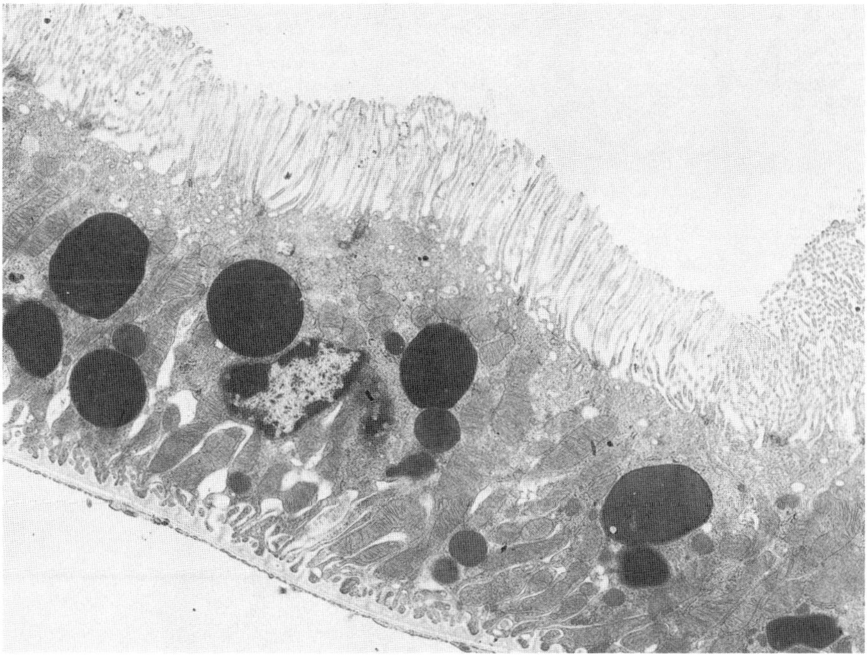

FIG. 11. Transmission electron micrograph of S_2 segment of rat proximal tubule. Note the shorter brush border, fewer apical endolysosomes, and numerous round, electron-dense phagolysosomes. ($\times$6,580.)

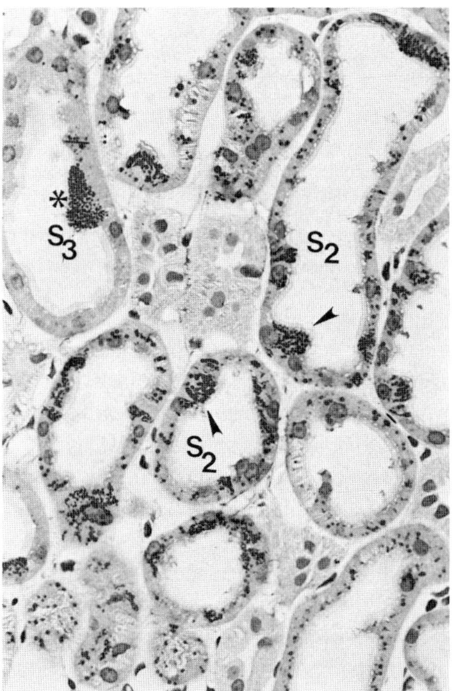

FIG. 12. Immunohistochemical staining of rat kidney for α_{2u}-globulin. Note the staining of protein droplets for α_{2u}-globulin within S_2 segments. Occasional clusters of α_{2u}-globulin droplets are observed in S_3 segments. (Glycol Methocrylate, $\times$280.)

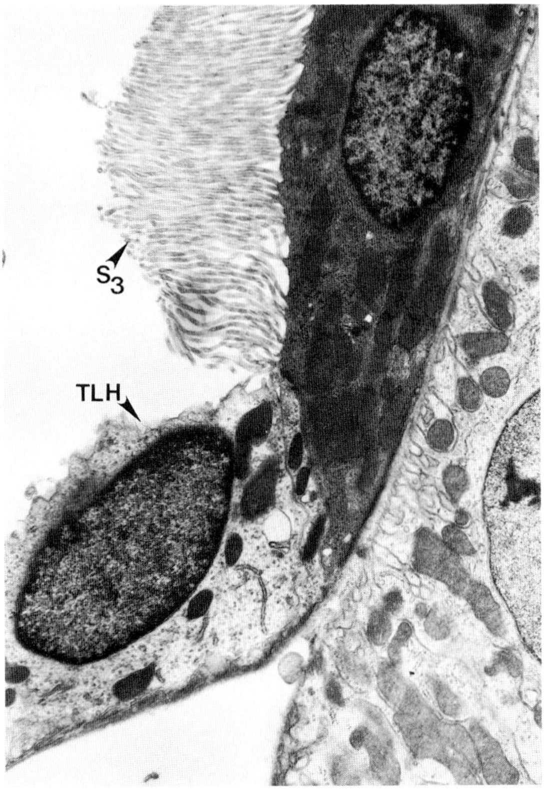

FIG. 13. Transmission electron micrograph of S_3 segment of rat proximal tubule at the junction with the thin limb of Henle (TLH). The brush border is tall, but the endocytic-lysosomal apparatus and mitochondria are less prominent than the S_1 or S_2 segments. The thin limb has only a few short microvillar projections and scanty mitochondria. (×11,520.)

also usually PAS positive, but are more specifically identified histochemically by acid phosphatase and β-galactosidase. Enzymatic markers for mitochondria include succinate dehydrogenase, α-glycerophosphate dehydrogenase, malate dehydrogenase (NADS), and β-hydroxybutyrate dehydrogenase. Peroxisomal enzymes studied are α-hydroxy acid oxidase and peroxidase. Glucose-6-phosphate dehydrogenase, malate dehydrogenase, and lactate dehydrogenase are a few of the many soluble cytoplasmic enzymes that have been examined. In general, the distribution of the histochemical activity of different enzymes along the proximal tubule reflects the abundance of the particular structure or organelle with which they are associated. The brush border, lysosomes, and basement membrane are stained by the PAS technique. A similar pattern of staining has been obtained using lectins, which are plant-derived substances that bind to oligosaccharides associated with glycoproteins and glycolipids at the cell surface.

The proximal tubule of the kidney reabsorbs approximately 50% to 60% of the glomerular filtrate and exhibits a plethora of cellular and transcellular mechanisms to effect the reabsorption of individual solutes and water. In general, essential nutrients (sugars, amino acids, and other neutral organic solutes), macromolecules (albumin and other proteins), and bicarbonate are extensively reabsorbed along the initial length of the proximal tubule. Although the tubular fluid to plasma (TF/P) chloride concentration ratio increases, it does not increase as fast as the TF/P inulin ratio, indicating net NaCl reabsorption. The potential difference is negative in the lumen of the early proximal tubule, which is due to sodium-coupled neutral organic solute reabsorption. In the late proximal tubule reabsorption of sodium chloride and secretion of organic acids and bases predominantly occurs. TF/P chloride ratio is increased and the potential difference in the lumen of these segments is positive. In addition to the morphological differences between the S_1, S_2, and S_3 segments of the proximal tubule, the early segments also display greater membrane surface areas, enhanced numbers of mitochondria, and greater rates of solute and water reabsorption. Maximal solute gradients cannot be achieved in the early segments, because the paracellular pathways are leaky to ions and other solutes. In the S_3 segment, transcellular solute transport rates are lower than in the S_1 and S_2 segments, but the paracellular pathways are less leaky and maximal solute concentration gradients can be achieved. This arrangement of transcellular transporters and paracellular permeabilities along the proximal tubule enables the kidney to more or less completely recover essential nutrients from proximal tubule fluid (45).

Delineation of specific transport mechanisms and permeabilities to specific proximal tubule segments is incomplete at this time. Lysosomal vacuolar apparatus and receptor-mediated endocytosis involved in the reabsorption and degradation of albumin and other low molecular weight proteins are most prominent in the S_1 segment under normal conditions but can be observed in the S_2 segment under proteinuric conditions (46). Cathespins B and L, the lysosomal proteolytic enzyme activities, are higher in S_1 than in S_2 or S_3, but increase in S_2 during proteinuric conditions. Transporters responsible for the secretion of organic acids are found in all proximal tubule segments, but are most prominent in the S_3 segment. Multiple sodium-glucose carrier transport processes have been distinguished by their kinetics and their location along the proximal tubule (45). An arrangement of glucose transport proteins with decreasing capacity, increasing affinity, and changing sodium-glucose stoichiometric ratio along the length of the proximal tubule ensures that while the S_1 segment reabsorbs glucose more rapidly, the S_3 segment can decrease the tubule fluid glucose concentration to a much lower level. Theoretically, a single uniform segment could not perform both rapid and complete solute absorption. Hence, similar heterogeneous distributions of transport proteins for other neutral solutes also likely exist on both the apical and basolateral membranes in the S_1, S_2, and S_3 segments. Proximal tubule transporters are currently being cloned and much is being learned about their molecular biology (47–49). Comparison of the structures of the glucose transporters cloned to date suggest families of multimeric proteins having multiple membrane-spanning domains. How these structures work to transport molecules is as yet unknown. Illustrations of the efficacy of the representative sugar and amino acid transport mechanisms are shown in Figs. 14 and 15, and the efficacy of an organic acid transport mechanism in Fig. 16.

The proximal tubule segments also contain the largest variety of transport mechanisms for sodium, potassium, chloride, bicarbonate, calcium, phosphate, and other ions and solutes. Both cellular and transcellular pathways are known. Examples of diffusion, facilitated transport, exchange diffusion, anion-cation cotransport, anion-anion and cation-cation countertransport, and active transport are known. Although the kinetics and stoichiometries of the putative transport proteins have been extensively investigated, less is known about the heterogeneity of their distribution in the S_3 proximal tubule segment. However, with the rapid advances in cloning of both organic and ion transport proteins we can expect rapid increases in our knowledge of the expression of specific messenger ribonucleic acids (mRNAs) for individual transport proteins in all nephron segments in the near future.

Because of the large volumes of fluid entering and being reabsorbed from the proximal tubule, its many and varied transport mechanisms, and its mitochondrial and cytoplasmic enzyme activities and associated high metabolic rate, the proximal tubule is a target for a wide variety of toxicants including metals, antibiotics, and halogenated hydrocarbons. Hexachlorobutadiene produces a well-defined lesion in the S_3 segment characterized by a loss of the brush border. Aminoglycosides produce characteristic lesions in S_1 and S_2 segments (19). Secretion of β-lactam antibiotics by the organic acid transporter is thought to be a principal contributing factor to the nephrotoxicity of these drugs to the proximal tubule (50). Cephaloridine is a substrate for the organic acid transporter and is transported from the blood into proximal tubule cells; however, the efflux of cephaloridine is very slow, suggesting that the nephrotoxicity of the drug is caused, in part, by its accumulation and retention within the cells of the proximal tubule (51). Many chemicals bind reversibly to α_{2u}-globulin in the male rat, disrupting lysosomal degradation of this slowly catabolized protein and thereby promoting its accumulation in renal cortical phagolysosomes (52,53). Contrast media also impair the handling of α_{2u}-globulin in the rat (54). Other drugs, like furosemide, are secreted into proximal tubule fluid and delivered downstream to the distal nephron in concentrations sufficient to disrupt nephron functions (55). The presence of glutathione in the renal cortex can act either to protect the proximal tubule from toxicants or to facilitate the formation of toxicants (51,56).

The Loop of Henle

The transition from the terminal S_3 segment of the proximal tubule to the thin limbs of Henle is abrupt, and marks the junction between the outer and inner stripe of the outer medulla (Fig. 13). The epithelium of the thin limb is low and fairly simple, with few organelles. Four types (I to IV) of epithelium have been described in this segment of the nephron in several animals, including the rat (25). The cell

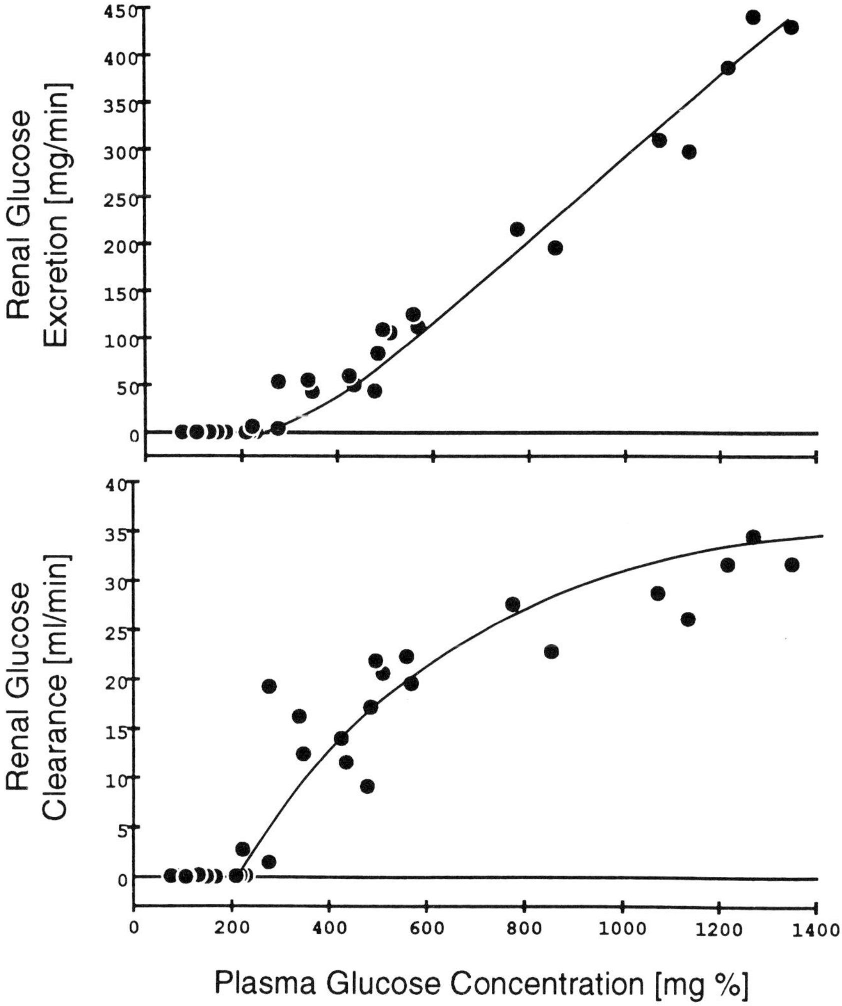

FIG. 14. Tubular reabsorption. The renal excretion of glucose by beagle dogs. In these studies groups of purpose-bred laboratory beagle dogs were infused intravenously with isotonic (5%) dextrose at rates of 0.3, 1.0, and 3.0 ml/kg per min for 60 min and blood and urine samples collected at 5- to 10-min intervals. In the *upper panel*, renal glucose excretion is presented as a function of plasma glucose concentration. Urinary glucose concentrations are below detection limits at plasma glucose concentrations lower than approximately 250 mg%, the plasma glucose concentration at which renal transport maximum (T_m) glucose is exceeded and glucose begins to "spill" into the urine. Above the T_m, the renal glucose excretion increases linearly with increasing plasma glucose concentration. The *lower panel* depicts the same data presented as the renal glucose clearance ($U_{Glu}V/P_{Glu}$). Once detectable concentrations of glucose appear in urine the renal glucose clearance rises rapidly as a function of the plasma glucose concentration, asymptotically approaching a value of approximately 35 ml/min. This value is equivalent to the glomerular filtration rate and, using this value, the renal transport maxima for glucose in the beagle dog is estimated to be approximately 90 mg/min.

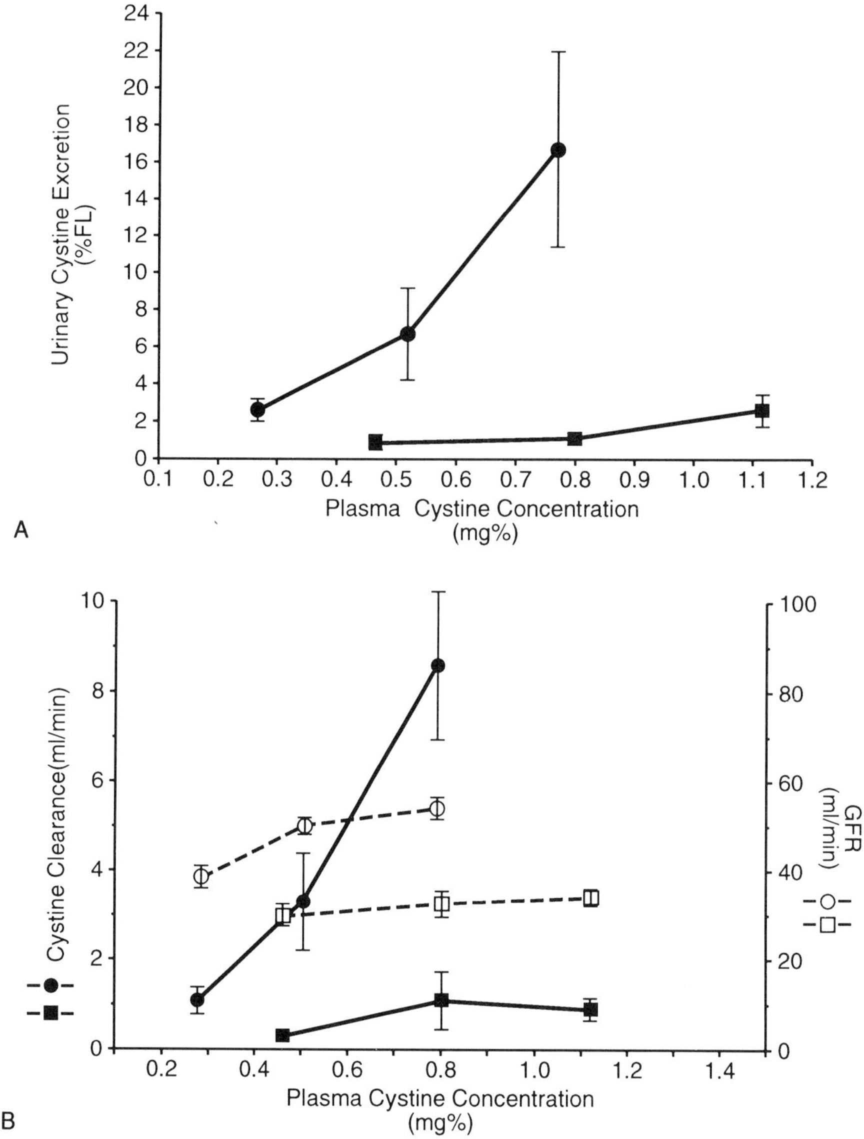

FIG. 15. Tubular reabsorption. The renal excretion of the cystine in normal mongrel dogs (*circles*) and dogs with diagnosed hereditary canine cystinuria resulting from a defective cystine transporter (*squares*) (71). In these studies, dogs were infused intravenously with isotonic solutions containing 0, 0.52, or 1.05 mM cystine (2 ml/min) to elevate plasma cystine concentrations. **A:** Urinary cystine excretion is increased in normal dogs only slightly (from 1% to 2% of the FL) at the highest plasma cystine concentration. However, in cystinuric dogs renal cystine excretion is increased to 15% or more of the FL. **B:** The same data is presented as renal cystine clearances ($U_{cys}V/P_{cys}$). The simultaneous measurements of glomerular filtration rate (GFR) are also presented. The differences in renal cystine clearance and cystine excretion in dogs with intact and defective cystine transport mechanisms illustrate the impact of proximal tubule reabsorption mechanisms on the composition of urine.

types vary in the numbers of interdigitations, cell height, and the number and location of tight junctions. Type I epithelium is found in the thin descending limb of short-looped nephrons. Type II epithelium forms the thin descending limb of long-looped nephrons in the outer medulla, which gives rise to type III epithelium in the inner medulla. Type IV epithelium forms the bends of the long loops and the entire thin ascending limb to the transition into the thick ascending limb at the boundary between the inner and outer medulla.

The cells of the thick ascending limb decrease in height as the tubule ascends from the inner stripe of the outer medulla to the cortex. There are extensive invaginations of the basolateral membrane that interdigitate with adjacent cells. Numerous elongated mitochondria are in close proximity to the plasma membrane, consistent with the high concentration of Na-K–ATPase involved in active transport. This segment is especially sensitive to ischemic damage because of its high energy demand for active transport and the limited availability of oxygen in this region. As the thick limb ascends, luminal microprojections and apical lateral invaginations become more prominent. Tamm-Horsfall protein is located along the luminal membrane of the thick ascending limb, but the functional significance of this protein is unknown.

Approximately 20% to 30% of the filtered Na and K and 15% to 20% of the filtered water are reabsorbed in the segments of the loop of Henle. The principal features of these segments are their differing permeabilities to water, electrolytes, and urea. The tubular fluid entering the thin descending limbs comes into osmotic equilibrium with the renal interstitium. Water is freely permeable of this epithelium and solutes (electrolytes and urea) may enter from the interstitium. The transport properties of the thin ascending limb are fundamentally different from those of the thin descending limbs. This epithelium is relatively impermeable to water. Sodium chloride, but not urea, is reabsorbed in the thin ascending limbs by passive diffusion and perhaps also by active transport. The differing transport and permeability properties of the thin limbs are thought to be a critical component of the mechanism responsible for the intermedullary axial osmotic gradient. The functional significance of these properties appears to be initiation of the conversion of the tubular fluid from a relatively pure NaCl solution to a relatively pure urea solution (57). The thick ascending limb is impermeable to water and is also the site of an avid Na-K-Cl cotransport mechanism. Reabsorption of solute is sufficient to increase the local osmotic concentration around these segments to crenate red blood cells passing down adjacent vasa recta and to render the fluid entering the distal tubule hypotonic to the cortical interstitium. The oxidative metabolism required to support Na-K-Cl cotransport in this segment is sufficient to reduce the local oxygen tension to near Q_{10} levels, putting this segment at risk of ischemic injury in the case of reductions in oxygen delivery or increases in metabolic demand. Amphotericin B toxicity in the thick ascending limb of Henle is prevented by inhibition of active sodium transport with ouabain, and the protective effect is attributed entirely to the decrease in oxygen demand for active transport (19).

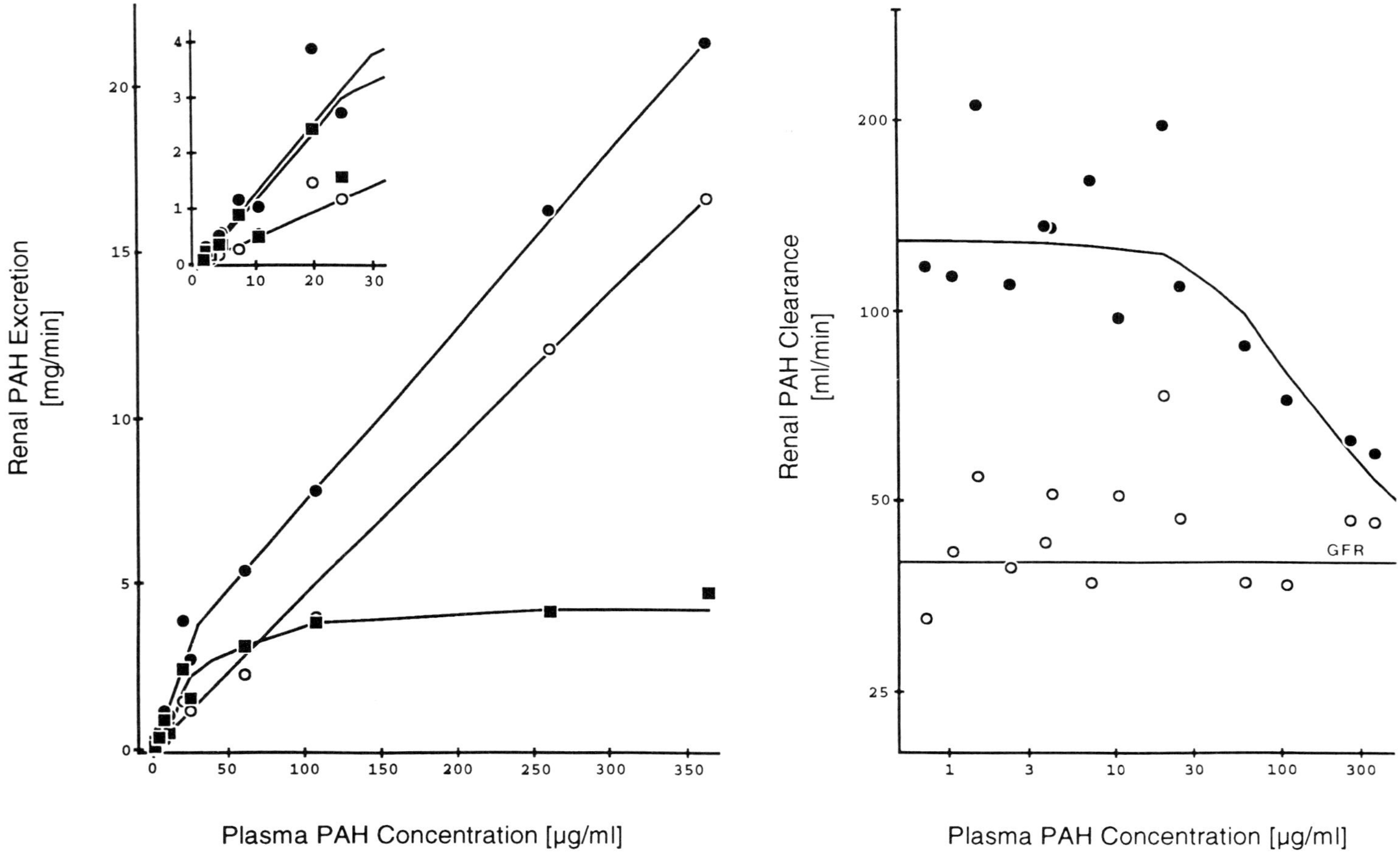

Renal PAH Excretion [mg/min]
Plasma PAH Concentration [μg/ml]
Renal PAH Clearance [ml/min]
GFR
Plasma PAH Concentration [μg/ml]

Distal Convoluted Tubule and Connecting Segment

The cells of the distal convoluted tubule are taller and have more prominent microprojections on the luminal surface than the cells of the ascending thick limb. The lateral cell margins are straight, in contrast to those of the thick ascending limb. These cells lack the well-developed brush border and the extensive endocytic apparatus characteristic of the pars convoluta of the proximal tubule (Figs. 4 and 10). Many small vesicles are present in the apical cytoplasm.

The connecting segment of the nephron represents a gradual transitional region between the distal convoluted tubule and the cortical collecting duct. Four types of cells have been described in this region: connecting tubule cells, intercalated cells, distal convoluted tubule cells, and principal cells. The connecting tubule cell is intermediate between the distal convoluted tubule cell and the principal cell of the collecting duct. The intercalated cell is of two configurations, types A and B, based on the number of vesicles in the apical cytoplasm. The functions of the different varieties of intercalated cells are unknown.

The distal convoluted tubule and connecting segment comprise those segments responsible for the "fine tuning" of renal water and solute excretion. Most of the remaining water and sodium are reabsorbed, and potassium is generally secreted into the tubular fluid in these segments. Again, there are described multiple mechanisms for electrolyte handling, including aldosterone-sensitive Na^+/K^+ exchange, thiazide-sensitive Na/Cl cotransport, and amiloride- sensitive sodium transport. The distal convoluted tubule has the highest activity of Na-K–ATPase of any segment of the nephron, indicating the importance of this segment in sodium reabsorption. Protons are secreted into the tubular fluid by these segments. Ammonia diffuses passively into the tubular fluid where it forms NH_4^+, which is excreted in the urine. The distal convoluted tubule and the connecting segment are sites of hormonal and neuronal regulation of electrolyte reabsorption. This is perhaps best illustrated by potassium, which is generally secreted but may be reabsorbed with chronically low

FIG. 16. Tubular secretion. The relationships between the renal filtration, secretion, and excretion (*left panel*), and the renal clearance (*right panel*) of *p*-aminohippuric acid (PAH) as a function of the plasma PAH concentration (*horizontal axis*) in purpose-bred laboratory beagle dogs. The *insert* is an enlargement of those relationships at plasma PAH concentrations <30 μg/ml. PAH (Mw 194.19) is freely filtered and the amount of PAH filtered is a linear function of the plasma PAH concentration (*open circles*). Secreted PAH also increases linearly at plasma PAH concentrations <30 μg/ml (*squares*). Above plasma concentrations of 30 μg/ml, the renal PAH secretion is virtually constant at approximately 4 mg/min, the apparent transport maximum (T_m) for PAH secretion in the beagle dog. Renal PAH excretion is the sum of PAH filtered and PAH secreted (*circles*) and is biphasic at the plasma PAH concentration at which T_m occurs. The renal clearance of PAH is constant at a value four to five times the glomerular filtration rate (GRF) at plasma PAH concentrations below that associated with T_mPAH; in this plasma concentration range the renal clearance of PAH approximates the renal plasma flow rate. At higher plasma PAH concentrations the renal PAH clearance decreases toward the GFR.

potassium intake. The distal tubule and connecting segment are sites of vasopressin-stimulated water reabsorption, which occurs through hormone-stimulated increases in water permeability of the apical epithelial membrane (58). The connecting segments coalesce with the tubules of other nephrons to form the final arcade of collecting ducts, which transport the final urine from the renal cortex into the renal pelvis.

The distal tubule and connecting segment appear not to be selectively damaged by most toxicants. However, compounds, such as amphotericin B, that influence the ability of the kidney to acidify urine probably exert this effect in these segments (20).

Collecting Ducts

The collecting duct can be divided into the cortical, outer medullary, and inner medullary collecting duct. Two main cell types are principal cells and intercalated cells (Fig. 17). The principal cells constitute 38% of the cortical collecting ducts, but increase to 90% in the inner medullary collecting duct. Principal cells have a light cytoplasm with relatively few organelles, with prominent infoldings of the basal, but not lateral, cell membrane. The surface is smooth with short, stubby microvilli and a single cilium (Fig. 18). Principal cells are thought to be the vasopressin-sensitive cells of the collecting ducts (58). Intercalated cells have a more electron-dense cytoplasm than that of principal cells, with tubulovesicles and numerous mitochondria and polyribosomes. Two types of intercalated cells, types A and B, have been distinguished in the cortical collecting duct based on the number of mitochondria, the morphology of tubulovesicles, and the number of surface microprojections. Carbonic anhydrase activity is high in intercalated cells, suggesting their role in urine acidification.

Further water and sodium reabsorption and potassium secretion/reabsorption occurs in the collecting ducts. Although the magnitude of the amounts reabsorbed are quite small, compared to the filtered loads, these segments contribute to the "fine-tuning" of renal water and solute excretion. In the cortical collecting duct, mineralocorticoid-stimulated potassium secretion and sodium reabsorption is mediated by the principal cells. Intercalated cells (type B) appear to mediate the reabsorption and secretion of bicarbonate, whereas other intercalated cells (type A) may be responsible for proton secretion. The outer medullary collecting duct participates in urine acidification via mineralocorticoid-stimulated proton secretion by intercalated cells. The inner medullary collecting duct has high permeability to urea and is the site of urea recycling into the inner medullary interstitium (59). Bicarbonate is also reabsorbed in this segment. Vasopressin-dependent water reabsorption also occurs in all collecting duct segments (58). The recently discovered atrial natruretic hormone prevents sodium reabsorption in both the cortical and terminal segments (60,61).

The collecting ducts appear to be relatively insensitive to most nephrotoxicants. Chronic administration of the antibiotic demeclocycline produces a water diuretic response that is due to a disruption of vasopressin-stimulated water reabsorption in

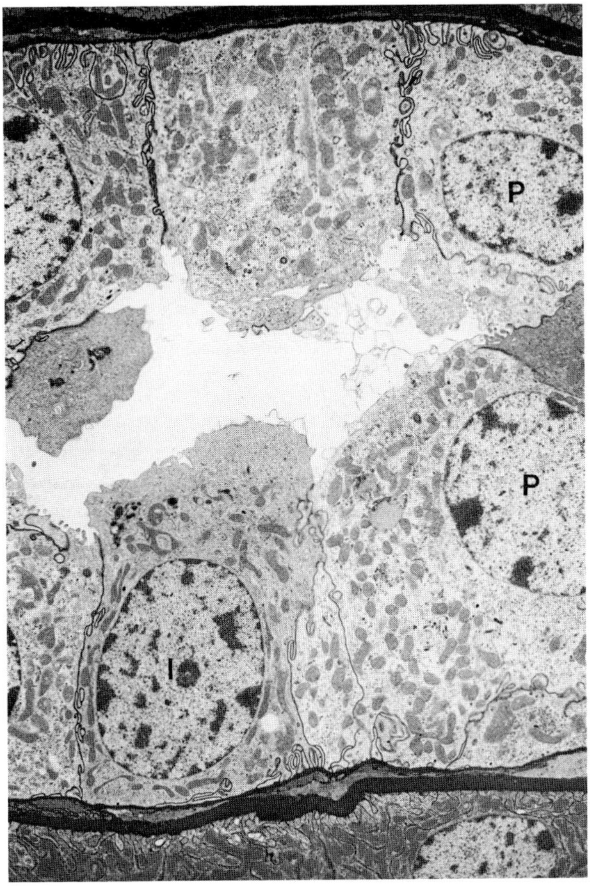

FIG. 17. Transmission electron micrograph of monkey collecting duct. Principal cells (P) with light cytoplasm and relatively few organelles. Mitochondria are sparse and scattered randomly in the cytoplasm. Intercalated cells (I) have a cytoplasm that is more electron dense than that of the principal cells. Basolateral infoldings of both cell types are minimal. (×6,300.)

the collecing duct (62). Damage due to outdated tetracyclines may occur in these segments (20). Chronic administration of vasopressin receptor antagonists causes up-regulation of vasopressin receptors in these segments and renders the kidney antidiuretic but functionally insensitive to exogenously administered vasopressin agonists or antagonists (63).

Renal Pelvis and Ureters

Once urine is excreted from the papilla tip it enters the complex epithelia-lined caverns of the renal pelvis. The epithelial cells lining the renal pelvis are similar to

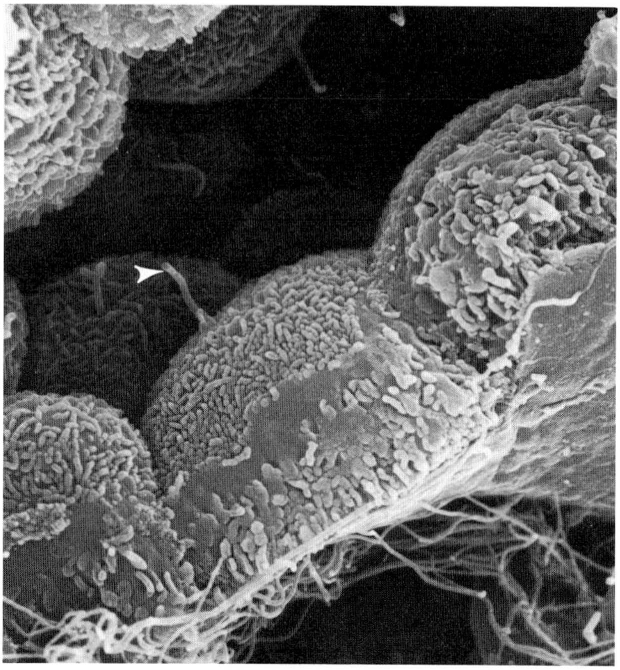

FIG. 18. Scanning electron micrograph of illustrating the liminal surface of monkey collecting duct. The principal cells have small stubby microprojections and a single cilium (*arrowhead*). (×7,605.)

those of the terminal collecting ducts (64). Urine in the pelvis surrounds the renal papilla and bathes the recesses of the pelvis (calyces) that extend into the cortex. The functions of the renal pelvis are not appreciated though an intact pelvis has been suggested to be necessary for maximal urine concentrating ability and for normal peristaltic contractions of the renal papilla. Urinary solutes (and possibly toxicants) are reabsorbed from the pelvis into the papilla (65,66). Urine is carried out of the renal pelvis through the ureters to the urinary bladder. The ureters are also under complex local reflex control and undergo rhythmic peristaltic contractions that appear to be triggered by the contractions of the renal pelvis (67). Ureteral contractions are necessary to propel urine toward the bladder and to prevent refluxing of urine back into the renal pelvis. Long thought to be inert conduits, the ureters are now appreciated to have electrolyte transport properties, too, though quantitatively these are quite small (68). The effects of toxicants on the renal pelvis and ureters are poorly described. Obstruction of the pelvis or ureters with calculus or disruption of ureteropelvic contractions can lead to retention of urine in the renal pelvis, increased pelvic pressure, and hydronephrosis.

Interstitium

The interstitium is composed of interstitial cells and extracellular matrix composed of sulfated and nonsulfated glycosaminoglycans. There is an increase in interstitial volume from 9% in the cortex to 30% to 40% in the papillary tip. In the cortex, interstitial cells can be identified as fibroblasts and mononuclear cells. In the medulla, there are three different types of interstitial cells: type 1, with lipid; type 2, with mononuclear characteristics; and type 3 cells, which are pericytes associated with the descending vas recta. The cells have an irregular shape with long cytoplasmic projections and are arranged in rows, with their long axis aligned perpendicularly to the long axis of the adjacent vasa recta and the loops of Henle. Numerous homogeneous and variably sized lipid droplets and a well-developed endoplasmic reticulum are present in the cytoplasm of type 1 cells.

The function of the interstitial cells has not been precisely established. The type 1 interstitial cells may provide structural support in the medulla. There appears to be a correlation between the lipid droplets of type 1 cells and the diuretic state of an animal. It has been suggested that type 1 cells synthesize prostaglandins, mainly PGE_2. However, the collecting duct cells are also a significant source of prostaglandins. Type 1 interstitial cells may have an endocrine antihypertensive function, and are believed to be responsible for the synthesis of glycosaminoglycans present in the matrix material of the interstitium. Little is known about the function of the type 2 and type 3 medullary interstitial cells.

Several renal anatomic, biochemical, and physiological properties contribute to the renal toxicity of the analgesic/antipyretic agent acetaminophen. Acetaminophen is filtered by the kidney and its nonionic form is reabsorbed and accumulates through diffusion trapping in the medullary interstitium during antidiuresis. Diuresis results in a reduction in the gradients favoring trapping of acetaminophen in the medulla and an increase in acetaminophen clearance. The nephrotoxicity of acetaminophen is linked to its accumulation in the medulla and its subsequent conversion to reactive intermediates within the kidney (19).

ACKNOWLEDGMENTS

The authors would like to acknowledge Tim Hart, Peter Bugelski, and Anne Klinker for their contributions of the transmission and scanning electron micrographs of the glomerulus and collecting duct, Reiner Beeuwkes III, Thomas Hastings Wilson, Christina Sarmousakis, and William Mann for permission to use previously unpublished data, and Diane J. Passerin for manuscript preparation.

REFERENCES

1. Smith H. *The kidney*. New York: Oxford University Press, 1951.
2. Guyton AC. Blood pressure control—special role of the kidneys and body fluids. *Science* 1991;252:1813–1816.

3. Powell JS, Adamson JW. Hematopoiesis and the kidney. In: Seldin DW, Giebisch G, eds. *The kidney: physiology and pathophysiology*. New York: Raven Press, 1985;847–866.
4. Slatopolsky E, Whyte MP. Renal regulation of extrarenal function: bone. In: Seldin DW, Giebisch G, eds. *The kidney: physiology and pathophysiology*. New York: Raven Press, 1985;823–846.
5. Kaplan NM. Renal regulation of extrarenal function: blood pressure. In: Seldin DW, Giebisch G, eds. *The kidney: physiology and pathophysiology*. New York: Raven Press, 1985;807–822.
6. Woodbury JW. Body acid-base state and its regulation. In: Patton HD, Fuchs AF, Hille B, Scher AM, Steiner R, eds. *Physiology and biophysics: circulation, respiration, fluids, metabolism, and endocrinology*. Philadelphia: WB Saunders, 1989;1114–1138.
7. Jackson EK, Branch RA, Margolius HS, Oates JA. Physiological functions of the renal prostaglandin, renin, and kallikrein systems. In: Seldin DW, Giebisch G, eds. *The kidney: physiology and pathophysiology*. New York: Raven Press, 1985;613–644.
8. Kriz W, Kaisling B. Structural organization of the mammalian kidney. In: Seldin DW, Giebisch G, eds. *The kidney: physiology and pathophysiology*. New York: Raven Press, 1985;265–306.
9. Lemley KV, Kriz W. Structure and function of the renal vasculature. In: Tisher CC, Brenner BM, eds. *Renal pathology with clinical and functional correlations*, vol II. Philadelphia: JB Lippincott, 1989;926–964.
10. Edwards RM. Segmental effects of norepinephrine and angiotensin II on isolated renal microvessels. *Am J Physiol* 1983;248:F526.
11. Edwards RM. Direct assessment of glomerular arteriole activity. *NIPS* 1988;3:216–219.
12. Edwards RM. Comparison of the effects of fenoldopam, SK&F R-87516, and dopamine on renal arterioles *in vitro*. *Eur J Pharmacol* 1986;126:167–170.
13. Wilkes BM, Susin M, Mento PF, Macica CM, Giradi EP, Boss E, Nord EP. Localization of endothelin-like immunoreactivity in rat kidneys. *Am J Physiol* 1991;260:F913–F920.
14. Carmines PK, Fleming JT. Control of the renal microvasculature by vasoactive peptides. *FASEB J* 1990;4:3300–3309.
15. Barajas L. Innervation of the renal cortex. *Fed Proc* 1978;37:1192–1201.
16. Beeuwkes R III, Ichikawa I, Brenner BM. The renal circulations. In: Brenner BM, Rector FC Jr, eds. *The kidney*, 2nd ed. Philadelphia; WB Saunders, 1976;249–288.
17. Beeuwkes R III, Bonventre JV. Tubular organization and vascular-tubular relations in the dog kidney. *Am J Physiol* 1975;229:695–713.
18. Beeuwkes RB III. The vascular organization of the kidney. *Annu Rev Physiol* 1980;42:531–542.
19. Walker RJ, Duggin GG. Drug nephrotoxicity. *Annu Rev Pharmacol Toxicol* 1988;28:331–345.
20. Hook JB, Hewitt WR. Toxic responses of the kidney. In: Klaassen CD, Amdur MO, Doul J, eds. *Casarett and Doull's toxicology: the basic science of poisons*, 3rd ed. New York; Macmillan, 1986; 310–329.
21. Kov V, Badr KF. Biological actions and pathophysiological significance of endothelin in the kidney. *Kidney Int* 1991;40:1–12.
22. Clapp WL, Tisher CC. Gross anatomy and development of the kidney. In: Tisher CC, Brenner BM, eds. *Renal pathology with clinical and functional correlations*, vol I. Philadelphia: JB Lippincott, 1989;67–91.
23. Kriz W, Kaisling B. Structural organization of the mammalian kidney. In: Seldin DW, Giebisch G, eds. *The kidney: physiology and pathophysiology*. New York: Raven Press, 1985;265–306.
24. Aukland K. Methods for measuring renal blood flow: total flow and regional distribution. *Annu Rev Physiol* 1980;42:543–555.
25. Tisher CC, Madsen DM. Anatomy of the kidney. In: Brenner BM, Rector RC Jr, eds. *The kidney*, vol I. Philadelphia: WB Saunders, 1991;3–75.
26. Tisher CC, Brenner BM. Structure and function of the glomerulus. In: Tisher CC, Brenner BM, eds. *Renal pathology with clinical and functional correlations*, vol I. Philadelphia: JB Lippincott, 1989;92–110.
27. Maddox DA, Brenner BM. Glomerular ultrafiltration. In: Brenner BM, Rector FC Jr, eds. *The kidney*, 4th ed. Philadelphia: WB Saunders, 1991;205–244.
28. Mene P, Simonson MS, Dunn MJ. Physiology of the mesangial cell. *Physiol Rev* 1989;69:1347–1424.
29. Valtin H. *Renal function: mechanisms preserving fluid and solute balance in health*. Boston: Little, Brown, 1983.
30. Lorenz JN, Weihprecht H, Schnermann J, Skott O, Briggs JP. Characterization of the macula densa stimulus for renin secretion. *Am J Physiol* 1990;259:F186–F193.

31. Forster RP, Maes JP. Effects of experimental neurogenic hypertension on renal blood flow and glomerular filtration rate in intact and denervated kidneys of unanesthetized rabbits with adrenal glands demedullated. *Am J Physiol* 1947;150:534–545.
32. Thurau K. Renal hemodynamics. *Am J Med* 1964;36:698–707.
33. Robertson CR, Deen WM, Troy JL, Brenner BM. Dynamics of ultrafiltration in the rat. III. Hemodynamics and autoregulation. *Am J Physiol* 1972;223:1191–1203.
34. Arendshorst WJ, Beierwalters WH. Renal tubule reabsorption in spontaneously hypertensive rats. *Am J Physiol* 1962;237:F38.
35. Haddy FJ, Scott JB. Metabolically linked vasoactive chemicals in the local regulation of blood flow. *Physiol Rev* 1968;48:688.
36. Dworkin LD, Brenner BM. The renal circulations. In: Brenner BM, Rector RC Jr, eds. *The kidney, Vol I*, Philadelphia: WB Saunders 1991;164–204.
37. Briggs JP, Skott O, Ofosu-Appiah O, Smart A. NaCl concentration dependence of macula densa mediated renin secretion. *Kidney Int* 1989;35:299.
38. Gerkens JF, Heidemann HT, Jackson EK, Branch RA. Effect of aminophylline on amphotericin B nephrotoxicity in the dog. *J Pharmacol Exp Ther* 1983;224:609–613.
39. Maunsbach AB. Observations on the segmentation of the proximal tubule in the rat kidney. Comparison of results from phase contrast fluorescence and electron microscopy. *J Ultrastruct Res* 1966;16:239–258.
40. Maunsbach AB. Ultrastructure of the proximal tubule. In: Orloff J, ed. *Handbook of physiology, section 8: renal physiology*. Washington, DC: American Physiological Society 1973;31–81.
41. Burnett VL, Short BG, Swenberg JA. Localization of $\alpha_2\mu$-globulin within protein droplets of the male rat kidney: immunohistochemistry utilizing perfusion-fixed GMA-embedded tissue section. *J Histochem Cytochem* 1989;37:813–818.
42. Bulger RE, Cronin RE, Doyban DC. Survey of the morphology of the dog kidney. *Anat Rec* 1979;194:41–66.
43. Bulger RE, Dobyan DC. Recent advances in renal morphology. *Annu Rev Physiol* 1982;44:147–179.
44. Jacobsen NO. Enzyme histochemical observations on the segmentation of the proximal tubules of the kidney of the female rat. *Histochemistry* 1975;43:11–32.
45. Berry CA, Rector FC Jr. Renal transport of glucose, amino acids, sodium, chloride, and water. In: Brenner BM, Rector FC Jr, eds. *The kidney*, 4th ed. Philadelphia: WB Saunders, 1991:245–282.
46. Olbricht CJ, Cannon JK, Garg LC, Tisher CC. Activities of cathespins B and L in isolated nephron segments from proteinuric and nonproteinuric rats. *Am J Physiol* 1986;250:F1055–F1063.
47. Hediger MA, Coady MJ, Ikeda TS, Wright EM. Expression cloning and cDNA sequencing of the Na^+/glucose co-transporter. *Nature* 1987;330:379–381.
48. MacLennan DH, Brandi CJ, Korczak B, Green NM. Amino-acid sequence of a Ca^{2+} + Mg^{2+}-dependent ATPase from rabbit muscle sarcoplasmic reticulum, deduced from its complementary DNA sequence. *Nature* 1985;316:696–700.
49. Kartner N, Ling V. Multidrug resistance in cancer. *Sci Am* 1989;260(March):44–51.
50. Tune BM. Mechanism of nephrotoxicity of beta-lactim antibiotics. *Contrib Nephrol* 1990;83:202–207.
51. Ford SM, Hook JB. Biochemical mechanisms of toxic nephropathies. *Semin Nephrol* 1984;4:88–106.
52. Borgoff SJ, Short BG, Swenberg JA. Biochemical mechanisms and pathobiology of $\alpha_2\mu$-globulin nephropathy. *Annu Rev Pharmacol Toxicol* 1990;30:349–367.
53. Lehman-McKeeman LC, Rivera-Torres MI, Cardill D. Lysosomal degredation of $\alpha_2\mu$-globulin and $\alpha_2\mu$-globulin-xenobiotic conjugates. *Toxicol Appl Pharmacol* 1990;103:539–548.
54. Donadio C, Tramonti G, Auner I, Giordani R, Lucchetti A, Calderazzi A, Deleide G, Lunghi F, Bianchi C. Nephrotoxicity and tubular effects of contrast media. *Contrib Nephrol* 1990;83:237–244.
55. Weiner IM. General pharmacological aspects of diuretics. In: Dirks JH, Sutton RAL, eds. *Diuretics: physiology, pharmacology and clinical use*. Philadelphia: WB Saunders, 1986;3–28.
56. Anders MW, Lash L, Dekant W, Elfarra AA, Dohn DR. Biosynthesis and biotransformation of glutathione S-conjugates to toxic metabolites. *CRC Crit Rev Toxicol* 1988;18:311–341.
57. Beeuwkes R III. Renal countercurrent mechanisms, or how to get something for (almost) nothing. In: Taylor CR, Johansen K, and Bolis L, eds. *A companion to animal physiology*. New York: Cambridge University Press, 1982;266–288.

58. Hays RM. Water transport in epithelia. In: Kinne RKH, ed. *Urinary concentrating mechanisms*, Comparative physiology series, vol 2. New York: Karger, 1989;1–30.
59. Knepper MA, Star RA. The vasopressin-regulated urea transporter in renal inner medullary collecting duct. *Am J Physiol* 1990;259:F393–F401.
60. Mejia R, Sands J, Stephenson JL, Knepper MA. Renal actions of atrial natriuretic factor: a mathematical modeling study. *Am J Physiol* 1989;257:F1146–F1157.
61. Nonoguchi H, Sands JM, Knepper MA. ANF inhibits fluid absorption in cortical collecting duct of rat kidney. *Am J Physiol* 1989;256:F179–F186.
62. Earley LE. Some aquaretic agents other than vasopressin analogs. In: Andreucci VE, Dal Canton A. eds. *Diuretics: basic, pharmacological, and clinical aspects*. Boston: Martinus Nijhoff, 1987; 188–195.
63. Caltabiano S, Kinter LB. Up-regulation of renal adenylate cyclase-coupled vasopressin receptors after chronic administration of vasopressin antagonists to rats. *J Pharmacol Exp Toxicol* 1991; 258:1046–1054.
64. Bonventre JV, Karnovsky MJ, Lechene CP. Renal papillary epithelial morphology in antidiuresis and water diuresis. *Am J Physiol* 1978;235:F69–F76.
65. Cirio A, Boivin R. Urea recycling from the renal pelvis in sheep: a study with [^{14}C]urea. *Am J Physiol* 1990;258:F1196–F1202.
66. Packer RK, Sands JM, Knepper MA. Chloride and osmotic water permeabilities of isolated rabbit renal papillary surface epithelium. *Am J Physiol* 1989;257:F218–F224.
67. Schmidt-Nielsen B. Function of the renal pelvis. In: Kinne RKH, ed. *Urinary concentrating mechanisms*, Comparative physiology series, vol 2. New York: Karger, 1989;103–140.
68. Welser B, Yagil Y, Jamison RL. Urea flux in the renal pelvis and ureter. *Kidney Int* 1988; 33:439(abstract).
69. Short BG, Burnett VL, Cox MG, Bus JS, Swenberg JA. Site-specific renal cytotoxicity and cell proliferation in male rats exposed to petroleum hydrocarbons. *Lab Invest* 1987;57:564–576.
70. Beeuwkes R III, Barger AC. *The human kidney: tubules, blood vessels, and vascular-tubular relations* (a film). New York: Robert P. Goldman Productions, 1975.
71. Tsan MF, Jones TC, Wilson TH. Canine cystinuria: intestinal and renal amino acid transport. *Am J Vet Res* 1972;33:2463–2468.

Toxicology of the Kidney, Second Edition,
edited by Jerry B. Hook and Robin S. Goldstein.
Raven Press, Ltd., New York © 1993.

2

Functional Assessment of the Kidney

Ernest C. Foulkes

Department of Environmental Health, University of Cincinnati College of Medicine, Cincinnati, Ohio 45267-0056

Ancient and medieval physicians routinely inspected urine and its sediments to diagnose systemic disease. Up to relatively recently, however, the lack of adequate concepts of the nature of renal function made it difficult to attribute urinary abnormalities to specific renal lesions. An example was the identification of cystine as an important constituent of renal stones (1), preceding the recognition of aminoaciduria as a reflection of tubular malfunction.

As is true of other fields of study, major advances in the elucidation of normal and abnormal renal function had to await the development of convenient and quantitative methods of analysis. Perhaps more than any other approach, it was the formulation of the concept of renal clearance and its application to the study of urea excretion by Moller et al. (2) in 1929 that enabled the rapid expansion of our understanding of normal and abnormal renal function. Clearance provides a quantitative measure and expression of renal function in a simple and physiologically meaningful manner. We need only look at Homer Smith's classic volume *The Kidney* (3) to appreciate the far-reaching advances made possible by the introduction of clearance calculations. Other techniques, however, have also found extensive use in the evaluation of renal function *in vivo*.

Function and metabolism of renal tissue obtained from intoxicated animals often yields important information on renal integrity *in vivo*. The same tissue preparations can also be used to study the mechanism of cytotoxic action of agents that directly affect renal function. Perhaps the best known of these preparations is the cortical slice, which actively transports various organic anions and cations in the direction of secretion. Slices from control animals have been used extensively in elucidation of secretory mechanisms, whereas those from experimental animals have served as probe for renal changes *in vivo*. Many investigators also studied metabolism of cortical homogenates and mitochondrial preparations, solute transport by isolated tissue fractions such as glomeruli (4), papillary slices (5), tubule fragments (6) and isolated, perfused tubules (7), function of renal cells in culture, and effects of toxicants on purified membrane vesicles (8). Each of these procedures has led to important insights into renal physiology and the mechanism of action of various nephrotoxicants, but full details lie beyond the scope of a chapter on evaluation of renal function. Similarly, renal histopathology will not be considered here.

The present chapter focuses on how toxicants affect the excretory role of the kidney, and does not deal with its metabolic and endocrine functions. For this reason, toxic effects interfering with systemic calcium metabolism by inhibiting renal hydroxylation of 25-α-hydroxy–vitamin D, or depressing hemopoiesis by reducing renal release of erythropoietin, will not be further considered here. We will therefore first define and discuss renal clearance, the concept that continues to provide the rationale for most renal function tests. Those solute clearances that have proven especially useful in the analysis of nephrotoxicity are tabulated and their application illustrated by selected examples taken from the toxicological literature. Next, other important approaches to the evaluation of renal function *in vivo* are presented. Finally, we will discuss some of the *in vitro* methods routinely employed in the evaluation of renal intoxication.

CLEARANCE-BASED STUDIES IN INTACT ORGANISMS

The Clearance Technique

Clearance techniques provide a convenient quantitative measure of renal function, and are usually based on simultaneous analysis of plasma and urine. The clearance concept possesses the great advantage of permitting assessment of renal function in terms of a physiologically meaningful quantity—the virtual volume of plasma cleared of a solute by the kidney in unit time. The significance of the term *virtual* here lies in the fact that the same clearance value would be calculated whether a solute is completely extracted from 100 ml plasma per unit time, or only 50% cleared from 200 ml. Clearance, in other words, only corresponds to a discrete physical volume if a single pass through the kidneys leads to complete removal of the solute under study. This is further discussed below in relation to Eq. 2.

Conventionally, renal clearance has been equated to urinary clearance. In this case, the amount of the plasma solute excreted in urine per minute is given by the product of urine flow V (in ml/min) and the concentration of the solute in urine (U). If P denotes the steady concentration of that solute in arterial plasma, then the expression UV/P describes the volume of plasma from which the solute has been extracted into the urine over a period of 1 min. This defines the urinary clearance (C) of a solute as summarized in Eq. 1:

$$C(\text{ml/min}) = UV/P \qquad [1]$$

Strictly speaking, of course, renal accumulation or metabolism of a plasma solute also constitutes renal clearance from plasma. Thus, the kidney readily filters plasma Cd-metallothionein but almost completely reabsorbs it at low concentrations; little is excreted in urine (9) and the reabsorbed protein is not returned to blood. A more general expression for renal plasma clearance in ml/min is therefore given by the product of renal plasma flow (*RPF*) and *E*, the percent extraction calculated as $(A-V)/A$, where *A* and *V* represent the arterial and venous plasma concentrations of the solute under study. Note that the simplifying assumption is implicitly made that solute fluxes between red cells and plasma do not affect *A* or *V*. The general formula for clearance is thus given by Eq. 2:

$$C = E \times RPF \quad [2]$$

Measuring clearance by determination of renal plasma flow and the $A-V$ difference is, of course, more invasive and less convenient than basing the calculation, when possible, on urinary excretion. In our further discussion of clearance we shall restrict ourselves, therefore to renal clearance as classically defined in terms of urinary excretion of plasma solutes. Note, therefore, that the clearance concept cannot be applied to urinary excretion of a solute like ammonia, which is synthesized in the kidney, or cadmium, whose excretion may result in part from release of metal sequestered for long periods of time in the kidney. It is important further to reiterate the statement above that only if the solute were completely removed from plasma during a single passage through the kidneys, i.e., if *E* in Eq. 2 equaled 100%, with subsequent excretion into the urine, would the calculated clearance correspond to a specific physiological parameter, namely the renal plasma flow. However, even for solutes like *p*-aminohippuric acid (PAH) that most closely approach these conditions, extraction from plasma seldom exceeds 90%.

The clearance of a solute like inulin, which is freely filterable at the glomerulus, and which is neither secreted nor reabsorbed in the tubules, by definition must equal the glomerular filtration rate (GFR). Note the demand for complete filterability of the quantity of solute expressed by *P* in Eq. 1. Thus, a major fraction of heavy metals in plasma is bound to plasma protein and can therefore not be filtered; accordingly, *P* in the expression *UV*/*P* must be corrected for nonfilterable metal for the clearance calculation to lead to a physiologically meaningful result. In practice, ultrafilterability of a solute circulating in plasma may be difficult to measure: First, properties of pores in synthetic ultrafiltration membranes may differ greatly from those of glomerular pores; a different charge distribution *in vitro* is likely to alter the filtration characteristics of ionic macromolecules from those observed *in vivo* (10). A second difficulty, sometimes overlooked, is related to the fact that anticoagulants, for instance by chelating heavy metals, may alter their filterability (11). Such an effect was reported in work on excretion of lead by the dog kidney (12).

Renal clearance of extracellular solutes that are not otherwise excreted or metabolized can be calculated from their plasma disappearance curves (13). Such techniques routinely utilize isotopically labeled compounds and are further discussed in the section Miscellaneous Techniques, below; they possess the advantage of not requiring either urine collections or prolonged equilibrating infusions. When urinary clearance is conventionally determined from the *U*/*P* ratio, the arterial plasma concentration of the solute should ideally have reached a steady state. For an exogenous solute, the classical clearance technique therefore requires as long as 1 hr of equilibrating infusion, often preceded by a priming injection. Alternatively, and more conveniently, reasonably stable plasma levels of solutes can be achieved by giving an intramuscular or subcutaneous depot injection. Even if absolute constancy is not achieved in this manner, a mean concentration can be computed provided the rate of change of plasma concentration is slow and constant.

The steady-state solute concentration, however achieved, must always lie well below the half-saturating concentration (K_m) of any nonlinear reabsorptive or secretory process in the renal tubule. A well-known illustration of this fact is the glucosuria of diabetes mellitus, which reflects not damage to the proximal tubules but saturation of their capacity to transport the excess sugar. Another prerequisite for significant clearance values is a urine flow sufficiently high to permit essentially complete collections during accurately timed clearance periods. Even carefully controlled experiments in the laboratory cannot always achieve such ideal conditions. As a result, renal clearance values seldom possess confidence limits of better than perhaps $\pm 10\%$. Such an accuracy may be adequate for most purposes; it implies, however, that as much as 20% depression of a renal solute clearance following exposure to a compound believed to act directly on the kidney does not necessarily indicate a nephrotoxic effect.

A special case is that of endogenous creatinine. This is normally produced at a constant rate as the end product of muscle metabolism and therefore circulates in plasma at a constant concentration; it is freely filtered at the glomerulus but neither reabsorbed nor effectively secreted in the tubule. Secretion has been reported in some species, but it is sufficiently small so that it does not significantly contribute to creatinine excretion except at low filtration rates. Like inulin clearance, that of creatinine can therefore serve as a convenient measure of the glomerular filtration rate. Creatinine possesses a great advantage over inulin in that its clearance can be measured without the need of an equilibrating infusion.

Measurement of the renal clearance of an exogenous solute by conventional techniques consumes relatively large amounts of this solute in order to reach and maintain the required steady plasma levels; this is especially true of determinations of maximum tubular transport activity (T_m) at high plasma concentrations (see the section Measurement of T_m, below). Factors of cost of the solute, time required for its equilibration, toxicity, radiation exposure in the case of labeled solutes, and metabolic breakdown or transformation as for instance by transamination of an infused amino acid into a competing amino acid, all constitute disadvantages of normal T_m measurements.

These problems can be minimized by use of a so-called arterial gradient infusion procedure in which the arterial plasma concentration of the solute in strongly diuresing animals is rapidly raised in a stepwise fashion. It can then usually be kept approximately constant for several minutes by decreasing the rate of infusion in a manner equal and opposite to the rate at which recirculation would have raised plasma levels at a constant infusion rate. It is possible in this manner to carry out a complete clearance determination in 3 to 4 min (14). The procedure has been successfully applied to dogs (15), rabbits (16), and rats (17), but has not been widely adopted, perhaps because of occasional difficulties encountered in maintaining constant plasma concentrations.

Simplified Clearance Determinations

Clearance determinations as discussed so far all require measurement of concentrations in carefully timed urine and plasma samples. Other techniques of assessing renal function, not directly based on the clearance concept, will be discussed in the section Additional Measures of Renal Function, below. In addition, useful approximations to relative solute clearance values can be obtained by simplified procedures. The best known of these simply takes the plasma level of urea, or preferably creatinine, as a measure of the glomerular filtration rate. Indeed, if creatinine excretion (UV in g/day) is constant then GFR ($= UV/P$) theoretically is inversely proportional to P_{Cr}, the creatinine concentration in plasma; any increase in P_{Cr} above a normal level of around 1 mg/dl should therefore reflect a corresponding fall in GFR. In practice the method is not very sensitive in the normal range of plasma creatinine levels (<1.4 mg/dl); a better correlation between measured creatinine clearance (C_{Cr}) and that predicted on the basis of P_{Cr} is obtained at higher plasma levels, i.e., lower C_{cr} values (18).

Because its rate of production is influenced by changes in protein metabolism, and its excretion by the rate of urine flow, the level of urea in plasma varies more widely than that of creatinine. Although it is therefore a less reliable indicator of glomeruler function than is plasma creatinine, plasma urea is frequently used to follow changes in GFR. This is illustrated in Fig. 1 for a group of lead (Pb) workers whose blood lead level reflects the length and severity of their exposure (19); a significant positive correlation was observed between blood lead and blood urea. Note that blood and plasma or serum urea are used interchangeably because this solute freely diffuses into and out of blood cells.

Considerable information can also be obtained on changes in clearance values by analysis of only randomly collected urine. This approach is also based on the characteristics of creatinine excretion as discussed above and consists of normalizing excretion of a solute by that of creatinine. A change in the solute/creatinine concentration ratio in urine then reflects a corresponding change in the excretion of the solute under study. This is illustrated in Table 1 by results obtained with rats exposed to cadmium oxide (CdO) dusts (MacDonald and Foulkes, unpublished). Clearly, the exposure was associated with increased protein excretion; no evidence for proximal tubular damage was seen in terms of reduced tubular reabsorption (i.e., increased normalized excretion) of amino acids, inorganic phosphate, or glucose. This finding suggests, therefore, that proteinuria here resulted from increased protein filtration rather than decreased tubular activity. Under other conditions of metal exposure a Fanconi-like syndrome may be produced, characterized by tubular aminoaciduria, phosphaturia, etc. (20); urinary solute/creatinine ratios will accord-

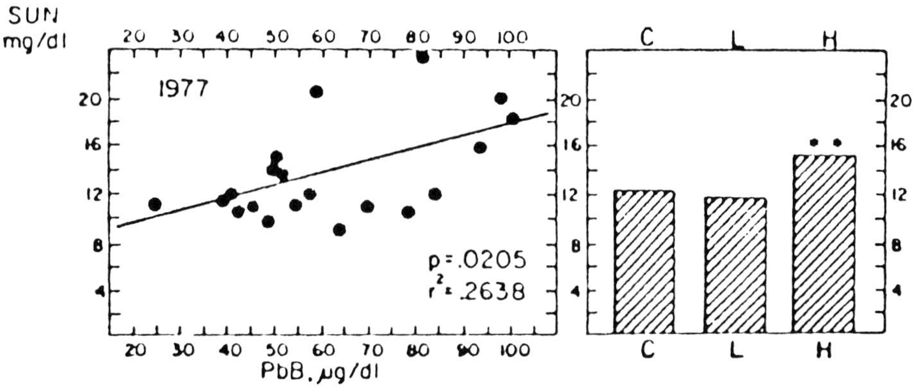

FIG. 1. Relationship between blood lead concentration as measure of exposure and serum urea nitrogen in a group of smelter workers (modified from Hammond et al., ref. 19). $^{**}p = .026$ for H (high exposure group); C (control group); $p = .072$ for L (low exposure group).

ingly rise. In all these instances, simple chemical analysis of urine suffices to monitor effects of nephrotoxins on renal clearances.

Normalization of urinary solute excretion on the basis of creatinine (or, to a lesser extent, on the basis of urinary specific gravity) possesses other advantages. Thus, as illustrated in Fig. 2, normalization significantly diminishes the large fluctuations often encountered in urinary solute concentrations. It also justifies, as discussed above, the analysis of spot samples of urine, thus avoiding the inconvenience of having to collect 24-hr urine samples. Because of diurnal variations in the GFR, the spot samples should be collected at the same time each day.

Gross changes in renal plasma flow, or a reduction in the efficiency (E) of extraction of secreted solutes from blood due to cytotoxic effects, can also be demonstrated by changes in the time required for excretion of a standard injected dose of compounds like ortho-iodohippurate, the dye phenol red (PSP) and x-ray contrast media like Diodrast. Each of these substances is efficiently extracted by the normal kidney, with a high value of E as defined in Eq. 2, so that their excretion provides a

TABLE 1. *Renal function after cadmium oxide (CdO) exposure in rats*

Excreted solute/mg creatinine	Control	Exposed
Protein (mg)	11.7 ± 1.0	19.5 ± 3.2*
Amino acids (mmol)	0.13 ± 0.01	0.14 ± 0.01
Inorganic PO_4 (umol)	21 ± 2	24 ± 3
Glucose (umol)	1.4 ± 0.2	1.6 ± 0.2

From MacDonald and Foulkes, unpublished.

All results represent the mean ± SE for six or more rats that had been exposed to CdO dust (200 μg/m^3), 35 hr/week, for 1 year.

*Significantly different from control ($p < .05$).

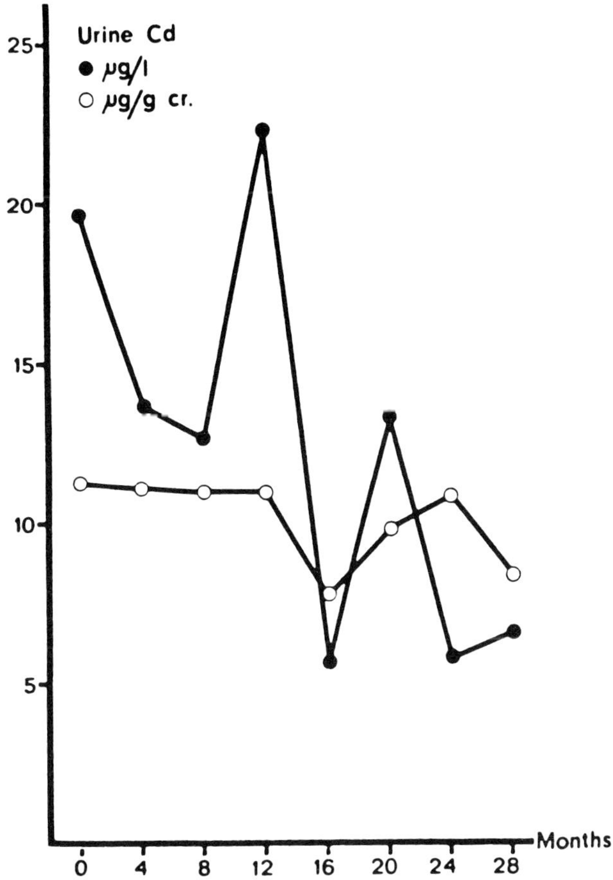

FIG. 2. Normalization of urinary Cd excretion. (From Piscator et al., ref. 52, with permission.)

composite measure of effective renal plasma flow, total tubular mass, and the functional integrity of the tubule cells; the technique is further considered in the section Miscellaneous Techniques, below. Additional information on changes in tubular mass and activity can be obtained from determination of maximum tubular capacity (T_m) as discussed below.

Double Indicator Dilution Techniques

A rapid and powerful approach to the study of renal function in control or poisoned animals is the double indicator dilution technique, introduced into renal studies by Chinard (21). It consists essentially of a rapid arterial bolus injection of a test solute, together with a glomerular and extracellular marker such as creatinine, followed by rapid collection of sequential urine or renal venous blood samples. Although the procedure is too invasive for routine or other than terminal functional assessment, it can provide extensive information on the integrity of solute transport processes and on their mechanisms, as well as on the site of action of various inhibitors.

Typical results obtained in this manner are illustrated in Fig. 3 for the amino acid aspartate injected into the renal artery of a rabbit, together with inulin as glomerular marker (22). On the left, in the control study, the recovery peak of the amino acid is obviously much smaller than that of inulin. In the absence of reabsorption, the peaks of the two solutes should have overlapped; the deficit of aspartate therefore reflects its greater than 90% reabsorption. In contrast, the much greater fractional excretion of aspartate in the presence of a competitive inhibitor of its reabsorption (glutamate) is clearly seen on the right side; the higher the inhibitor concentration, the more closely the recovery curve of aspartate approaches that of inulin. The finding also illustrated in Fig. 3 that the mean transit time (t) of aspartate equals that of inulin even in the presence of the inhibitor led to the conclusion that the inhibitor acts at the brush border membrane (22). The method has also been applied to the study of function at the basolateral membrane of the tubular epithelium, by measurement of artery to vein transit curves (23).

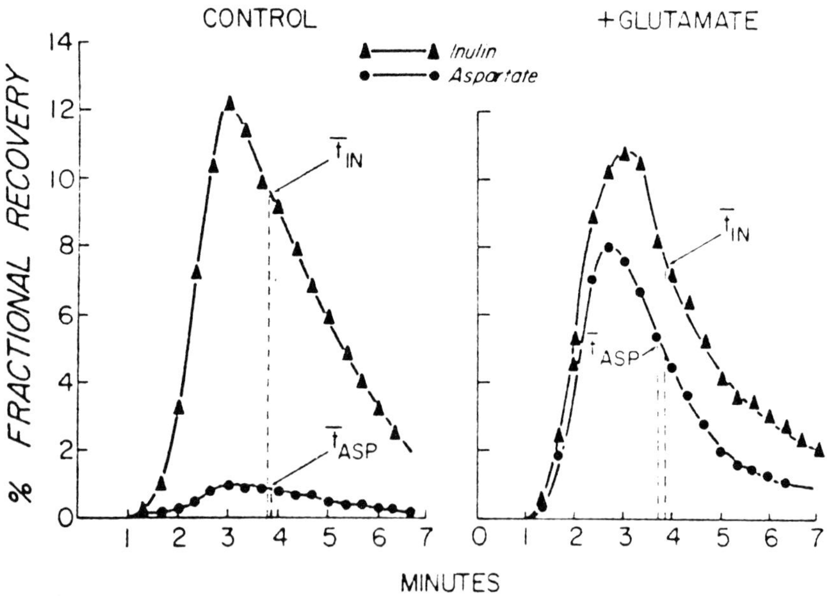

FIG. 3. Double indicator dilution analysis of aspartate reabsorption. Recoveries of inulin and aspartate in successive urine samples are shown following their injection as arterial bolus, under control conditions (*left*), and after administration of a competing amino acid (*right*); $\bar{t}$=mean artery-urine transit time. (From Foulkes, ref. 22, with permission.)

The indicator dilution technique possesses the disadvantage of requiring arterial injection and ureteral cannulation in the anesthetized animal. On the other hand, it is rapid and consumes relatively little solute, thus permitting convenient and repeated measurements of relative clearances. Care must be taken in all renal transit experiments to use sufficiently low bolus concentrations of the test solute so that even at its peak plasma concentration renal transport mechanisms do not become saturated. Saturation of a reabsorptive system will, by definition, increase the fractional excretion of its substrate. As example of the important use to which such observations can be put, reference may be made to the report that at high bolus concentrations of metallothionein (MT) the characteristics of its transit from artery to urine approach those of inulin (24). The implications of this finding are that MT is freely filterable and that it is normally reabsorbed by a saturable mechanism. In addition, obviously little nonfiltered MT can have been transported directly from blood into urine (secretion), a conclusion further confirmed by the similar renal vascular transit curves of inulin and of MT.

Free Water Clearance and Renal Concentrating Ability

One of the most important functions of the normal kidney is its ability to respond to changes in the state of hydration by excreting dilute or concentrated urine. Thus, aquatic mammals like the beaver produce very dilute urine in order to remove excess water; in contrast, desert mammals obliged to conserve water may excrete urine of the consistency of toothpaste. Appropriate water excretion or retention provides a very sensitive measure of general renal integrity.

The simplest measure of the ability of the kidney to conserve water is provided by the osmolality of urine excreted by a water-deprived subject. The osmolality of plasma changes relatively little and averages close to 300 mOsm; analysis of the osmolar concentration of urine thus leads directly to the (U/P)osmol ratio. Simple and convenient osmometers are available for such determinations. Human urine may range from osmolalities below 100 mOsm to a maximum of perhaps 1,800, i.e., to a urine sixfold more concentrated than plasma. The rat, in contrast, can readily concentrate its urine nine- to-tenfold.

A more quantitative measure of urine concentrating ability is the clearance of free water (C_{H_2O}), derived in turn from the osmolal clearance, (UV/P)osmol. The latter in effect represents the volume that would be required to excrete total urinary solute in isosmotic solution, i.e., at a concentration of 300 mOsm. If filtrate were excreted as such, the osmolal clearance would equal the GFR. If the urine is more dilute than the filtrate, the dilution may be visualized as that volume of filtrate from which solute was removed without reabsorption of water; this volume is defined as the free water clearance (C_{H_2O}), or free water excretion, and is given by Eq. 3, where V stands as usual for the urine volume excreted per unit time:

$$C_{H_2O} = V - (UV/P)\text{osmol} \qquad [3]$$

Dilution of urine, i.e., reabsorption of solute without water, primarily occurs in the so-called diluting segment in the thick ascending loop of Henle. The water permeability of this segment is very low and as NaCl is reabsorbed the remaining fluid is rendered dilute. Additional solute reabsorption occurs in the more distal nephron and contributes to a high interstitial solute concentration in the medulla. In the presence of antidiuretic hormone, water can move out of the lumen along the osmotic gradient, so that the final osmolality of the urine reflects the osmolal concentration in the medulla. Excretion of concentrated urine, by analogy with the formation of dilute urine discussed above, implies that a certain volume of solute-free water must have been removed from the isosmotic filtrate, in addition to the large fraction of filtered water and solute normally reabsorbed isosmotically in the proximal tubule. In this case, the clearance of solute-free water is negative, and appropriately referred to as negative free water clearance; it is calculated as $(UV/P)\text{osmol} - V$.

Several intrarenal factors are involved in the production of concentrated urine, including especially the attainment and maintenance of high interstitial osmolality in the medulla as a result of solute filtration and reabsorption, and of the countercurrent concentrating mechanism, which depends in turn on normal medullary blood flow. Urinary concentrating ability can therefore not be associated with a specific aspect of renal function but serves rather as reflection of its general integrity, and can thus prove useful for screening purposes. This is illustrated in Table 2 by renal function measurements performed in workers employed in the production of lead and Cd-containing pigments; note that, in this population, only urine concentrating ability revealed significant renal damage. Urine osmolality has also been measured in the study of effects of nephrotoxicants in animals; we have used it extensively to follow the progression of metal intoxication in the rat (25,26).

TABLE 2. *Renal effect of exposure to Pb and Cd*[a]

	Mean value observed	Average normal	Percent abnormal
Plasma creatinine (mg/dl)	1 ± 0.2	<1.4	0
Creatinine clearance (ml/min × 1.73 m^2)	130 ± 32	Age-dependent	0
β_2-microglobulin (μg/24 hr)	148 ± 170	<370	8
Urine osmolality	802 ± 140	>800	52

Modified from Greenberg et al., ref. 50.

[a]These workers had been exposed for 11 to 37 years; urine osmolality was measured after overnight water deprivation.

Measurement of T_m

The maximum capacity of the renal tubule actively to reabsorb or secrete a solute is referred to as the T_m for this solute. Determination of a T_m value consists essentially of a regular clearance measurement performed at sufficiently high solute concentrations in plasma so that a further increase does not lead to additional active transport. In other words, the clearance is measured at saturating solute levels. Under those conditions, and given the definition of filtered load of a freely filterable solute as the product of glomerular filtration rate and plasma concentration ($GFR \times P$), T_m equals ($GFR \times P - UV$) for a solute undergoing net reabsorption, and ($UV - GFR \times P$) for a solute showing net secretion.

Determination of T_m customarily requires measurement of excretion at several high plasma concentrations, in order to assure that saturation has indeed been achieved. A complication arises from the fact that active transport is often accompanied by nonsaturable passive solute movement, occurring along paracellular pathways or through the cells (27). Accordingly, a correction may have to be applied for such passive fluxes, as determined from the slope of net reabsorption against plasma concentration at high levels. Excessively high levels should be avoided, both because of possible pharmacological effects, and because some solutes at high concentrations may depress their own net transport (the so-called self-depression of transport).

It is clear that T_m normally reflects the total mass of transporting tissue, and should therefore be independent of changes in renal blood flow. Reducing the blood supply to a kidney would not alter T_m values but would only correspondingly increase the plasma concentrations required to saturate the tubules. Removal of one kidney, in contrast, would initially reduce T_m values by 50%. Inhibitory or toxic changes leading to a decreased tubular ability to transport solutes at saturating levels would also decrease the T_m for these solutes. To normalize T_m values, they are often expressed per unit mass of functioning nephrons as reflected by the glomerular filtration rate (Table 3); the expression T_m/GRF is given in concentration units (i.e., mg per min/ml per min = mg/ml). The reduced efficiency (E) of PAH extraction in Table 3 presumably resulted from cytotoxic effects, although theoretically it could also have been caused by a redistribution of renal blood flow away from tubular regions. In any case, major circulatory changes appear to have occurred, as revealed by the decrease in *RPF*. The fall in T_m of glucose could be interpreted in terms of a severely impaired tubular ability to transport glucose. Such a conclusion is, however, not supported by the normal value of T_m/GFR; this suggests, instead, that circulatory or other changes may have, for instance, reduced the number of filtering glomeruli without change in T_m per functioning nephron.

Even if, however, the T_m for glucose should be depressed following intoxication, this would not necessarily lead to glucosuria at normal plasma levels. As is generally true of any enzyme inhibition study, the degree of substrate saturation of an enzyme determines whether an inhibitory effect can be observed. In renal terms, attention must therefore be paid to the ratio of load/T_m. If the load of a solute filtered

TABLE 3. *Acute effect of Cd on renal function in rabbits*

	Control	Poisoned
C_{Cr} (ml/min)	13.5 ± 1.8	3.6 ± 1.1
RPF (ml/min)	70.3 ± 11.4	34.2 ± 6.8
E_{PAH} (%)	84 ± 4	38 ± 9
FF	0.23 ± 0.01	0.12 ± 0.03
T_m gl (mg/min)	39 ± 8	14 ± 2
T_m gl/GFR (mg/ml)	2.9 ± 0.6	3.8 ± 0.6
FE_{AA} (%)	3 ± 1	27 ± 5

Modified from Gieske and Foulkes, ref. 51.

C_{Cr}, creatinine clearance = GFR; RPF, total renal plasma flow = C_{PAH}/% extraction of PAH (E_{PAH}); *FF*, filtration fraction = C_{Cr}/RPF; T_m gl, maximum tubular glucose reabsorption; FE_{AA}, fractional excretion of filtered amino acids = C_{AA}/C_{Cr}.

All values represent means ± SD from 13 or more rabbits.

in a single nephron is reduced sufficiently by a fall in the single nephron filtration rate, essentially normal reabsorption at low plasma levels might proceed in spite of inactivation of a major fraction of carriers responsible for reabsorption.

General Comments

The concept of renal clearance provides the rationale for most evaluations of renal excretory function in the living animal; this holds true for the classical clearance technique as well as for the modifications and simplifications described above. Implicitly, therefore, clearance remains basic for the evaluation of the extent to which toxicants alter renal function. Although some of the *in vitro* techniques available for the study of renal function, such as the slice technique to be discussed below, have found use in assessing nephrotoxicity, their major application is in work aimed at elucidating basic mechanisms of renal function and of their perturbation by toxicants.

Table 4 summarizes the main clearance-based procedures described so far. Note that suitable choice of a test solute may permit one to isolate to some extent functions of a specific nephron portion. For instance, toxic effects on the proximal tubule will result in altered clearances of such solutes as glucose or amino acids, whereas changes in free water clearance are likely to be correlated with damage to the diluting segment in the more distal nephron. Additional procedures pointing to changes in function of particular nephron segments will be considered in the sections Enzymuria and Miscellaneous Techniques, below. Other tests, in contrast, may possess little specificity. Thus, urine concentrating ability is a sensitive measure of total renal integrity rather than of function in a specific portion of the nephron. Finally, various renal functions may exhibit different sensitivities to a toxicant, so that evidence for their inhibition may be found at different stages of intoxication. This is seen particularly clearly in Fig. 4 from the work of Nomiyama and Nomiyama (28), which illustrates the time of appearance of certain signs of intox-

TABLE 4. *Clearance-based techniques for assessment of renal function*

Compound	Conditions	Purpose and significance	Remarks
1. Inulin	Exogenous	Measure of GFR	Other nonreabsorbed or nonsecreted compounds like ^{51}Cr-EDTA may be used
2. Urea	Endogenous	Approximate measure of GFR	Reduced at low urine flow; see also 3.
3. Creatinine	Endogenous or exogenous	Measure of GFR	*P* changes inversely with GFR and thus provides a rough measure of GFR
4. Glucose, amino acids	Normal *P*	Increased excretion due to proximal malfunction	Rise in urinary concentration ratio to creatinine reflects changed fractional reabsorption
5. Glucose	High *P*	Determination of T_m, a measure of proximal integrity or active tubular mass	T_m may change with GFR, and may therefore be normalized by GFR
6. PO_4 (inorganic)	Normal *P*	Measure of tubular reabsorption	—
7. PAH (PSP, etc.)	Low *P*	Measure of effective RPF	100% extraction from peritubular plasma assumed; may be reduced by transport inhibition
	High *P*	T_m reflects active proximal tubular mass	Reduced by fall in perfused mass, transport inhibition
8. Total osmoles	Endogenous	Required to calculate free water clearance	(*U*/*P*) measures concentrating ability
9. Solute-free water	Antidiuresis	Negative clearance measures concentrating ability	Influenced by antidiuretic hormone, changes in filtered load, reabsorption, and blood flow
	Water diuresis	Estimate of distal solute reabsorption	—
10. Na		Clearance Na/GFR or *U* (Na/creatinine) reflects fractional reabsorption	Affected by Na intake, changes in extracellular volume, GFR, etc.
11. Plasma proteins	Low MW	Increased by inhibition of proximal reabsorption (tubular proteinuria)	Excretion expressed/g creatinine or /24 hr; *P* usually ignored
	High MW	Not appreciably filtered by normal glomerulus (glomerular proteinuria)	Excretion expressed as *U*, or as above

GFR, glomerular filtration rate; MW, molecular weight; *P*, plasma concentration; *PAH*, *p*-aminohippurate; PSP, phenol red; RPF, renal plasma flow; *U*, urine concentration.

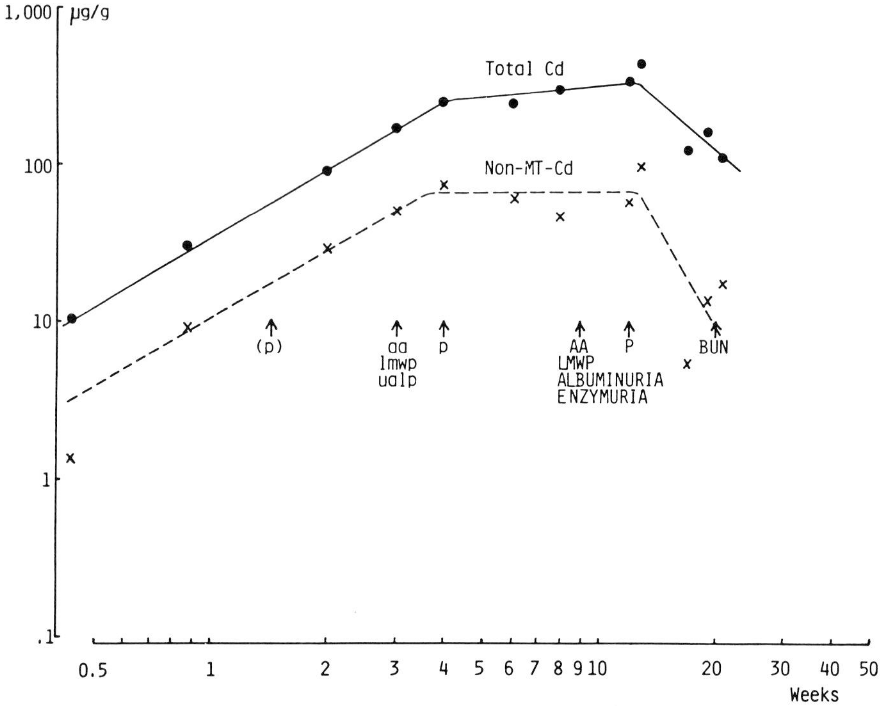

FIG. 4. Appearance of functional lesions in Cd-poisoned rabbits. Concentrations of total Cd, and nonmetallothionein Cd (non-MT-Cd) are shown in µg/g cortex (fresh weight). p, proteinuria; aa, aminoaciduria; lmwp, low molecular weight proteinuria; ualp, urinary alkaline phosphatase; BUN, blood urea nitrogen; lowercase letters describe small changes. (From Nomiyama and Nomiyama, ref. 28, with permission.)

ication following chronic exposure of rabbits to cadmium. Note also that even though Cd levels especially in the nonmetallothionein fraction, believed to contain the toxic species of the metal, approached maximum values already after 4 weeks of exposure, signs of malfunction were not fully developed until much later.

Such an initiation delay, as pointed out by Yuile (29), raises the likelihood that an effect of a toxicant on, e.g., membrane transport, results indirectly from its action at some other site, and is not being exerted directly on the membrane carrier system under study. It is likely, for instance, that the immune system is involved in the delayed onset of acute renal failure following Hg administration (30). Similarly, the slow onset of aminoaciduria following acute loading of the rabbit kidney with Cd (31) can readily be explained on the basis of an indirect action of the metal. Indeed, 12 hr or longer elapse after the loading, with significant fall of Cd concentration from its peak value in the kidney, before the T_m of aspartate reabsorption declines. On the basolateral side, passive extrusion and active uptake of cycloleucine proved to be equally sensitive to Cd intoxication, raising the possibility here too that effects may arise from some nonspecific action of the metal; perhaps the primary effect is some change in blood flow distribution or in cell geometry due to cell swelling, etc. (32). This hypothesis is strengthened by the fact that basolateral movement of another solute, PAH, is also equally sensitive to cadmium in either direction.

In summary, the choice from among the clearance-based techniques cited in Table 4 should be based on such considerations as the duration of exposure, the nature and dose of nephrotoxicant used, and the need to focus on a particular nephron segment. Where possible, the results should be complemented by parallel analysis with histopathological or other techniques.

ADDITIONAL MEASURES OF RENAL FUNCTION

General

Other simple techniques are available for assessing renal function by analysis of urine, without the need for collecting and analyzing plasma as required for clearance measurements. Thus, much can be learned from the physical appearance of urine, or its volume and specific gravity. Renal failure may be manifested by oliguria, i.e., excretion of relatively large volumes of inappropriately dilute urine; this results from the inability of the diseased kidney to concentrate the urine, even though the volume of filtrate may be much reduced. In anuric renal failure urine excretion falls, usually because of tubular blockage (hyaline casts).

Essentially qualitative conclusions can be drawn from inspection of urine sediments. Semiquantitative information on urine composition can be gathered with the use of indicator papers, especially for glucose, protein, or the presence of blood. Analysis of enzyme activity in urine also yields insight into renal integrity. These, and some additional procedures, are reviewed in this section.

Enzymuria

Enzymuria, the measurement of enzyme excretion in urine, provides another useful tool for assessing renal function *in vivo*. A distinction must be made between excretion of plasma enzymes and the release of enzymes from renal parenchyma. Identification of nonrenal enzymes in urine points to increased protein filtration, i.e., to glomerular damage; this presupposes that the enzymes are not normally filterable. Appearance of enzymes of renal origin, of course, reflects intrarenal changes, and can readily be demonstrated in the isolated, saline-perfused kidney (33). Proteinuria without significant excretion of tubular enzymes suggests the presence of glomerular lesions. A massive increase in, e.g., hepatic enzymes in plasma due to liver necrosis could conceivably also lead to their appearance in urine.

Under optimal conditions, meaningful results can be obtained from measurement of enzyme excretion in urine; certain precautions, however, need to be taken. First, the urine must be free of bacterial contamination and host cells, whose presence may severely influence the results obtained. Second, the urine should be assayed as soon after collection as possible; if necessary, urine samples can be stored in the frozen state, but only after preliminary control measurements have shown that freezing does not affect the particular enzyme activity under study. Third, the possibility must be considered that urine may contain enzyme inhibitors. Such inhibitors can sometimes be removed by dialysis, or their influence is minimized by measuring activity in maximally diluted urine samples.

It is important to emphasize that enzyme activities are not distributed evenly along the nephron. Alkaline phosphatase, for instance, although present in the highest concentration in the proximal convoluted portion of the human nephron (34), is found also in all other nephron sections. Further, enzyme distribution patterns along the nephron differ from species to species. As a result, increased excretion of a particular enzyme cannot readily identify the localization of functional lesions. In the work of Ellis et al. (35), for instance, a transient increase in *N*-acetylglucosaminidase was reported in the urine of dogs 4 days after injection of ethylenimine, a papillary poison; alkaline phosphatase rose only at a later stage in the experiment. It is unlikely, however, that glucosaminidase could serve as marker enzyme for papillary damage. Zhou et al. (26) reported large increases in urinary excretion of this enzyme in rats exposed to cadmium, primarily a proximal tubular poison.

Information on the nature of the damage can be derived also by considering the subcellular origin of enzyme activity recovered in the urine. Thus, high concentrations of alanine aminopeptidase, alkaline phosphatase, and maltase are associated with proximal brush border, and may thus be excreted at an early stage of cell intoxication. In contrast, excretion of the mitochondrial enzyme glutamate dehydrogenase presumably reflects profound cell destruction. Loss of a cytosolic enzyme such as lactic dehydrogenase may result from lesser degrees of cellular injury. Additional information on the origin of urinary enzymes can sometimes be gained by separation of various isoenzymes, as described by Sternberg et al. (36). These authors reported that one of the urinary isoenzymes of aspartate aminotransferase in the Hg-poisoned rat could not be identified in plasma and, therefore, presumably originated in the kidney. Isoenzyme analysis may also help determine the subcellular source of an enzyme excreted in urine.

Perhaps because of slow changes in the extent of cellular damage following exposure to a toxicant, or as a result of the loss of all enzyme available in a particular cell type, activity of a particular enzyme in urine may be raised only transiently, and different enzymes may be found at different stages of exposure. To that extent, enzymuria does not differ from other measures of renal malfunction (see Fig. 4). The relationship in these experiments between increases in urinary excretion and the duration of exposure, and consequently the total dose of cadmium administered, need not represent a direct dose-effect relationship. This follows, as noted in the section General Comments, above, from the fact that the concentration of the presumed toxic species of Cd, the so-called nonmetallothionein Cd, reached a steady state already after 4 weeks, whereas maximum enzymuria was observed only after 9 weeks. Such a delayed response is therefore likely to reflect an initiation delay of metal action (31) rather than a relationship between effect and total dose administered and/or retained after 9 weeks.

Despite the problems of detailed interpretation, analysis of enzyme activity has proven popular and useful. The techniques are generally relatively simple, and possess the advantage of being noninvasive. The most commonly measured enzymes are probably the lysosomal *N*-acetylglucosaminidase, the cytosolic lactate dehydrogenase, and the brush border alkaline phosphatase. These and some of the numerous other enzymes that have been measured in urine as a reflection of renal damage are listed in Table 5. Note that this list does not include lysozyme, whose ready filterability makes it difficult to distinguish renal from extrarenal enzyme in urine. The table does identify, where possible, the principle nephron segment from which urinary enzyme may have originated, but some activity is present in all segments. Precise distribution of activity along the nephron also varies somewhat between species; no segment of origin is specified when no general preferential distribution could be established.

Acute intoxication of rabbits with uranium causes them to excrete a peak of catalase activity in urine (37), but the specificity and rationale of this effect are not entirely clear; no catalase excretion has been noted in chronically exposed human subjects. For certain other enzymes, however, increased urinary excretion can serve as a sensitive probe for renal damage. As in the case of other measures of renal malfunction it is important to reemphasize that the time of appearance of different enzymes during exposure to a given toxicant may vary, and that the nature of the enzymes excreted in urine may differ for various toxicants. It is generally advisable, therefore, not to rely on only one technique for evaluating renal damage, and to confirm conclusions drawn from enzyme assays by other procedures.

TABLE 5. *Some urinary enzymes used in assessment of renal lesions*

Enzyme	Principal nephron segment involved	Subcellular localization
Alkaline phosphatase	Proximal	Brush border
Alanine aminopeptidase	Proximal	Brush border
Maltase	Proximal	Brush border
Lactate dehydrogenase	*	Cytoplasm
Glutamate dehydrogenase	Proximal, distal	Mitochondria
Acid phosphatase	*	Lysosomes
N-acetylglucosaminidase	*	Lysosomes
Galactosidase	*	Lysosomes

*No clear preferential distribution.

Urinary Sediments

Sediments collected by centrifugation of fresh urine samples and inspected under the microscope either directly or after suitable staining can provide much qualitative information on renal integrity. In particular, evidence is routinely sought in this manner for erythrocytes (intrarenal bleeding), leukocytes (inflammation, rejection), bacteria, tubule cells (tubular damage), tubular casts resulting from inappropriate presence of protein in the tubule, and crystals of various relatively insoluble solutes. The subject of sediment analysis has been extensively covered in many publications and need not be further considered here.

Miscellaneous Techniques

The renal functions evaluated by several of the clearance techniques discussed in the section Clearance-Based Studies in Intact Organisms, above can be assigned to a particular nephron segment. Additional tests for damage at specific sites may be devised on the basis of the known localization of different functions. Thus, acidification of urine occurs primarily in the distal tubule whose functional integrity therefore is important in determining the ability of an organism to excrete an acid load. Normal impermeability of the collecting duct epithelium to urea in absence of antidiuretic hormone, and unchanged potassium secretion, helped localize the toxic action of uranyl acetate to more proximal portions of the rabbit nephron (38).

Urinary excretion of a low molecular weight protein like β_2-microglobulin is attributed to inhibition of its normal tubular reabsorption (tubular proteinuria). On the other hand, excretion of significant amounts of larger plasma protein molecules such as albumin results primarily from glomerular damage (glomerular proteinuria).

Renal function *in vivo* has been studied with the aid of x-ray contrast media such as Diodrast. This is a compound normally secreted by the tubular anion transport system, and the rate of its renal accumulation and subsequent excretion following acute injection can be conveniently followed by x-ray techniques. More recently the use of external gamma scanners with radioactive compounds labeled with 99_mTc or ^{131}I, such as for instance iodohippurate, has proven useful. An older technique attempted to provide similar information simply by measuring the fractional excretion of a secreted dye (PSP) in urine following a standard time lapse after an intravenous bolus injection. Major variables influencing the renal handling of these indicator substances are renal blood flow, glomerular filtration rate, and the ability of the tubule to transport the compound.

Following the intravenous injection of labeled compounds like iodotrizoate and ^{51}Cr–ethylenediaminetetraacetic acid (EDTA), which are freely filterable but restricted to the extracellular space, the rate of fall of their plasma concentration can be used to calculate GFR (13). Several such isotope procedures are used clinically for diagnostic purposes, and are described in detail in the literature on nuclear medicine.

STUDIES ON RENAL FUNCTION *IN VITRO*

Isolated Perfused Kidney

For certain purposes, the analysis of renal clearances by the isolated perfused kidney offers advantages over the often unavoidable use of intact animals. This is true, for instance, when studying the mechanism of excretion of very toxic substances whose systemic administration might poison the experimental animals. For assessing renal function *in vivo*, however, the isolated perfused organ has had only limited significance.

This limitation arises in the first place from technical difficulties. Thus, for many years, few preparations were capable of normal physiological function such as essentially complete fractional reabsorption of filtered Na and osmolal concentration of urine above that of the perfusion fluid. It was only more recently that study, especially of the metabolic requirements of the kidney, led to perfused preparations still exerting their normal physiological functions (39). They have been used, for instance, to analyze effects of cadmium (40) and other metals on the kidney. Like many other *in vitro* procedures, however, the isolated perfused kidney will continue to find greater application in the study of mechanisms of toxic action rather than in the assessment of renal function in exposed animals.

Solute Transport by Cortical Slices and Tubule Fragments

The use of thin tissue slices for the study of solute transport phenomena was introduced many years ago (41). Subsequently, Cross and Taggart (42) adapted the technique to the study of PAH transport in renal cortex. Since that time, the slice preparation has been used extensively both in the analysis of tubular transport mechanisms and their inhibition by toxic compounds *in vitro*, as well as for assessment of remaining tubular function in poisoned animals; no insight is obtainable on glomerular function. Before citing some instances where evaluation of function in cortical slices has proven the power of this technique in toxicology, it is appropriate to consider the important limitations of the slice preparation.

First, the active solute accumulation in slices is usually expressed in terms of a slice/medium (S/M) concentration ratio (mg per gram tissue/mg per ml incubation medium); it would be more informative to express this quantity instead in mg per ml intracellullar water/mg per ml medium. Second, the S/M value as determined after relatively prolonged incubation represents not a rate measurement but a steady state. Changes in the S/M ratio could arise from altered rates of influx and/or efflux, and determination of initial rates of solute uptake, for instance, could in many cases yield more meaningful results than can measurement of the steady state. Third, there is every reason to believe that solute transfer in slices represents primarily events at the basolateral side of tubular epithelial cells, and that the technique can therefore provide only very limited information on tubular reabsorption (43). A major reason for this conclusion is the long diffusion pathway along the tubule from medium to reabsorbing cell, coupled with the fact that in the normal slice continued salt and water reabsorption leads to collapse of tubular lumina. As a result, the luminal cell border in slices is relatively inaccessible from the medium.

The active accumulation by slices of organic anions like PAH or organic cations like *N*-methylnicotinamide thus primarily involves the basolateral aspect of the cells. In the case at least of PAH, basolateral transport has also been identified as the step-limiting tubular secretion *in vivo* (44). For these reasons, important aspects of tubular secretion can be conveniently studied in slices, and determination of the S/M ratio of PAH and similar solutes *in vitro* may provide a useful measure of tubular function *in vivo*.

In contrast, slices cannot unambiguously serve for the analysis of luminal transport processes such as reabsorption of amino acids. Tubular fragments are more useful than slices for evaluating solute transport at the brush border. This preparation was introduced by Burg and Orloff (6) and consists essentially of short segments of tubules obtained by collagenase digestion of renal cortex. Comparison of transport in slices and tubule fragments suggests that in the latter both sides of the cells are exposed to the medium (45). The method possesses no particular advantage for the estimation of general renal integrity *in vivo*.

Interpretation of slice data may be complicated if preliminary treatment of an animal with nephrotoxicants stimulates rather than depresses subsequent solute accumulation *in vitro* (e.g., 46). Such a result could arise from differential effects of intoxication on solute uptake and extrusion in slices (47). Nevertheless, there are many instances of dose-related depression of solute accumulation by slices from poisoned animals. An example of such an effect is illustrated in Table 6, abstracted from the work of Kluwe and Hook (48). Here, mice received increasing intraperitoneal doses of chloroform, and their renal function was evaluated 24 hr later. Note that results reflecting glomerular function *in vivo* (BUN) paralleled those provided by analysis of secretory activity (PAH accumulation) in slices. In other words, the *in vitro* assay here permitted evaluation of renal integrity *in vivo*; apparently chloroform in this study had interfered with both glomerular and tubular function. Of course, slices cannot serve for screening potentially nephrotoxic compounds when these first have to be metabolically activated in, e.g., the liver.

Metabolism in slices and other *in vitro* preparations such as tubular fragments, glomerular suspensions, or tissue biopsies may also serve as sensitive indicator of cytotoxic effects, whether manifested by inhibition or specific enzymes, changes in patterns and control of metabolism (e.g., increased gluconeogenesis, decreased oxidative phosphorylation), loss of ability to maintain normal tissue water and electrolyte content *in vitro*, etc. In addition, enzymatic or chemical analysis of freshly obtained samples of tissue can provide information on possible lesions *in vivo*. The great advantage of slices for the assessment of renal function lies in the ease with which they permit testing of specific renal transport systems, especially those involved in renal secretion. In summary, therefore, slice studies, like use of other *in vitro* systems (see the next two sections), often provide useful alternative approaches to the assessment of renal function *in vivo*.

TABLE 6. *Demonstration* in vivo *and* in vitro *of dose-dependent nephrotoxic effects of $CHCl_3$ injected into mice*

	$CHCl_3$ (ml/kg)			
	0	.03	.10	.30
BUN (mg/dl)	22 ± 2	20 ± 2	30 ± 2	102 ± 10
PAH (S/M)	12.6 ± 0.6	12.1 ± 1.0	11.0 ± 1.0	4.9 ± 0.4

Values represent means ± SE for six mice, and are based on Kluwe and Hook, ref. 48 (Fig. 4).

Effects of Nephrotoxicants on Isolated Membranes

Over the last decade, results obtained with purified preparations of brush border or basolateral membrane fragments have contributed significantly to the study of epithelial solute transport (e.g., 8). Because such fragments usually form closed vesicles, they have permitted detailed investigation *in vitro* of mechanisms of normal transmembrane solute transport and of the effects of certain inhibitors. It is likely that study of such mechanisms will continue to be the major area of application of vesicle preparations, but to the extent that their activity correlates with function *in vivo*, they have also been used to assess function in the intact organ.

An example of such use is the demonstration that the ability of brush border vesicles to react with Cd-metallothionein parallels the changes in tubular reabsorption of this protein in cadmium-treated rabbits (49). The vesicle preparation, however, is less suitable for general evaluation of renal function than for elucidation of specific mechanisms of action.

Use of Other Tissue Preparations

As described elsewhere in this volume many other *in vitro* preparations have been applied to the study of renal function. As described for vesicles above, such techniques are more likely to prove useful in the exploration of basic mechanisms, and for preliminary screening of potentially toxic compounds, rather than for assessment of renal intoxication *in vivo*. Among such techniques may be cited those utilizing renal cells in culture, and others based on perfusion of isolated portions of single renal tubules under various conditions. Cell cultures will in all likelihood serve as useful tools for identifying some possible nephrotoxic agents *in vitro* and in elucidating their mechanism of action, but they will not be further considered in this chapter.

CONCLUSIONS

As described in this chapter, extensive advantage has historically been taken of the relative convenience of renal function measurements for the diagnosis of disease. With the multitude of tests now available it has become possible to focus on specific aspects of renal function, and thus frequently to localize functional lesions along the nephron. Not all these procedures lend themselves, of course, to screening purposes. As a first step in surveying groups of experimental animals or human populations for the occurrence of renal malfunction the following tests are therefore recommended: serum creatinine (or blood urea) and urinary protein, primarily as measures of changes in glomerular filtration rate; urine glucose (dipstick) to reflect tubular function; and urine concentrating ability (measured by urinary osmolality or specific gravity after 12 hr of water deprivation) as a general measure of renal integrity. Microscopic analysis of urine sediments may also prove useful. On the basis of these simple and minimally invasive tests, further procedures may then be chosen if necessary to provide more detailed information on kidney damage in selected individuals.

REFERENCES

1. Wollaston WH. On cycstic oxide: a species of urinary calculus. *Phil Trans* 1810;100:223–230; cited in Morton LT, *A medical bibliography: an annotated check-list of texts, illustrating the history of medicine,* (4th ed.) Aldershot, UK: Gower, 1983.
2. Moller E, McIntosh JF, Van Slyke DD. Relationship between urine volume and the rate of urea excretion by normal adults. *J Clin Invest* 1929;6:427–465.
3. Smith H. *The kidney*. New York: Oxford University Press, 1950.
4. Mackenzie S, Scriver CR. Transport of L-proline and alpha-aminoisobutyric acid in the isolated rat kidney glomerulus. *Biochim Biophys Acta* 1971;241:725–736.
5. Lowenstein LM, Smith I, Segal S. Amino acid transport in the rat renal papilla. *Biochim Biophys Acta* 1968;150:73–81.
6. Burg MB, Orloff J. Oxygen consumption and active transport in separated renal tubules. *Am J Physiol* 1962;203:327–330.
7. Burg MB, Grantham J, Abramow M, Orloff J. Preparation and study of fragments of single rabbit nephrons. *Am J Physiol* 1966;210:1293–1298.
8. Murer H, Kinne R. The use of isolated membrane vesicles to study epithelial transport processes. *J Membr Biol* 1980;55:81–95.
9. Nomiyama K, Foulkes EC. Reabsorption of filtered cadmium metallothionein in the rabbit kidney. *Proc Soc Exp Biol Med* 1977;156:97–99.
10. Brenner B, Bohner M, Baylis C, Deen W. Determinants of glomerular permselectivity: insights derived from observations in vivo. *Kidney Int* 1977;12:229–237.
11. Foulkes EC. Mechanisms of renal excretion of environmental agents. In: Lee DHK, ed. *Handbook of physiology, section 9: reactions to environmental agents*. Washington, DC: American Physiological Society, 1977;495–502.
12. Vander AJ, Taylor DL, Kalitis K, Mouw DR, Victery W. Renal handling of lead in dogs: clearance studies. *Am J Physiol* 1977;233:F532–F538.
13. Tepe PG, Tauxe WN, Bagchi A, et al. Comparison of measurements of glomerular filtration rate by single sample, plasma disappearance slope/intercept and other methods. *Eur J Nucl Med* 1987; 13:28–31.
14. Foulkes EC. On the mechanism of chlorothiozide-induced kaliuresis in the rabbit. *J Pharmacol Exp Ther* 1965;150:406–413.
15. Banks RO, Foulkes EC. Quantitation of urinary precession of water, potassium and other solutes. *Am J Physiol* 1971;220:1325–1331.
16. Foulkes EC, Blanck S. Mechanism of inhibition of renal amino acid reabsorption in rabbits by heavy metals. *Toxicol Appl Pharmacol* 1982;64:103–107.
17. Linder G, Foulkes EC. Kinetics of renal aspartate reabsorption and its inhibition by metals in the intact rat kidney. *Environ Res* 1985;36:241–247.
18. Cockroft DW, Gault MH. Prediction of creatinine clearance from serum creatinine. *Nephron* 1976;16:31–41.

19. Hammond PB, Lerner SI, Gartside PS, et al. The relationship of biological indices of lead exposure to the health status of workers in a secondary lead smelter. *J Occup Med* 1980;22:475–484.
20. Chesney RW. Etiology and pathogenesis of the Fanconi syndrome. *Miner Electrolyte Metab* 1980; 4:303–316.
21. Chinard FP. Relative renal excretion patterns of *p*-aminohippurate (PAH) and glomerular substances. *Am J Physiol* 1956;185:413–417.
22. Foulkes EC. Cellular localization of amino acid carriers in renal tubules. *Proc Soc Exp Biol Med* 1972;139:1032–1033.
23. Silverman M, Aganon MA, Chinard FP. Specificity of monosaccharide transport in dog kidney. *Am J Physiol* 1970;218:743–750.
24. Foulkes EC. Renal tubular transport of cadmium metallothionein. *Toxicol Appl Pharmacol* 1978; 45:505–512.
25. Wang X-P, Foulkes EC. Specificity of acute effects of Cd on renal function. *Toxicology* 1984; 30:243–247.
26. Zhou JY, Foulkes EC, Jones M. Delayed nephrotoxic effects of cadmium and their reversibility by chelation. *Toxicology* 1990;64:235–243.
27. Foulkes EC, Blanck S. Non-saturable amino acid reabsorption in kidneys of normal and mercury-poisoned rabbits. *Proc Soc Exp Biol Med* 1988;189:223–228.
28. Nomiyama K, Nomiyama H. Tissue metallothionein in rabbits chronically exposed to cadmium with special reference to the critical concentration of cadmium in the renal cortex. In: Foulkes EC, ed. *Biological role of metallothionein*. Amsterdam: Elsevier/North Holland, 1982;47–67.
29. Yuile CL. Animal experiments. In: Hodge HC, et al., ed. *Handbook of experimental pharmacology*. Berlin: Springer-Verlag, 1973;165–196.
30. Bernaudin JF, Druet E, Druet P, Masse R. Inhalation or ingestion of organic or inorganic mercurials produces auto-immune disease in rats. *Clin Immunol Immunopath*. 1981;20:129–135.
31. Foulkes EC, Blanck S. Acute cadmium uptake by rabbit kidneys: mechanism and effects. *Toxicol Appl Pharmacol* 1990;102:464–473.
32. Foulkes EC, Blanck S. Cadmium inhibition of basolateral solute fluxes in rabbit renal tubules and the nature of basolateral cycloleucine uptake. *Toxicol Appl Pharmacol* 1991;108:150–156.
33. Lockwood TD, Bosman HB. The use of urinary *N*-acetylglucosaminidase in human renal toxicology. I. Partial biochemical characterization and excretion in humans and release from isolated perfused rat kidney. *Toxicol Appl Pharmacol* 1979;49:323–336.
34. Calcamuggi G, Cestonaro G, Emanuelli G, et al. L'impiego degli enzimi urinari per la valutazione del danno renale. *Minerva Med* 1978;69:1–16.
35. Ellis BG, Price RG, Topham JC. The effect of papillary damage by ethyleneimine on kidney function and some urinary enzymes in the dog. *Chem Biol Interact* 1973;7:131–142.
36. Sternberg M, Szlamka I, Moisy M, Rebeyrotte P, Lagrue G. Comparison of the urinary excretion of aspartate aminotransferase, lactic dehydrogenase, alkaline and acid phosphatase, and beta-galactosidase during nephrotoxic serum glomerulonephritis and mercuric chloride tubulonephritis in the rat. *Z Klin Chem Klin Biochem* 1974;12:543–550.
37. Katz EJ, Holt LG, Schwartz S. The effect of uranium exposure on urinary catalase excretion. In: Tannenbaum A, ed. *Toxicology of uranium*. New York: McGraw-Hill, 1951;283–289.
38. Bowman FJ, Foulkes EC. Effects of uranium on rabbit renal tubules. *Toxicol Appl Pharmacol* 1970;16:391–399.
39. Gronow GHJ, Cohen JJ. Substrate support for renal functions during hypoxia in the perfused rat kidney. *Am J Physiol* 1984;247:F618–F631.
40. Diamond GL, Cohen JJ, Weinstein SL. Renal handling of cadmium in the perfused rat kidney and effects on renal function and tissue composition. *Am J Physiol* 1986;251:F784–F798.
41. Stern JR, Eggleston LV, Hems R, Krebs HA. Accumulation of glutamic acid in isolated brain tissue. *Biochem J* 1949;44:410–418.
42. Cross RJ, Taggart JV. Renal tubular transport: accumulation of PAH by rabbit kidney slices. *Am J Physiol* 1950;161:181–190.
43. Silbernagl S, Foulkes EC, Deetjen P. Renal transport of amino acids. *Rev Physiol Biochem Pharmacol* 1975;74:105–167.
44. Foulkes EC. The kinetics of PAH secretion in the rabbit. *Am J Physiol* 1963;205:1019–1024.
45. Murthy L, Foulkes EC. Movement of solutes across luminal cell membranes in kidney tubules of the rabbit. *Nature* 1967;213:180–181.
46. Hirsch GH. Differential effects of nephrotoxic agents on renal transport and metabolism by use of in vitro techniques. *Environ Health Perspect* 1976;15:89–99.

47. Hirsch GH, Pakuts AP. Renal cortical slice uptake and runout of *N*-methylnicotinamide and *p*-aminohippurate after potassium dichromate treatment. *Can J Physiol Pharmacol* 1974;52:465–468.
48. Kluwe WM, Hook JB. Potentiation of acute chloroform nephrotoxicity by the glutathione depletor diethyl maleate and protection by the microsomal enzyme inhibitor piperonyl butoxide. *Toxicol Appl Pharmacol* 1981:59:457–466.
49. Selenke W, Foulkes EC. The binding of cadmium metallothionein to isolated renal brush border membranes. *Proc Soc Exp Biol Med* 1981;167:40–44.
50. Greenberg A, Parkinson DK, Fetterolf DE, et al. Effects of elevated lead and cadmium burdens on renal function and calcium metabolism. *Arch Environ Health* 1986;41:69–76.
51. Gieske TH, Foulkes EC. Acute effects of cadmium on proximal tubular function in rabbits. *Toxicol Appl Pharmacol* 1974;27:292–299.
52. Piscator M, Foulkes EC, Hammond PB. Early detection of renal disease. In: Radford EP, Underhill DW, eds. *New and sensitive indicators of health impacts of environmental agents*. Pittsburgh: University of Pittsburgh, 1986;99–114.

Toxicology of the Kidney, Second Edition,
edited by Jerry B. Hook and Robin S. Goldstein.
Raven Press, Ltd., New York © 1993.

3

Overview of Clinical Nephrotoxicity

William M. Bennett and George A. Porter

Division of Nephrology and Hypertension, Department of Medicine, Oregon Health Sciences University, Portland, Oregon 97201-3098

DRUG-RELATED RENAL SYNDROMES

The clinical manifestations of toxic nephropathy are protean, corresponding to the presenting symptoms and signs of renal disease in general. It is convenient for the clinician to categorize renal disease in syndromes that correspond to how the patient presents to the doctor (1). It should be recognized that toxicants are in the differential diagnosis of most of these syndromes and further, that a single therapeutic agent or nephrotoxicant may cause more than one clinical picture, depending on the nature of the toxicant, dose, duration of exposure, as well as a variety of host factors, such as age, sex, hepatic and renal drug metabolism phenotype, etc. In this chapter, an overview will be provided, which will serve as a framework for the specific information on individual nephrotoxicants, which make up the rest of this book. The major clinical syndromes in nephrology produced by drugs and chemicals are tabulated in Table 1.

Acute Renal Failure

One of the most frequent ways that nephrotoxic renal damage is manifested clinically is by acute deterioration of renal function over a matter of days to weeks. The severity of this renal failure depends on the nature and dose of the toxicant as well as a wide variety of individual host factors. It should be emphasized that acute renal failure can be present with relative preservation of urine flow (>500 ml/24 hr), so-called nonoliguric acute renal failure. In fact, most clinically relevant nephrotoxicants, such as aminoglycoside antibiotics, *cis*-platinum, cyclosporine, and radiocontrast media produce a nonoliguric type of acute renal failure. The precise pathophysiology of the renal failure may differ depending on the particular mechanism of toxic injury. Examples will be given in the following sections.

TABLE 1. *Clinical syndromes in nephrology produced by drugs and chemicals*

Syndrome	Clinical examples
Acute renal failure	
Direct tubular injury	Aminoglycosides, radiocontrast agents, chemotherapeutic drugs, amphotericin B, cephaloridine, heavy metals
Prerenal azotemia due to impaired perfusion	Nonsteroidal anti-inflammatory drugs (NSAIDs), angiotensin-converting enzyme (ACE) inhibitors, cyclosporine, diuretics
Acute interstitial nephritis	Penicillins, sulfonamides, phenytoin, diuretics, allopurinol, NSAIDs, many miscellaneous drugs
Acute obstructive uropathy	High-dose methotrexate, acyclovir, methysergide
Chronic renal failure	Analgesic-associated nephropathy, lead nephropathy, cyclosporine, nitrosoureas, intravenous drug abuse
Nephrotic syndrome	Gold, penicillamine, captopril, NSAIDs, heroin
Hyperkalemia	Beta blockers, NSAIDs, ACE inhibitors, potassium-sparing diuretics, cyclosporine
Hyponatremia	NSAIDs, chlorpropamide, thiazide diuretics
Nephrogenic diabetes insipidus	Lithium, demeclocycline, clofibrate

Direct Tubular Injury with Tubular Necrosis

Aminoglycoside antibiotics are widely used in the treatment of serious gram-negative infections. Some 10% to 15% of therapeutic courses are complicated by renal dysfunction due to proximal tubular injury. This injury is reported even when peak and trough drug levels are maintained in the therapeutic range (2).

The aminoglycosides are cationic with molecular weights of approximately 500. They are excreted by the kidney quantitatively with a clearance only slightly less than the glomerular filtration rate (GFR). Since there is little evidence for metabolism of the aminoglycosides, trough serum levels are a reflection of renal excretory capacity. A small fraction of filtered aminoglycosides binds to anionic phospholipid receptors on the proximal tubular epithelium, where a high-capacity transport system internalizes the drug into tubular cells. By interfering with critical intracellular biochemical processes, aminoglycosides ultimately produce cell necrosis (3). The drug is concentrated in the renal cortex to values 10 to 20 times concomitant serum levels. The elimination half-life of aminoglycosides, which is normally 2 hr, is markedly prolonged as renal function falls. Thus, maintenance-dose intervals should be extended in patients with existing renal dysfunction when aminoglycosides are required. Because the therapeutic efficacy of aminoglycosides is strongly correlated with peak serum levels, it is important to give an adequate initial loading dose independent of renal function. Among the clinically available aminoglycosides, the spectrum of nephrotoxicity is gentamicin > tobramycin > amikacin > netilmicin.

Nonoliguric renal insufficiency is the most common manifestation of aminoglycoside nephrotoxicity. Less common are a variety of isolated tubular syndromes, e.g., nephrogenic diabetes insipidus and Fanconi syndrome. Severe oliguric renal failure requiring dialysis is rare from aminoglycosides alone. A drug-induced concentrating defect characterized by polyuria and secondary thirst stimulation may precede the detectable rise in blood urea nitrogen and serum creatinine in patients given more than 5 to 7 days of aminoglycoside treatment (4). Granular casts and mild proteinuria occur frequently, but are not of diagnostic assistance. Enzymuria regularly develops between the second and fourth day of administration of aminoglycosides to both infected patients and human volunteers. In particular, the quantity of β_2-microglobulin and proximal tubular brush border enzymes, namely alanine aminopeptidase and *N*-acetyglucosaminidase, increase significantly. Whether such enzymuria represents evidence of nephrotoxicity or is simply a marker of ami noglycoside treatment with proximal tubular drug uptake remains controversial.

The renal histologic picture associated with aminoglycoside nephrotoxicity is one of patchy proximal tubular necrosis. In addition, in patients who satisfy the clinical criteria for aminoglycoside nephrotoxicity, cellular autophagocytosis has been observed using electron microscopy. Prominent cytosegresomes, containing whorled material referred to as "myeloid bodies," are observed in the proximal tubular lumen and urine (5).

A variety of clinical risk factors that predispose to the development of aminoglycoside nephrotoxicity have been identified. They are summarized in Table 2.

Since aminoglycosides are often necessary for the best antibiotic management of a critically ill patient, therapy should be optimally prescribed. Loading doses should be sufficient to achieve high peak levels to maximize bacterial killing, and maintenance doses should be based on calculated or measured renal function (6). Extending the interval between doses is safer than reducing the size of individual doses in patients with renal insufficiency. Correctable risk factors should be minimized, and in high-risk patients, the less-nephrotoxic congeners should be considered. Elevation of the trough level, indicating drug accumulation, usually precedes a rise in the less-sensitive serum creatinine measurement.

Other common examples of direct tubular injury are nephrotoxicity due to amphotericin B and *cis*-platinum.

Amphotericin B is a polyene antibiotic with excellent activity against a broad spectrum of fungi responsible for human infection. It has been estimated that renal function becomes impaired in more than 80% of patients given this drug (7). This nephrotoxicity is dose related and probably inevitable in cumulative doses greater than 5 g in adults. Patients at high risk include elderly patients, particularly those with depleted extracellular volume.

The usual clinical presentation of amphotericin B nephrotoxicity is characterized by defects in urinary concentrating ability and distal-type renal tubular acidosis. Occasionally, this condition will lead to nonoliguric renal failure with frank azotemia. Modest proteinuria associated with a relatively normal urinary sediment is the initial finding. In addition, the presence of a magnesium-wasting syndrome

TABLE 2. *Risk factors for aminoglycoside nephrotoxicity*

High dose and long duration of drug treatment
Recent courses of aminoglycoside therapy
Age greater than 60 years
Volume depletion
Potassium depletion
Magnesium depletion
Existing renal dysfunction
Liver disease

has now been recognized to be a prominent feature of amphotericin nephrotoxicity. Repetitive courses of amphotericin B may cause permanent impairment of renal function (8).

Recently, sodium loading has been reported to be useful in the prevention of amphotericin nephrotoxicity. Using a sodium supplementation approach, Branch (9) has reduced the incidence of amphotericin-associated renal impairment from 67% to 12%.

Nephrotoxicity is a well-recognized problem with the use of platinum derivatives. Cisplatin is a useful agent that improves tumor response rates in patients with disseminated testicular cancer (10). Dose-limiting nephrotoxicity is manifested by increases in serum creatinine and drops in creatinine clearance. Renal dysfunction tends to be cumulative, even if acute falls in GFR are prevented by hydration (11).

After cisplatin administration, there is early reduction of both GFR and effective renal plasma flow. Extracellular fluid volume depletion, prior renal impairment, and increased age tend to be special risk factors for renal dysfunction. Renal magnesium wasting is present in a high percentage of patients treated with cisplatin. Total body magnesium depletion is implicated in the frequently associated hypokalemia and hypocalcemia (12). Recent reports have emphasized renal sodium wasting with polyuria, hyponatremia, and volume depletion. In as many as 10% of patients treated with cisplatin, the tubular dysfunction is severe enough to produce orthostatic hypotension. In some of these patients, the renin-angiotensin system did not respond to the drug-induced, decreased, effective circulating volume (13). Carboplatin has also caused renal sodium wasting (14). Repeated cycles of platinum therapy, particularly with high doses, can also lead to chronic structural and functional abnormalities in the tubules.

Good hydration and forced diuresis will minimize the acute changes in renal hemodynamics attributable to cisplatin, although tubular uptake of the drug is not prevented. Magnesium and potassium losses should be anticipated with vigorous replacement. Concomitant nephrotoxicants, such as aminoglycosides, amphotericin, and nonsteroidal anti-inflammatory drugs should be avoided. Carboplatin may be indicated in patients with reduced renal function and those who are unable to tolerate high-volume hydration regimens.

Prerenal Azotemia

Renal hemodynamics may be compromised in certain predisposed patients by a variety of drugs. A common example would be the use of nonsteroidal anti-inflammatory drugs (NSAIDs) in patients in whom renal perfusion is dependent on vasodilatory prostaglandins such as PGE_2 and PGI_2. In such circumstances, inhibition of cyclooxygenase by the NSAID results in intrarenal vasoconstriction and decreased renal perfusion.

Certain subsets of patients are particularly prone to the development of oliguric acute renal failure when treated with NSAIDs. These include patients with congestive heart failure, chronic renal insufficiency, cirrhosis with ascites, systemic lupus erythematosus, intravascular volume depletion, elderly patients with significant atherosclerotic disease, and those treated with diuretics (15,16). All of these conditions may be associated with a decrease in renal perfusion and activation of the renin-angiotensin system. Angiotensin II constricts both the afferent and efferent glomerular arterioles. Constriction of the efferent arteriole increases intraglomerular capillary hydrostatic pressure, enhancing glomerular filtration rate during periods of decreased renal perfusion. Angiotensin II is also a potent stimulator for the renal synthesis of prostaglandin E_2, which, through its vasodilatory effect, augments renal perfusion. Thus, blockade of prostaglandin synthesis can result in an acute decline in renal blood flow and glomerular filtration rate. The hemodynamic nature of NSAID-induced acute renal failure is supported by the abrupt onset of oliguria, avid sodium and water retention, and rapid reversibility after discontinuation of the prostaglandin inhibitor. Compared with other forms of acute renal dysfunction, these patients recover baseline renal function within 2 to 3 days after the NSAID is discontinued. All available NSAIDs have been implicated as causes of acute renal failure, although there is some evidence that sulindac may have relatively less effect on renal prostaglandin synthesis than the other NSAIDs, and may thus be the agent of choice in patients at risk for renal insufficiency (17).

Likewise, angiotensin-converting enzyme inhibitors may cause acute, usually reversible renal failure in patients whose GFR is dependent on the presence of angiotensin's vasoconstrictor effect on the postglomerular efferent arteriole. Examples of such patients include those with bilateral renal artery stenosis, renal artery stenosis in a solitary kidney, transplant artery stenosis, severe intrarenal vascular disease, or patients with congestive heart failure. If such patients have volume depletion due to concurrent diuretics, they are at particular risk. Renal function rapidly improves with volume repletion. Potent diuretics per se may also produce a prerenal type of acute renal failure.

Interstitial Nephritis

Many drugs can cause rises in BUN and creatinine in the context of other evidence of systemic hypersensitivity such as fever, eosinophilia, and a diffuse skin rash. However, a renal hypersensitivity response may be present without any systemic manifestations. In these cases, the diagnosis depends on clinical suspicion and a confirmatory renal biopsy showing acute interstitial inflammation with lymphocytes and eosinophils. The urinary sediment shows microhematuria, pyuria, and urinary eosinophils. Withdrawal of the offending drug usually results in renal functional improvement, which can be hastened by a 10-to 14-day course of steroid therapy. Acute renal failure is nonoliguric and can be severe enough to necessitate dialysis. Common offending drugs are allopurinol, cimetidine, sulfonamides, penicillins, rifampicin, and phenytoin. NSAIDs may rarely produce a distinctive clinical picture of progressive nonoliguric acute renal failure, plus nephrotic syndrome. Glomerular pathology is most consistent with minimal-change nephropathy, since there are few electron-dense deposits and negative immunofluorescence. Interestingly, this unusual complication can occur after many months of therapy with NSAIDs. The renal dysfunction and proteinuria are usually reversible following drug discontinuation and steroid therapy.

Obstructive Nephropathy

Drug-induced intrarenal and extrarenal obstruction can cause acute renal failure. Intrarenal obstruction may occur when insoluble crystalline material deposits within tubular lumens. Examples include uric acid crystal deposition, particularly in acid urine. This usually occurs after cancer chemotherapy with tumor lysis. Alkaline diuresis, adequate hydration, and allopurinol can be given prophylactically with good results. Intrarenal obstruction may also be caused by high-dose methotrexate, rapidly infused acyclovir, and triamterene. Extrarenal obstruction due to methysergide-induced retroperitoneal fibrosis may require surgical relief. Obviously, the alert clinician must consider drug-induced obstructive nephropathy when evaluating patients with acute renal failure.

Chronic Renal Failure

This clinical syndrome usually presents with nonspecific symptoms such as nocturia, weakness, fatigue, nausea, or vomiting. Since renal functional reserve is large and disease processes proceed slowly, patients may be asymptomatic until 85% to 90% of renal function is lost. With primary involvement of glomeruli or blood vessels, hypertension and proteinuria are usually noted, whereas tubulointerstitial disease is often characterized by normal blood pressure and absence of proteinuria. Obviously, these distinctions are simply rules of thumb since most chronic renal diseases involve all parenchymal elements at end stage. It is not unusual to have advanced renal disease discovered during the workup of unexplained anemia or even on a routine chemistry screen.

Chronic Tubulointerstitial Nephritis

The association between chronic interstitial nephritis and ingestion of large amounts of analgesic drugs was first noted in 1953 (18). The number of cases reported is generally thought to be a gross underestimate of the true incidence of this preventable form of renal disease. Furthermore, discontinuance of ingestion after renal insufficiency develops often results in stabilization or improvement in renal function (19). It is widely believed that a combination of drugs causes the renal disease. Difficulties in relating the disease to a single drug result from the fact that combination analgesic therapy is the rule for most patients. The most distinct manifestation of the abuse of analgesics is renal papillary necrosis. Although prolonged use of aspirin alone has been reported as a cause of analgesic-associated nephropathy (20), it is likely that a combination of drugs is usually necessary to produce nephropathy. Acetaminophen is the major metabolite of phenacetin in man. Reports of association of this drug, both alone and with aspirin, with papillary necrosis are now known (21).

Clinically, the patient usually presents with the chronic complaints that require analgesics, that is, headache, back pain, or with some manifestation of chronic renal failure. Depression and gastrointestinal symptoms are prominent. The typical patient is a woman who is middle aged and somewhat defensive about consumption of analgesics. To obtain accurate histories, repeated questioning and family interviews may be necessary. Anemia and pyuria occur commonly, and acute infection or obstruction may be present if a papilla is sloughed. In view of the potential scope of this problem physician and patient education must be given high priority if this common form of chronic renal failure is to be eliminated.

Arteriolar Nephrosclerosis

This pathologic picture is most often seen in patients with long-standing hypertension. Clinical manifestations include slowly progressive renal failure with proteinuria of moderate proportions (1 to 2 g/day—nephrosis is rare). Hyperuricemia is common either as a cause or result of the vascular disease. The glomeruli and interstitium show the effects of chronic ischemia. Lead nephropathy is known to produce similar clinicopathologic features (22). Patients can be exposed to lead in homemade whiskey made in stills coated with lead. Lead can also be ingested by children from paint or toys or in rain water from porches painted with lead-containing paints. Cable jointers and battery workers are often exposed industrially. Pathologic descriptions in patients dying from chronic lead nephropathy are nonspecific, but severe nephrosclerosis predominates. Treatment is directed at removal of the source of lead and, in some cases, chelation therapy.

Chronic Glomerulonephritis

This slowly progressive syndrome of proteinuria, hypertension, and declining renal function is not commonly due to drugs, since most agents are not ingested over the long periods of time required. Immunologic renal injury induced by the intravenous injection of heroin may progress to chronic renal failure with progressive glomerular obliteration. The typical patient is an intravenous drug abuser in the second to fourth decade who has injected himself with heroin for 1 to 10 years. Some 70% to 75% of patients with proteinuria progress to end-stage renal insufficiency within 4 years despite steroid or cytotoxic drug therapy. Heroin or its injection vehicle may be directly toxic, or more likely, may sensitize the addict who subsequently develops immune complex nephropathy (23).

Progressive renal insufficiency requiring management for end-stage renal disease has been reported in cardiac allograft recipients treated with cyclosporine (24). Because these patient have excellent function of their allografts and have no other causes for renal disease, cyclosporine is almost certainly implicated. Although many of these patients had large initial doses, it is disturbing that disease progression has been noted despite dose reduction and strict maintenance of "therapeutic" blood levels. When biopsies have been performed, chronic tubulointerstitial fibrosis in a striped pattern and glomerulosclerosis have been observed. The striped pattern of fibrosis has been attributed to an arteriolar lesion, the arterioles being presumed to be a primary target for the drug in these patients. This type of change is less common in patients given doses less than 5 mg per kg, but it may still occur. In some patients treated for autoimmune uveitis, these same chronic histopathologic findings have been observed (25).

Nephrotic Syndrome

Nephrotic syndrome is the combination of massive proteinuria, hypoproteinuria, edema, and hyperlipoproteinemia. The most common causes of this syndrome are disease processes that affect glomerular permeability. Common drugs that produce nephrotic syndrome, albeit rarely, include Tridione, tolbutamide, and probenecid, as well as intravenous heroin abuse. In addition, environmental substances known to produce allergy or used to desensitize allergic patients are sometimes associated with nephrotic syndrome. Pathologic correlates of these clinical entities are sparse.

The nephrotic syndrome produced by gold therapy is characterized pathologically by membranous nephropathy (26). Although gold can be seen in the proximal tubules on ultrastructural examination, electron-dense deposits are noted within the glomerular basement membrane. In addition, IgG and other immunoglobulins are found on immunofluorescent examination. Gold-induced injury to tubular cells likely triggers an antigen-antibody complex reaction with some tubular component as the antigen. The nephrotic syndrome usually recedes when gold treatment is stopped. Penicillamine and captopril may also be associated with membranous nephropathy.

Disturbances of Body Fluids: Osmolality and Volume

Fluid and electrolyte disorders are among the most common conditions evaluated by a consulting nephrologist or internist. In this are, drug-induced or aggravated disease ironically has contributed much to the understanding of normal renal physiology.

Hyponatremia and Hypo-osmolality of Body Fluids

This disturbance is common in hospitalized patients and can result from many drugs that have an ability to impair renal water excretion. These effects may be independent of the primary pharmacologic action of the drug. The ability of some drugs, such as chlorpropamide, to impair water excretion has even been used therapeutically to treat diabetes insipidus (27). Prostaglandins also antagonize the effects of antidiuretic hormone (ADH). Consequently, prostaglandin blockade by NSAIDs can enhance ADH action resulting in a decrease in free-water excretion leading to the development of hyponatremia. A full review of the drugs that impair water excretion and their mechanisms of action is beyond the scope of this chapter.

Diabetes Insipidus and Hyperosmolality

This is most often nephrogenic when produced by drugs. However, central diabetes insipidus can be simulated under appropriate circumstances by the effects of ethanol and phenytoin. Drug-induced states of nephrogenic diabetes insipidus have been reviewed (28). Therapeutic advantage may be gained by using these drugs to treat severe states of hypo-osmolality. Lithium, fluoride from halogenated anesthetic metabolism, and demeclocycline are known causes.

Acid-Base Disturbances

Virtually any disturbance of hydrogen-ion balance, metabolic or respiratory, can be produced by, or related to, a drug or toxicant. The following section will catalogue such disorders, using as examples common entities that clinicians frequently see.

Metabolic Acidosis

Metabolic acidosis may be conveniently divided into two types. When there is a difference between measured cations and anions of greater than 12-14 mEq/l, an "anion gap" is said to exist. Retention of unmeasured anions implies an excess of nonvolatile acids and is most commonly observed in diabetic ketoacidosis and acute renal failure. Overdoses of such toxicants as methanol, ethylene glycol, and salicylate may produce metabolic acidosis in which large anion gaps are measured.

Lactic acidosis is a cause of metabolic acidosis produced by accumulations of lactate (>7 mm/l). Phenformin, an oral hypoglycemic agent, increases anaerobic metabolism of glucose by peripheral tissues with excess production of lactate. Clinical lactic acidosis most often occurs in diabetic patients with impaired renal function.

Renal tubular acidosis is a form of metabolic acidosis, usually without an increase in unmeasured anions. The kidney is unable to acidify the urine in response to systemic acidosis. The proximal type or type 2 renal tubular acidosis is associated with a decreased capacity of the nephron to reabsorb filtered bicarbonate, leading to "bicarbonate leak." Often, proximal reabsorptive defects for amino acids, glucose, and phosphate are associated (Fanconi syndrome). The full-blown picture may be produced by exposure to outdated tetracycline. Bicarbonate wasting without the multiple dysfunction of the proximal tubule is a common finding in patients treated with acetazolamide, a potent carbonic anhydrase inhibitor. This may lead to metabolic acidosis, hypercalciuria, nephrolithiasis, and hypokalemia. In this type of acidosis, the urinary pH is inappropriately high. Bicarbonaturia, however, occurs only when acidosis is mild to moderate. At this level, the serum bicarbonate is above the reduced nephron reabsorptive capacity. The amount of bicarbonate necessary to raise serum bicarbonate to normal and sustain it is generally large.

Distal or type 1 renal tubular acidosis is characterized by alkaline urine and bicarbonaturia persisting despite severe degrees of systemic acidosis. The dysfunction is thought to be due to an inability of the distal nephron segments to generate or maintain steep luminal-to-peritubular fluid hydrogen-ion gradients. Amphotericin B is known to produce this type of physiological defect in man. A fall in hydrogen-ion excretion and a rise in urine pH usually precede overt acute renal failure. Maintenance of adequate diuresis and bicarbonate during therapy may minimize toxicity. If therapy with amphotericin B can be stopped before azotemia occurs, recovery of renal function is the rule. Hypokalemia, despite systemic acidosis, is a prominent feature of amphotericin B distal renal tubular acidosis, and early $KHCO_3$ replacement is warranted.

Metabolic Alkalosis

Metabolic alkalosis may be produced by mineralocorticoid excess. Such patients characteristically have expansion of the extracellular fluid volume, hypokalemia, and alkalosis. The volume expansion causes "escape" from sodium-retaining effects of these steroids, making clinical edema uncommon. Habitual heavy users of licorice can reproduce such a syndrome because licorice has mineralocorticoid-like properties.

Hyperkalemia

Elevation of serum potassium may be produced by drugs, particularly in patients with preexisting renal disease. Among the commonly used therapeutic agents, angiotensin converting enzyme inhibitors frequently produce hyperkalemia via inhibition of angiotensin formation with secondary impairment of aldosterone secretion.

In addition to their effects on glomerular filtration rate, NSAIDs can have prominent effects on tubular function, especially with regard to renal handling of sodium, water, and potassium. Prostaglandins stimulate the production of renin, which subsequently leads to enhanced secretion of aldosterone. Decreased production of renal prostaglandins has been implicated in the pathogenesis of hyperkalemia in patients with hyporeninemic hypoaldosteronism (29). It is not surprising, then, that predisposed patients may develop hyperkalemia when treated with NSAIDs. This has been most commonly reported with indomethacin, but may occur with all NSAIDs. High-risk patients are characterized by preexistent renal insufficiency, vascular disease, diabetes mellitus, and mild hyperkalemia. Other drug-associated causes of hyperkalemia are potassium-sparing diuretics, beta blockers, and large doses of heparin.

Drug-induced renal disease is increasingly common, and it is vital for the clinician to recognize these nephrotoxic syndromes, since they are usually reversible. The spectrum of drug-related nephrotoxicity is broad, and virtually any primary renal disorder can be mimicked. Drugs may lead to acute and chronic renal failure, interstitial nephritis, nephrotic syndrome, obstructive uropathy, and altered tubular function. Multiple pathogenetic mechanisms are involved including direct renal toxicity, altered hemodynamics, hypersensitivity reactions, and altered hormone metabolism. The key to the diagnosis and treatment of drug-related renal syndrome is generally dependent on early recognition of the action of the offending agent and discontinuing the agent (30).

INCIDENCE/OUTCOME

The incidence of in-hospital acute renal failure (ARF) attributed to drug nephrotoxicity is currently estimated at one in five cases (31). The interpretation of this estimate in contemporary terms is complicated since it was derived during a period of significant change in the clinical pattern of ARF. With improved technology for both the diagnosis and treatment of ARF, plus the extended longevity of the American population, today's hospitalized patient with ARF is older (>59), if oliguric, having a multifactorial etiology and an expected death rate of >50% (32). The presence of nonoliguria imparts a lower mortality and is more likely to be due to a single etiology, i.e., drug induction (33).

Recently, the Societé de Nephrologie (34) conducted a 1-year survey of all patients with ARF to determine the frequency and causes of drug-induced acute renal injury. This survey has yielded the most comprehensive data by far regarding the epidemiology of drug-induced nephrotoxicity. Of the 2,175 cases of ARF, 398 (18.3%) were considered to be drug induced. Table 3 provides a summary of the distribution of the cases of ARF according to offending agent. As with previous reports concerning specific drug etiologies, antibiotics were most frequently encountered, with analgesics and NSAIDs sharing the second spot. Glafenin, an analgesic that is available in Europe but not in the United States distorted the data when compared to reports from North America (Table 4). More importantly, two-thirds of Glafenin cases represented acute ingestions associated with suicidal attempts. If these patients ($n = 79$) are excluded for purposes of calculating an incidence to compare with recent reports in the United States literature, the contribution of either antibiotics (7.8%) or contrast agents (2.9%) is still less than reported by either Rasmussen and Ibels (31) or Hou et al. (32). The new category of offending agent is NSAIDs, compounds that raised great concern within the nephrology community when one member was released as an over-the-counter preparation (35).

The significant contribution that NSAIDs provided to the overall incidence of drug-induced nephrotoxicity, summarized in Table 3 is in keeping with recent reports concerning the nephrotoxic potential of this group of compounds (36). Over half of the patients presented with nonoliguric ARF (NOARF), many having antibiotics or Glafenin as the causative agent. Of particular interest was the outcome of patients who survived the episode of ARF (mortality was 12.7%—50 patients) and only 28.6% of all patients required acute dialysis support during the episode of ARF. Table 3 summarizes the outcome of the 398 patients. Most impressive is the unexpectedly high percentage of patients who were left with permanent renal damage, i.e., 23.3%. This latter observation led the authors to speculate that "drug-induced acute renal failure" is an underestimated cause of chronic renal failure (34). In an earlier report, Pru et al. (37) had stated that up to 16% of patients surviving

TABLE 3. *Distribution of drug-induced acute renal failure (ARF)*

Drug	No. of patients	%	
Antibiotics	136	34.2	
Glafenin	79	19.8	} 35.4
NSAIDs	62	15.6	
Contrast media	50	12.6	
Diuretics	18	4.5	
Chemotherapy	14	3.5	
Others	39	9.8	
Clinical presentation			
Oliguric	175	44.8	
Nonoliguric	216	55.2	
Outcome			
Recovery complete	190	47.7	
Residual renal impairment	153	38.4	
Death	50	12.6	
Lost to follow-up	5	1.3	

Adapted from Société de Nephrologie, ref. 34.

severe ATN were left with chronic renal failure (CRF), nearly 50% requiring chronic dialysis. In the case of the French study, only 2 (2%) of the patients required dialysis support. One final comment regarding this pivotal study: nearly 15% of the 398 patients were classified as prerenal azotemia, a category of renal presentation that is often excluded in reports concerning ARF. Which category of drug was associated with this group of patients is not reported but diuretics would probably be a prime candidate.

To summarize this 1-year experience, nearly one in five patients who were diagnosed as having ARF were categorized as drug induced. Over 50% presented as NOARF, but almost one in four suffered significant renal sequelae.

The estimated incidence of 20% drug-induced ARF in hospitalized patients is in marked contrast to the extremely low incidence of outpatient drug-induced renal disease requiring hospitalization reported by Beard et al. (38), i.e., 1:300,000 person/year. Part of the explanation for this low incidence may rest in the authors' exclusion of chronic preexisting renal disease. In the study from France (34), 74 of 398 or nearly 19% of their cases occurred in patients with preexisting renal disease. Clearly, the difference is not traceable to a low offending drug exposure, since an accompanying summary of outpatient medication provided ample exposure to antibiotics, chemotherapeutics, and NSAIDs, but not contrast agents.

As noted from the study conducted by the Societé de Nephrologie, a surprisingly large percentage of patients who suffered an episode of ARF were left with permanent renal impairment. An earlier report from the European Dialysis and Transplant Association (39) allows a similar conclusion. In evaluating its 1982 data, the association plotted a direct correlation between the number of ARF patients per million and new ESRD patients per million. The conclusion was that the more dialysis skill available, the greater the number of patients with ARF that can be treated. However, it is also possible that this correlation is compatible with the proposition that ARF, successfully treated, leaves a significant portion of people with residual renal damage, which contributes to the ESRD patient pool.

A myriad of risk factors, along with certain acute insults, have been suggested as contributing to the incidence of ARF. The study by Rasmussen and Ibels (31) is particularly relevant since they were one of the first groups to apply multivariant

TABLE 4. *Incidence of ARF due to nephrotoxins*

Authors (ref. no.)	Date	*n*	% ARF due to Antibiotics	% ARF due to Contrast agents	Total
Anderson et al. (123)	1977	92	16%	4%	20%
Suki et al.	1975	82			27%
Galpin et al. (124)	1978	43	33%	9%	42%
Rasmussen and Ibels (31)	1982	143	11%	11%	22%
Hou et al. (32)	1983	129	7%	12%	19%
Societé de Nephrologie (34)	1985	2,175	6%	2%	18%*

*6% due to NSAID.

analysis to characterizing significant contributions to clinical deterioration, the hope being that by identifying those factors that significantly contributed, a strategy to modify or prevent the occurrence of ARF would result. Of the six risk factors evaluated, only preexisting hypertension and renal disease were found to contribute; age >59 years, gout/hypouricemia, diabetes, and diuretics could not be implicated. Of the six acute insults evaluated, aminoglycosides, pigmenturia, and dehydration all had a significant contribution, whereas no weighted contribution was identified for sepsis, radiocontrast media, or liver disease.

More recently, Shusterman et al. (40) have reported on the influence of risk factors on outcome of hospitalized ARF. These authors used a case-control study design and calculated the odds ratio. Based upon logistic regression, volume depletion, aminoglycoside use, congestive heart failure, radiocontrast exposure, and septic shock contributed to the development of ARF in the hospital. Thus, although several of these factors are beyond the physician's control, e.g., sepsis, volume depletion, and congestive heart failure, the decision to give aminoglycosides and to administer radiocontrast media rest with the physician and, thus, may be modified or eliminated. We will examine these and other nephrotoxic drugs to better understand how, why, and when they induce renal injury, and how this may be prevented, modified, or at the very least recognized early in its course.

STRUCTURE/FUNCTION

Vulnerability of the Kidney to Toxic Injury

As a vital organ, the kidney performs several unique functions that can be impaired by drug-induced renal injury including: (a) regulation of the body's fluid volume, a major contributor to the control of blood pressure; (b) regulating the pH of the body, in concert with the lungs, through the excretion of fixed, nonvolatile acids and the conservation of body base; (c) excretion of waste products and, equally important, the conservation of critical body constituents, e.g., electrolytes and other body nutrients; (d) detoxification of certain drugs, and (e) synthesis and release of hormones, such as renin and erythropoietin, and the conversion of vitamin D_3 to the 1,25-dihydroxy form.

To perform these functions requires the integration of many physiological actions of the kidney. Analysis of these actions provide insights as to the vulnerability of the kidney to drug-induced injuries.

One-fifth of the resting cardiac output goes to the kidneys, of which 10% undergoes glomerular filtration. Electrolyte reabsorption accounts for the principal oxygen consuming work performed by the kidneys. Regulation of plasma volume and the generation of vasoactive humoral agents, e.g., renin and prostaglandins, play a key role in blood pressure regulation, which is signaled by changes in blood flow resistance.

Mechanism of Nephron Injury

In the glomerulus, renal blood flow, in concert with net glomerular hydrostatic pressure, acts on the endothelial surface area of the glomerulus to create an ultrafiltrate of plasma. Two aspects of the endothelial surface warrant comment. The filtration area has been assigned a prominent role in a novel concept proposed to explain sustained, progressive loss of renal function following acute injury or insult. The concept, known as "hyperfiltration-injury," is experimentally anchored in the work of Hostetter et al. (41), who demonstrated that loss of a nephron unit causes the remaining nephrons to hypertrophy, with a rise in single-nephron filtration rate due to an elevated glomerular hydrostatic pressure. The latter results from preferential vasoconstriction of efferent compared to afferent arteriolar resistance. Progressive nephron loss induces glomerular hypertension in the remaining nephrons eventuating in the pathologic state of glomerulosclerosis characterized by faulty blood pressure regulation and the diminution of renal excretory capacity.

The hyperfiltration-injury concept is attractive as it provides an explanation for the well-recognized phenomena of progressive deterioration of renal function after the acute insult has been eliminated. It also provides an approach to preventative treatment using maneuvers that cause reversal of glomerular hypertension. Such maneuvers involve the idea of a "renal reserve." As part of the early definition of human renal function (42), it was noted that a meat-enriched meal caused a predictable rise in the GFR. Building on this concept, Bosch et al. (43), having measured the increase in GFR following a proscribed amount of red meat, labeled it the "renal reserve," i.e., a patient's functional renal adaptive capacity. The renal reserve has been assessed in a variety of patients with chronic renal failure (44). An implication of the meat effect on GFR can be related to the hyperfiltration injury concept. Animals with experimentally induced hyperfiltration have a predictable rate of deterioration of renal function that can be delayed by reducing glomerular hypertension by converting enzyme inhibition or restricting dietary protein (45). By understanding the vulnerability of the endothelial surface, new principles of management with potential maneuvers to prevent chronic renal failure are emerging.

The negative charges of endothelial filtration surface can be modified sufficiently to cause renal injury. These fixed negative charges are responsible for variations in the sieving coefficient of neutral versus charged particles (46). In particular, electrostatic attachment of positively charged ligands can either alter the permeability coefficient of the glomerulus (K_f), or act as "planted" antigens. Thus, cationic proteins may sequestrate in either the vascular or mesangial cells of the glomerulus to become "planted" antigens. Subsequently, a circulation antibody may attach to the "planted" antigens causing *in situ* immune complex formation (47). An example of this form of injury is the linear immunophoretic deposits noted in anti–glomerular basement membrane (GBM) disease. A group of environmental toxicants implicated as causing an anti-GBM lesion in the kidney are short-chain hydrocarbons resulting from the refinement of crude oil (48).

When the complex biochemical composition of the glomerulus (49) is exposed to the wide spectrum of antigenic compounds to which the body is exposed over a lifetime, it is not surprising that a variety of glomerular injury patterns have been identified. This is not the only form of immunologically mediated glomerular injury recognized. Additional mechanisms include "circulating antigen-antibody complexes," which are formed elsewhere in the body but undergo filtration arrest in the glomerulus. The glomerulonephritis associated with systemic lupus erythematosus is an example of this; heavy metals also induce this lesion by forming circulating complexes (50). Once bound to tissue, the complexes fix complement with subsequent activation of the complement cascade triggering the *in situ* inflammatory response.

Another mechanism of glomerular damage is cell-mediated injury. Macrophages, either leukocytes or monocytes, attach to glomerular cells resulting in a local inflammatory response due to release of cytokines, thromboxanes, and leukotrienes. This tissue damage may be augmented by a contribution from activated platelets or intrinsic glomerular cells. The therapeutic implications include both techniques, which modify the inflammatory response as well as eliminating drugs that potentiate inflammation. For example, nonsteroidal anti-inflammatory agents, because of the selective inhibition on cyclooxygenase, create a circumstance in which activation of endogenous prostaglandin production would now favor proinflammatory factors.

In the tubular cell, the renal tubules, like the glomerulus, are also vulnerable to drug-induced kidney disease. There are several tubular processes for which drug exposure can cause a unique loss of function. The medullary countercurrent multiplier system, which probably evolved as an adaption to terrestrial existence (51), provides a mechanism of eliminating waste products while minimizing body water losses. The reabsorption and recycling of small molecular weight compounds, in particular urea, are critical to the process. Since this process is dependent on the permeability of collecting and medullary duct cells, plus the luminal to medullary interstitial concentration gradients, it follows that drugs and/or their metabolites can accumulate in the medullary interstitium. Furthermore, depending upon the chemical properties of the accumulated drugs, an inflammatory response can occur through activation of mediators similar to those involved in glomerular injury. Chronic analgesic nephropathy is an example of such injury. Mudge (52) has proposed that the analgesic-induced chronic interstitial nephritis results from the accumulation of salicylate metabolic intermediate APAP. Conversely, an opposite effect during osmotic diuresis when the capacity of the distal concentration-dilution mechanism is severely curtailed results in an increased risk of either volume depletion or selective electrolyte losses. Carbenicillin is an example of a drug capable of such an "osmotic" effect since it induces substantial electrolyte depletion. Other examples of drugs that interfere with the regulation of body fluid volume are included in Table 5.

The organic acid and base transport systems of the proximal tubule are an important route of elimination for nonfilterable molecular species. Several commonly used drugs undergo such transport (Table 6). Some drugs' mechanism of action is dependent upon the transport, e.g., loop diuretics (53), whereas for others proximal

TABLE 5. *Drug-induced alterations of body water balance*

I. Polyuria
A. Centrally mediated
Alcohol
Diphenylhydantoin
Norepinephrine
Lithium
B. Renally mediated
Lithium
Gentamicin
Tetracycline
Colchicine
Fluoride
Amphotericin
Diuretics
II. Water retention
A. Centrally mediated
Nicotine
Carbamazepine
Narcotics
Vincristine
Clofibrate
Opiates
Histamine
Isoproterenol
Thioridazine
B. Renally mediated
Cyclophosphamide
Vasopressin
Sulfonylureas
Biquanides
Nonsteroidal anti-inflammatory agents

tubular transport represents a major route of drug elimination from the body, e.g., penicillin. Drugs transported by the organic ion system can cause renal injury either directly, e.g., cellular accumulation and/or high urinary concentrations, or indirectly, e.g., as competitive inhibitors to block the elimination of endogenously produced toxic end metabolites.

The process of urinary acidification can either prevent or contribute to toxic renal injury. Since urinary acidification involves sequential steps located along the course of the nephron, it is not surprising that abnormalities of acidification are found in a variety of drug-induced renal disease. Chronic lithium nephropathy is an example of a drug-induced acidification defect (54). Other examples of drug-induced injury in which renal tubular acidosis is a prominent feature are summarized in Table 7.

Large molecular weight substances that enter the proximal tubule are recaptured by the process of pinocytosis. Pinocytotic vesicles, once formed, will fuse with proximal tubular lysosomes, the combination allowing the digestive enzymes of the lysosomes to exert their proteolytic action on the material contained within the pinocytotic vesicle, thus insuring reclamation and recycling within the body. Ami-

TABLE 6. *Drugs eliminated through organic transport*

Organic acid system	Organic base system
Para-aminohippurate	Isoproterenol
Phenylbutazone	Tetraethylammonium
Salicylate	Quinidine
Cephalothin	Morphine
Sulfonamides	Procaine
Salyrgan	Tolazoline
Chlorothiazide	Macanylamine
Furosemide	Piperidine
Penicillin	
Methotrexate	
Probenecid	

noglycoside antibiotics undergo pinocytotic reabsorption in the proximal tubule. However, unlike proteins, the aminoglycoside arrests proteolytic digestion, creating a pathologic appearance that resembles lysosomal storage disease (55). From experimental data, it is speculated that this interruption of digestion accounts for the proximal tubular necrosis that characterizes the more severe renal injury associated with aminoglycoside nephrotoxicity (56).

Finally, toxin-induced renal disease can cause excessive urinary loss of vital anions or cations. Examples of clinical conditions are summarized in Table 8. Often

TABLE 7. *Drug-induced acid/base disturbances*

I. Metabolic acidosis
Anion-gap acidosis
Non–anion-gap acidosis
Phenformin
Acetazolamide
Methanol
Tetracyclines (old)
Salicylates
Amphotericin B
Ethylene glycol
Toluene
Paraldehyde
Analgesic
Ethanol abuse
Lithium
II. Metabolic alkalosis
Chloride dependent
Non–chloride dependent
Licorice
Bicarbonate
Carbenoxolone
Carbenicillin
Diuretics
Mannitol

TABLE 8. *Drug-induced electrolyte disturbances*

I. Sodium	
	Hyponatremia—drugs that impair water excretion
	Hypernatremia—saline
II. Potassium	
	Hypokalemia
	Diuretics
	Antibiotics
	Tocolytic agents
	Licorice
	Hyperkalemia
	Potassium supplements
	Potassium-sparing diuretics
	Selected antihypertensive drugs
III. Calcium	
	Hypocalcemia
	Aminoglycoside antibiotics
	Hypercalcemia
	Thiazide diuretics
	Vitamin D supplements
IV. Phosphorus	
	Hypophosphatemia
	Parenterol nutrition
	Hyperphosphatemia
	Cytotoxic drugs

such losses coexist with either defects in the urinary concentrating-diluting mechanism or renal acidosis.

SITES OF NEPHRON INJURY

Classification

Nephrotoxicity can be categorized according to offending agents (8), by clinical syndrome (1), or by proposed site of nephron injury (57). Each approach has its advocates and unique utility. From the standpoint of the emergency room physician, toxicologists, and clinical pharmacologists, since the suspect drug is often known but the effects are in question, a tabulation of the various groups of drugs and their renal effects is very appropriate. Using such a classification one would have categories such as analgesics; anesthetics; anti-infectives, including antibiotics; antifungal and antiviral compounds; biologic agents; cardiovascular drugs, including antihypertensives; antiarrythmics and diuretics; cytotoxic chemotherapeutic agents; image enhancing agents; immunosuppressive drugs; and cycotropic agents. We have recently published such a tabulation (8). Conversely, for the physician seeing a patient with a particular constellation of signs and symptoms suggesting renal disease, classification using clinical syndromes is more useful. In 1977, we proposed that drug-related syndromes could be a useful technique for identifying patients with nephrotoxicity (1). Over the years, this approach has been modified and expanded.

Table 1 summarizes our most recent classification of drug-related clinical syndromes (30). In addition to defining the clinical syndrome, the common causative agents, based upon the frequency of occurrence, are included.

Defining the site of drug-induced nephron damage has depended in large part on recognition of distinctive clinical patterns of presentation. In some cases, this can be supplemented by animal experiments (58). Since there are several suitable methods for estimating GFR and RBF, drugs inducing a dominantly glomerular injury are easier to characterize. However, since there is no satisfactory technique for assessing global renal tubular function, more indirect and inferential approaches are required. The first involves matching changes in plasma electrolytes as they reflect site-specific alteration in tubular function (59). An example would be the renal concentrating effect that characterizes chronic analgesic nephropathy, since the pathologic lesion involves the medullopapillary portion of the kidney. Conversely, the type II renal tubular acidosis (RTA), bicarbonate wasting, that has been reported with exposure to heavy metals is consistent with the proximal tubular pathology characteristic of such exposure (22). If a drug-induced injury were limited to the proximal tubule, the altered tubular function would consist of a reduced reabsorption of a wide variety of filtered items, e.g., glucose, bicarbonate, phosphate, uric acid, amino acids. These alterations would be detected by glucosuria (with normal blood glucose concentration), increased fractional excretion[1] of phosphorus, a fractional excretion of uric acid >10%, and aminoaciduria. For a drug whose injury involves the distal nephron changes in both reabsorption, e.g., sodium, and secretion, e.g., potassium and hydrogen, the alterations would be detected by an increased FE of sodium and elevated plasma potassium and distal (type I) RTA. Finally, for drug-induced damage of the medullopapillary portion of the nephron, a decreased reabsorption of both sodium and water would result in a concentrating defect combined with an increased FE of sodium. The specificity of these patterns of findings decrease from the proximal tubule to the medullopapillary site. Unfortunately, the sensitivity of these observations is sufficiently low that alternate techniques for assessing tubular injury have been pursued.

Another approach for evaluating tubular injury is by determining the presence of "tubular proteinuria" (60). Basically, this involves the precise measurement of low molecular weight proteins that undergo filtration but fail to be reabsorbed due to tubular cell dysfunction (61). An example of this approach is the use of β_2-microglobulin (β_2-MG) excretion with increasing body burden of cadmium (62,63). Furthermore, Price (64) has concluded that the clearance of β_2-MG is a sensitive measure of tubular function provided one is careful to prevent urinary proteolytic digestion by maintaining a pH >5.5 in the sample. The excretion of Tamm-Horsfall protein (THP) has also been proposed as a measure of tubular injury (65,66); however, the technical aspects of measuring THP preclude its widespread use at present.

Urinary enzymes have attracted recent attention as a possible biomarker of renal tubular injury because of the known differences in enzyme distribution in various segments of the nephron (67). Unfortunately, to date, few studies have been re-

[1]Fraction excretion $+ uX/pX - uCR/pCR \times 100$.

ported correlating enzymuria with histological confirmed tubular damage (68). In part, this may be traced to the variety of nonpathologic factors that are known to increase the urinary excretion of certain enzymes (69). The basis for linking enzymuria with tubular disease rests on the premise that the bulk of large molecular weight enzymes (>70 K/d) reach the nephron lumen by cellular release rather than filtration (70). On a practical basis, only a limited number of urinary enzymes have proven useful in detecting renal injury. *N*-acetyl-β-glucosaminidase (NAG) is an example of a urinary enzyme that has been used both for screening for chemical exposure in the workplace (71) and the detection of nephrotoxic injury associated with the injection of contrast media (72). Another enzyme that has been reported to correlate with various drugs that have effects on the kidney is alanine aminopeptidase (AAP) (73,74). A third urinary enzyme that is emerging as useful in specific situations is γ-glutamyl transpeptidase (GGT), particularly with respect to cisplatin-induced acute renal failure (75). Although enzymuria is much more sensitive than proteinuria as a biomarker of tubular disease (70,76), there still remain several unresolved questions as to site specificity and quantitation that need to be answered before universal acceptance will be possible.

Recently, urinary monoclonal antibodies to renal cell membrane have been developed and offer a sensitive, specific, available biomarker for assaying tubular injury (77). Encouraging results for patients with a wide variety of drug and chemical-induced nephropathies, e.g., cisplatin, contrast media, cadmium, and hydrocarbons, have been reported recently (78). Confirmation and extension of the clinical conditions studied will improve application and acceptance of this technology.

ASSESSMENT OF KIDNEY FUNCTION

Estimation of Glomerular Filtration Rate

Serum Creatinine and Creatinine Clearance

The clinical diagnosis of toxic renal insults is often delayed because of the insensitivity of current tests used to assess renal damage. The standard test of renal function used by most clinicians is the serum creatinine, which related only indirectly to the glomerular filtration rate. Creatinine is generated by conversion, nonenzymatically, of muscle creatine and phosphocreatine. Daily muscle production of creatinine is a relatively constant fraction of the total creatine pool and as such is produced in proportion to total muscle mass. Thus, the serum creatinine is less in women than men because of the reduced muscle mass in the latter. Endogenous creatinine (molecular weight 113 d) is excreted by the kidney by glomerular filtration and tubular secretion. The latter occurs by the same secretory pathway as other cations in the proximal tubule. Thus, the clearance of creatinine as measured by the standard clearance formula in Eq. 1,

$$C_{\mathrm{Cr}} = U_{\mathrm{Cr}} \frac{(\mathrm{mg/dl}) \times \text{urine flow (ml/min)}}{\text{serum creatinine (mg/dl)}} \tag{1}$$

overestimates the true glomerular filtration rate, as measured by a more ideal marker such as inulin, which is neither secreted or reabsorbed following filtration at the glomerulus. However, there are substances in normal plasma that are measured as creatinine in the colorimetric assays usually performed by many laboratories. Such noncreatinine chromagens found in blood include glucose, acetoacetate, and uric acid, among others, and may cause as much as a 20% rise in the serum creatinine measurement. As the glomerular filtration rate falls, due to renal disease, noncreatinine chromagens make up an increasingly smaller percentage of serum creatinine as measured by colorimetric techniques (79). Since noncreatinine chromagens do not act as interfering substances in urine, the clearance of creatinine using colorimetric analysis is a reasonable approximation of glomerular filtration rate in health, since the noncreatinine chromagens in serum or plasma offset the tubular secretory component of urinary creatinine. With progressive renal disease, the ratio of secreted creatinine to filtered creatinine rises and, together with the decreasing contribution of noncreatinine chromagens to the serum values, results in creatinine clearances that overestimate the actual glomerular filtration rate (80). With autoanalyzer and imidohydrolase enzyme techniques, noncreatinine chromagens are less of an interpretive problem. However, variability can still be present due to ingestion of cooked meat (exogenous creatinine load) (81), extrarenal elimination, which increases with renal disease (82), and interference from drugs competing for creatinine secretion (83). Factors affecting the serum creatinine value other than renal function are shown in Table 9.

Although the creatinine clearance is not an ideal filtration marker, it is widely used because of the ease of assay and the lack of a requirement for administration of an exogenous marker by infusion. With a timed urine and a blood and urine creatinine measurement, creatinine clearance can be calculated from the above formula. For practical purposes, it is difficult to collect an accurately timed urine and, thus, repeat creatinine clearances may have a coefficient of variation approaching

TABLE 9. *Factors affecting serum creatinine besides renal function*

Increase	Decrease
Cooked meat meal	Muscle wasting
Increase creatinine intake	Malnutrition
Tubular cell secretion inhibitors	Reduced muscle mass (women, elderly)
Trimethoprim	
Cimetidine	
Noncreatinine chromogens	
Glucose	
Acetoacetate	
Fructose	
Uric acid	
Ascorbic acid	
Cephalosporins (cephalothin, cefoxitin, cefamandole, cefazolin)	
Methyldopa	

15% to 20%. Thus, creatinine clearance, as performed in clinical practice, should be considered only approximately equal to the glomerular filtration rate. Since creatinine clearance exceeds inulin clearance at all levels of renal function, a normal or near normal creatinine clearance may be obtained even when GFR is reduced to 25% of normal. In addition, there may be adaptation and increased filtration in nondiseased nephrons in response to loss of other nephrons. These compensatory changes may give a false impression that renal disease is absent when in fact considerable nephron damage is present.

Since there is a reciprocal relationship between creatinine clearance and the serum creatinine, the serum value alone is widely used as a renal function test. Because of increase muscle mass and thus creatinine production, normal values are 10% to 15% higher in men than women. Often creatinine production drops with age and reduced nutrition, resulting in unchanged serum creatinine values, despite reduction of glomerular filtration rate. It is well to remember the relationship between serum creatinine and GFR, even as estimated by creatinine clearance (Fig. 1), such that a drop in GFR of greater than 50% to 70% may occur before the serum creatinine rises outside the normal range. To use the serum creatinine as an index of

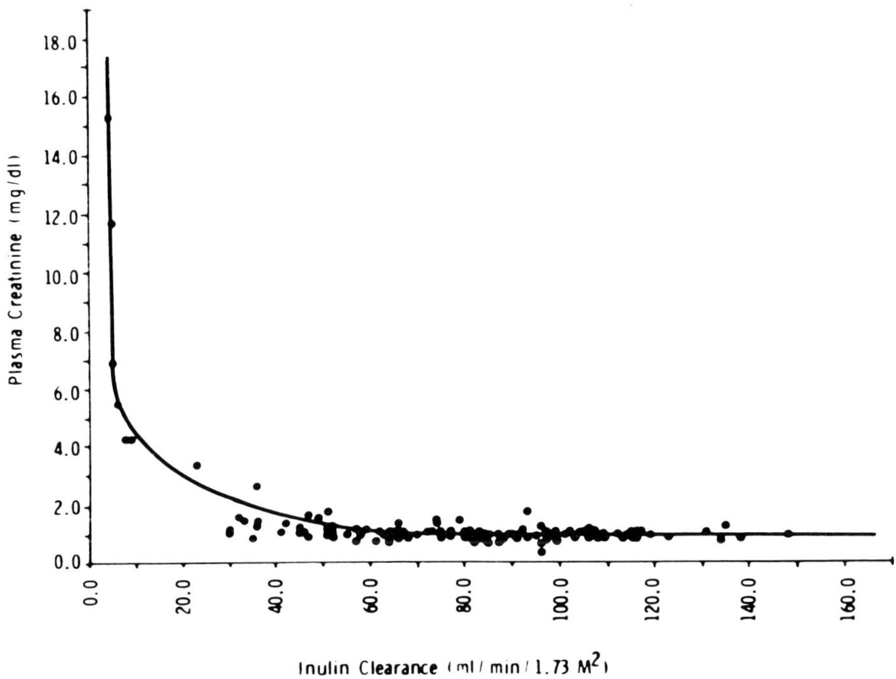

FIG. 1. The relationship between serum creatinine and glomerular filtration rate, as estimated by creatinine clearance.

GFR, one has to assume constant creatinine generation and insignificant, unchanging extrarenal elimination and tubular secretion. With renal disease, these assumptions break down such that a "normal" serum creatinine cannot be used per se to exclude a toxic renal insult.

Using population-based formulae based on age, body size, and gender, it has been possible to estimate creatinine clearance from a serum creatinine value without urine collection. The formula of Cockcroft and Gault (84) is particulary useful and compares favorably to a simultaneously measured creatinine clearance in nonedematous, nonpregnant patients (85). The formula is

$$C_{Cr} = \frac{(140 - \text{age}) \cdot (\text{weight in kg})}{72 \cdot \text{serum creatinine}} \qquad (2)$$

The answer should be multiplied by 0.85 in women. These formulae are only useful in a steady state with unchanging creatinine generation and distribution. The creatinine clearance will be overestimated in cases of obesity or edema since the measured body weight exceeds lean body mass. Other formulae and nomograms have similar limitations. The clinical validity of creatinine clearance estimates has been confirmed in independent studies utilizing comparisons with measured inulin and endogenous creatinine clearances (86).

Although blood urea and urea clearance have historically been advocated to monitor renal function, they have more limitations than does creatinine. Renal handling of urea is dependent on urine flow rate and urea clearance is variably less than inulin clearance, due to net tubular reabsorption. Further, urea production is highly variable depending on protein intake and protein catabolic rate. A normal blood urea does not exclude renal disease, nor does an elevated value indicate a reduced glomerular filtration rate.

At present then, despite the lack of sensitivity and other problems, the serum creatinine is the standard test used to diagnose and monitor toxic insults to the kidney.

Isotopic Measurement of Glomerular Filtration Rate

Because of the imperfections of endogenous creatinine as a filtration marker, various isotopes have been used to measure GFR. Radiation exposure, although a concern, is low since the whole body radiation dose with an isotopic clearance is less than a chest x-ray. To be strictly comparable with the standard inulin clearance, such isotopes would have to be administered by constant infusion, which is unwieldy for clinical purposes. However, the use of the plasma disappearance after intravenous injection of isotopic filtration markers, such as ^{125}I-iothalamate (87), ^{99m}Tc–diethylenetriaminepentaacetic acid (DPTA) (88) or ^{51}Cr–ethyldiaminetetraacetic acid (EDTA) (89) gives an accurate appraisal of glomerular filtration rate. Subcutaneous injections of ^{125}I-iothalamate, combined with epinephrine to produce local vasoconstriction, yield stable plasma iothalamate concentrations, allowing timed urine collections for GFR calculations (90). Although the use of isotopic methodology allows an accurate GFR measurement, expense and inconvenience have limited widespread acceptance by practitioners. For research studies designed to detect renal dysfunction due to drugs and chemicals, actual GFR measurements are preferable to creatinine clearance or estimates from serum creatinine because of markedly improved sensitivity. Even with isotopic methodology, measured clearances may overestimate inulin clearance when GFR is low; however, this is seldom of clinical relevance.

Recently, the use of unlabeled radiocontrast agent detected by high performance liquid chromatography has been proposed for GFR measurement after subcutaneous injection similar to the isotopic iothalamate techniques (91).

Estimation of Renal Plasma Flow

Like the classic determination of glomerular filtration rate with inulin, effective renal plasma flow (ERPF) can be measured by the clearance of a marker, *para*-aminohippurate (PAH) after intravenous constant infusion if low plasma concentrations of PAH are maintained. To serve as a substance whose clearance will reflect renal plasma flow, there should be minimal recirculation following a single pass of marker containing blood through the kidney. The only way to validate a low recirculation rate is to measure PAH in renal venous blood. Thus, PAH clearance, particularly if renal extraction is to be characterized, cannot be used in routine practice. The clearance of the radiopharmaceutical ^{131}I-orthoiodohippurate by plasma disappearance after intravenous injection can be used to closely approximate ERPF. This is usually done in conjuction with isotopic GFR measurement. Expense and inconvenience limit the utility of isotopic ERPF studies to research settings in which information on the effects of drugs on renal hemodynamics can be compared to suitable control information using the same or similar patients.

Kidney structure and function can be also assessed by the use of radionuclide renography. By combing images obtained with a gamma scintillation camera and time-activity curves, both quantitative and qualitative information can be obtained. In addition to the formal quantitative isotopic measure of GFR and ERPF discussed above, the initial uptake of such isotopes as ^{99m}Tc-DPTA and ^{131}I-iodohippurate in the first 6 to 10 min after injection is useful. Some authors have found that such ^{99m}Tc-DPTA isotope uptake correlates well with measured creatinine clearance (92). Separate kidney images and the percent of overall function coming from each kidney can also be helpful in diseases where renal function may be unequally represented, e.g., renovascular disease, obstruction, and ureterovesical reflux. Since a well-equipped nuclear medicine department is necessary to perform these investigations, drug nephrotoxicity is seldom the indication for physicians to order these tests in practice. Static nuclear medicine images have largely been replaced by more sensitive and specific imaging techniques, such as computed tomography, ultrasound, and magnetic resonance imaging. Gallium 67 scans have been used for the diagnosis of interstitial inflammatory disease due to drugs, but these studies lack specificity and even if positive, are of little value in separating toxic insults from other causes of renal dysfunction.

Renal Reserve

As nephrons are lost due to injury and disease, remaining nephrons display increased function such that overall reduction in glomerular filtration rate is less than what might be expected from the loss of renal mass. An example of renal reserve is the drop of GFR to only 60% to 70% of prenephrectomy values in healthy organ donors. In this situation, serum creatinine is often unchanged, emphasizing the insensitivity of this test in detection of significant loss of renal function. The capacity to increase glomerular filtration rate after a protein load has been suggested as an index of the ability of the kidney to withstand further insults (intact renal reserve). A "normal" filtration rate might mask the loss of this reserve capacity, such that further insults or protein loads would result in rapid appearance of clinical renal insufficiency. Although the concept of renal reserve has some experimental basis, some patients with advanced renal disease demonstrate abrupt increases in GFR following protein loading. This is somewhat inconsistent with the idea that a diseased kidney operates using its reserve capacity and remaining healthier nephrons for filtration. The concept of a renal reserve capacity does tend to emphasize the fact that major parenchymal renal disease can be present even if conventional glomerular function studies are normal.

Examination of Urine and its Constituents

Although specificity is often lacking, a carefully performed urinalysis can provide vital information at little cost to the clinician evaluating a patient for drug-induced disease. Furthermore, disease activity can easily be followed over time. Specific gravity of the urine in the absence of glucose, protein, and radiographic contrast dyes gives an acceptable estimate of a directly measured urinary osmolarity. If the patient's state of hydration is known, the urinary specific gravity or osmolality can be a general guide to the renal tubular capacity for normal concentration and dilution. Formal concentration and dilution tests are seldom utilized in clinical practice because of difficult standardization and inconvenience. Inability to concentrate the urine in a setting of extracellular volume depletion or dehydration may be an early clue to toxic tubular injury. Conversely, preservation of concentrating ability despite a low measured or estimated GFR may suggest that the cause of renal dysfunction is "prerenal." Similarly, the urinary pH can be used if the patient's physiological circumstances are known, to ascertain the kidneys' ability to excrete the body's daily acid load. In the face of systemic acidosis, a urinary pH above 6 may indicate renal tubular dysfunction.

The qualitative presence of proteinuria, blood pigments, leukocytes, and glucosuria may be useful in documenting the renal effects of some drugs and toxins. Positive qualitative and/or dipstick tests should be followed up with more specific and quantitative studies to eliminate the substantial number of false positives when these sensitive studies are used for screening. Quantification of urinary protein is useful for separating glomerular diseases (>2 g per 24 hr) from tubulointerstitial processes (<1.5 g per 24 hr). There is a close correlation between 24-hr urinary protein excretion and the ratio of protein to creatinine in a random urine (93). A normal ratio is 0.1, whereas a ratio of 2 equates with 2 g of protein per 24 hr. Dipstick concentrations of protein in a single urine sample are inadequate because of the wide inter- and intrapatient variation in urine volume. Also, the presence of nonalbumin proteins in the urine may be missed by dipstick methodology. This applies to immunoglobulin light chains in multiple myeloma. Sensitive assays are now available to detect small amounts of urinary albumin excretion. So-called microalbuminuria is a predictor of subsequent renal disease in diabetic nephropathy. Its use as an indicator of toxic nephropathy has not been explored.

Microscopic examination of the urine sediment may provide the clinician with useful information about possible nephrotoxic renal disease. In addition to red blood cells and white blood cells, increased numbers of tubular cells may be noted in tubular necrosis, due to drugs or toxins. Eosinophilia is quite specific for acute interstitial nephritis, which is most often due to drugs and chemicals. Casts containing a matrix of Tamm-Horsfall mucoprotein form in the acidic environment of the distal nephron. Granular casts may contain aggregates of serum proteins, including darkly pigmented casts containing hemoglobin or myoglobin. Patients with tubular necrosis due to hemoglobinuria or myoglobinuria will often excrete large numbers of these pigmented casts. Red cells, white cells, and tubular cells may appear in the casts of patients with glomerulonephritis, interstitial nephritis, and tubular cell injury, respectively. Calcium oxalate crystalluria in patients with acute renal failure may be a clue to ethylene glycol of methoxyflurane-induced acute renal failure.

Urinary electrolyte concentrations vary greatly with intake and thus are of limited value in the diagnosis and management of toxic renal disease. When intake and volume status are known, inappropriately high urinary sodium concentrations may indicate renal tubular dysfunction. Likewise, in hypokalemic states, a high urinary potassium may indicate a renal source of potassium loss.

The presence in the urine of low molecular weight proteins, such as β_2-microglobulin and retinol-binding protein, which are filtered at the glomerulus and catabolized by the proximal tubule, indicates tubular disease or damage. Serial evaluations in patients receiving a drug or chemical may provide an early sensitive indicator of tubular cell damage. Correlation of these and other sensitive indicators of tubular cell integrity, such as enzymuria with functional and structural evidence of renal damage, are not available in patients exposed to drugs and chemicals. Until these types of studies are done, nephrotoxicity will continue to be defined by GFR estimations. Thus, it is imperative that new drugs with nephrotoxic potential in preclinical testing not be considered safe until long-term experience provides evidence that cumulative renal damage is absent with long-term, low-dose or repeated exposures.

Structural Assessment of the Kidney

The kidney may be imaged by a wide variety of techniques, such as ultrasound, computed tomography, and magnetic resonance imaging. Although these techniques all provide useful information for the clinician, they have no specific use in nephrotoxic renal disease. Definition of overall kidney size is a rough guide as to functional reserve. Small, contracted kidneys are associated, in general, with more chronic disease processes. The end-stage kidney, due to toxic nephropathy, cannot be distinguished from other causes of this process by imaging procedures. Cysts and renal masses are best delineated by computed tomography or magnetic resonance imaging. The prognosis of many acute renal insults may be gauged by computed tomography scanning to exclude renal cortical mass loss; loss of corticomedullary differentiation on magnetic resonance imaging is a sensitive indicator of a moderate to severe insult to the kidney, but provides no information about the cause of damage. Thus, renal imaging can provide useful general information, but specific details are only ascertained by renal biopsy.

Percutaneous renal biopsy needs to be performed by an experienced operator. The overall complication rate is 2% to 3%, mainly as bleeding, perirenal hematoma, or rarely, arteriovenous fistula. The primary indication for the procedure is renal failure, acute or chronic, of unknown cause. Biopsy is also helpful in defining the pathological processes involved in patients with proteinuria, hematuria, or nephrotic syndrome. Valuable prognostic information, particularly about the amount and type of interstitial involvement in a disease process, may help determine the aggressiveness or type of therapeutic approach. There are few data on a systematic morphological approach to patients with toxic renal injury.

RISK FACTORS—DRUG-INDUCED RENAL FAILURE

Based upon experimental findings our understanding of drug-induced renal disease has expanded rapidly; despite this, it is still important to identify the patient groups that are at significant risk for toxin-induced renal injury. The clinical manifestations of drug-induced renal injury may be a sudden, acute deterioration of renal function or a chronic insidious loss. The different time course may simply represent dosage exposure to toxins, as it has been reported that the rapidity with which experimental renal failure occurs is dependent on the rate at which the nephrotoxin is administered (94). Although this has not been proven for human renal disease, if true it provides an explanation for why it has been so difficult to confirm the role of suspected environmental toxicants.

Because of the frequency and well-defined clinical course of acute renal failure, much of our knowledge regarding risk factors in renal failure comes from analysis of these patients. In particular, when multivariant analysis was applied to a group of patients with acute renal failure, a defined frequency for both predisposing insults (Table 10) and clinical risk factors (Table 11) was achieved (31).

TABLE 10. *Frequency of combined acute insults in patients without previous renal disease (n = 121)*

Acute insult	↓ BP	S	AG	RM	P	LD	↓ ECV
Hypotension (↓ BP)*	33						
Sepsis (S)	29	0					
Aminoglycoside (AG)*	4	10	1				
Radiocontrast media (RM)	12	1	0	1			
Pigmentoria (P)*	12	2	0	1	5		
Liver disease (LD)	2	3	1	0	0	0	
Dehydration (↓ ECV)*	20	14	9	8	11	1	1
Multiple insults	79	30	10	9	11	1	

From Rasmussen and Ibels, ref. 31.
*Significant insult in causing ARF based on discriminant multiple linear regression analysis.

Hypotension was the most frequent single predisposing insult, with pigmenturia second. However, for the majority of patients acute renal failure occurs in the setting of multiple, simultaneous insults. Hypotension, dehydration, and sepsis cause abnormal body fluid volume regulation, which can be monitored as changes in blood pressure. The other predisposing insults of significance are drugs or chemicals used to establish a diagnosis or treat a coexisting disease. Antibiotics continue to be the most frequent cause of drug-induced renal failure in hospitalized patients (32).

The patient risk factors summarized in Table 10 indicate that although it is more common for a single risk factor to be recognized than a single acute insult, the pattern of multiple risk factors coexisting in the same patient occurs in the majority of patients who develop acute renal failure.

Age above 60 has been a consistent risk factor in several studies (95–99). It is reasonable to view age as biomarker of increased renal vulnerability due to the measurable decline in GFR that occurs with each decade beyond the age of 50 (100). In searching for an explanation for this decline in renal function, it has been suggested that progressive atherosclerotic lesions, which accompany aging, could induce the progressive decline through a diminished renal blood flow (101). An

TABLE 11. *Frequency of combined risk factors in patients with ARF (n = 143)*

Suspected risk factors	A	↑ BP	↑ UA	DM	RD	D
Age >59 years (A)	30					
Hypertension (↑ BP)*	29	4				
Gout/hyperuricemia (↑ UA)	21	18	4			
Diabetes (DM)	11	6	4	1		
Renal disease (RD)*	18	12	12	6	4	
Diuretics (D)	29	27	21	8	13	0
Multiple risks	108	63	37	14	13	

From Rasmussen and Ibels, ref. 31.
*Significant risk contributing to ARF based on discriminant multiple linear regression analysis.

alternate explanation uses the failure of mature kidneys to respond to hypertrophic growth factors as its central theme. In patients who act as live donors of a kidney, it has been observed that following unilateral nephrectomy, the retained kidney undergoes both functional and structural hypertrophy (102). However, for live donors 50 years or older, little or no functional increase occurs, which suggests that their stimulus of growth is blunted and ineffective. Whether or not renal cell regeneration is a lifelong physiological process that deteriorates with aging remains an interesting speculation.

Preexisting renal disease is a very significant patient risk factor. Conceptually, the added burden of a hyperfiltering nephron would intensify the vulnerability of the tubular processes previously outlined. In addition, for drugs that depend upon intact renal function for elimination (103), abnormal accumulation and excess blood levels will add to the nephrotoxic insult.

The sex of a patient has not been verified as a significant risk factor for humans. This is not the case for experimental nephrotoxicants where the animal's sex clearly influences susceptibility to drug or chemical insults (104).

Disease states that predispose to drug-induced renal injury include systemic hypertension, diabetes mellitus, liver disease vasculitis, and systemic lupus erythematosus (SLE) (97). These conditions may share the existence of glomerular hypertension, an observation that has been confirmed in experimental studies where glomerular dynamics are determined using micropuncture techniques (41).

Aminoglycoside antibiotics are an example of a drug whose prior exposure increases the risk of renal injury. A critical accumulation of the drug, which has been reported to occur in those patients who eventually develop aminoglycoside nephrotoxicity, is consistent with this observed risk (105). Exactly how this critical accumulation induces risk is unclear but may be due to unusual tissue binding and/or delayed drug elimination.

To evaluate risk factors in states of chronic drug exposure is problematic. One group of patients of interest are those with chronic lithium administration. Observations on these patients indicate that 10 to 20 years of low-dose treatment are probably required for chronic lithium nephropathy to develop. Lokkegaard et al. (106) correlated a small decline in glomerular filtration rate with the duration of lithium treatment. The derived regression line intersected the 95% confidence limits for age-matched control glomerular filtration rates with the duration of lithium administration. This is important since the report by Benz (107), which found that no correlation existed between lithium-induced nephropathy and sex, diagnosis, duration of treatment, serum lithium levels, type of lithium preparation used, or combined lithium-neuroleptic treatment, was derived from a patient population whose average duration of treatment was only 5 years. A defect in maximum urinary concentrating capacity occurs in 30% to 100% of patients receiving chronic lithium treatment (107) and is inversely correlated with the duration of lithium treatment (108). Importantly, approximately 10% of patients receiving long-term lithium therapy will demonstrate measurable reductions in glomerular filtration with a larger fraction showing mild renal tubular acidosis. Chronic interstitial nephritis has been reported (108,109) in patients receiving long-term lithium therapy without acute lithium intoxication. To assign these changes to lithium seems premature since similar pathologic changes have been noted in renal biopsies from patients with affective disorders not receiving lithium (108). Additional risk factors for chronic lithium nephropathy include dose frequency, but not accumulative dose and volume depletion, irrespective of its cause (110).

Intrinsic to determining relative risk from the various factors discussed is the lack of any verifiable cause and effect. For chronic renal impairment, the long duration of environmental exposure that is probably required before clinically evident renal dysfunction is manifested further complicates the interpretation. Adding to this uncertainty is the absence of a convenient clinical measure of total tubular function as a companion to the measurement of glomerular filtration rate. The lack of a universally accepted measure of tubular function severely curtails our ability to detect early nephron changes.

At present, Table 10 contains the list of commonly identified patient risk factors that seem to be consistent between patient populations developing acute renal failure. Furthermore, in certain cases the toxicant possesses unique features that will assist in the identification and the prevention of drug-induced renal injury.

PREVENTION/MODIFICATION

Experimentally, many approaches to modifying or preventing drug-induced nephrotoxicity have been tried (111). Such techniques may vary from concomitant administration of specific drugs or chemicals through modifying drug dosage amounts or schedules to changing dietary content. To date, only a few such strategies have undergone clinical trial. The use of risk stratification is very important when developing a clinical management program directed at prevention. Obviously, patient characteristics that cannot be changed include age, sex, and coexisting disease; on the other hand, volume or electrolyte depletion, hypotension, and concomitant nephrotoxic drugs can be actively treated or eliminated prior to administering a potentially injurious drug or chemical.

Clinically tested methods for preventing or modifying drug-induced ARF include (a) volume expansion/osmotic diuresis, (b) loop diuretics, and (c) calcium channel antagonists. Of the three approaches, volume expansion has had the greatest accumulated experience. The basis by which mannitol might prevent drug-induced ARF probably involves its action to reduce proximal tubular reabsorption of sodium and water, thus inducing an osmotic diuresis. The net effect of such limited proximal reabsorption would be to decrease the concentration of drug available for tubular cell uptake. Furthermore, the increased flow in the distal nephron and collecting duct system would limit reabsorption in this region. Much of the early clinical experience with mannitol involved its use in patients undergoing aortic surgery (112). In a similar application we reported a reduced incidence of postoperative acute renal failure in a group of patients undergoing prosthetic valve replacement (113). Two problems exist with the interpretation of these results. The first was that we employed a series of historic controls to compare the change in incidence of

ARF, but more importantly, we demonstrated that by introducing mannitol into the perfusate, a substantial reduction in the rate of hemolysis occurred that could also account for the reduced incidence of ARF. More recently, there has been interest in the use of mannitol to prevent contrast associated nephropathy in high-risk patients (114). Again, the results are inconclusive with the majority of investigators remaining skeptical. Anto et al. (115) evaluated mannitol prophylaxis in high-risk patients undergoing contrast studies and reported a decline in the incidence of contrast-associated nephropathy from 70% to 22%, a very significant difference. However, there are two problems with accepting the authors' conclusions that this effect was totally due to mannitol pretreatment. First, they employed historic controls, which always poses the problem of comparability. Second, and probably of greater importance, during the mannitol series postprocedure urine output was matched for the first day, thus preventing any volume depletion that can be induced due to the osmotic load presented during contrast studies. Additional uncontrolled studies that claim a beneficial role for mannitol in the prevention of nephrotoxicity have been reported for cisplatin (116) and amphotericin (117).

The use of loop diuretics is based on the concept that converting oliguric ARF to nonoliguric ARF improves patient survival by reducing the problem of fluid management (118). This approach has been extended to prevent CAN by Oguagha et al. (119), who reported a decrease in incidence (18% compared to 70%) when furosemide was given 1 hr prior to the procedure. A similar result was reported by Beroniade (120), who used furosemide to induce a postprocedure diuresis. Once again both studies used historic controls for comparison. The use of calcium channel blockers to prevent drug-induced ARF is very recent. Although there are much experimental data to support such an approach (121), few clinical studies have been reported. Recently, Neumayer et al. (122) found that 3 days of pretreatment with the calcium channel blocker nitrendipine, followed by the injection of contrast media, reduced the magnitude of the decline in GFR in patients preselected to be at high risk. As with other proposed techniques for preventing ARF, this one will have to await confirmation.

In summary, the best prevention is avoidance of potentially nephrotoxic drugs or chemicals, especially in patients at high risk. However, in many circumstances that is not practical, since often patients are critically ill and no alternative approaches are available. Under such circumstances, it is crucial to eliminate the situations known to predispose to nephrotoxicity, e.g., volume repair, restoration of blood pressure, and electrolyte replacement. It must also be emphasized that careful monitoring of renal function, usually by serial serum creatinines, is essential since most cases of drug-induced renal injury present as nonoliguric ARF.

REFERENCES

1. Bennett WM, Plamp C, Porter GA. Drug-related syndromes in clinical nephrology. *Ann Intern Med* 1977;87:582–590.

2. Matzke G, Lucarotti R, Shapiro HS. Controlled comparison of gentamicin and tobramycin nephrotoxicity. *Am Nephrol* 1983;3:11–17.
3. Humes HD. Aminoglycoside nephrotoxicity. *Kidney Int* 1988;33:900–911.
4. Bennett WM. Aminoglycoside nephrotoxicity. *Nephron* 1983;35:73–77.
5. Mandal A, Bennett WM. Transmission electron microscopy of urinary sediment in the assessment of aminoglycoside nephrotoxicity in the rat. *Nephron* 1988;49:45–53.
6. Bennett WM. Guide to drug dosage in renal failure. *Clin Pharmacokinet* 1988;15:326–354.
7. Bennett JE. Treatment of cryptococcal, candidal and coccidioidal meningitis. In: Remington RS, Swartz MN, eds. *Current clinical topics in infectious disease*, vol 2. New York: McGraw-Hill, 1981;54–67.
8. Porter GA, Bennett WM. The effect of drugs on the kidney. In: Petersdorf R, Adams RD, Bromwall E, et al., eds. *Harrison's principles of internal medicine*. New York: McGraw-Hill, 1985;57–76.
9. Branch RA. Prevention of amphotericin B-induced renal impairment: a review on the use of sodium supplementation. *Arch Intern Med* 1988;148:2389–2394.
10. Lochrer PJ, Einhorn LD. Drugs, five years later: cisplatin. *Ann Intern Med* 1984;100:704–713.
11. Madias NE, Harrington JT. Platinum nephrotoxicity. *Am J Med* 1978;65:307–314.
12. Blachley JD, Hill JR. Renal and electrolyte disturbances associated with cisplatin. *Ann Intern Med* 1981;95:628–632.
13. Hutchison FN, Perez EA, Gandara DR, et al. Renal salt wasting in patients treated with cisplatin. *Ann Intern Med* 1988;108:21–25.
14. Wagstaff AJ, Ward A, Benfield P, et al. Carboplatin: a preliminary review of its pharmacodynamic and pharmacokinetic properties and therapeutic efficacy in the treatment of cancer. *Drugs* 1989; 37:162–190.
15. Blackshear JL, Davidman M, Stillman MT. Identification of risk for renal insufficiency from nonsteroidal anti-inflammatory drugs. *Arch Intern Med* 1983;143:1130–1134.
16. Clive DM, Stoff JS. Renal syndromes associated with nonsteroidal anti-inflammatory drugs. *N Engl J Med* 1984;310:563–572.
17. Ciabattoni G, Cinotti GA, Pierucci A, et al. Effects on sulindac and ibuprofen in patients with chronic glomerular disease: evidence for the dependence of renal function on prostacyclin. *N Engl J Med* 1984;310:279–283.
18. Spuler O, Zollinger HU. Die chronische-interstitielle nephritis. *Z Klin Med* 1953;151:1–50.
19. Murray T, Goldberg M. Analgesic abuse and renal disease. *Annu Rev Med* 1975;26:537–550.
20. Murray R, Lawson D, Linton A. Analgesic nephropathy: clinical syndrome and prognosis. *Br Med J* 1971;1:479–482.
21. Bennett WM, DeBroe ME. Analgesic nephropathy—a preventable renal disease. *N Engl J Med* 1989;320:1269–1271.
22. Bennett WM. Lead nephropathy. *Kidney Int* 1985;28:212–220.
23. Rao TKS, Nicastri AD, Friedman EA. Natural history of heroin-associated nephropathy. *N Engl J Med* 1974;290:19–23.
24. Myers BD, Ross J, Newton L, et al. Cyclosporine-associated chronic nephropathy. *N Engl J Med* 1986;311:699–705.
25. Palestine AG, Austin HA, Balow JE, et al. Renal histopathologic alterations in patients with cyclosporine for uveitis. *N Engl J Med* 1986;314:129–398.
26. Lee JC, Dushkin M, Eyring EJ, Engleman EP, Hopper J Jr. Renal lesions associated with gold therapy. Light and electron microscopic studies. *Arthritis Rheum* 1965;8:1–13.
27. Miller M, Moses AM. Mechanism of chlorpropamide action in diabetes insipidus. *J Clin Endocrinol Metab* 1970;30:488–496.
28. Singer I, Forrest JN Jr. Drug-induced states of nephrogenic diabetes insipidus. *Kidney Int* 1976; 10:82–95.
29. Norby LH, Weidig J, Ranwell P. Possible role for impaired renal prostaglandin production in the pathogenesis of hyporeninaemic hypoaldosteronism. *Lancet* 1979;2:1118.
30. Cooper K, Bennett WM. Nephrotoxicity of common drugs used in clinical practice. *Arch Intern Med* 1987;147:1213–1218.
31. Rasmussen HH, Ibels LS. Acute renal failure: multivariate analysis of causes and risk factors. *Am J Med* 1982;73:211–218.
32. Hou SH, Bushindky DA, Wish JB, Cowen JJ, Harrington JT. Hospital-acquired renal insufficiency: a prospective study. *Am J Med* 1983;74:243–248.

33. Frankel ML, Weinstein AM, Stenzel KH. Prognostic patterns in acute renal failure: the New York Hospital 1981–1982. *Clin Exp Dialysis Apheresis* 1983;7:145–167.
34. Societé de Nephrologie. Kleinknecht D (coordinator), Laudais P, Goldfarb B. Drug-associated acute renal failure. A prospective multicentre report. *Proc EDTA-ERA* 1985;22:1002–1007.
35. Ad Hoc Committee—NKF. Statement on the release of ibuprofen as an over-the-counter medicine. *Am J Kidney Dis* 1985;6:4–6.
36. Pirson Y, Van Ypersele de Strihou C. Renal side effects of nonsteriodal anti-inflammatory drugs: clinical relevance. *Am J Kidney Dis* 1986;8:338–344.
37. Pru C, Ebben J, Kjellstrand C. Chronic renal failure after acute tubular necrosis. *Kidney Int* 1982; 21:176.
38. Beard K, Perera DR, Jick H. Drug-induced parenchymal renal disease in outpatients. *J Clin Pharmacol* 1988;28:431–435.
39. Report on acute (reversible) renal failure. *Proc EDTA-ERA* 1983;20:64–67.
40. Shusterman N, Strom BL, Murray TG, Morrison G, West SL, Maisten G. Risk factors and outcome of hospital-acquired acute renal failure. *Am J Med* 1987;83:65–71.
41. Hostetter TH, Rennke HG, Brenner BM. The case for intrarenal hypertension in the initiation and progression of diabetic and other glomerulopathies. *Am J Med* 1982;72:375–380.
42. Smith HW, Goldring W, Chasis H, Ranges HA, Bradley SE. The application of saturation methods to the study of glomerular and tubular function in the human kidney. *J Mt Sinai Hosp* 1943;10:59–87.
43. Bosch JP, Saccaggi A, Lauer A, Ronco C, Belledonne M, Glabman S. Renal functional reserve in humans: effect of protein intake on glomerular filtration rate. *Am J Med* 1983;75:943–950.
44. Bosch JP, Lew S, Glabman S, Lauer A. Renal hemodynamic changes in humans: response to protein loading in normal and diseased kidneys. *Am J Med* 1986;81:809–815.
45. Blantz RC, Konnen KS, Tucker BJ. Angiotension II effects upon the glomerular microcirculation and ultrafiltration coefficient of the rat. *J Clin Invest* 1976;57:419–434.
46. Brenner BM, Hostetter TH, Humes HD. Glomerular permselectivity: barrier function based on discrimination of molecular size and change. *Am J Physiol* 1978;234:F455–F460.
47. Batsford SR, Takamiya H, Vogt A. A model of in situ immune complex glomerulonephritis in the rat employing cationized ferritin. *Clin Nephrol* 1980;14:211–224.
48. Ravnskov U. Possible mechanism of hydrocarbon associated glomerulonephritis. *Clin Nephrol* 1985;23:294–298.
49. Glassock RJ. Clinical, immunologic, and pathologic aspects of human glomerular disease. In: Schrier RW, ed. *Renal and electrolyte disorders*, 3rd ed. Boston: Little, Brown, 1986;591–657.
50. Albini B, Glurich I, Andres GA. Mercuric chloride-induced immunologically mediated diseases in experimental animals. In: Porter GA, ed. *Nephrotoxic mechanisms of drug and environmental toxins*. New York, London: Plenum, 1982;413–423.
51. Smith HW. *From fish to philosopher*. Boston: Little, Brown, 1953;136–152.
52. Mudge GH. Analgesic nephropathy: renal drug distribution and metabolism. In: Porter GA, ed. *Nephrotoxic mechanisms of drugs and environmental toxins*. New York: Plenum, 1982;209–225.
53. Porter GA. Diuretics and renal disease. In: Bennett WM, ed. Drugs and renal disease, 2nd ed. New York: Churchill-Livingstone, 1986;102–116.
54. Batlle D, Gaviria M, Grupp M, Arruda JA, Wynn J, Kurtzman NA. Distal nephron function in patients receiving lithium therapy. *Kidney Int* 1982;21:477–486.
55. Tulkens PM. Experimental studies on nephrotoxicity of aminoglycosides at low doses: mechanisms and perspectives. *Am J Med* 1986;80(6B):105–114.
56. Houghton DC, Campbell-Boswell MV, Bennett WM. Myeloid bodies in the renal tubules of humans: relationship to gentamicin therapy. *Clin Nephrol* 1987;10:140–145.
57. Mujais RA, Batlle JB. Functional correlations of tubulo-interstitial damage. *Semin Nephrol* 1988; 8:94–99.
58. Porter GA. Extrapolation of animal data to man: the concordance between toxicity screening and clinical consequences. In: Bach PH, Lock EA, eds. *Nephrotoxicity in the experimental and clinical situation*. Darducht, Boston, Lancaster: Naiturus Nijhoff, 1987; 613—642.
59. Cogan MG. Tubulo-interstitial nephropathies: a pathophysiologic approach. *West J Med* 1980; 132:134–141.
60. Peterson PA, Evrin PE, Berggard I. Differentiation of glomerular, tubular, and normal proteinuria: determinations of urinary excretion of β_2-microglobulin, albumin and total protein. *J Clin Invest* 1969;48:1189.

61. Dennis V, Robinson RR. Proteinuria. In: Seldir DW, Giebisch G, eds. *The kidney: physiology and pathology*. New York: River Press, 1985; 1805.
62. Friberg L, Procator M, Norelberg GF, Kjellstrom T, eds. *Cadmium in the environment*. Cleveland: CRC Press, 1974.
63. Goyer R. Cadmium nephropathy. In: Porter GA, ed. *Nephrotoxic mechanism of drugs and environmental toxins*. New York/London: Plenum 1982; 305.
64. Price RG. Urinary enzymes, nephrotoxicity, and renal disease. *Toxicology* 1982;23:99.
65. Thornby C, Dawnay A, Cattell WR. Human Tamm-Horsfall glycoprotein: urine and plasma levels in normal subjects and patients with renal disease determined by a fully validated radioimmunoassay. *Clin Sci* 1985;68:529.
66. Lynn KL, Marshall RD. Excretion of Tamm-Horsfall glycoprotein in renal disease. *Clin Sci* 1985;68:253.
67. Harrison DJ, Kharbanda RK, Cunningham DS, et al. Distribution of glutathione S transferase isoenzymes in human kidney: Basis for possible markers of renal injury. *J Clin Pathol* 1989; 42:624.
68. Partman RJ, Kissane JM, Roleson AM, et al. Use of β-microglobulin to diagnose tubulointerstitial renal lesions in children. *Kidney Int* 1986;30:91.
69. Plummer DT, Naarazar S, Obatomi DK, Haslam JD. Assessment of renal injury by urinary enzymes. *Uremia Invest* 1985;9:97.
70. Dubach UC, LeHir M. Clinical evaluation of the diagnostic use of urinary enzymes. *Contrib Nephrol* 1984;42:74.
71. Meyer BR, Fischbein A, Rosenman K, et al. Increased urinary enzyme excretion in workers exposed to nephrotoxic chemicals. *Am J Med* 1984;76:989.
72. Rahimi A, Edmondson RP, Jones NF. Effect of radiocontrast media on kidneys of patients with renal disease. *Br Med J* 1981;282:1194–1195.
73. Mondarf AW. Urinary enzymatic markers of renal damage. In: Whelton A, Neu HC, eds. *The aminoglycosides: microbiology, clinical use and toxicology*. New York and Basel: Marcel Dekker, 1982;283.
74. Davey PG, Cowley DM, Geddes AM, Terry J. Clinical evaluation of β-microglobulin, muramidase, and alanine aminopeptidase as markers of gentaminicin nephrotoxicity. *Contrib Nephrol* 1984;42:100–106.
75. Gordon JA, Gattone VH, Schoolwerth AC. α-Glutamyl transpeptidase excretion in cisplatin-induced acute renal failure. *Am J Kidney Dis* 1986;8:18–25.
76. Palmieri L, Ronca G, Cioni L, Puceini R. Enzymuria as a marker of renal injury and disease: studies of N-acetyl-β-glucosaminidase, alanine aminopeptidase, and lysozyme in patients with renal disease. *Contrib Nephrol* 1984;42:123.
77. Mutti A, Lucertini S, Valcaer PP, et al. Urinary excretion of brush border antigens: early indicator of toxic nephropathy. *Lancet* 1985;2:914.
78. Mutti A, Lucertini S, Fornari M, et al. Urinary excretion of brush border antigen revealed by monoclonal antibodies in subjects occupationally exposed to heavy metals. *Proceedings of the International Conference on Heavy Metals in the Environment*. Edinburgh: CEP Consultants, 1986.
79. Doolan PD, Alpen EL, Thiel GB. A clinical appraisal of the plasma concentration and endogenous clearance of creatinine. *Am J Med* 1962;32:65.
80. Shemesh O, Golbetz H, Kriss JP, Myers BD. Limitations of creatinine as a filtration marker in glomerulopathic patients. *Kidney Int* 1985;28:830.
81. Mayersohn M, Conrad KA, Achari R. The influence of a cooked meat meal on creatinine plasma concentration and creatinine clearance. *Br J Clin Pharmacol* 1983;15:227.
82. Mitch WE, Collier VU, Walser M. Creatinine metabolism in chronic renal failure. *Clin Sci* 1980;58:327.
83. Young DS, Pestaner LC, Gibberman V. Effects of drugs on clinical laboratory tests. *Clin Chem* 1975;21:1.
84. Cockroft DW, Gault MH. Prediction of creatinine clearance from serum creatinine. *Nephron* 1976;16:31.
85. Parker RA, Bennett WM, Porter GA. Clinical estimation of creatinine clearance without urine collection. *Dialysis Transpl* 1980;9:251.
86. Luke DR, Halstenson CE, Opsahl JA, Matzke GR. Validity of creatinine clearance estimates in the assessment of renal function. *Clin Pharmacol Ther* 1990;48:503–508.

87. Maher FT, Nolan NG, Elverback LR. Comparison of simultaneous clearances of ^{125}I-labeled sodium iothalamate and of inulin. *Mayo Clin Proc* 1971;46:690.
88. Dubovsky EV, Russell CD. Quantification of renal function with glomerular and tubular agents. *Semin Nucl Med* 1982;12:308.
89. Brochner-Mortenson J. Routine methods and their reliability for assessment of glomerular filtration rate in adults. *Dan Med Bull* 1978;25:181.
90. Israelit AH, Long DL, White MG, Hull AR. Measurement of glomerular filtration rate utilizing a single subcutaneous injection of ^{125}I-iothalamate. *Kidney Int* 1973;4:326.
91. Dalmeida W, Suk WN. Measurement of GFR with nonradioisotopic radiocontrast agents. *Kidney Int* 1988;43:725.
92. Gates GF. Split renal function testing using T_c-99_M-DPTA: a rapid technique for determining differential glomerular filtration. *Clin Nucl Med* 1983;8:400–407.
93. Schwab S, Christensen R, Dougherty R, Klahr S. Quantification of proteinuria by use of protein to creatinine ratios in single urine samples. *Arch Intern Med* 1987;147:943–944.
94. Aviv A, John E, Bernstein J, Goldsmith DI, Spitzer A. Lead intoxication during development: its late effects on renal function and blood pressure. *Kidney Int* 1980;17:430–443.
95. Kumar R, Hill CM, McGeown MG. Acute renal failure in the elderly. *Lancet* 1973;1:90–91.
96. Eliahou HE, Boichis H, Bott-Kanner G, Bavell V, Bar-Noach N, Modan B. An epidemiologic study of renal failure: acute renal failure. *Am J Epidemiol* 1975;101:281–286.
97. McMurray SD, Luft FC, Maxwell DR, Hamburger DH, Kleit S. Prevailing patterns and predictor variables in patients with acute tubular necrosis. *Arch Intern Med* 1978;138:950–955.
98. Byrd L, Sherman RL. Radiocontrast-induced acute renal failure. A clinical and pathophysiologic review. *Medicine (Baltimore)* 1979;58:270–279.
99. Porter GA, Kloster FE, Herr RJ, Starr A, Griswald HE, Kimsey J, Lenertz H. The relationship between alterations in renal hemodynamics during cardiopulmunary bypass and postoperative renal function. *Circulation* 1966;34:1005–1021.
100. Davies DF, Shock NW. Age changes in glomerular filtration rate, effective renal plasma flow and tubular excretory capacity in adult males. *J Clin Invest* 1950;29:496–507.
101. Avendano LH, Lopez-Novoa JM. Glomerular filtration and renal blood flow in the aged. In: Macias-Nunez IF, Cameron JS, eds. *Renal function and diseases in the elderly*. London: Butterworth, 1987;27–48.
102. Boner G, Sherry J, Riselbach RE. Hypertrophy of the normal human kidney following contralateral nephrectomy. *Nephron* 1972;9:364–372.
103. Bennett WM, Aronoff G, Morrison G, Golper TA, Pulliam J, Wolfson M, Singer IW. Drug prescribing in renal failure: dosing guidelines for adults. *Am J Kidney Dis* 1983;3:155–193.
104. Porter GA, Bennett WM, Gilbert DN. Unraveling tissue accumulation of gentamicin. *Clin Pharmacol Ther* 1977;23:445–452.
105. Schentag JJ, Jusko WJ. Renal clearance and tissue accumulation of gentamicin. *Clin Pharmacol Ther* 1977;22:364–370.
106. Lokkegaard H, Andersen NF, Henriksen E, Bartels PD, Branm M, Baastrup PC, Jorgensen HE, Larsen M, Munch O, Rasmussen K. Renal function in 153 manic-depressive patients treated with lithium for more than 5 years. *Acta Psychiatr Scand* 1985;71:347–355.
107. Bendz HD. Kidney function in lithium-treated patients: a literature survey. *Acta Psychiatr Scand* 1983;68:303–324.
108. Walker RG, Bennett WM, Davis BM, Kincaid-Smith P. Structural and functional effects of long-term lithium therapy. *Kidney Int* 1982;21:513–519.
109. Hestbeck J, Hansen HE, Andersen A, Olsen S. Chronic renal lesions following long-term treatment with lithium. *Kidney Int* 1977;12:205–203.
110. Plenge P, Mellerup ET, Bolury TG, Bury C, Hetmar O, Ladefoged J, Larsen S, Rafaelson OJ. Lithium treatment: Does the kidney prefer one daily dose instead of two? *Acta Psychiatr Scand* 1982;66:121–128.
111. Bennett WM, Wood CA, Houghton DC, Gilbert DN. Modification of experimental aminoglycoside nephrotoxicity. *Am J Kidney Dis* 1986;8:292–296.
112. Doberneck PC, Schwartz FD, Barry KG. A comparison of the prophylactic value of 20% mannitol, 4% urea and 5% dextrose on the effects of renal ischemia. *J Urol* 1963;89:300–307.
113. Porter GA, Kloster FE, Herr RJ, Starr A, Griswold HE, Kimsey J. Renal complication associated with valve replacement surgery. *J Thorac Cardiovasc Surg* 1967;53:145–152.
114. Vari RC, Natarajan LP, Whitescarver SA, Jackson BA, Ott CE. Induction, prevention and mechanisms of contrast media-induced acute renal failure. *Kidney Int* 1988;33:699–707.

115. Anto HR, Chou SY, Porush JG, Shapiro WB. Infusion intravenous pyelography and renal function. Effects in patients with chronic renal insufficiency. *Arch Intern Med* 1981;141:1652–1656.
116. Pera MF, Zook BC, Harder HC. Effects of mannitol or furosemide diuresis on the nephrotoxicity and physiologic disposition of Cis-dichlorodiamine-platinum II in rats. *Cancer Res* 1979;39:1269–1276.
117. Hellebusch AA, Salma F, Eadie E. The use of mannitol to reduce the nephrotoxicity of amphotericin B. *Surg Gynecol Obstet* 1973;134:241–246.
118. Levinsky NG, Bernard DB. Mannitol and loop diuretics in acute renal failure. In: Brenner BM, Lazarus JM, eds. *Acute renal failure*, 2nd ed. New York; Churchill-Livingstone, 1988;841–856.
119. Oguagha C, Porush JC, Chou SY. Prevention of acute renal failure (ARF) following infusion intravenous pyelography (IVP) in patients with chronic renal insufficiency (CRI) by furosemide (F). *Abstract of the 8th International Congress of Nephrology*. Athens: University Studio, 1981;290.
120. Beroniade VC. Prevention of acute renal failure secondary to radiocontrast agents. *Abstract of the 8th International Congress of Nephrology*. Athens: University Studio, 1981;380.
121. Heyman SN, Brezis M, Greenfeld Z, Rosen S. Protective role of furosemide and saline in radiocontrast-induced acute renal failure in the rat. *Am J Kidney Dis* 1989;14:377–385.
122. Neumayer HH, Junge W, Kufner A, Wenning A. Prevention of radiocontrast-media-induced (CM) nephrotoxicity by the calcium antagonist (CA) nitrendipine: a prospective randomized clinical trial. *Am Soc Nephrol* 1989;72A.
123. Anderson RJ, Linas SL, Berns AS, Schrier R. Non oligunicacute renal failure. *N Engl J Med* 1977;296:1134–1137.
124. Galpin JE, Shinaberger JH, Stanely TM. Acute interstitial nephritis due to renal failure. *Am J Med* 1978;65:756–765.

Toxicology of the Kidney, Second Edition,
edited by Jerry B. Hook and Robin S. Goldstein.
Raven Press, Ltd., New York © 1993.

4

Morphological Features of Acute Renal Failure

Steen Olsen and *Kim Solez

*University Institute of Pathology, Aarhus Kommunehospital, Aarhus C, Denmark; and *Department of Pathology, University of Alberta, Edmonton, Alberta, Canada T6G 2R7*

Acute renal failure (ARF) is defined as a sudden decrease of renal function leading to retention of nitrogenous waste products in the blood. Although this situation was formerly considered to be synonymous with acute anuria or oliguria, it is now clear that ARF as defined above may be present despite continued urine output within the normal range, or even in situations with polyuria. There is no general agreement on how severe the renal failure should be, but as an arbitrary definition it can be proposed that ARF is present if renal function expressed as creatinine clearance suddenly becomes reduced to the range of 10 to 20 ml/min or below.

Defined in this way, ARF may be prerenal, renal, or postrenal, a classification of value for the clinician, since these possibilities should always be kept in mind as the first step toward a precise diagnosis.

Prerenal ARF is present if (due to factors operative outside the kidney) the glomerular filtration pressure is decreased to a level not compatible with the formation of an ultrafiltrate. This situation may be due to acute obstruction of both renal arteries (or one in case of a single functioning kidney), but by far the most frequent cause is hypotension or hypovolemia. It is important to realize that this form of prerenal ARF is restricted to the period during which the low blood pressure is operative. If renal failure continues despite normalization of systemic blood pressure, the ARF is no longer prerenal but renal. In *postrenal* ARF there is obstruction of the urinary tract, again bilateral, or unilateral if there is only one functioning kidney.

In the present context only *renal (parenchymal)* ARF is discussed. This type is caused by disease within the kidney proper. Even with this restriction, ARF is not a single disease, but comprises a rather extensive list of diseases defined by morphology or etiology (1). Some are characterized by lesions localized to renal vasculature and glomeruli, whereas in others the main lesions affect the tubulointerstitial structures. Within the framework of this book, the tubulointerstitial diseases are the most important since they include most toxic or drug-induced conditions. The following review will deal with morphological alterations characteristic of the main types of tubulointerstitial diseases associated with ARF in man as well as some experimental models of ARF. Pathogenesis will be discussed comparatively briefly with emphasis on possible relationship to morphological changes. For a detailed presentation of the pathophysiology of experimental ARF, the reader is referred to the chapter by Abbate, Macconi, and Remuzzi.

MAIN TYPES OF ACUTE RENAL FAILURE IN MAN

Toxic Acute Tubular Necrosis

Toxic acute tubular necrosis (toxic ATN) can be defined as a disease characterized histopathologically by extensive necroses of the tubular cells (2). This necrosis does not typically involve all tubules as in cortical necrosis or extensive infarction, but is usually selective in the sense that some tubular segments appear more vulnerable than others. It can be distinguished from bilateral cortical necrosis because this condition is characterized by widespread necrosis and glomerular capillary and/or arteriolar thrombosis. Toxic ATN is most often due to poisoning and the effect is dose dependent and immediate in contrast to allergic acute interstitial nephritis, which may have a more insidious onset. Ischemic ARF is distinguished from toxic ATN by its lack of extensive tubular cell necrosis.

Etiology

In the prebiopsy period, poisoning with "corrosive sublimate" (mercuric chloride) was the most common cause. Many other agents, however, have been reported to give rise to toxic ATN when ingested accidentally or in attempts to commit suicide or to induce abortion: uranyl nitrate, arsenic, cadmium, potassium dichromate, phosphorus, dioxane, *cis*-dichlorodiamine platinum (an antineoplastic agent), some antibiotics taken in doses higher than recommended for therapeutic use, such as gentamicin and kanamycin, and antibiotics now not prescribed for systemic use, such as bacitracin and others.

Clinical Features

The clinical features are quite varied, depending upon other organs affected by the specific poison and irritative symptoms and signs from the site of ingestion (mouth, esophagus, airways, etc.). The symptomatology associated with each specific poison will not be discussed here. Oliguria or anuria occurs with rapidly progressive renal failure shortly after ingestion of the poison. If the patient is kept alive with dialysis, recovery is possible, but the prognosis depends on the severity of renal lesions as well as on the other organ manifestations.

Histopathology

Grossly, the kidneys are swollen, with a wide cortex which is pale in contrast to the dark medulla.

The light microscopy is not well known from renal biopsies. Based on a number of autopsy cases, mainly from patients poisoned by mercuric chloride, and few biopsies (3–5) the following description can be given.

If the patient dies a few days after ingestion of the poison, there is extensive necrosis of tubular epithelium, followed by desquamation. In most extreme cases, the tubules consist of basement membranes surrounding masses of necrotic epithelial cells. The most severe lesions are present in the proximal tubules. The cells lining the distal parts of the nephron and the collecting ducts are either normal or only moderately degenerated. Masses of necrotic proximal cells, however, form extensive casts in these parts of the tubules and particularly in the collecting ducts. If the patient survives these first days, proximal epithelium regenerates (with the appearance of many mitoses) and appears as a flat layer of basophilic cells. At 2 weeks, necrotic masses of proximal epithelium that had not been exfoliated in the early stage undergo calcification, but calcification may also occur at an earlier time.

Organic mercury compounds formerly used as diuretics have given rise to renal toxicity with a histopathologic picture resembling that described above (6). As a general rule, however, organic compounds are much less toxic than inorganic.

Other direct nephrotoxic substances produce a similar histologic picture. Proximal tubules are much more vulnerable than distal (Fig. 1). It has repeatedly been maintained that different poisons affect specific parts of the proximal nephron. Care should be taken in interpreting such data since they are based on kidneys investigated at autopsy, where autolysis may severely interfere with the microscopic picture.

Electron microscopic data have not been published. The same applies to immunofluorescence microscopy.

Ischemic Acute Tubular Nephropathy

The ischemic type of ARF can be induced by a large number of clinical conditions. Among the most frequent are extensive trauma or burns, shock associated with surgical operations, pancreatitis and inflammation of the biliary tract, incompatible blood transfusions, rhabdomyolysis, septicemia, dehydration, septic abortion, postpartum hemorrhage, and reaction to drugs or poisons (morphine derivatives, barbiturates, sedatives, and many others). It derives its name from the fact that many cases occur as a sequel to shock or hypovolemia, but in some patients, ARF with an identical morphology develops without overt clinical shock. In some of these patients the clinical setting makes it probable or at least possible that a period of circulatory shock had been present, although not observed. However, it cannot be excluded that the pathogenetic mechanism leading to this type of ARF can

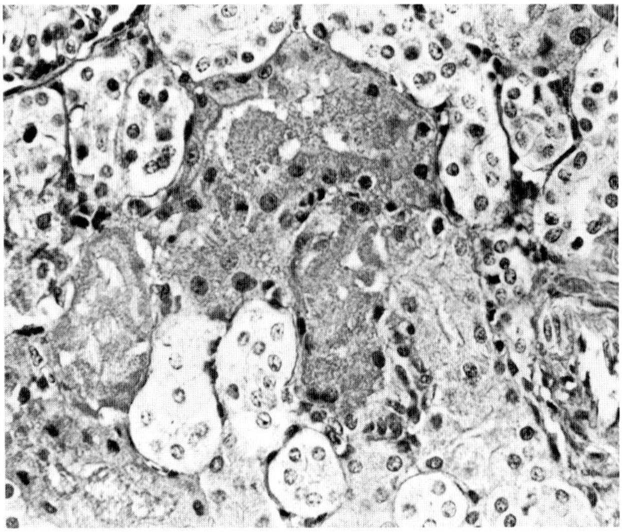

FIG. 1. Toxic acute tubular necrosis due to kanamycin. In the central part of the picture a group of necrotic proximal tubules surrounded by preserved distal tubules. (PAS ×300.)

be triggered without preceding shock. It follows from this that the disease cannot be defined by observed shock at the onset of the disease, nor by etiology. As a working definition, we propose that the term *ischemic acute tubular nephropathy* be used for cases of ARF developing in association with one of the etiologies mentioned above if the morphological picture in the renal biopsy shows mild lesions, i.e., no extensive necrosis and no severe interstitial, glomerular, or vascular lesions. If no biopsy is available, a case of ARF may be due to another category of disease such as acute interstitial nephritis or acute glomerulonephritis, although the clinical setting may often speak convincingly in favor of one of the possibilities mentioned.

Ischemic ARF has formerly been identified by many different terms, some of them reflecting assumptions about pathogenesis or histopathology now considered to be obsolete, others using overtly restrictive etiologic terms. Examples are crush syndrome, vasomotoric nephrosis, traumatic anuria, hemoglobinuric nephrosis, transfusion kidney, lower nephron nephrosis, acute tubulointerstitial nephritis, and others. The term *acute tubular necrosis* is today the most widely used designation. The reason why we have not used it in the present context is that extensive tubule cell necrosis is in fact *not* present, and we wish to avoid confusion with the direct toxic type. The term *acute tubulointerstitial nephritis* has been used much in Scandinavian countries. This name should be reserved for the acute interstitial nephritis associated with an allergic drug reaction or systemic infections.

Clinical features

Ischemic ARF may develop as a continuation of prerenal ARF when normal renal function does not return following normalization of the circulatory status. Complete anuria or, more often, oliguria develops and the patient fails to excrete nitrogenous waste products. The serum creatinine rises rapidly. As mentioned above, some patients are not oliguric or anuric, but excrete a normal or even increased amount of urine. The urine osmolality is less than 350 mOsm/kg H_2O. Urine sodium concentration is comparatively high, indicating a deficient tubular reabsorption of sodium. Renal failure may last from a few days to several weeks. Oliguria was formerly often followed by a polyuric stage, probably due to overloading with fluids. This is rare today.

The disease is usually followed by complete normalization of renal function, but some patients have mild permanent impairment of renal function. The prognosis is considered to be excellent for uncomplicated ARF but many patients have multiorgan failure with resulting high mortality (7–12).

Histopathology

Soon after introduction of the percutaneous renal biopsy, a number of studies appeared describing the light microscopic histopathology of ischemic ARF (13,14). The following presentation is based mainly upon systematic and blind semiquantitative investigations of a large series with clinicopathological correlations, reported by Solez and coworkers (15).

The glomeruli are normal. Subtle changes such as bloodless and contracted capillaries have been described, but not documented as different from controls. The same applies to an assumed increase in height of parietal epithelium. The arteries and arterioles do not display changes associated with ARF, but may show nonspecific lesions often seen in renal arteries, such as arteriolosclerosis.

Accumulations of leukocytes (polymorphs as well as mononuclear cells) are present in the vasa recta of the outer medulla. They have a differential approximately equal to that of peripheral blood.

The interstitial tissue may be edematous. Morphometry has shown that the relative interstitial cortical volume is increased although not as marked as in acute interstitial nephritis (1). Mild focal infiltration with mononuclear leukocytes is usually present. It should be stressed that marked interstitial inflammation is *not* compatible with the diagnosis of ischemic ARF but is the hallmark of acute interstitial nephritis.

The tubules display marked alterations. These do *not* include extensive tubule cell necrosis, which attracted attention in earlier autopsy pathology. The most impressive lesion of the proximal tubules is an attenuation of the periodic acid-Schiff (PAS)–positive brush border (Fig. 2). This alteration belongs to a small group of

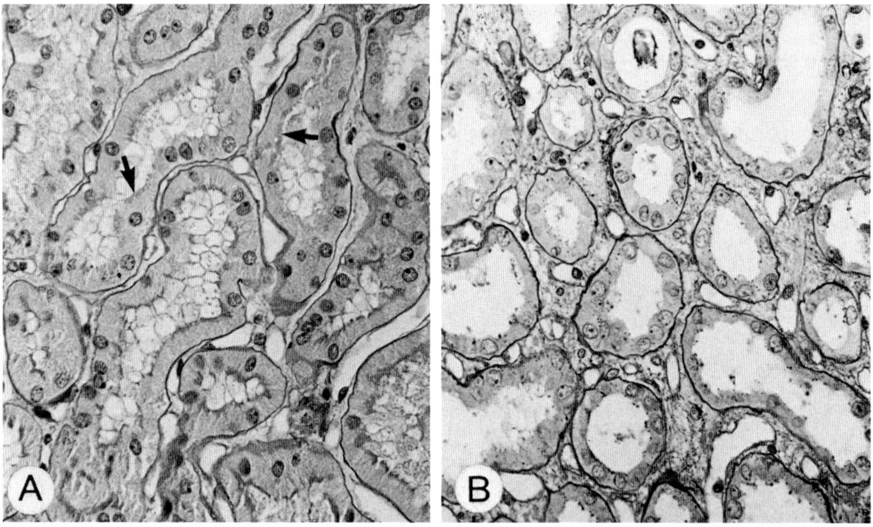

FIG. 2. A: Brush border (*arrows*) in proximal tubules from a normal human kidney. (PAS ×312.) **B:** Absence or attenuation of brush border in proximal tubules from a biopsy of an 18-year-old woman with ischemic ARF of 16 days' duration that followed an episode of sepsis treated with gentamicin. Note that there is no extensive necrosis. (PAS ×257.) (From Solez et al., ref. 15, with permission.)

lesions that are more marked in ischemic ARF than in controls and more severe in the active phase than following recovery (15). The normal, strong reaction for alkaline phosphatase in the brush border is abolished or markedly reduced (13, 16). The proximal tubules are distended, with comparatively low epithelium, and this, together with the brush border loss, causes many proximal tubules to resemble distal tubules (Fig. 3). The lumina are usually empty without casts. Hydropic change may occur to a severe degree, but this alteration is probably due to treatment with hypertonic intravenous solutions and is not related to the ARF proper. The distal tubules including the thick ascending limbs of Henle are dilated and lined with flattened epithelium. Casts of various types are numerous. Some are PAS positive and homogeneous, probably formed by the Tamm-Horsfall protein secreted in this part of the nephron. Other casts are brown and granular. These are very characteristic of ischemic ARF. They are faintly positive with PAS staining and positive with benzidine. They are very frequent in cases of ARF due to hemolysis or myolysis and are probably derived from the heme group (17). Casts are also frequent in the collecting ducts.

Frank tubular necrosis is, as mentioned, not present (Figs. 2 and 3). Desquamation of single cells occurs, however, rather often. The cells are not immediately replaced by adjacent cells, giving rise to small defects in the lining of epithelial cells. This lesion is also (like brush border disappearance) significantly less severe in recovery than in active ARF, which makes these two lesions particularly good

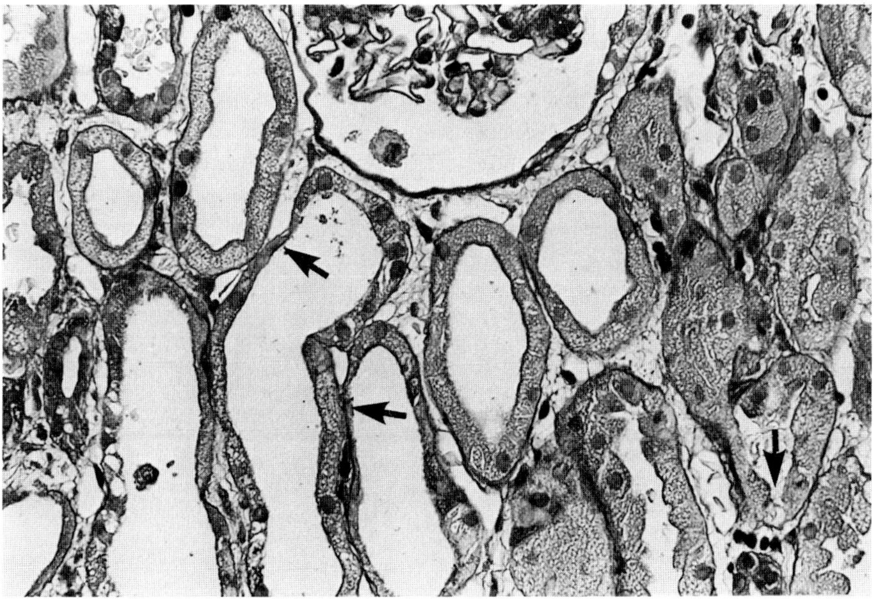

FIG. 3. Patchy loss of individual tubular cells (*arrows*). Dilatation and "distalization" of proximal tubules. From a case of ischemic ARF. (PAS ×480.)

candidates for being linked to the pathogenesis of renal functional failure. In areas with focal mononuclear infiltration, the leukocytes may invade the tubules (focal tubulitis [18]), but this lesion is much less prominent than in acute interstitial nephritis.

None of the single lesions described is specific. The lesions' combination in a renal biopsy in absence of other parenchymal alterations (such as severe interstitial cell infiltration or impressive glomerular or vascular lesions) is, however, strongly indicative of ischemic ARF.

In autopsy specimens, most of the lesions described above can be seen. Autolysis, which affects proximal tubules the most, may make it difficult to identify the subtle but very important alterations of brush border disappearance and single cell desquamation. From normal animal kidneys fixed immediately by perfusion and from intravital microscopic studies it is known that proximal lumina are open *in vivo*. They are collapsed in autopsy and biopsy specimens from normal persons and most renal diseases, but appear open and dilated in biopsy as well as autopsy material from patients with ischemic ARF.

Fluorescence microscopy does not reveal any constant or significant deposits, and intravascular fibrin is only present in cases associated with disseminated intravascular coagulation.

Electron microscopy supports the light microscopic observation that no widespread tubular necrosis is present. The use of transmission electron microscopy

(TEM) with systematic, semiquantitative and quantitative methods (19–21) has permitted a detailed and precise description of ultrastructural changes (Figs. 4 to 7). Classical cell necroses with disruption of outer and inner cell membranes are very rare, and do not occur significantly more frequently than in control biopsies. Apoptosis or shrinkage necrosis is a normal phenomenon, probably reflecting programmed cell death in cellular turnover. This type of necrosis also occurs in ischemic ARF with the same frequency as in controls. The so-called nonreplacement phenomenon described light microscopically by Solez et al. (15), can also be seen by electron microscopy (Fig. 5). It appears as defects in the epithelial lining of the tubules. These defects correspond usually to missing single cells, but in the medulla more than one cell can be missing, or still located *in situ*, but loosened from the basement membrane. When the desquamated cells are seen close to the defect, they appear to be viable, without signs of necrosis. That at least some of these desqua-

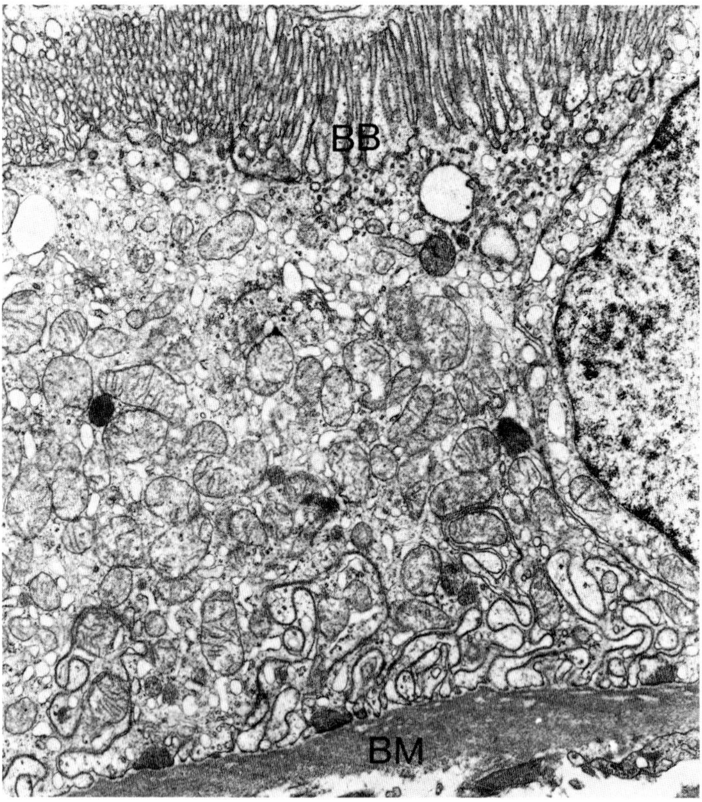

FIG. 4. Electron micrograph of normal proximal tubule for comparison with Figs. 5 and 6. Note the well-developed brush border and the meandering basolateral infoldings in the basal part of the cytoplasm. (×7,200.)

mated cells are viable is supported by studies of shed tubular cells in the urine. They are clearly viable since they exclude vital dyes and can be grown in cell culture (22). The basement membrane is always intact below the site where one or more cells are missing. These changes are much more marked in the straight tubules in the medulla and the medullary rays than in the convoluted tubules in the cortex.

Another impressive ultrastructural change of the renal tubules in ischemic ARF is a simplification of the luminal and basolateral cell surfaces (Fig. 5). It has been documented by scanning electron microscopy (SEM) (23) as well as by a blinded, semiquantitative technique on TEM (19). Most proximal tubules show some degree of disappearance of the brush border, and many have only a few areas left, which allows the identification of the tubule as proximal. The internalization of luminal villi as seen in some experimental models (24) is not a feature observed in human ischemic ARF, and loosened or disrupted villi are seldom seen in the lumen in its maintenance phase. The simplification of the luminal cell surface may be so marked in proximal tubules that they take on the appearance of distal tubules. That this must often be the case is documented indirectly by a change in the ratio of apparent distal/proximal tubular cross sections, from 0.38 in controls to about 0.54 in ischemic ARF.This spurious low relative number of proximal tubular profiles has been called

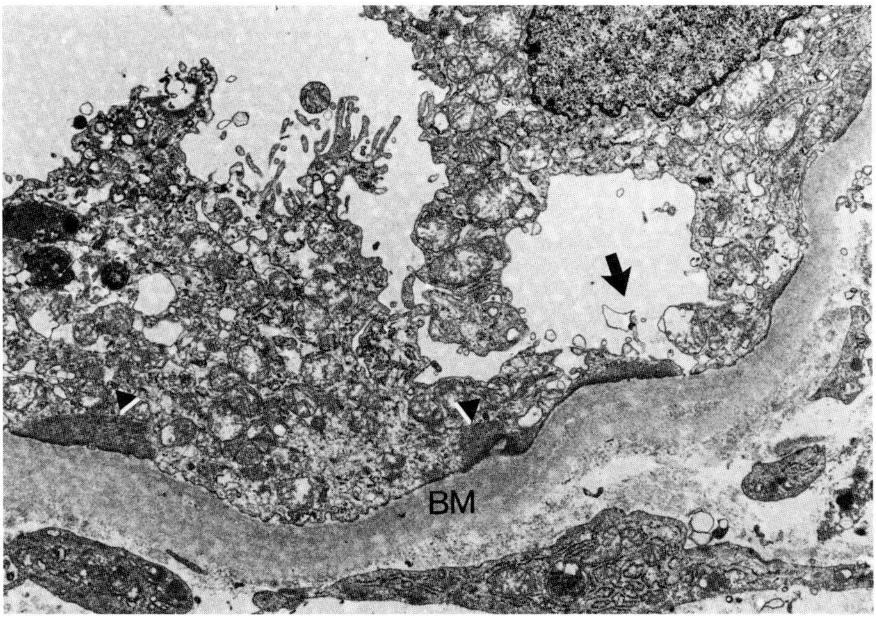

FIG. 5. Electron micrograph of proximal tubule from a case of ischemic ARF. One cell is missing and the defect is incompletely covered by the adjacent tubular cells (*arrow*). There is almost total disappearance of the brush border and the basolateral infoldings. Note also the prominent actin bundles (*arrowheads*). Compare with Fig. 4. BM. ($\times$6,300.)

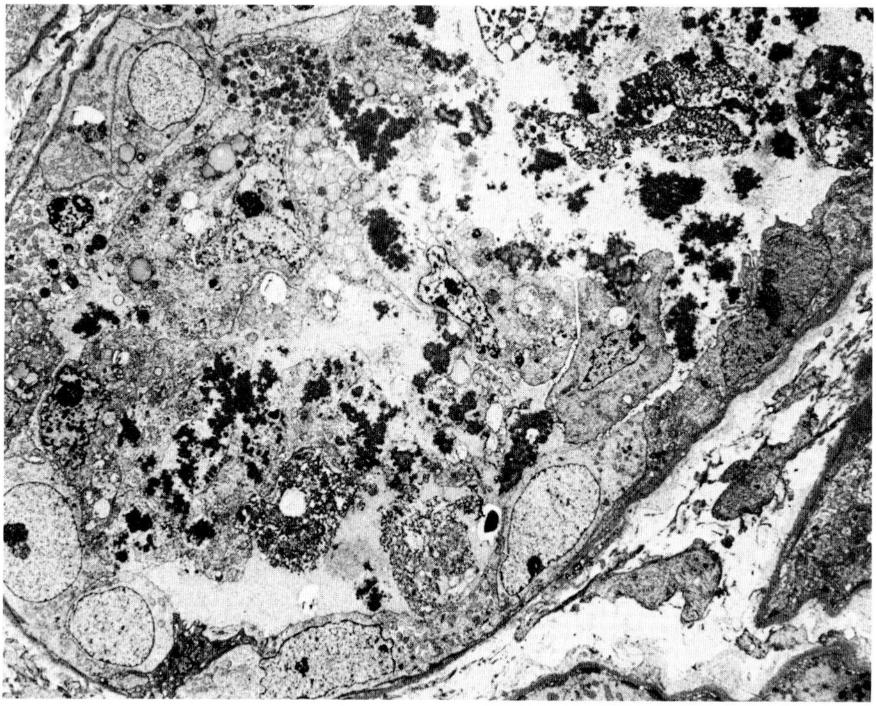

FIG. 6. Electron micrograph of distal tubule from a case of ischemic ARF due to postpartum hemorrhage (6 days). The lumen is distended, the epithelial cells flat, not necrotic. In the lumen there is a pigmented cast with inclusion of desquamated epithelial cells and cell debris. (×2,240.)

"distalization." Using SEM, the disappearance of proximal brush border can be seen directly (23). The extensive basolateral infoldings can, by the same semiquantitative technique on TEM, be demonstrated to be greatly reduced so that the basal cell membrane becomes totally flat, following the basement membrane closely. This basal cell surface simplification is present in proximal as well as distal tubules, and in the convoluted as well as the straight parts. Taking into consideration the important functions these cell surface amplifications have for the normal tubular function (transport of water and solutes), it is clear that their disappearance in ARF must necessarily have serious functional consequences.

Renal tubular epithelial cells contain actin fibrils like most other cells. Actin fibrils are particularly rich in the basal part of the cells, where they are condensed into broad bundles, attached at both ends to the basal cell membrane, and probably to the adjacent basement membrane. They are predominantly circularily oriented in a plane perpendicular to the axis of the tubule. They are presumed to have a function in adjusting the size of the lumen, and hence the luminal pressure. In ischemic ARF, these actin bundles are significantly hypertrophic compared with controls,

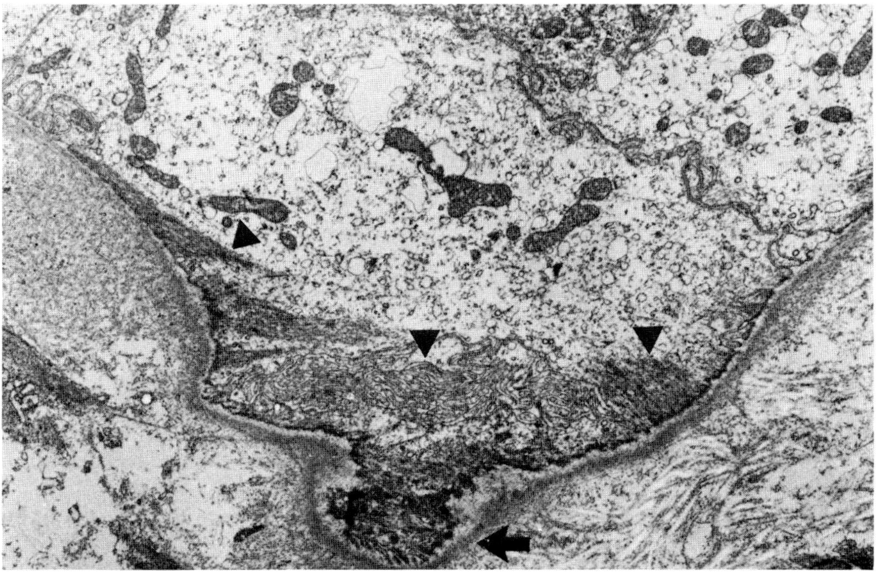

FIG. 7. Electron micrograph from a case of ischemic ARF showing prominent bundles of actin fibrils (*arrowheads*). They appear to constrict the circumference of the tubular basement membrane with formation of a small diverticle (*arrow*). (×5,100.)

and diverticular pouches of the basement membrane are often seen between their attachment points, giving the impression that they contract the circumference of the tubule in response to a decreased luminal content (Fig. 7) (25).

Special Types of ARF, Possibly Related to Ischemic ARF

Tubular casts are, as discussed above, part of the histopathological picture in ischemic ARF. In some types of ARF *crystalline casts* are predominant. This is the situation in poisoning with ethylene glycol (used as antifreeze solution) (26,27). In this disease distal tubules and collecting ducts contain a multitude of doubly refractile oxalate crystals. Such crystals may also occur in some cases of ischemic ARF, but in ethylene glycol poisoning they are numerous, reflecting the fact that oxalic acid is a metabolite of ethylene glycol. Tubular degeneration and possibly also tubular necrosis may also be present, and it is uncertain whether these lesions or tubular obstructions are responsible for the renal failure. No systematic studies of renal biopsies including electron microscopy have been published. Tubular calcium oxalate crystals are also a characteristic finding in ARF due to halogenated anesthesics such as methoxyflurane (formerly much used as an anesthesic) and halothane (28–31) as well as to oral and intravenous cholangiographic materials (32). Oxalate crystals can be demonstrated by polarization microscopy in formalin-fixed, paraffin-embedded tissue if the section is stained with hematoxylin and eosin, but not in sections stained with PAS or silver methenamine, stains often used for renal biopsy studies.

Concretions of sulfonamide were found in the distal tubules in many cases of ARF occurring in the early years following the introduction of sulfonamide therapy.

If the serum concentration of uric acid is markedly increased as in diseases with rapid breakdown of nucleic acid (leukemia and lymphoma during treatment with chemotherapy and radiation), huge numbers of uric acid crystals may occur in the distal tubules and collecting ducts.

The *hepatorenal syndrome* is not well defined and the term has been used for different types of renal disease associated with hepatic or biliary disorders. The ischemic type of ARF may develop following surgery on the liver and biliary tract, or in association with severe hepatic disease. In such cases, bile-stained casts are present together with lesions of ischemic ARF discussed above. The term *hepatorenal syndrome* has also been used for a special type of renal failure characterized by *low sodium urinary excretion*. Apart from lesions characteristic for ischemic ARF, the tubules in this condition contain large greenish crystals (probably leucine) as well as bile-stained casts and there is a focal leukocyte infiltration around these casts (33–36).

ARF associated with *increased blood concentration of calcium* probably has the histopathology of ischemic ARF, but few structural data are available.

Patients with *multiple myeloma* have a high incidence of ARF. The renal histopathology is that known from myeloma cast disease; and hyperuricemia, which is often present, may give rise to uric acid crystals. The renal failure may be due to obstruction of tubules by the characteristic casts of light chains, to associated hypercalcemia or hyperuricemia (37).

Allergic Acute Interstitial Nephritis

Acute interstitial nephritis (AIN), also called acute tubulointerstitial nephritis, is usually due to an allergic reaction to drugs. AIN can also be associated with generalized infections, and this etiology was in fact the first to be recognized (38). In some infections, an interstitial inflammation of the kidney is caused by the presence of the responsible microorganisms in the renal parenchyma (virus infections, *Leptospira*, various bacteria causing pyelonephritis); in others the circumstances point toward an allergic reaction like that following drugs. AIN can rarely be caused by various immune reactions of poorly known nature, or it may occur under circumstances where etiology and pathogenesis are totally unknown (2). The following discussion of AIN will deal mainly with drug-induced allergic AIN, the form most frequent by far today.

Etiology

Drug-induced allergic AIN can follow administration of a great number of drugs belonging to various chemical or pharmacological classes. Among *antibiotics*, those of the β-lactam class are by far the most frequent, methicillin being one of the first documented causes and still probably the most common offender. Penicillin, ampicillin, and the cephalothins are also often reported to be responsible. Other antibiotics and chemotherapeutics that may be responsible include sulfonamides, chloramphenicol, rifampicin, and others.

Nonsteroidal anti-inflammatory drugs (NSAIDs) are also often reported as responsible for AIN. The long list of other agents include thiazide diuretics, cimetidine, allopurinol, and many others (39–42).

Clinical Features

Clinical features include renal failure together with general symptoms of uremia and systemic symptoms of allergy.

The acute renal failure occurs usually following 1 or 2 weeks of administration of the responsible drug. Fever and a skin rash may herald the disease and soon the renal function begins to deteriorate. The ARF is most often oliguric, but nonoliguric cases have been reported. Hemodialysis will often be necessary. When the responsible drug is withdrawn, renal function begins to increase after a few days or weeks. Most patients recover, but permanent reduction of renal function may occur. The latent period as well as the skin rash testify to the allergic nature of the disease, and other features pointing in the same direction are blood eosinophilia and eosinophiluria.

Histopathology

Light microscopy (43) of renal biopsies shows a marked interstitial infiltrate consisting predominantly of mononuclear cells (Fig. 8). Large and small lymphocytes are most numerous, but plasma cells may also be present. The infiltrate is patchy and most marked in the inner cortex and the outer medulla. In spite of the assumed allergic character of the disease, eosinophils are usually scarce, but a few reported cases had dominance of eosinophils.

There may be small accumulations of histiocytes giving the inflammation of granulomatous character, and in rare cases multinuclear giant cells may occur. Morphometry has shown that the relative interstitial volume of the cortex is strongly increased, which is due to the presence of leukocytes as well as to interstitial edema (1).

Lymphocytes are present between tubular epithelial cells and in the lumina ("tubulitis"), particularly in areas with marked interstitial infiltration, but they may also occur in otherwise normal tubules in cortical areas without interstitial infiltration. Using silver methenamine staining of the basement membranes, some tubular cross sections appear normal, even in the presence of tubulitis, but some show thinning or even focal absence of the basement membrane. Other tubular profiles are more severely damaged, with epithelial desquamation and extensive defects of the tubular basement membrane. The presence of accumulations of epithelial-like cells in the

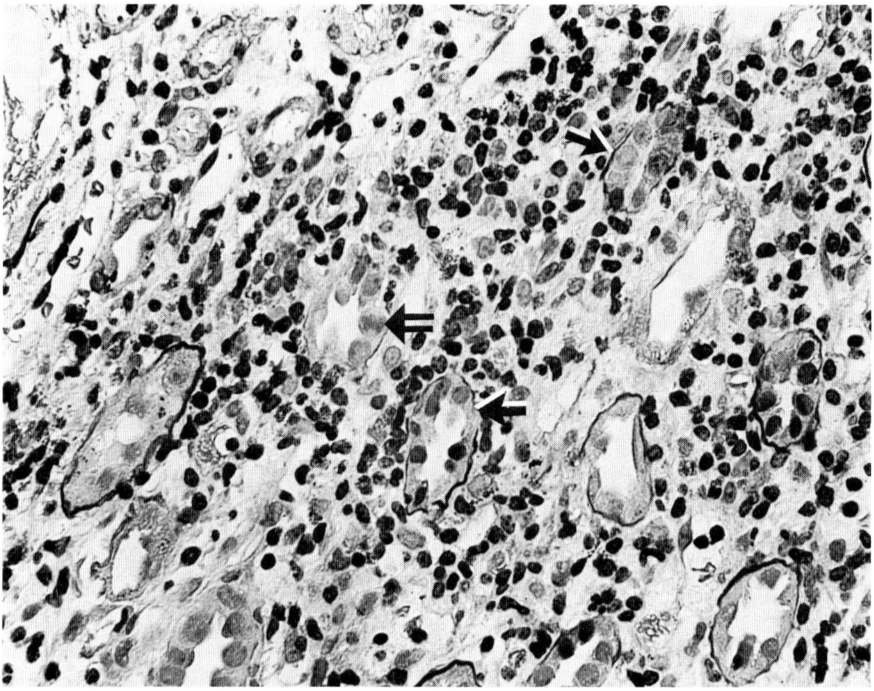

FIG. 8. Acute interstitial nephritis. There is severe interstitial infiltration with lymphocytes. The basement membranes of the tubules are deficient (*arrows*) or almost totally absent (*double arrow*). (PAS ×240.)

interstitium and of scattered fragments of basement membranes constitute the remnants of totally destroyed tubules. The identification of the tubular segment most severely affected can be difficult, but use of immunohistochemical methods has shown that tubulitis predominantly affects distal tubules (43a).

The glomeruli and vessels are normal.

Few cases have been rebiopsied following recovery with reduced renal function. Such biopsies show tubular atrophy and interstitial fibrosis.

Immunofluorescence microscopy fails in most cases to show immunoglobulins or complement in the tubular or glomerular basement membranes. A linear fluorescense with antibody against IgG has, however, been reported in few biopsies (43).

Electron microscopy (44) shows severe tubular damage in regions with interstitial cellular infiltration. This tubular damage seems to follow a three-phase sequence. The first phase is migration of lymphocytes through the tubular basement membrane.This passage must be very fast since the location of a lymphocyte in a defect in the basement membrane in this early phase has never been documented. Many lymphocytes are, however, situated between normally appearing tubular epithelial cells, indicating that no direct "killer" effect is exerted on epithelial cells. In the second phase, the tubular basement membrane becomes focally extremely thin or may even be lacking in some parts of the periphery. The epithelial cells are nevertheless intact in such tubules although some are loosened from the basement membrane. The thinned and later defective basement membrane may be due to diminished synthesis from the epithelial cells. The last stage is a rupture of the tubule with necrosis of epithelial cells now situated in the interstitial tissue. At this stage, which can be seen in areas severely infiltrated with mononuclear cells, the renal parenchyma presents a chaotic appearance with a mixture of small and large lymphocytes, histiocytes, and plasma cells together with fragments of tubular basement membranes and of the remnants of necrotic tubular cells. Some of these constituents are phagocytosed by macrophages. Outside of areas infiltrated with mononuclear cells, the tubules are intact. They display, however, marked changes of the same type as in ischemic ARF: reduction of proximal brush border and proximal as well as distal basolateral infoldings.

The glomeruli are ultrastructurally normal except in the few cases where an associated glomerulonephritis is present. As discussed above, some cases of AIN are associated with a nephrotic syndrome. In such patients, the glomerular ultrastructure has shown podocyte effacement as in minimal change disease, but few or no deposits.

Primary Renal Allograft Dysfunction

In primary allograft dysfunction, normal function does not begin immediately after opening of the anastomoses, but may be delayed for hours, days, or even several weeks. It is a matter of dispute if this condition per se is associated with unfavorable graft survival, but if rejection (which may be difficult to diagnose in the graft without function) or other graft complications do not occur, excellent long-term function may eventually be attained. Owing to clinical similarity to ischemic ARF in the native kidney, it has been implied that the primary graft dysfunction is the counterpart to this disease. It is, thus, assumed that renal ischemia sustained before harvesting or during preservation or implantation is responsible for this graft ARF.

Investigating a series of renal allograft recipients treated with steroid/azathioprine immunosuppression, we were able to demonstrate marked morphological differences between native ischemic ARF and primary graft dysfunction (45). Transplant ARF showed significantly less thinning and absence of proximal tubular brush border and less variation in size and shape of cells in individual tubular cross sections. There were also fewer casts and a significantly greater number of oxalate crystals in transplant ARF. The latter condition showed sites of tubular injury affecting short tubular segments, characterized by presence of necrotic tubular epithelial cells, a finding seldom seen in native ischemic ARF. By electron microscopy, in transplant

ARF there were no significant alterations in proximal and distal basolateral infoldings of cell surfaces, which contrasted sharply with marked reduction in basolateral infoldings observed in native, ischemic ARF. The volumes of basal actin filament bundles, which were increased in native ARF, were significantly reduced in transplant dysfunction.

It is not possible at the moment to explain these differences but they suggest that the two conditions may each have a different pathogenesis.

EXPERIMENTAL ACUTE RENAL FAILURE

Toxic Models

Mercuric Chloride

Administration of 1.5 to 5 mg/kg of $HgCl_2$ to rats results in necrosis of the proximal tubules. No change can be seen by light microscopy during the first few hours, but after about 12 hr epithelial necrosis is evident in the proximal tubules, mainly the pars recta (S_3). All nephrons are involved and necrotic debris fills out the lumina also of the lower segments of the nephron. Injection of trypan blue or sodium ferrocyanide as tracers during this period demonstrates that the tubular walls are leaky, letting the tracer permeate to the interstitium and the intertubular vessels. Between the 2nd and the 5th day there is beginning reconstitution of the tubular epithelium by proliferation from the distal end of the necrotic part. During the necrotic period, the seemingly undamaged tubular basement membranes form the scaffold upon which the new tubular epithelium is built (46–49).

There are few changes in the distal tubules, which may, however, show some degree of degeneration. The glomeruli are normal, including pore size and foot process width as measured by morphometry on SEM and TEM (50).

Uranyl Nitrate

Uranium nephrotoxicity has been studied experimentally since the beginning of the century and the severe tubular damage caused by this heavy metal was recognized early. Tubular necrosis is limited to the pars recta of the proximal tubule, and can be seen 2 days after a single dose. As demonstrated by Flamenbaum et al. (51), there is a fall in cortical blood flow, which can be detected as early as 3 to 6 hr after injection, i.e., long before frank necrosis occurs. Renal failure appears insidiously 2 to 3 days after injection. It seems therefore that renal failure is better correlated to histological necrosis than to the early decrease in blood flow. The severity of histological lesions and of the renal failure are both clearly related to the injected dose (52–56).

In contrast to mercuric chloride nephropathy, the toxic action of uranyl nitrate is also associated with glomerular abnormalities (52). There is marked reduction in the number and size of endothelial fenestrae and this is an early lesion appearing after few hours. Later on there is podocyte swelling and fusion of foot processes. Uranyl nitrate–damaged tubules regenerate more slowly than mercuric chloride–damaged tubules and just as the onset of renal failure is more insidious, the renal failure tends to persist for a longer period in the uranyl nitrate model. Although there are similarities between the renal effects of mercury and uranium such as the location of the tubular necrosis and detachment of tubular epithelial cells, there are, thus, also distinct differences.

Cis-*platinum*

Cis-dichlorodiamine platinum is a potent antineoplastic agent. It is, however strongly nephrotoxic. In humans a single dose of 2 mg/kg body weight will cause ARF in 25% to 33% of patients, and nephrotoxicity is more severe if greater or frequent repetitive doses are administered. In rats injections of *cis*-platinum causes an ARF that is nonoliguric and of the high urinary sodium type. The renal failure develops within a few days after injection. Morphologically there are few lesions the first days, but later loss of proximal brush border, focal cellular necrosis, and sloughing and cellular casts occur. After 5 to 6 days there is extensive and severe tubular necrosis, most severe in the straight portion of the proximal tubule (S_3) and thus most marked in the outer medullary region where *cis*-platinum concentration is also highest. In surviving animals, tubular necrosis is followed by regeneration as in $HgCl_2$ poisoning (57–61).

The extensive tubular necrosis present in this model makes backleak probable, and evidence derived from dye markers or radioactive inulin injection support this mechanism. There is, however, also reduced renal blood flow, and this as well as other experimental data suggest preglomerular vasoconstriction.

Gentamicin

Gentamicin, an aminoglycoside, is a valuable and widely used antibiotic. It is, however, nephrotoxic, and is currently estimated to be associated with renal complications in about 10% of patients treated. The characteristic clinical manifestation is nonoliguric ARF beginning 7 to 10 days after initiation of therapy.

Gentamicin is filtered by the glomerulus and enters proximal tubule cells via the luminal surface and binding to brush border microvilli (62,63). The degree and histologic type of gentamicin nephrotoxicity is different in male and female patients and experimental animals. In male Fischer rats, gentamicin produces widespread necrosis of the straight part of the proximal tubules when 10 times the maximum dose recommended for man is given (Fig. 9) (64). The degree of necrosis correlates with serum creatinine (65). It is interesting that renal function returns to normal even if administration of gentamicin is continued, presumably because regenerating proximal tubular cells are resistant to the effect of the drug. After 1 month, sequelae

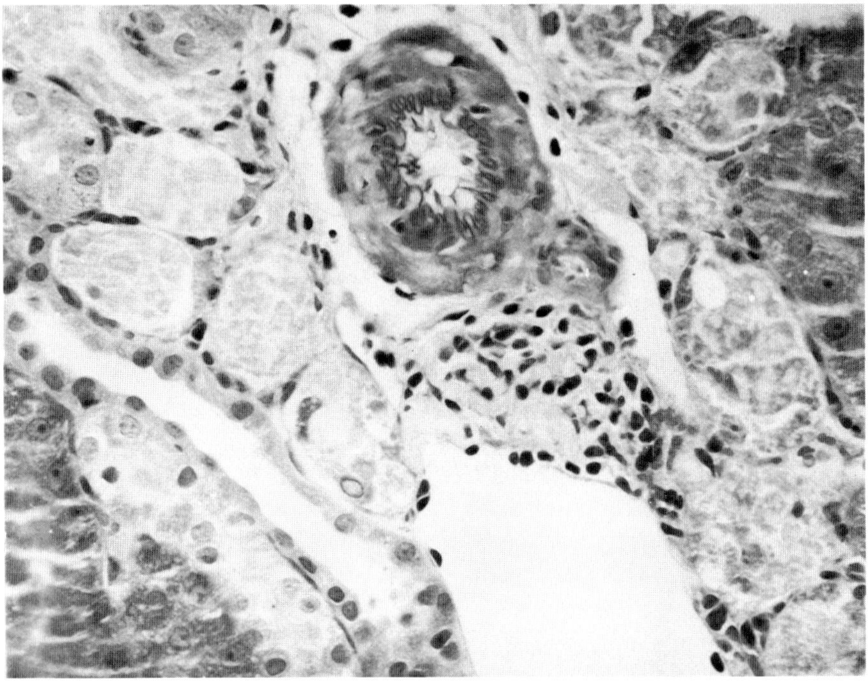

FIG. 9. Tubular necrosis with tubular disruption and small mononuclear cell infiltration in the corticomedullary junction in a gentamicin-treated male rat. The smooth muscle cells of the artery are vacuolated. (H&E ×425.) (From Kourilsky et al., ref. 65, with permission.)

of the tubular necrosis can be seen in the form of patchy interstitial fibrosis and inflammation, and tubular atrophy (66–69). Experiments with castration and testosterone administration indicate that the susceptibility of male rats to gentamicin is due to the action of testosterone. Although the nephrotoxicity in male rats in this model using large doses is a direct, dose-dependent toxic effect, the female rat suffers from acute interstitial nephritis of probable immunologic origin (Fig. 10) (70).

In the female Lewis rat, using doses giving serum levels of gentamicin comparable to those obtained in clinical practice, Tolkoff-Rubin et al. (71) found obvious signs of necrosis or damage in proximal tubule cells manifested by nuclear pyknosis, karyolysis, and sloughing of some of the cells. Some animals had interstitial nephritis. Peak injury was observed 7 to 10 days after therapy. The lesions were dose dependent and low doses were only associated with cytoplasmic vacuolization in some tubules (71).

Brush border enzymes have been demonstrated in the urine of subjects given gentamicin. Histologically, there is brush border loss in proximal tubules in experimental animals as well as in man. Morphometric investigations have shown that basolateral cell surface infoldings are considerably decreased in rats treated with

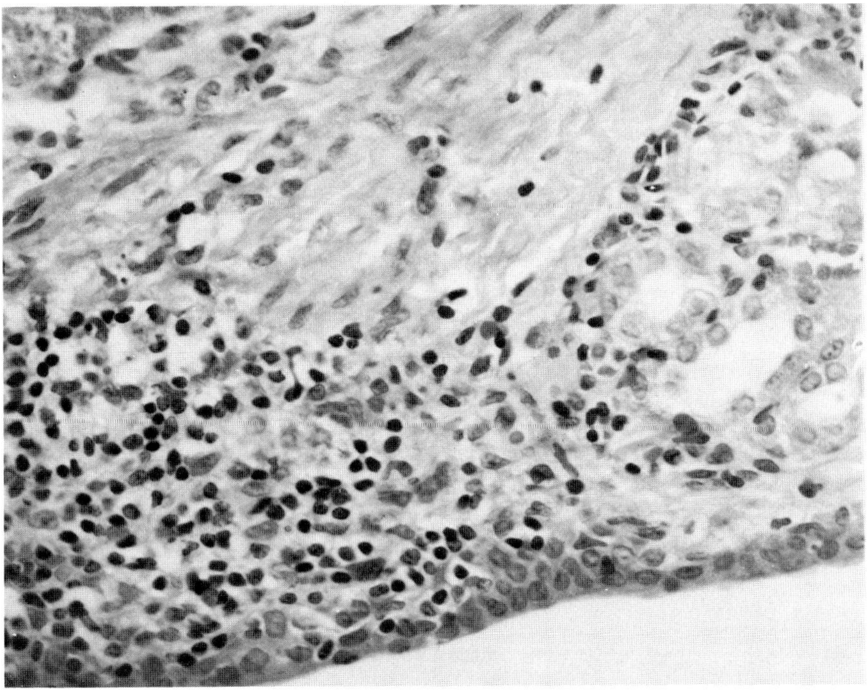

FIG. 10. Mononuclear infiltrate under the renal pelvic epithelium of a gentamicin-treated female rat. The cause of this pelvic inflammation, which is uncommon in untreated female rats, is unknown. (H&E ×320.)

gentamicin, and this is related to the degree of renal failure (72). In this respect (but not with respect to tubular necrosis present in gentamicin rats) gentamicin toxicity resembles ischemic ARF in man.

Conflicting reports have been published about the glomerular morphology in gentamycin nephrotoxicity. One group (73) has found reduction in size and number of glomerular, capillary endothelial fenestrae by SEM, which may explain a decreased glomerular ultrafiltration coefficient (K_f) described earlier. Another group (74) did not confirm this observation. It is possible that the apparent decrease in fenestral number and size may be artificial, caused by perfusion with saline before perfusion fixation.

In both experimental animals and man, peculiar "myeloid bodies" are seen in proximal tubular epithelium (75). They probably represent altered lysosomes. Although not entirely specific, they are markers of gentamicin administration but their presence is probably not related to clinical tubular toxicity. The same applies to the vacuolization of smooth muscle cells in the arterial wall, which is more prominent in rats treated with gentamicin than in controls (Fig. 9). This lesion has been described in patients who have received amphotericin, but the change is not specific (64,76).

Ischemic Models

Arterial Occulsion

Acute postischemic renal failure can be produced in the rat by clamping the renal pedicle for 1 hr (77). There is considerable variation in the time course and severity of renal failure produced, and the type of anesthesia used, as well as the presence or absence of a contralateral kidney, influences functional outcome. Histopathologically this model is characterized by severe and widespread proximal tubular necrosis (Fig. 11). Careful investigations of the morphological events have been performed by Venkatachalam et al. (78,79). By electron microscopy, swelling of tubular epithelial cells can be seen already while the clamp is in place. Within minutes after release of the clamp brush border microvilli are partially shed into the tubular lumen. Other microvilli still attached to the cells, swell, and become club-shaped. Eventually such microvilli coalesce and become incorporated with apical

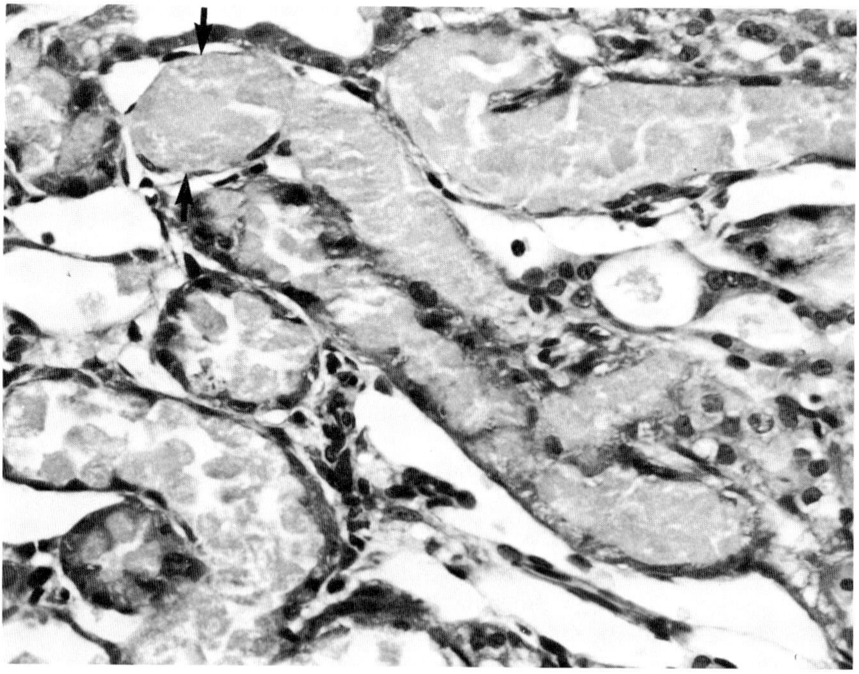

FIG. 11. Extensive necrosis of proximal tubules (between *arrows*) 48 hr after 1 hr of pedicle clamping in a rat. (H&E ×400.) (From Solez, ref. 88, with permission.)

cytoplasm of the cells. Shed microvilli swell, fill the tubular lumina, and travel down the nephron where they impact the descending limb of the loop of Henle. By 24 hr most distal lumina are distended and contain casts seeming to obstruct the flow of tubular fluid, an assumption that has been confirmed by measurements of intratubular pressure by micropuncture studies. Tubular cell necrosis and extensive casts make it likely that leakage as well as obstruction are operative in producing renal failure, but vasoconstriction may also be operative, and after 2 weeks, when tubular epithelial damage and casts are no longer present, impairment of renal function may be the most important cause of impairment of the renal function.

The extensive tubular necrosis characteristic of this rat model makes it different from ischemic ARF in man. By clamping the pedicle for 1 hr and removing the contralateral kidney in the rabbit, Solez and coworkers (80) were able to produce a model of ARF morphologically and physiologically more similar to ischemic ARF in man. In this model acute oliguria is not associated with extensive tubular necrosis, but hyaline casts were seen as an early change. By 1 week, renal failure is still present, but casts have almost disappeared. In these rabbits there was a significant correlation between serum creatinine and the extent of accumulation of leukocytes in the vasa recta of the renal medulla, a lesion also known from ARF in man. This led the authors to investigate the vasa recta with colloid carbon as a marker. The carbon particles were selectively trapped in damaged endothelium in the vasa recta within 2 hr after release of the pedicle clamp. This capillary damage could be prevented by treatment with clonidine (an antihypertensive agent), which also lessened the severity of the ARF (81).

In the glomeruli, morphological abnormalities have been demonstrated by SEM in pedicle-clamping models in both rats and rabbits (Fig. 12). These lesions, which are restricted to the podocytes and can be demonstrated while the clamp is still in place, may eventually increase or disappear (82).

Norepinephrine Infusion

Infusion of norepinephrine causes anuria and abolishment of renal blood flow while the infusion is given (83,84). Following infusion of 2 hr to dogs, the renal failure is irreversible and 8 weeks after, the renal blood flow and glomerular filtration is less than 5% of normal (85). Histologically there is extensive tubular necrosis to a degree similar to cortical necrosis in man. In contradistinction to the tubular necrosis in toxic models and the pedicle clamp model, the necrosis affects all segments of the proximal tubule as well as the distal tubules, and medullary hemorrhagic necrosis has also been demonstrated. In the glomeruli there is flattening of podocyte processes and lessening of the area covered by filtration slits (86).

Reduction of the infusion time to 40 min results in almost completely reversible ARF (87). The necrosis is still marked, but present predominantly in proximal tubules. There is marked formation of casts.

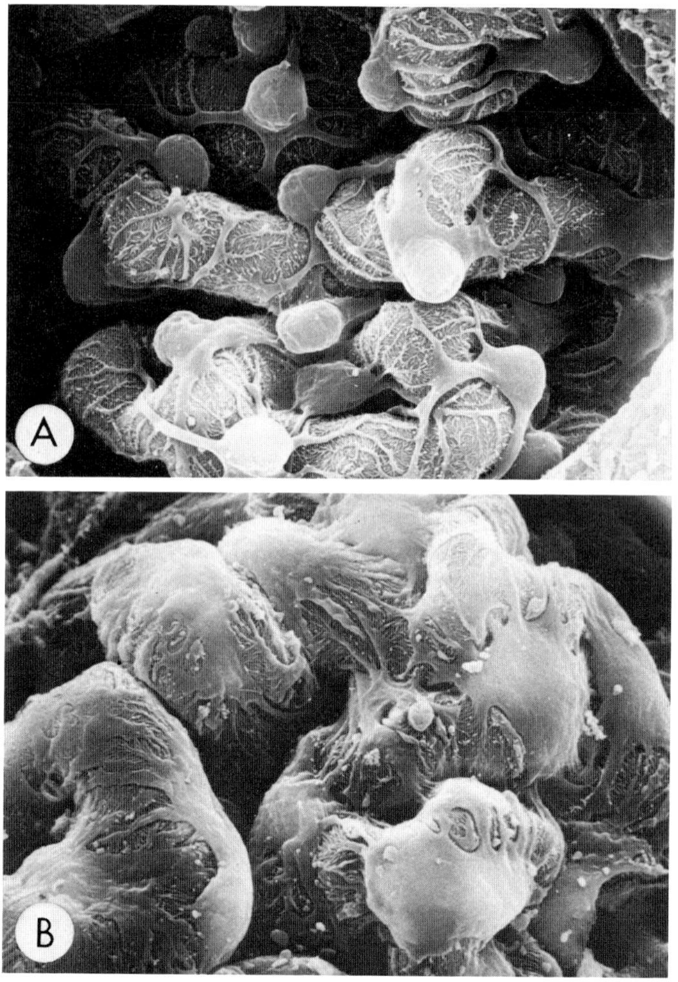

FIG. 12. A: Scanning electron micrograph of a normal rabbit glomerulus. The podocyte cell bodies hang off the capillary loops in a berry-like fashion. Most of the capillary surface is covered by foot processes and podocyte processes narrower than 1 μm. (×1,500.) **B:** Scanning electron micrograph of a rabbit glomerulus 2 hr after a 1- hr period of pedicle clamping. Cell bodies are flattened and indistinguishable from the sheetlike cytoplasmic processes that emanate from them and cover most of the capillary surface. Few foot processes and podocyte processes narrower than 1 μm are seen. (From Solez et al., ref. 82, with permission.)

IMPACT OF HISTOPATHOLOGY ON CONCEPTS OF PATHOGENESIS OF ISCHEMIC ARF IN MAN

Studies of animal models as well as of ischemic ARF in man have led to general recognition of four main pathogenetic factors that alone or in concert might explain the renal failure in ischemic ARF: (a) backleak of tubular fluid, (b) tubular obstruction, (c) arteriolar vasoconstriction, and (d) decreased glomerular ultrafiltration coefficient (88,89). We will first discuss the possible significance of these factors for ischemic ARF in man and subsequently add a few remarks on what can be learned from animal models. The discussion will concentrate upon interpretations of morphological data in terms of pathogenesis. A detailed discussion of pathogenesis taking into consideration the immense body of pathophysiological data is presented in the chapter by Abbate, Macconi, and Remuzzi.

Backleak of Tubular Fluid

The idea that tubular fluid leaks back through damaged tubular walls was natural at a time when extensive tubular necrosis was considered to be present not only in direct nephrotoxic ARF but also in the ischemic type. The significant correlation between interstitial edema and tubular dilatation demonstrated by Bohle et al. (90) and Solez et al. (91), might support this contention, but it could also have alternative explanations. Masses of extravasated tubular fluid may occasionally be seen in the interstitium in renal biopsies and it should be recalled that Oliver et al. (5) by microdissection detected tubular disruption, which may, however, have been overestimated due to artifacts from the preparation of the tissue and its dissection as well as postmortem autolysis.

Although, as demonstrated above, tubular cell necrosis is not characteristic for ischemic ARF, some morphological lesions may still support the contention that backleak may be operative, at least as an additional factor. The demonstration that about 5% of the distal tubular cells in the convoluted tubules in the cortex are shed without substitution by adjacent cells (and even more in the medullary portions of the proximal and distal tubules) (21) makes it possible that tubular fluid under pressure may leak through these denuded areas of the tubular basement membrane. The mild focal tubulitis with break of the basement membranes may also contribute to backleak.

Tubular Obstruction

Tubular obstruction may be of causative importance for the renal failure due to increased pressure in the tubular system, which must counteract glomerular filtration and facilitate tubular backleak. There is also experimental evidence that obstruction may lead to afferent vasoconstriction and consequently to decreased ultrafiltration.

Morphological lesions suggest that tubular obstruction takes place. Casts of various composition constitute an important part of the histopathological picture in ischemic ARF in man, and dilatation of the tubular lumina can be explained as resulting from increased intratubular pressure. There is, on the other hand, also evidence against the importance of obstruction for the renal failure. Steinhausen (92) has experimentally demonstrated that hemoglobin casts can easily be expelled from the tubular system. It is of course uncertain if this is also the case in man. More significant is the fact that casts are still present at a time when the patient has just recovered from ARF.

It is, however, very difficult to judge the importance of casts seen in the biopsy specimens. A single cast in a distal convoluted tubule may appear in many tubular cross sections, giving the appearance of many casts. The functionally most important casts may be those in terminal collecting ducts acting as common terminal outlets for several nephrons, and these ducts are seldom seen in biopsies (93).

Arteriolar Vasoconstriction

The renal blood flow is reduced to about 25% to 50% of normal in patients with ischemic ARF and there is a preferential reduction of blood flow to the cortex (94–97). Renal arteriograms in patients with ARF show constriction of arcuate and segmental arteries. These and other data led several investigators to consider vasoconstriction as a "final common pathway" responsible for the renal failure, as testified by the revival of the old term *vasomotor nephropathy*. Supported by micropuncture experiments, Thurau and Boylan (98) proposed a detailed hypothesis involving disturbance of the tubuloglomerular balance. The concept involves the assumption of a primary defect in tubular reabsorption of sodium, chloride, or both. As long as this defect is operative, the sodium concentration at the macula densa is increased. From experimental work it is known that the sodium or chloride concentration at this site is a signal for local renin release and, consequently, for preglomerular vasoconstriction caused by activation of angiotensin. The glomerular filtration will be diminished until tubular reabsorption normalizes.

Morphological studies have so far not been able to provide evidence for arteriolar constriction or increased local activity of the renin-angiotensin system in the juxtaglomerular apparatus, but the part of the hypothesis involving tubules is supported by structural data. Normal tubular reabsorption of sodium and chloride is facilitated by the immense amplification of cellular surfaces due to the proximal brush-border and the basolateral infoldings present in the proximal convoluted tubule and thick ascending limb of Henle, situated proximal to the macula. The extreme simplification of these surfaces demonstrated by SEM and TEM in ischemic ARF must necessarily reduce ion transport. It is clear that these ultrastructural data are highly compatible with the hypothesis of Thurau and Boylan, and it is conceptually possible that initial damage to the nephron caused by ischemia or toxic influences may affect the turnover of the cell membrane, for example by suppression of its synthesis (89). The strong, selective vulnerability of the thick ascending limb in the medulla and the medullary rays, documented experimentally by the group from Harvard (99, with further references), is highly compatible with the morphological demonstration of a particularly marked reduction of cell surface amplifications in this part of the nephron in ischemic ARF in man (21). As long as this abnormality exists, the sodium resorption will be diminished. Against this hypothesis it might be argued that the morphological alterations could be secondary phenomena appearing as sequelae to a markedly decreased ultrafiltrate. However, a reduction of tubular cell surfaces is not seen in another form of ARF, distinctly different from native kidney ARF, namely transplant ARF (45). This shows that decreased glomerular filtration, which certainly occurs in transplant ARF, does not necessarily cause a simplification of cell surfaces.

Another difficulty with the Thurau and Boylan hypothesis is that it does not adequately explain why renal vasoconstriction in patients with ischemic ARF can be reversed pharmacologically without improvement of renal function (100).

Decreased Glomerular Ultrafiltration Coefficient

Data from several experimental models have provided evidence for reduction of the glomerular ultrafiltration coefficient, but so far there is no evidence for this pathogenetic factor in human ischemic ARF. There is flattening of podocytes in early biopsies from patients with primary graft dysfunction and this lesion is correlated to the eventual severity of the postischemic ARF (101), but as discussed above, primary graft dysfunction probably has a pathogenesis different from ischemic ARF in the native kidney. Morphometric investigation of glomerular ultrastructure in human biopsies from patients with native ischemic ARF have shown normal basement membrane thickness, capillary diameter, endothelial pores and foot process width (Olsen et al., unpublished). From the available data, no support can be found for decreased ultrafiltration coefficient as an important factor in ischemic ARF in man.

Animal models of ARF differ in many ways from the disease as it is encountered in human patients. Many studies have used animal models in which the reduction in glomerular filtration is much more modest than in ARF in man. Micropuncture studies, which have served to clarify single nephron function in experimental ARF, have mainly employed such "soft" insults, whereas collection for micropuncture is more difficult and less accurate from "hard" insults with more marked reduction of renal function. Of even greater importance is that the histological changes in animals are substantially greater than in ischemic ARF in man. From the discussion above, it will be clear that *almost all experiments resulted in marked and extensive tubular necroses, making the models similar to the rare, direct, toxic form of ARF but not to the common ischemic type*. When Solez et al. (15) compared rabbits with glycerol-induced renal failure with patients suffering from ischemic ARF, they found that tubular necrosis was approximately 10 times greater in rabbits than in man at comparable times after onset. Tubular necrosis is even more severe in rats with experimental renal failure than in rabbits. In ARF produced in the rabbit by clamping one renal pedicle for 1 hr and removing the other kidney, there is oliguria and a histological picture very similar to that encountered in man (81). However, even this model is in some ways unlike typical ischemic ARF in man. In the rabbits, the renal failure is often not severe and many animals survive with dialysis. Those rabbits that develop severe ARF die by the 4th day. Thus, it is difficult to compare the morphological lesions in these animals with the lesions in renal biopsy specimens, almost all of whom have renal failure severe enough to require dialysis, but who are biopsied more than 4 days after the onset of the disease.

These marked differences between animal models and ischemic ARF in man suggest that the pathophysiology may be entirely different in the two situations. Our knowledge of renal physiological parameters in ischemic ARF in man is, however, incomplete and it is clear that we are at the moment still in a phase of mounting arguments for and against various hypotheses to explain the renal dysfunction observed.

REFERENCES

1. Olsen S. Renal histopathology in various forms of acute anuria in man. *Kidney Int* 1976;10:S2–S8.
2. Churg J, Cotran RS, Sinniah R, Sakaguchi H, Sobin LH. *Renal disease: classification and atlas of tubulo-interstitial diseases*. Tokyo, New York: Igaku-Shoin, 1984.
3. Solez K. Acute renal failure. In: Heptinstall RH, ed. *Pathology of the kidney*. Boston: Little, Brown, 1992;1235–1314.
4. Schreiner GE, Maher JF. Toxic nephropathy. *Am J Med* 1965;38:409–449.
5. Oliver J, MacDowell M, Tracy A. The pathogenesis of acute renal failure associated with traumatic and toxic injury: renal ischemia, nephrotoxic damage and the ischemuric episode. *J Clin Invest* 1951;30:1307–1439.
6. Freeman RB, Maher JF, Schreiner GE, Mostofi FK. Renal tubular necrosis due to nephrotoxicity of organic mercurial diuretics. *Ann Intern Med* 1962;57:34–43.
7. Beaman M, Turney JH, Rodger RSC, McGonigle RSJ, Adu D, Michael J. Changing pattern of acute renal failure. *Q J Med* 1987;62:15–23.
8. Myers BD, Moran SM. Hemodynamically mediated acute renal failure. *N Engl J Med* 1986; 314:97–105.
9. Cameron JS. Acute renal failure—the continuing challenge. *Q J Med* 1986;5:337–343.
10. Gillum DM, Dixon BS, Yanover MJ, Kelleher SP, Shapiro MD, Benedetti RG, Dillingham MA, Paller MS,Goldberg JP, Tomford RC, Gordon JA, Conger JD. The role of intensive dialysis in acute renal failure. *Clin Nephrol* 1986;25:249–255.
11. Wheeler DC, Feehally J, Walls J. High risk acute renal failure. *Q J Med* 1986;61:977–984.
12. Kennedy AC. Long-term follow-up of renal function after recovery from acute tubular necrosis. In: Andreucci, ed. *Acute renal failure*. Boston: Nijhoff, 1984;481–485.
13. Brun C. *Acute anuria*. Copenhagen: Munksgaard, 1954.
14. Iversen P, Brun C. Aspiration biopsy of the kidney. *Am J Med* 1951;11:324–330.
15. Solez K, Morel-Maroger L, Sraer JD. Morphology of 'acute tubular necrosis' in man: analysis of 57 renal biopsies and comparison with the glycerol model. *Medicine* 1979;58:362–376.
16. McManus JFA. *Medical diseases of the kidney*. Philadelphia: Lea & Febirger, 1950;87–94.
17. Zollinger HU. *Anurie bei Chromoproteinurie*. Stuttgart: Thieme, 1952.
18. Olsen TS, Sommer Hansen E, Jepsen FL. The prevalence of focal tubulointestitial lesions in various renal diseases. *Acta Pathol Microbiol Scand* 1981;A89:137–145.
19. Olsen TS, Hansen HE, Olsen HS. Tubular ultrastructure in acute renal failure: alterations of cellular surfaces (brush border and basolateral infoldings). *Virchows Arch[A]* 1985;406:91–104.
20. Olsen TS, Olsen HS, Hansen HE. Tubular ultrastructure in acute renal failure in man: epithelial necrosis and regeneration. *Virchows Arch[A]* 1985;406:75–89.
21. Olsen TS, Hansen HE. Ultrastructure of medullary tubules in ischemic acute tubular necrosis and acute interstitial nephritis in man. *APMIS* 1990;98:1139–1148.
22. Racusen LC, Fivusch BA, Li YL, Slatvik I, Solez K. Dissociation of tubular cell detachment and tubular cell death in clinical and experimental "acute tubular necrosis." *Lab Invest* 1991;64:546–556.
23. Jones DB. Ultrastructure of human acute renal failure ("ATN"). *Lab Invest* 1982;46:254–264.
24. Venkatachalam MA, Berhard DB, Donohoe JF, Levinsky NG. Ischemic damage and repair in the rat proximal tubule. Differences among the S_1, S_2, and S_3 segments. *Kidney Int* 1978;14:31–49.

25. Olsen TS, Olsen HS, Hansen HE. Hypertrophy of actin bundles in tubular cells in acute renal failure. *Ultrastruct Pathol* 1984;7:241–250.
26. Pons CA, Custer RP. Acute ethylene glycol poisoning: a clinico-pathologic report of eighteen fatal cases. *Am J Med Sci* 1946;211:544–552.
27. Hagemann PO, Chiffelle TR. Ethylene glycol poisoning. A clinical and pathologic study of three cases. *J Lab Clin Med* 1948;33:573–584.
28. Aufderheide AC. Renal tubular calcium oxalate crystal deposition. *Arch Pathol* 1971;92:162–166.
29. Cousins MJ, Mazze RI, Kosek JC, Hitt BA, Love FV. The etiology of methoxyflurane nephrotoxicity. *J Pharmacol Exp Ther* 1941;190:530–541.
30. Mazze RI, Cousins MJ, Kosek JC. Dose-related methoxyflurane nephrotoxicity in rats: a biochemical and pathological correlation. *Anesthesiology* 1972;36:571–587.
31. Cotton JR, Schwartz MM, Lindley JD, Hunsicker LG. Acute renal failure following halothane anesthesia. *Arch Pathol Lab Med* 1976;100:628–629.
32. Mudge GH, Meier FA, Krook Ward K. Pathogenesis of renal impairment induced by radio contrast media. In: Solez K, Whelton A, eds. *Acute renal failure*. New York: Marcel Dekker, 1984;361–388.
33. Papper S. Hepatorenal syndrome. In: Andreucci, ed. *Acute renal failure*. Boston: M. Nijhoff, 1984;233–250.
34. Mandal AK, Lansing M, Fahmy A. Acute tubular necrosis in hepatorenal syndrome: an electron microscopic study. *Am J Kidney Dis* 1982;2:363–374.
35. Solez K. The pathology and pathogenesis of human "Acute tubular necrosis." In: Solez K, Whelton A, eds. *Acute renal failure*. New York: Marcel Dekker, 1984;17–42.
36. Wilkinson SP, Hirst D, Day EW, Williams R. Spectrum of renal tubular damage in renal failure secondary to cirrhosis and fulminant hepatic failure. *J Clin Pathol* 1978;31:101–107.
37. DeFronzo RA, Humphrey RL, Wright JR, Cooke CR. Acute renal failure in multiple myeloma. *Medicine* 1975;54:209–218.
38. Councilman WT. Acute interstitial nephritis. *J Exp Med* 1898;3:393–420.
39. Olsen S, Solez K. Pathology of drug nephrotoxicity in humans. In: Whelton A, Neu HC, eds. *The aminoglycosides*. New York: Marcel Dekker, 1982;355–385.
40. Porter GA, Bennett WM. Nephrotoxin-induced acute renal failure. In: Brenner BM, Stein JH, eds. *Acute renal failure*. New York: Churchill Livingstone, 1980;123–162.
41. Michielsen P, De Schepper PJ. Renal disease due to drugs. In: Meyler L, Peck HM, eds. Drug induced diseases. *Excerpta Medica* 1972;4:261–324.
42. Appel GB, Kunis CL. Acute tubulo-interstitial nephritis. In: Cotran RS, ed. *Tubulo-interstitial nephropathies*. New York: Churchill Livingstone, 1983;151–185.
43. Colwin RB, Fang LST. Interstitial nephritis. In: Tisher CC, Brenner BM, eds. *Renal pathology*. Philadelphia: Lippincott, 1989;Ch. 24.
43a. Iványi B, Marcussen N, Kemp E, Olsen TS. The distal nephron is preferentially infiltrated by inflammatory cells in acute interstitial nephritis. *Virchows Arch [A]* 1992;420:37–42.
44. Olsen TS, Wasseff NF, Olsen HS, Hansen HE. Ultrastructure of the kidney in acute interstitial nephritis. *Ultrastruct Pathol* 1986;10:1–16.
45. Olsen TS, Burdick JF, Keown PA, Wallace AC, Racusen LC, Solez K. Primary acute renal failure ("acute tubular necrosis") in the transplanted kidney. *Morphol Pathogen Med* 1989;68:173–187.
46. Zalme RC, McDowell EM, Nagle RB, McNeil JS, Flamenbaum W, Trump BF. Studies on the pathophysiology of acute renal failure. II. A histochemical study of the proximal tubule of the rat following administration of mercuric chloride. *Virchows Arch [B]* 1976;22:197–216.
47. McDowell EM, Nagle RB, Zalme RC, McNeil JS, Flamenbaum W, Trump BF. Studies on the pathophysiology of acute renal failure I. Correlation of ultrastructure and function in the proximal tubule of the rat following administration of mercuric chloride. *Virchows Arch [B]* 1976;22:173–196.
48. Oken DE, Landwehr DM, Kirschbaum BB. On the pathogenesis of murine experimental acute renal failure. In: Seybold D, Gessler V, eds. *Acute renal failure*. Basel: Karger, 1982;1–8.
49. Hostetter TH, Wilkes BM, Brenner BM. Mechanisms of impaired glomerular filtration in acute renal failure. In: Brenner BM, Stein JH, eds. *Acute renal failure*. New York: Churchill Livingstone, 1980;52–78.
50. Bulger RE, Dobyan DC, Eknoyan G. Absence of glomerular endothelial pore size differences in ARF in rats induced by mercuric chloride or gentamicin. *Kidney Int* 1983;23:201.
51. Flamenbaum W, Mc Neil JS, Kotchen TW, Saladino AJ. Experimental acute renal failure induced by uranyl nitrate in the dog. *Circ Res* 1972;31:682–698.

52. Avashti PS, Evan AP, Hay D. Glomerular endothelial cells in uranyl nitrate-induced acute renal failure in rats. *J Clin Invest* 1980;65:121–127.
53. Evan AP, Gattone VH, Luft FC. Glomerular filtration barrier in ischemic and nephrotoxic acute renal failure. In: Solez K, Whelton A, eds. *Acute renal failure*. New York: Marcel Dekker, 1984;119–133.
54. Stein JH, Gottschalk J, Osgood RW, Ferris TF. Pathophysiology of a nephrotoxic model of acute renal failure. *Kidney Int* 1975;8:27–41.
55. Kleinman JG, Neil JS, Flamenbaum W. Uranyl nitrate acute renal failure in the dog: early changes in renal function and hemodynamics. *Clin Sci* 1975;48:9–16.
56. Sudo M, Honda N, Hisida A, Najase M. Renal hemodynamics in uranyl acetate-induced renal failure of rabbits. *Kidney Int* 1977;11:35–43.
57. Dobyan DC, Levi J, Jacobs C, Kosek J, Weiner MW. Mechanism of Cis-platinum nephrotoxicity. II. Morphologic observations. *J Pharmacol Exp Ther* 1980;213:551–556.
58. Leonard BS, Eccleston E, Jones D, Todd P, Walpole A. Antileucemic and nephrotoxic properties of platinum compounds. *Nature* 1971;234:43–45.
59. Choie DD, Longnecker DS, Del Campo AA. Acute and chronic cisplatin nephropathy in rats. *Lab Invest* 1981;44:397–402.
60. Chopra S, Kaufman JS, Jones TW, Hong WK, Gehr MK, Hamburger RJ, Flamenbaum W, Trump BF. Cis-diamine-dichlor-platinum-induced acute renal failure in the rat. *Kidney Int* 1982;21:54–64.
61. Safirskin R, Winston J, Goldstein M, et al. Cisplatin nephrotoxicity. *Am J Kidney Dis* 1986;8:356–367.
62. Collier VU, Lietman PS, Mitch WE. Evidence for luminal uptake of gentamicin in the perfused rat kidney. *J Pharmacol Exp Ther* 1979;210:247–251.
63. Lipsky JJ, Cheng L, Sacktor B, Lietman PS. Gentamicin uptake by renal tubule brush border membrane vesicles. *J Pharmacol Exp Ther* 1980;215:390–393.
64. Olsen TS, Solez K. Pathology of drug nephrotoxicity in humans. In: Whelton A, Neu H, eds. *The aminoglycosides*. New York: Marcel Dekker, 1982;355–385.
65. Kourilsky O, Solez K, Morel-Maroger L, Whelton A, Duhoux P, Sraer J-D. The pathology of acute renal failure due to interstitial nephritis in man. *Medicine (Baltimore)* 1982;61:258–268.
66. Cuppage FE, Setter K, Sullivan LP, Reitzes EJ, Melnykovych AO. Gentamicin nephrotoxicity. II. Physiological, biochemical and morphological effects of prolonged administration to rats. *Virchows Arch [B]* 1977;24:121–138.
67. Luft FC, Rankin LI, Sloan RS, Yum MN. Recovery from aminoglycoside nephrotoxicity with continued drug administration. *Antimicrob Agents Chemother* 1978;14:284–287.
68. Gilbert DN, Houghton DC, Bennett WM, Plamp CE, Reger K, Porter GA. Reversibility of gentamicin nephrotoxicity in rats. *Proc Soc Exp Biol Med* 1979;160:99–103.
69. Bennett WM, Gilbert DN, Elliott WC, Houghton DC, Porter GA. Gentamicin nephrotoxicity—morphologic and pharmacologic features. *West J Med* 1977;126:65–68.
70. Whelton A, Solez K. Sex and the gentamycin-damaged kidney. In: Solez K, Whelton A, eds. *Acute renal failure*. New York: Marcel Dekker, 1984;221–233.
71. Tolkoff-Rubin NE, McCluskey RT, Bhan AK, Rubin RH, Haddad EP. Renal damage due to aminoglycoside administration in the Lewis rat. In: Solez K, Whelton A, eds. *Acute renal failure*. New York: Marcel Dekker, 1984;249–259.
72. Mondorf AW, Scherberich JE, Falkenberg FW, Sachse HJ, Gaul C, Schoeppe W. Brush border enzymes and drug nephrotoxicity. In: Solez K, Whelton A, eds. *Acute renal failure*. New York: Marcel Dekker, 1984;287–298.
73. Avasthi PS, Evan AP, Huser JW, Luft FC. Effect of gentamicin on glomerular ultrastructure. *J Lab Clin Med* 1981;98:444–454.
74. Schor N, Ichikawa I, Rennke HG, Troy JL, Brenner BM. Pathophysiology of altered glomerular function in aminoglycoside treated rats. *Kidney Int* 1981;19:288–296.
75. Houghton DC, Campbell-Boswell MV, Bennett WM, Porter GA, Brooks RE. Myeloid bodies in the renal tubules of humans: relationship to gentamicin therapy. *Clin Nephrol* 1978;10:140–145.
76. Bullock WE, Luke RG, McHall CE, Bhathena D. Can mannitol reduce amphotericin-B nephrotoxicity? *Antimicrob Agents Chemother* 1976;10:555–563.
77. Koletsky S, Gustafson GE. The effects of temporary cessation of renal blood flow in rats. *J Clin Invest* 1947;26:1072–1078.
78. Venkatachalam MA. Pathology of acute renal failure. *Contemp Issues Nephrol* 1980;6:79–107.

79. Venkatachalam MA, Jones DB, Rennke HG, Sandstrom D, Patel Y. Mechanism of proximal tubule brush border loss and regeneration following mild renal ischemia. *Lab Invest* 1981;45:355.
80. Solez K, D'Agostini RJ, Stowowy L, Freedman MT, Scott WW, Siegelman SS, Heptinstall RH.Beneficial effect of propranolol in a histologically appropriate model of postischemic acute renal failure. *Am J Pathol* 1977;88:163–192.
81. Solez K, Freshwater MF, Su C-T. The effect of propranolol on postischemic acute renal failure in the rat. *Transplantation* 1977;24:148–151.
82. Solez K, Racusen LC, Whelton A. Glomerular epithelial cell changes in early postischemic acute renal failure in rabbits and man. *Am J Pathol* 1981;103:163 173.
83. Knapp R, Hollenberg NK, Busch GJ, Abrams HL. Prolonged unilateral acute renal failure induced by intra-arterial norepinephrine infusion in the dog. *Invest Radiol* 1972;7:164–173.
84. Moskowitz PS, Korobkin M, Rambo ON. Diuresis and improved renal hemodynamics produced by prostaglandin E_1 in the dog with norepinephrine-induced acute renal failure. *Invest Radiol* 1975;10:284–299.
85. Cronin RE, Erickson AM, DeTorrente A, McDonald KM, Schrier RW. Norepinephrine-induced acute renal failure. *Kidney Int* 1978;14:187–190.
86. Cox JW, Baehler RW, Sharma H, O'Dorisio T, Osgood RW, Stein JH, Ferris TF. Studies on the mechanism of oliguria in a model of unilateral acute renal failure. *J Clin Invest* 1974;53:1546–1558.
87. Cronin RE, Erikson AM, DeTorrente A, McDonald KM, Schrier RW. Norepinephrine-induced acute renal failure. *Kidney Int* 1978;14:187–190.
88. Solez K. Pathogenesis of acute renal failure: *Int Rev Exp Pathol* 1983;24:277–333.
89. Olsen S. Acute tubular necrosis and toxic renal failure. In: Tisher CC, Brenner BM, eds. *Renal pathology*. New York: Lippincott, 1989;Ch. 22.
90. Bohle A, Jahnecke J, Myer D, Schubert GE. Morphology of acute renal failure. *Kidney Int* 1976;10:S9–S16.
91. Solez K, Morel-Maroger L, Sraer J-D. Morphology of "acute tubular necrosis" in man. *Medicine (Baltimore)* 1979;58:362–376.
92. Steinhausen M. Intravital microscopic observations of acute renal failure as a tool for simultaneously analyzing structure and function. In: Solez K, Whelton A, eds. *Acute renal failure*. New York: Marcel Dekker, 1984;169–176.
93. Venkatachalam MA. Pathology of acute renal failure. In: Brenner BM, Stein JH, eds. *Acute renal failure*. New York: Churchill Livingstone, 1980;79–107.
94. Hollenberg NK, Epstein M,Rosen SM, Basch RI, Oken DE, Merrill JP. Acute oliguric renal failure in man: evidence for preferential renal cortical ischemia. *Medicine* 1968;47:455–474.
95. Munk O. *Renal circulation in acute renal failure*. Oxford: Blackwell, 1958.
96. Reubi FC, Vorburger C. Renal hemodynamics in acute renal failure after shock in man. *Kidney Int* 1976;10:S137–S143.
97. Epstein M, Schneider NS, Befeeler B. Effect of intrarenal furosemide on renal function and intrarenal hemodynamics in acute renal failure. *Am J Med* 1975;58:510–516.
98. Thurau K, Boylan JW. Acute renal success. The unexpected logic of oliguria in acute renal failure. *Am J Med* 1976;61:308–315.
99. Epstein FH, Brown RS. Acute renal failure, a collection of paradoxes. *Hosp Pract* 1988;23:171–194.
100. Ladefoged L. Winkler K. Hemodynamics in acute renal failure. *Scand J Clin Lab Invest* 1970; 26:83.
101. Solez K, Racusen LC, Whelton A. Glomerular epithelial cell changes in early post-ischemic acute renal failure in rabbits and man. *Am J Pathol* 1981;103:163–173.

Toxicology of the Kidney, Second Edition,
edited by Jerry B. Hook and Robin S. Goldstein.
Raven Press, Ltd., New York © 1993.

5

Pathophysiology of Acute Renal Failure

Mayer Brezis and *Franklin H. Epstein

*Department of Medicine, Hadassah University Hospital, Mount Scopus, Jerusalem, Israel; and *Department of Medicine, Beth Israel Hospital, and the Harvard Center for the Study of Kidney Diseases, Harvard Medical School, Boston, Massachusetts 02215*

The vulnerability of the kidney to toxins differs in many ways from other forms of organ toxicity. Liver injury from isoniazid or phenothiazines is idiosyncratic and possibily genetically predetermined, whereas hepatic failure from acetaminophen and cardiac damage from anthracyclines are clearly dose dependent. By contrast, in most cases of nephrotoxin-induced acute renal failure, the occurrence is neither idiosyncratic nor simply related to excessive dosage. The renal response to potentially nephrotoxic drugs is often primarily determined by associated physiological and hemodynamic conditions prevailing at the time of exposure. For instance, aminoglycoside nephrotoxicity is poorly correlated with either plasma or kidney tissue levels of the drug, but is markedly augmented by concomitant volume depletion or liver cirrhosis (1). Similarly, acute renal failure following the administration of radiocontrast material is at best loosely related to the amount injected, whereas it is most easily induced in patients with preexisting diabetic nephropathy (2) or in the presence of low cardiac output (3). Likewise, amphotericin (4) or *cis*-platinum (5) given in doses sufficient to produce kidney insufficiency, may be entirely innocuous if intravascular volume is concurrently expanded by saline infusion. This unique and complex relationship between organ physiology and susceptibility to nephrotoxins has been a major obstacle in the development of experimental models of acute renal failure that would faithfully reproduce the clinical picture. Too frequently, researchers have been tempted to study in healthy animals the response of the kidney to a single insult, intensive enough to conveniently generate reproducible renal failure. The relevance of such studies to human acute renal failure should be considered cautiously, since at the bedside combinations of multiple factors rather than single insults are generally operative. This chapter will first review the lessons learned from "single-insult" models of acute renal failure (ARF) and then examine differences between clinical nephrotoxic ARF and these models; it will next describe the more recently developed "multiple-insults" models, and finally propose the theory of renal medullary hypoxia as a key for the synergistic interaction between kidney hypoperfusion and nephrotoxicity.

LESSONS FROM "SINGLE-INSULT" MODELS OF EXPERIMENTAL ACUTE RENAL FAILURE

The pathogenesis of the suppression of kidney function in acute renal failure has been attributed to several mechanisms demonstrated in experimental models and involving tubular, vascular, and/or glomerular effects (Fig. 1; see refs. 6–9 for review). Tubular injury may contribute to the reduction in glomerular filtration rate (GFR) by obstruction with casts, cellular debris, or cell swelling, or by increasing reabsorption of luminal fluid through damaged epithelium (backleak). Alternatively, hemodynamic effects can impair GFR by a decrease in glomerular blood flow coupled to a reduction in total renal blood flow, or by a decrease in the glomerular ultrafiltration coefficient (K_f) resulting from a reduction in filtering area.

Tubule Effects

Increased Permeability (Backleak)

Kidney micropuncture observations first documented abnormal back diffusion of glomerular filtrate in frogs poisoned with mercury. Later, considerable backleak was reported in other toxic nephropathies, from uranium, gentamicin, and *cis*-platinum. Substantial tubular backleak has generally been found in models of severe ARF, using large doses of toxins, and frequently associated with oligoanuria and

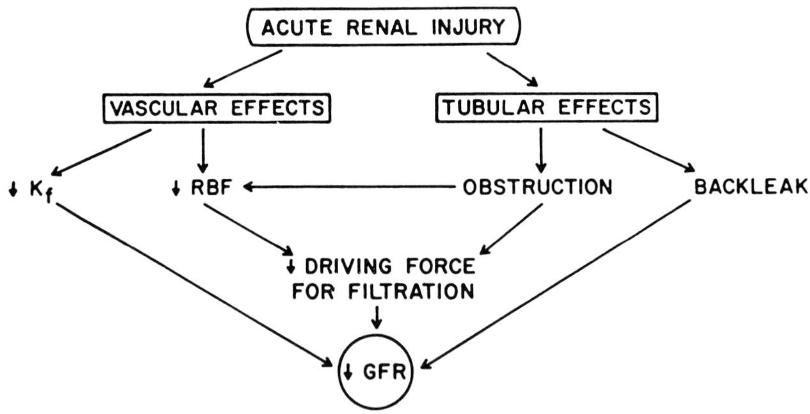

FIG. 1. Schematic representation of the mechanisms considered to initiate or maintain the defect in glomerular filtration rate (GFR) in acute renal failure. Different experimental models have been shown to have various preferential effects. Available data suggest that increasing severity of the injury causes a shift from the left (↓ K_f, ↓ RBF) to the right arms (obstruction and backleak). K_f, glomerular ultrafiltration coefficient; RBF, renal blood flow. (From Hostetter et al., ref. 6, with permission.)

morphological evidence of extensive necrosis. By contrast, abnormal back diffusion through tubules has been, as a rule, negligible in milder forms (often nonoliguric) of toxic nephropathy usually associated with little histological damage.

In most experimental models, GFR is reduced long before gross disruption of tubular epithelia is seen. The correlation between tubular necrosis and renal failure is often poor (as reported in humans). In fact, amelioration of renal function by chronic salt loading does not prevent tubular cell necrosis, further evidence against a major role for backleak as a cause of uremia.

A special instance of backleak, despite morphological integrity, has been documented in a model of amphotericin-induced ARF. This is probably due to a specific ionophore-like action of polyene antibiotics to induce abnormal membrane permeability (10). Increased permeability triggers a compensatory increase in the rate of active electrolyte transport, associated with a rise in oxygen demand, leading to an imbalance between oxygen delivery and consumption, precipitating hypoxic cell necrosis in zones of limited oxygen availability and high oxygen demand, as in the renal medulla. Thus, in isolated perfused kidneys, it was possible to show that the polyene antibiotics amphotericin and nystatin induce extensive injury to the medullary thick ascending limb, a nephron segment with limited oxygen supply. This damage was prevented if reabsorptive transport was inhibited by ouabain (11). Under these circumstances, cell death appeared to be mediated by increased oxygen demand for transport activity. If this mode of injury were to be operative *in vivo*, tubular damage would be predicted to follow intrarenal gradients of oxygenation and to be maximal in regions of lowest oxygen availability. Very recent studies in our laboratory have confirmed this pattern (Heyman et al., unpublished data).

Backleak may therefore contribute to some of the apparent decrease in GFR in most severe toxic nephropathies and/or participate in the synergism between toxic and hypoxic insults, as discussed below.

Tubular Obstruction

Elevated intratubular pressure has been demonstrated by micropuncture in several, but not all, models of toxic ARF, including *cis*-platinum, gentamicin, and lysine infusions. The absence of a demonstrable increase in intratubular pressure cannot be viewed as strong evidence against significant obstruction complicated by glomerular constriction. Intraluminal obstruction has also been suggested with cyclosporine and radiocontrast material, because intraluminal deposits of microliths were seen in cyclosporine-treated rats and diatrizoate was found to precipitate proteins derived from renal tubular suspensions (9). Ethylene glycol nephrotoxicity may at least in part relate to intratubular precipitation of oxalate crystals.

The observation that maneuvers that enhance solute excretion rate (mannitol, furosemide) sometimes exert a beneficial effect on the course of ARF has been construed as indirect evidence for the role of obstructing cell debris and casts that are presumably dispersed by high urine flow. However, additional effects of these forms of treatment include extracellular volume repletion, renal vasodilatation, decreased cell swelling, and decreased oxygen demand for transport, all of which might also affect the course of renal failure. In fact, furosemide may aggravate gentamicin nephropathy and possibly radiocontrast-induced ARF if volume depletion is allowed to occur. Because acid urine augments the intraluminal precipitation of some toxins (uric acid, myoglobin, hemoglobin, methotrexate), alkaline diuresis may be beneficial by reducing tubular obstruction in some forms of ARF.

In humans, tubular obstruction has been inferred from the morphological picture of luminal casts and tubule dilatations in some severe forms of toxic ARF or intratubular precipitations of crystals of uric acid, oxalate, sulfonamides, or methotrexate. The exact role played by tubular obstruction in human ARF remains uncertain.

Vascular Effects

Reduction and Redistribution of Renal Blood Flow

A reduction by more than 50% in renal blood flow is the rule during the *initial* phase of experimental toxic ARF. During the *established* phase, GFR is characteristically depressed out of proportion to a moderate decline in renal blood flow. Reduction of blood flow is more pronounced in the superficial cortex than in the deeper portions of the kidney after uranium nitrate or mercuric chloride but not after *cis*-platinum administration (9).

In human ARF, decreased renal and particularly cortical perfusion corroborates the common observation of cortical pallor at autopsy. The moderate decrease in renal blood flow, however, cannot itself account for the marked reduction in GFR typical of toxic nephropathy.

Decreased Glomerular Ultrafiltration Coefficient (K_f) and Changes in Glomerular Vascular Resistances: Role of Tubuloglomerular Feedback

A regulatory mechanism that lowers GFR whenever the solute delivery or solute concentration at the macula densa is raised has been well documented in normal kidneys and termed tubuloglomerular feedback (Figs. 2 and 3). Tubuloglomerular feedback has been shown to persist after experimentally induced renal damage. Defective reabsorption of NaCl at any site proximal to the macula densa may trigger feedback reduction of the GFR, and dysfunction of the medullary thick ascending limb is particularly prone to induce such an effect, as there is little room for correcting the concentration of intraluminal electrolytes by enhanced tubular reabsorption between this site and the macula densa. Impaired function of the thick ascending limb has been observed in a variety of models of ARF. A defective urinary concen-

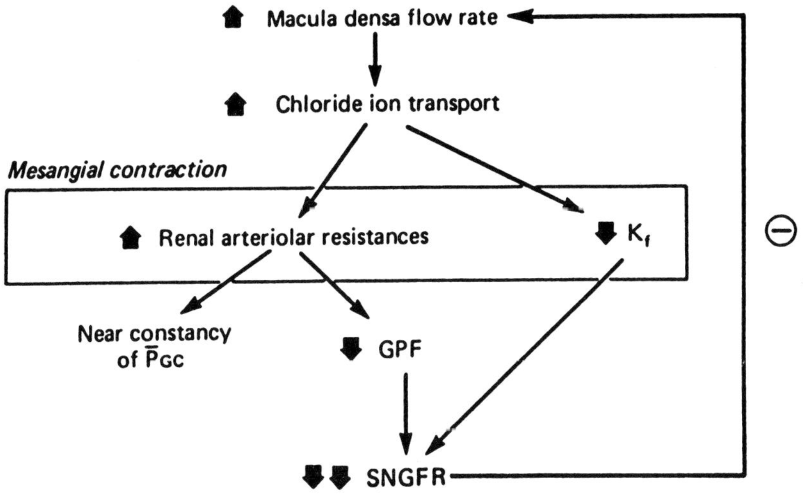

FIG. 2. Schematic representation of the signal and effector mechanism involved in tubuloglomerular feedback. $\bar{P}_{GC}$, glomerular capillary pressure; GPF, glomerular plasma flow; SNGFR, single nephron glomerular filtration rate. (From Ichikawa, ref. 12, with permission.)

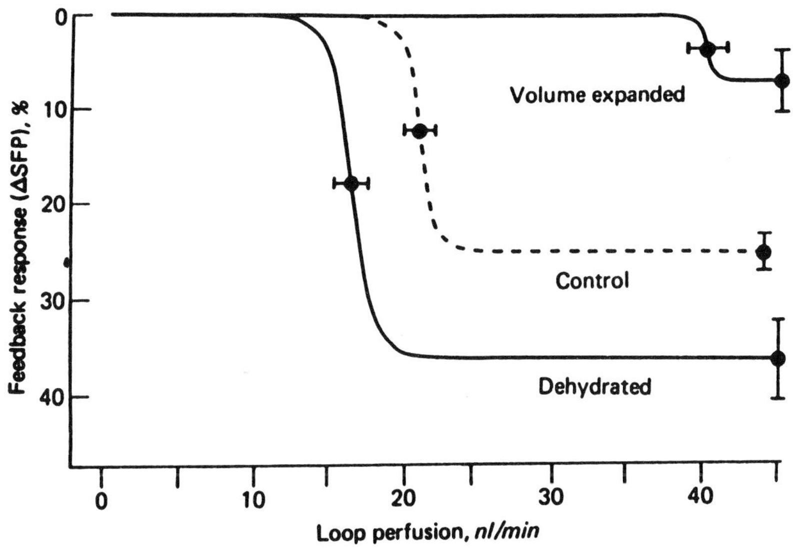

FIG. 3. Magnitude of tubuloglomerular feedback response (expressed as percent decline in stop flow pressure, ΔSFP, estimate of glomerular ultrafiltration pressure) as function of solute delivery rate to the macula densa (represented by loop perfusion rate). Feedback response is profoundly affected by the state of the extracellular volume, maximal in dehydrated animals and minimal in volume expanded animals. (From Persson, ref. 13, with permission.)

trating mechanism, with the production of isotonic urine, is indeed the earliest, most consistent, and most lasting tubular defect of ARF, both in animals and in humans (8).

Despite extensive investigation, the humoral mediation of tubuloglomerular feedback remains unclear. Renin-angiotensin, adenosine, prostaglandins, endothelin, and calcium may participate in the modulation or transmission of feedback signals. As shown in Fig. 3, the integrity of the feedback control can be greatly modified by the physiological state of extracellular volume. Maximal in dehydrated animals, the tubuloglomerular feedback is almost eliminated during volume expansion. Correspondingly, both in experimental animals and in humans, most nephrotoxic effects are greatly potentiated by concomitant volume depletion, while volume expansion protects.

A decline in the ultrafiltration coefficient (K_f), most likely reflecting glomerular capillary constriction (possibly secondary to activation of tubuloglomerular feedback), has been reported in a variety of nephrotoxic models of ARF (uranyl nitrate, mercury, gentamicin, *cis*-platinum). Since adenosine potentiates tubuloglomerular feedback, it is of interest to note that theophylline, an adenosine antagonist, attentuates radiocontrast-induced intrarenal vasoconstriction, myoglobinuric renal damage, and amphotericin B nephrotoxicity, even though the precise role of tubuloglomerular feedback remains controversial (9).

The role of activated tubuloglomerular feedback may predominate in certain phases of ARF, whereas it might be overwhelmed by tubule effects (backleak and obstruction) later or under different conditions. Examination of two models of gentamicin-induced ARF suggest that divergent outcomes with renin-angiotensin blockade might relate to the severity of the injury inflicted (Table 1). Protection with inhibition of the renin-angiotensin axis appears at an earlier stage and in milder forms of injury. When extensive tubular necrosis is present, diminution of tubuloglomerular feedback no longer protects from the effects of backleak or obstruction.

TABLE 1. *Comparison of divergent effects of captopril on renal function in two models of gentamicin-induced acute renal failure (ARF)*

Reference	14	15
Doses of gentamicin	40 mg/kg	80 mg/kg
Rat strain	Munich-Wistar	Sprague-Dawley
Decrease in GFR (% of control)	58%	23%
Histologic changes	Increase in lysosomes; changes in brush border; no significant tubule cell necrosis	Extensive tubule cell necrosis
Effect of captopril (same dose) on GFR	Prevention of ARF	Aggravation of ARF

From Brezis et al., ref. 8, with permission.
GFR, glomerular filtration rate.

DIFFERENCES BETWEEN CLINICAL NEPHROTOXIC ARF AND EXPERIMENTAL MODELS

From the previous section, it is evident that the extensive laboratory investigations using "single-insult" experimental models have allowed a detailed analysis of the potential intrarenal mechanisms leading to failure of glomerular filtration (see Fig. 1). It is too often forgotten, however, that important differences exist between these models and the clinical picture of ARF usually seen in human patients. The following dissimilarities can be described (see Table 3).

Incidence

Although the "single-insult" models are usually designed to obtain reproducible and predictable ARF, at the bedside the administration of the potential nephrotoxin to a patient usually carries a relatively small risk. Nephrotoxicity occurs in less than 1% of the general population given radiocontrast material, 10% to 26% in the case of aminoglycoside treatment, and about 20% or less during *cis*-platinum therapy (8,16). Experimental models of nephrotoxic renal failure with a "success" rate of only 20% would be viewed as inefficient and unreliable by most investigators. In general, in order to achieve a 100% rate of ARF, researchers have simply increased the dose of the nephrotoxin until clear-cut toxicity was reliably produced. Under these circumstances, the changes produced may not accurately reflect the pathophysiology of ARF in man.

Number of Insults

By definition, "single-insult" models use only one insult, intense enough to generate by itself acute renal failure in an otherwise healthy animal. For instance, gentamicin, 80 mg/kg/day for 10 days injected into an intact rat will invariably cause ARF. By contrast, in human ARF the majority of patients have more than one insult identified, or they have preexisting renal disease (Fig. 4). The acute insults most frequently involved in patients are volume depletion, aminoglycoside use, radiocontrast exposure, NSAID exposure, septic shock, and pigmenturia. Since in man these insults augment the risk of ARF rather than predictably induce it, it may be more appropriate to define them as acute risk factors. For instance, the use of aminoglycoside in any patient increases sixfold the chance of developing ARF (Table 2). The combination of risk factors increases the likelihood of renal failure proportionally (18). The interaction between multiple factors appears to be central in the pathogenesis of human ARF.

Chronic Risk Factors

Epidemiological studies of occurrence of human ARF have clearly indicated the important role of chronic premorbid conditions in the development of kidney failure

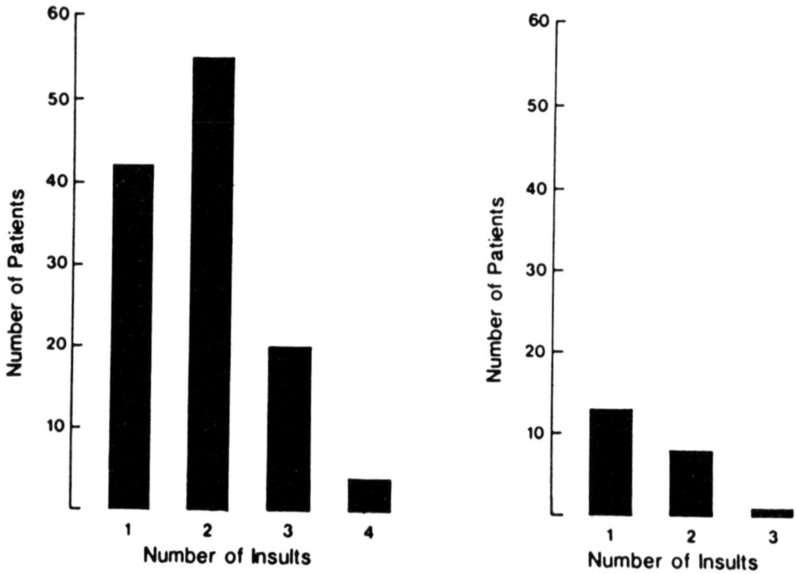

FIG. 4. Distribution of the number of insults potentially involved in the pathogenesis of ARF identified per patient in 121 patients without preexisting renal disease (*left*) and in 22 patients with preexisting renal disease (*right*). (From Rasmussen and Ibels, ref. 17, with permission.)

TABLE 2. *Acute and chronic risk factors associated with the development of ARF*

Acute risk factors
Volume depletion (×10)
Aminoglycoside use (×6)
Radiocontrast exposure (×5)
NSAID exposure
Septic shock (×>100)
Dehydration
Hypotension
Pigmenturia
Chronic risk factors
Preexisting renal disease
Hypertension
Congestive heart failure (×9)
Diabetes mellitus (in combination with volume depletion, ×100)
Age (with aminoglycoside)
Liver cirrhosis (with aminoglycoside or NSAID)

Adapted from Brezis et al., ref. 8, with permission.

Odds ratios for the increased chances of ARF in the presence of a particular risk factor are indicated in parentheses, when available.

NSAID, nonsteroidal, anti-inflammatory drugs.

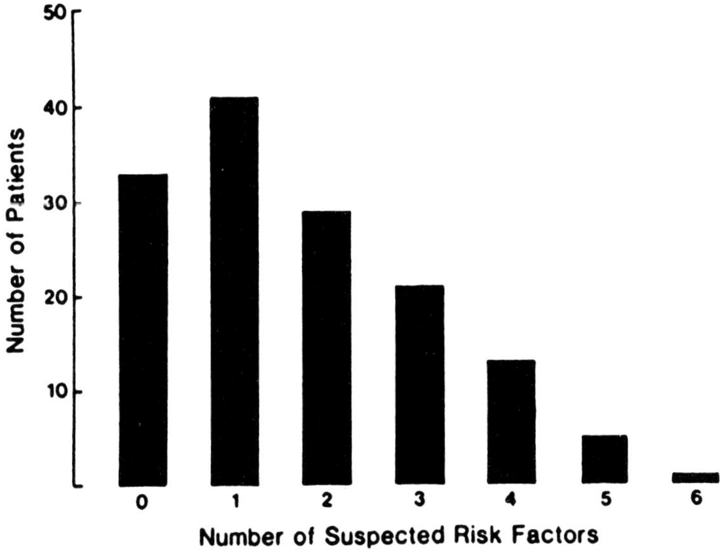

FIG. 5. Distribution of the number of chronic risk factors potentially involved in the pathogenesis of ARF identified per patient in a study involving 143 patients. (From Rasmussen and Ibels, ref. 17, with permission.)

(Fig. 5; Table 2). For instance, congestive heart failure was associated with a ninefold higher incidence of ARF in the case-control study by Shusterman et al. (18). Chronic hypertension, preexisting renal disease and diabetes mellitus have also been proposed as independent risk factors for the development of ARF. Diabetes mellitus and volume depletion act in synergy to increase a hundredfold the chance of ARF. An additional recognized condition is advancing age (with aminoglycosides or NSAID). This interplay between the acute and chronic risk factors listed in Table 2, so characteristic of human ARF, is not reproduced in "single-insult" experimental models of ARF.

Drug Dosage and Dose-Dependency of Nephrotoxicity

In animal studies, the dose of nephrotoxin selected is commonly one that will reliably induce ARF. The largest dose that does not produce extrarenal toxicity is usually employed. For instance, to achieve renal failure in rats, gentamicin is given at the daily dose of 40 mg/kg or more for several days, because 4 mg/kg produces little nephrotoxicity (14). The ratio of body surface area (BSA) to body mass is approximately five times higher in a 300-g rat (estimated BSA $0.04 m^2$) than in a 70-kg man (BSA $1.7 m^2$). Thus the gentamicin dosage of 40 mg/kg/day in the rat would be roughly equivalent in man to 8 mg/kg/day, more than twice the recommended dose for this antibiotic and likely to cause severe nephrotoxicity and toxicity in man.

Clinical studies, however, have repeatedly shown that aminoglycoside-associated ARF occurs in 10% to 20% of patients even when the most careful precautions are taken to use therapeutic doses and when plasma levels are carefully monitored to avoid the toxic range (1,19). In such patients, the presence of comorbid conditions such as liver cirrhosis or volume depletion, are far more predictive of a nephrotoxic outcome of aminoglycoside therapy than the drug levels measured in blood (1,21). In fact, in several studies, no relationship could be found between aminoglycoside concentrations and the occurrence of ARF (1,20). In radiocontrast nephropathy, a relationship between the volume of radiocontrast material injected and the occurrence of ARF has often either not been observed (22,23), or found to be far weaker than the association between radiocontrast-mediated ARF and the presence of dehydration, low cardiac output, or diabetic nephropathy (2,24,63).

Although the doses of other nephrotoxicants such as *cis*-platinum or amphotericin used in animals are closer to the dosage used in humans, they are also deliberately set at the level that will reproducibly induce ARF in *all* treated animals. It is therefore questionable whether or to what extent these "single-insult" convenient models actually represent the clinical problem since they do not incorporate the peculiar synergism between drug administration (usually nontoxic) and a specific coexisting pathophysiological circumstance, so typical of human ARF.

Morphology

In most experimental models using a single insult, renal histology shows prominent cortical injury, usually with frank necrosis of proximal tubular epithelium. High-dose gentamicin, uranyl nitrate, mercuric chloride, and potassium dichromate cause extensive damage to proximal tubules. Similarly, glycerol (to induce rhabdomyolysis), norepinephrine (infused into the renal artery), and complete ischemia (clamping the renal artery) produce generalized proximal tubular necrosis.

By contrast, in human ARF, focal single-cell necrosis scattered throughout the kidney and along the nephron is the rule. Discrete lesions are more frequent in distal than proximal tubules, often concentrated in the outer medulla. Even biopsies from patients with aminoglycoside-associated ARF have shown only focal necrosis indistinguishable from nontoxic ARF, sharply contrasting with the confluent proximal tubular necrosis typically observed in experimental high-dose gentamicin nephropathy.

One instructive exception to this rule is the case of patients accidentally exposed to large doses of heavy metals (e.g., mercuric chloride or bismuth) or organic solvents (e.g., carbon tetrachloride). Renal morphology in these instances shows extensive necrosis of the proximal tubules in the cortex. The massive toxicity seen in the renal cortex, where the mechanism of cell injury is indiscriminate and dose dependent, resembles toxic liver damage, as from CCl_4. "Single-insult" experimental models more closely simulate this type of overdosage ARF, now rare, than the common form of ARF associated with multiple risk factors (including nephrotoxic drugs) encountered in clinical wards. The morphology of ARF is more extensively reviewed in this volume in the chapter by Olsen and Solez.

Pathophysiological Mechanisms

Although the pathophysiology of human ARF remains uncertain, it appears that in "single-insult" models of ARF, toxic cell injury predominates in the proximal tubule. Experimental work in the isolated perfused kidney has demonstrated that proximal tubules readily express striking morphological alterations whenever mild to moderate adenosine triphosphate (ATP) depletion is achieved by either hypoxic or toxic exposure (25). This may underlie the prominence of cortical proximal tubular damage reported in high-dose single insult nephrotoxic models of ARF. By contrast, the distal tubule, and in particular the medullary thick ascending limbs, appear relatively more resistant to energy depletion but are exquisitely vulnerable to an imbalance between O_2 supply and demand (25). Medullary zones of lowest O_2 availability could therefore render the kidney susceptible to nephrotoxins that might interfere with intrarenal oxygen balance, at doses far lower than those necessary to produce proximal tubular damage. Nephrotoxicity would be expressed only, or mainly, under conditions already associated with compromised intrarenal hemodynamics such as salt depletion or renal hypoperfusion.

To understand better the synergism between risk factors in clinical ARF, "multiple insult" models of ARF will now be reviewed.

DEVELOPMENT OF "MULTIPLE-INSULTS" MODELS OF ARF

Because of the important deviations of "single-insult" models from the clinical syndrome of ARF, efforts have been made by several laboratories to design "multiple-insults" models that would more closely reflect human ARF (Table 3). These models use as a principle the combination of multiple factors that would not by themselves have caused any significant renal injury.

Radiocontrast Nephrotoxicity

Although radiological contrast materials have long been recognized as a cause of human ARF, the mechanism of kidney injury remains unclear, because of the scarcity of adequate animal models. Until recently, in "single-insult" models, animals injected with a radiocontrast agent either manifested only a slight and transient fall in renal function or died from the adverse extrarenal effects. In 1988, Vari et al. (26) in the rabbit and Heyman et al. (27) in the rat, showed that it is necessary to precondition the animal by salt depletion and indomethacin for the injection of radiocontrast agents to provoke a syndrome of ARF that resembles clinical radiocontrast nephropathy. Renal injury was minimal when insults were applied sep-

TABLE 3. *Comparison between clinical nephrotoxic ARF and two modalities of experimental ARF ("single-insult" and "multiple-insults")*

	Clinical ARF	"Single-insult" models	"Multiple-insults" models
Incidence	<1% to 30%	100%	<100%
Number of acute insults	Usually ≥2	1	≥2
Chronic risk factors	Frequently present	None	Sometimes present
Drug dosage	Usually therapeutic	Toxic	Minimally toxic
Dose dependency	Often tenuous	Strong	—
Morphology	Focal tubular necrosis, interstitial edema, vasa recta congestion and infiltration	Prominent cortical injury—proximal tubular necrosis	Prominent outer medullary injury—necrosis of S_3 and/or mTAL
Pathophysiological mechanism	?	Toxic cell injury predominant on one nephron segment, usually the proximal tubule	Interference with medullary oxygen balance

mTAL, medullary thick ascending limb.

arately. The combination of the insults produced remarkable kidney failure. In the rat, severe morphological injury was confined to the outer medulla and included necrosis of medullary thick ascending limbs and tubular casts. These changes were most marked in the deepest areas of the outer medulla, away from vasa recta in zones remote from oxygen supply. The nature of medullary thick limb injury was similar to selective lesions observed in isolated kidneys perfused with cell-free medium, shown to derive from an imbalance between high oxygen demand by actively transporting tubules and the meager oxygen supply to the renal medulla (28–30). In this model, furosemide administered before the contrast agent and in combination with aggressive saline infusion (to avoid concomitant volume depletion) protected renal function and morphology (31). Oxygen microelectrodes inserted into the kidney have confirmed a remarkable decline in medullary pO_2, already low at baseline, from 25 to 10 mm Hg ($p<.001$) after radiocontrast injection (64). This effect could derive from active medullary vasoconstriction or from a sludging or erythrocytes (made more rigid by radiocontrast) within the renal medullary microcirculation (32) at a time when osmotic diuresis imposes an added workload for tubular reabsorption on the distal nephron.

In a variation on these models, an infusion of angiotensin II in the rat could substitute for salt depletion, and, in combination with indomethacin and radiocontrast material, also produced ARF with selective medullary injury (33). Most recently, radiocontrast agents were found to stimulate the release of endothelin, a potent vasoconstrictor peptide (34). Furthermore, inhibition of the endothelial-derived relaxing factor nitric oxide, in Heyman's model, markedly exaggerated the medullary hypoxic injury observed after radiocontrast administration (35). These observations suggest that interference of radiocontrast with medullary O_2 balance is especially likely to produce tubular injury and renal failure when associated with systemic vasoconstriction and kidney hypoperfusion, as present in man during salt depletion or low cardiac output.

Aminoglycoside Nephrotoxicity

To elude the artificiality of high-dose "single-insult" model (see Table 3), Zager (36–38) attempted to mimic the clinical association of gentamicin nephropathy with comorbid conditions, by combining in rats, endotoxemia, liver injury, or renal hypoperfusion with gentamicin treatment. Although high doses were used (80 to 120 mg/kg), gentamicin alone did not produce renal injury, probably because it was given only once. By contrast, when administered in combination with gram-negative bacteremia (*Pseudomonas* or *Escherichia coli*) or with endotoxemia (achieved by injecting an endotoxin), the same dose of gentamicin induced ARF, associated with noticeable tubular necrosis. The endotoxemia by itself caused only minimal renal damage, suggesting a synergism between aminoglycoside therapy and a systemic abnormality to produce ARF. In a different model, liver necrosis (induced by acute ligation) was found to predispose to gentamicin nephrotoxicity (37). In yet another model, renal hypoperfusion was created by a suprarenal partial aortic constriction and combined with a single gentamicin injection. Renal hypoperfusion or gentamicin alone produced minimal injury and no azotemia. In combination, however, extensive tubular necrosis occurred as well as severe renal failure, suggesting a synergism between gentamicin and renal ischemia to elicit nephrotoxicity (38).

A remarkable finding in these models is the site of morphological injury. Although gentamicin characteristically causes tubular necrosis in the initial, cortical segments of the proximal tubule (S_1 and S_2) in "single-insult" models (39), in the combination protocols described above, severe injury was observed in the outer medulla, sometimes exclusively in the terminal segment of proximal tubule (S_3), in a zone recognized for its greatest vulnerability to ischemic damage (40). This difference in the site of damage between "single-insult" and "multiple-insult" models suggest dissimilar pathophysiological mechanisms for the development of ARF. The cortical proximal tubule manifests a noticeable susceptibility to prolonged administration of aminoglycosides in high doses. When associated with compromised renal hemodynamics, however, the vulnerable target is shifted toward the deeper zones of the kidney, known for their propensity to hypoxic damage (see below) as if aminoglycoside therapy might interfere under certain circumstances with medullary oxygen balance.

Cyclosporine

Recent experimental and clinical observations have shown a marked potentiation of cyclosporine nephrotoxicity by salt depletion. "Single-insult" models have successfully induced renal failure by high-dose cyclosporine and have focused on the damage in the renal cortex. By contrast, models combining moderate dose of cyclosporine with salt depletion (41,42) have identified the earliest signs of injury in the outer medulla and in the medullary rays, in zones of lowest oxygen availability. Cyclosporine might, at least in part by vasoconstriction, exacerbate renal medullary susceptibility to oxygen deprivation, and therefore manifest its nephrotoxicity especially in conditions associated with renal hypoperfusion.

Amphotericin

Unpublished work from our laboratory (by Heyman et al.) indicates a prominent augmentation of amphotericin nephrotoxicity in salt-depleted rats. Importantly, severe tubular injury is concentrated in medullary thick ascending limbs and medullary rays, suggesting again a synergism between toxic and hypoxic insults initially affecting the renal zones of hypoxia in the pathogenesis of amphotericin-associated renal failure.

As summarized in Table 4, both clinically and experimentally, the evidence is growing that in many instances of nephrotoxic ARF, additive or synergistic interactions with renal hypoperfusion predispose the kidney to the deleterious effect of a nephrotoxin. As illustrated in Table 3, the "multiple-insults" models may therefore more closely resemble the clinical syndrome of ARF associated with nephrotoxins. A common denominator of these models, compared to "single-insult" models, is a shift of the injury site from the cortex toward the deeper zones of the kidney, in the outer medulla. This region is characterized by low ambient levels of oxygen and a tenuous balance between oxygen supply and demand, which may render the kidney

TABLE 4. *Evidence for additive or synergistic interaction of hypoperfusion and nephrotoxins*

	References	
	Clinical	Experimental
Exogenous toxins		
Aminoglycosides	1,17	36–38
Amphotericin	4,54	52
Cyclosporin A	53	41,42
Contrast agents	2,22–24	3,26,27
Cis-platinum	5,16	16
Methotrexate	16	
Nonsteroidal anti-inflammatory agents	55	
Captopril	56	
Bacterial endotoxin		57
Endogenous toxins		
Myoglobinuria	58	59
Multiple myeloma	60	
Hypercalcemia	61	46

Modified from Brezis et al., ref. 8, with permission.

especially susceptible to combined hypoxic and toxic insults. Central to this suggested mechanism is therefore the question of renal medullary hypoxia, its basis, its regulatory modalities, and its pathophysiological implications.

THEORY OF RENAL MEDULLARY HYPOXIA AS A KEY TO THE SUSCEPTIBILITY OF THE KIDNEY TO HYPOPERFUSION WITH OR WITHOUT CONCOMITANT NEPHROTOXIC EXPOSURE

In the clinical setting of hypotension, the kidney appears to have a distinct susceptibility to injury. The reason for this is not readily apparent, since renal blood flow is normally high and O_2 supply exceeds by far the requirement for O_2 utilization (Table 5). This overall balance, however, conceals remarkable regional hypoxia, predominantly in the outer medulla. Gradients of O_2 availability within the kidney relate to the countercurrent exchange of O_2 within the medulla, to the relatively low medullary blood flow, and to the high metabolic requirements of the medullary thick ascending limb, all of which are necessary to provide efficient concentration of the urine. Renal medullary hypoxia is thus a characteristic property of concentrating kidneys and has indeed been observed in a number of mammalian species, including man.

Renal blood flow, nearly a quarter of the cardiac output, is principally directed to the renal cortex, which receives therefore one of the highest rates of tissue perfusion in the body. This apparent overabundance is designed to maximize flow-dependent renal functions such as glomerular filtration and tubular reabsorption. By contrast, in the medulla, blood flow and oxygen supply are restricted by a tubulovascular anatomy specially designed for urinary concentration (Fig. 6). Medullary hypoxia is therefore the obligatory price paid for an efficient urinary concentrating mechanism.

The cortex and medulla of the mammalian kidney are strikingly disparate in anatomy, function, and metabolism. The filtering renal cortex with its oversupply of oxygen contrasts sharply with the concentrating medulla, working constantly on the verge of anoxia. This duality is particularly important to consider when studying

TABLE 5. *Comparison of balance of O_2 delivery and O_2 consumption in several organs*

Region or organ	O_2 delivery (ml/min/100 g)	Blood flow rate (ml/min/100 g)	O_2 consumption (ml/min/100 g)	O_2 consumption/ O_2 delivery (%)
Hepatoportal	11.6	58	2.2	18
Kidney	84.0	420	6.8	8
Renal outer medulla	7.6	190	6.9	79
Brain	10.8	54	3.7	34
Skin	2.6	13	0.38	15
Skeletal muscle	0.5	2.7	0.18	34
Heart	16.8	84	11.0	65

From Brezis et al., ref. 8, with permission.

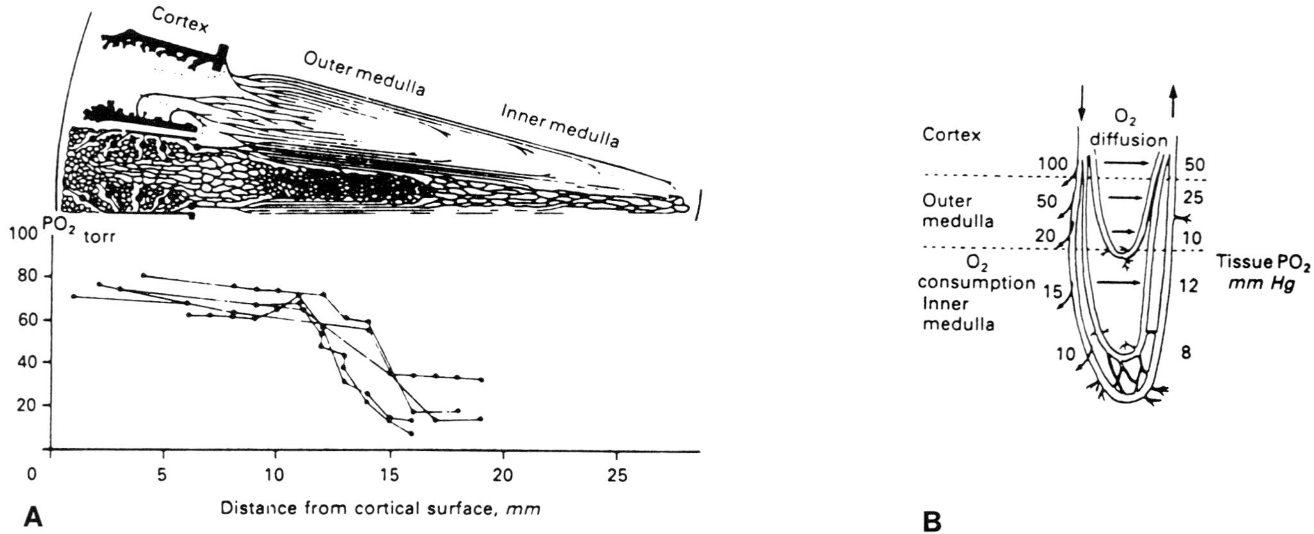

FIG. 6. Heterogeneity of renal oxygenation. **A:** Renal tissue oxygen tension in different parts of the kidney. The upper part illustrates schematically the renal vascular pattern. **B:** Countercurrent exchange of oxygen in the vasa recta. Diffusion of oxygen between arterial and venous limbs minimizes the dissipation of the corticomedullary gradient of tissue oxygen tension. (From Brezis et al., ref. 8, with permission.)

nephrotoxicity. On the one hand, the kidney is predisposed to injury from many drugs and toxins because of its high blood flow, its vast expanse of electrically charged surfaces for glomerular filtration, and its complex mechanisms for tubular secretion and reabsorption of a variety of substances. Injury from many cellular toxins may therefore be expected to become manifest first in the renal cortex, as observed in "single-insult" models of ARF. On the other hand, the kidney is also predisposed to nephrotoxicity because of its efficient concentrating mechanism including, within the renal medulla, a system of countercurrent multiplication resulting in the accumulation of certain solutes to levels far above their concentration in plasma. In the renal medulla, where some drugs are concentrated by this mechanism, they may interact with hypoxia to express their toxicity.

The synergism between renal hypoperfusion and toxic insults may derive from several factors: (a) when urine flow is reduced, there may be increased accumulation of hydrophilic toxic substances (such as crystals) in urine and renal parenchyma; (b) drug toxicity may interfere with renal autoregulation and preservation of the circulation to strategic areas of the kidney (e.g., inhibitors of prostaglandin synthesis); (c) drug-induced membrane damage or mitochondrial uncoupling can cause an increase in inefficient O_2 consumption at the same time that oxygen delivery is compromised, thus exacerbating anoxic injury (e.g., polyene antibiotics); (d) toxic substances and O_2 deprivation may interact at the mitochondrial level to produce depletion of adenosine triphosphate (ATP) (e.g., aminoglycosides).

What are the renal structures most at risk from medullary hypoxia? A series of experimental studies in the rat *in vitro* and *in vivo* have identified renal structures particularly susceptible to O_2 deficiency, within the loop of Henle (27–29). These include the medullary thick ascending limb, the thin descending limb, and the pars recta (S_3) of the proximal tubule, all localized in the outer medulla, a region normally characterized by relatively low oxygen tension. These nephron segments are metabolically active and also remote from sources of O_2 supply, i.e., from vasa recta. The medullary thick ascending limbs of the superficial nephrons (originating from glomeruli located in the outer cortex), which are positioned away from the vasa recta, are more vulnerable than are those of the deep nephrons (originating from juxtamedullary glomeruli), which are adjacent to vascular bundles. Collecting tubules, although distant from O_2 sources, are relatively resistant to hypoxia, probably because of their large capacity for anaerobic metabolism.

Important and instructive adjuncts to these susceptible medullary structures are, in the cortex, the medullary rays, which appear comparably vulnerable to hypoxic injury. The medullary rays are longitudinal elements extending from the corticomedullary junction toward the superficial cortex, formed by S_3 segments of proximal tubules, cortical thick ascending limbs and collecting ducts. Because the blood supply to this region is, to a large extent, from a venous ascending effluent of the outer medullary capillary network, the low tissue pO_2 of the medulla is reflected in the cortex, in the medullary rays, as if they were functionally cortical expansions from the medulla. Medullary rays show preferential vulnerability to ischemic injury (62). Moreover, injury to medullary rays, consisting of tubular degeneration and fibrosis, has been observed in several models of nephrotoxic ARF, such as in hypercalcemia (46), cyclosporine toxicity (42), and most recently amphotericin toxicity (Heyman et al., unpublished). Apparently the "stripe fibrosis" described in human cyclosporine nephropathy corresponds to medullary ray damage. These cortical lesions in medullary rays are probably not specific for cyclosporine and may rather relate to prolonged renal vasoconstriction compromising regions of lowest O_2 availability both in cortex and medulla.

The vulnerability of the medullary thick ascending limb (mTAL) to hypoxia is most strikingly demonstrated in the isolated perfused rat kidney model (28). It is the result of an imbalance between the meager supply of oxygen and the active metabolic demand in this nephron segment. Thus, inhibition of electrolyte transport with furosemide or ouabain reduces or eliminates hypoxic injury to the mTALs (30). By contrast, when sodium pump activity is augmented by the ionophore effect of polyene antibiotics (e.g., amphotericin), medullary hypoxic damage is markedly exaggerated (11). Following the same principle, tubular necrosis is strikingly prevented when glomerular filtration ceases and consequently the distal delivery of electrolytes for reabsorption in this nephron segment stops (30). These observations emphasize the close interdependence between metabolic workload and tubular vulnerability to hypoxic injury in the mTAL.

Medullary hypoxia can be modulated by a variety of pharmacological or physiopathological maneuvers, as summarized in Table 6. Increased tubular transport activity (e.g., by amphotericin) and increased GFR (e.g., in renal compensatory hypertrophy) are associated with augmented medullary hypoxic injury to mTALs in isolated perfused kidneys and also lead to a greater propensity to mTAL injury *in vivo* (43). A preferential decrease in medullary blood flow is probably responsible, at least in part, for potentiation of mTAL hypoxic damage during inhibition of prostaglandin synthesis by NSAIDs, both *in vitro* and *in vivo* (27,44). Under the action of angiotensin II (which vasoconstricts postglomerular efferent arterioles) renal blood flow is decreased while GFR is relatively preserved, leading to a reduction in renal (and medullary) oxygen delivery while tubular work tends to remain high. Angiotensin II predisposes to medullary hypoxic injury, both in the perfused kidney and in intact rats (33). Radiocontrast materials and an excess of calcium exacerbate mTAL hypoxic injury in perfused kidneys and can produce a similar lesion *in vivo* (27,45,46). Nonsteroidal anti-inflammatory drugs, radiocontrast agents, and angiotensin II all reduce medullary pO_2 measured by oxygen microelectrodes (unpublished work).

Relief of medullary hypoxia is consistently achieved by inhibition of tubular transport activity. Furosemide protects mTALs from hypoxic injury in perfused kidneys and *in vivo*, and increases medullary pO_2 (11,30,47; and unpublished data). Reduction in GFR also prevents medullary hypoxic injury, as shown both in isolated kidneys (made nonfiltering by elevation of perfusate oncotic pressure) and *in vivo* (by the recurrent observation that collapsed tubules are protected from damage). Metabolic inhibition reduces mTAL hypoxic injury by diminution of oxygen demand (25,48,49). Locally released substances may relieve medullary hypoxia by

TABLE 6. *Modulation of medullary hypoxia by pharmacological or physiopathological maneuvers (data collected from studies in isolated perfused rat kidneys and in vivo)*

Medullary hypoxia exacerbated	Medullary hypoxia relieved
Polyenes (e.g., amphotericin) (11)	↓ Tubular transport (11,30,47) (e.g., furosemide)
Renal hypertrophy (43)	↓ GFR (30,47)
Angiotensin II (33)	Metabolic inhibition (25,48,49)
NSAIDs (44)	PGE_2 (44), thromboxane (unpublished)
Radiocontrast agents (27)	Adenosine (50,51)
Calcium (45,46)	Nitric oxide (35)

several mechanisms. Prostaglandin E_2 and adenosine alleviate medullary hypoxia both by inducing medullary vasodilatation and by reducing mTAL transport activity (44,50,51). Recent work suggests that the endothelial-derived relaxing factor, nitric oxide, participates in the balance of renal medullary oxygenation and could play an important role in the prevention of medullary hypoxic injury (35).

It appears that several systems of defense are available to the kidney in order to avoid medullary hypoxic damage. Figure 7 describes a hypothetical scheme of an integrated neurohumoral control system governing the delicate homeostasis of medullary oxygenation. Medullary O_2 deficiency would trigger a number of mechanisms that will tend to restore O_2 balance either by reduction of transport work or by medullary vasodilatation. Diminution of GFR by activation of tubuloglomerular feedback (secondary to mTAL hypoxic malfunction) would contribute importantly to the restitution of medullary metabolic balance. The local secretion of paracrine agents such as prostanoids, adenosine, or nitric oxide may induce medullary vasodilatation or diminish tubular work. The net result would be a restoration of medullary oxygen balance at the expense of a reduction in kidney function.

It is likely that such an important and precisely regulated homeostasis control system involves multiple mechanisms operating in parallel, some apparently redundant, and some others yet unrecognized. Excessive or deficient activation of these self-defense systems may have far-reaching consequences upon renal function and/or morphology. Importantly, this scheme may explain why the demonstration of the renal toxicity of some nephrotoxins encountered in clinical practice requires the coexistence of conditions that partially or completely compromise these defense systems. This multiplicity of defense mechanisms may underlie the synergistic interplay seen both in man and in experimental animals between renal hypoperfusion and toxic insults to produce kidney injury far more significant than each insult imposed separately.

The hypothesis advanced here is that structures of the renal medulla, including particularly the straight portion of the proximal tubule and the thick ascending limb, manifest a special vulnerability that derives from the precarious balance of renal medullary oxygenation. Injury proximal to the macula densa and therefore at a strategic site for the regulation of renal function, may have major consequences for kidney function. Medullary oxygenation homeostasis, defended by a remarkably

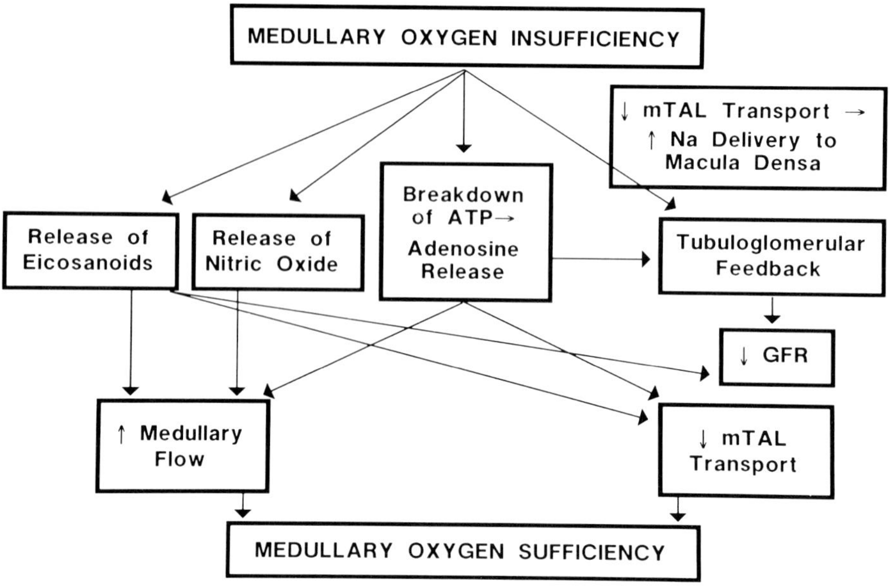

FIG. 7. Regulatory pathways involved in the homeostasis of renal medullary oxygenation. mTAL, medullary thick ascending limb; GFR, glomerular filtration rate. (From Brezis et al., ref. 8, with permission.)

well-orchestrated humoral and paracrine system, becomes susceptible to coordinated attack from multiple fronts, such as during the combined insults of renal hypoperfusion and exposure to nephrotoxins (Fig. 8). This principle is central to understanding and preventing the nephrotoxicity of drugs and for adequate screening of new therapeutic agents with potential toxicity to the kidney.

CONCLUSIONS

This chapter has reviewed our current understanding of the pathophysiology of ARF. Experimental models of ARF using single insults have demonstrated multiple mechanisms of nephron damage leading to failure of glomerular filtration, including tubular backleak, luminal obstruction, vasoconstriction, and feedback inhibition of GFR. Important differences emerge, however, between "single-insult" models and clinical ARF, as in the former overly toxic dosages are purposely administered to healthy animals to regularly induce ARF, whereas in the latter combined risk factors and preexisting conditions act together to cause kidney failure. Recently developed "multiple-insults" models of ARF disclose the target of renal damage to reside most often in the outer medulla, a zone of precarious oxygen balance, suggesting a synergism between hypoxic and toxic insults affecting renal homeostatic mechanisms before leading to medullary injury.

In human ARF, indirect evidence strongly suggests medullary involvement.

RENAL HYPOPERFUSION ↘ NEPHROTOXINS ↙

MEDULLARY HYPOXIA

↓

ACUTE RENAL FAILURE

FIG. 8. Hypothetical scheme of the synergistic interaction between renal hypoperfusion and nephrotoxins in the development of ARF.

First, failure of the urinary concentrating mechanism, manifested by isotonicity of the urine, is the earliest and most predictive impairment of tubule function in ARF. Second, the typical urine sediment of ARF shows many brown casts essentially composed of precipitated Tamm-Horsfall protein released by and exclusively synthesized by thick ascending limbs. Finally, the histology of human ARF has stressed the frequent finding of mononuclear cell infiltration in the vasa recta (presumed reaction to focal injury in outer medulla) and a predominance of injury to tubules in the medulla and medullary rays.

The loop of Henle appears therefore to express a unique susceptibility derived from the fragile homeostasis of renal medullary oxygenation, readily disrupted by the combined insults of kidney hypoperfusion and exposure to nephrotoxins. This modality of renal injury provides an important basis for the prevention of ARF. Optimal hydration and volume repletion are crucial whenever possible before and during exposure to a potential toxin. In patients with uncorrected renal perfusion (despite best hydration) such as in chronic nephropathies or congestive heart failure, exposure to toxins should be either avoided or as limited as possible. Timely and efficient uncoupling of the pernicious combination of hypoxic and toxic insults is the best way to prevent ARF.

ACKNOWLEDGMENTS

This work was supported by NIH grants DK18078 and DK39249, and by a grant from the United States–Israel Binational Science Foundation. The authors are grateful to Dr. S. Heyman for his criticism and to Mrs. S. Nelson for her excellent assistance.

REFERENCES

1. Moore RD, Smith CR, Lipsky JJ, et al. Risk factors for nephrotoxicity in patients treated with aminoglycosides. *Ann Intern Med* 1984;100:352.

2. Manske CL, Sprafka JM, Strony JT, Wang Y. Contrast nephropathy in azotemic diabetic patients undergoing coronary angiography. *Am J Med* 1990;89:615–620.
3. Margulies KB, McKinley LJ, Cavero PG, Burnett JC Jr. Induction and prevention of radiocontrast-induced nephropathy in dogs with heart failure. *Kidney Int* 1990;38:1101–1108.
4. Heideman JT, Gerkens JF, Spickard WA, et al. Amphotericin nephrotoxicity decreased by salt repletion. *Am J Med* 1983;75:476.
5. Ozols RF, Corden BJ, Jacob J, et al. High-dose cisplatin in hypertonic saline. *Ann Intern Med* 1984;100:19.
6. Hostetter TH, Wilkes BM, Brenner BM. Mechanisms of impaired glomerular filtration in acute renal failure. In: Brenner BM, Stein JH, eds. *Contemporary issues in nephrology, vol 6: Acute renal failure*. New York: Churchill Livingstone, 1980;52–77.
7. Hostetter TH, Brenner BM. Renal circulatory and nephron function in experimental acute renal failure. In: Brenner BM, Lazarus JM, eds. *Acute renal failure*, 2nd ed. New York: Churchill Livingstone, 1988;67–89.
8. Brezis M, Rosen S, Epstein FH. Acute renal failure. In: Brenner BM, Rector FJ, eds. *The kidney*, 4th ed. Philadelphia: WB Saunders, 1991;993–1061.
9. Stein J, Levinsky NG, Epstein FH. Acute renal failure. In: Tannen RL, ed. *American Society of Nephrology: a 25 year perspective*. Washington, DC: American Society of Nephrology, 1992;[still in press].
10. Cheng JT, Witty RT, Robinson RR, Yarger WE. Amphotericin B nephrotoxicity: increased renal resistance and tubule permeability. *Kidney Int* 1982;22:626–633.
11. Brezis M, Rosen S, Silva P, Spokes K, Epstein FH. Polyene toxicity in renal medulla: injury mediated by transport activity. *Science* 1984;224:66.
12. Ichikawa I. Hemodynamic influence of altered distal salt delivery on glomerular microcirculation. *Kidney Int* 1982;22:S1090–S1113.
13. Persson AEG, Boberg U, Hahne B, Muller-Suur R, Norlen BJ, Selen G. Interstitial pressure as a modulator of tubuloglomerular feedback control. *Kidney Int* 1982;22:S122–S128.
14. Schor N, Ichikawa I, Rennke HG, et al. Pathophysiology of altered glomerular function in aminoglycoside-treated rats. *Kidney Int* 1981;19:288.
15. Luft FC, Aronoff GR, Evan AP, et al. The renin-angiotensin system in aminoglycoside-induced acute renal failure. *J Pharmacol Exp Ther* 1982;220:433.
16. Garnick MB, Mayer RJ, Abelson HT. Acute renal failure associated with cancer treatment. *In*: Brenner BM, Lazarus JM, eds. *Acute renal failure*, 2nd ed. New York: Churchill Livingstone, 1988;621–657.
17. Rasmussen HH, Ibels LS. Acute renal failure. Multivariate analysis of causes and risk factors. *Am J Med* 1982;73:211–218.
18. Shusterman N, Strom BL, Murray RG, Morrison G, West SL, Maislin G. Risk factors and outcome of hospital-acquired acute renal failure. *Am J Med* 1987;83:65–71.
19. Smith CR, Lipsky JJ, Laskin OL, et al. Double-blind comparison of the nephrotoxicity and auditory toxicity of gentamicin and tobramycin. *N Engl J Med* 1980;302:1106.
20. Bennett WM, Plamp CE, Gilbert DN, et al. The influence of dosage regimen on experimental gentamicin nephrotoxicity: dissociation of peak serum levels from renal failure. *J Infect Dis* 1979; 140:576.
21. Leehey DJ, Braun BI, Lentino JR. Pharmacokinetic dosing increases efficacy but does not decrease nephrotoxicity associated with aminoglycosides. *J Am Soc Nephrol* 1990;1:323.
22. Eisenberg RL, Bank WD, Hedgcock MW. Renal failure after major angiography. *Am J Med* 1980;68:43.
23. D'Elia J, Gleason R, Alday M, et al. Nephrotoxicity from angiographic contrast material: a prospective study. *Am J Med* 1982;72:719.
24. Taliercio CP, Vlietstra RE, Fisher LD, Burnett JC. Risks for renal dysfunction with cardiac angiography. *Ann Intern Med* 1986;104:501–504.
25. Brezis M, Shanley P, Silva P, Spokes K, Leaf S, Epstein FH, Rosen S. Disparate mechanisms for hypoxic cell injury in different nephron segments. Studies in the isolated perfused rat kidney. *J Clin Invest* 1985;76:1796–1806.
26. Vari RC, Natarajian LA, Whitescarver SA, Jackson BA, Ott CM. Induction prevention and mechanisms of contrast media induced acute renal failure. *Kidney Int* 1988;33:699–707.
27. Heyman SN, Brezis M, Reubinoff CA, et al. Acute renal failure with selective medullary injury in the rat. *J Clin Invest* 1988;82:401–412.

28. Brezis M, Rosen S, Silva P, Epstein FH. Selective vulnerability of the thick ascending limb to anoxia in the isolated perfused kidney. *J Clin Invest* 1984;73:182–189.
29. Brezis M, Rosen S, Silva P, Epstein FH. Renal ischemia: a new perspective. *Kidney Int* 1984; 26:375–383.
30. Brezis M, Rosen S, Silva P, et al. Transport activity modifies thick ascending limb damage in isolated perfused kidney. *Kidney Int* 1984;25:65–72.
31. Heyman S, Brezis M, Greenfeld Z, et al. Protective role of furosemide and saline in radiocontrast induced acute renal failure. *Am J Kidney Dis* 1989;14:377–385.
32. Nygren A, Ulfendahl JR, Hansell P, Erikson U. Effects of intravenous radiocontrast material on cortical and medullary blood flow in the rat kidney. *Invest Radiol* 1988;23:753–761.
33. Brezis M, Greenfeld Z, Shina A, et al. Angiotensin II augments medullary hypoxia and predisposes to acute renal failure. *Eur J Clin Invest* 1990;20:199–207.
34. Clark BA, Heyman SN, Spokes K, West C, Epstein FH. Rise in plasma endothelin produced by radiocontrast agents. *J Am Soc Nephrol* 1990;1:412.
35. Brezis M, Heyman SN, Spokes K, Epstein FH, Rosen S. Role of nitric oxide in renal medullary oxygen balance. *J Clin Invest* 1991;88:390–395.
36. Zager RA, Prior RB. Gentamicin and gram-negative bacteremia. A synergism for the development of experimental nephrotoxic acute renal failure. *J Clin Invest* 1986;78:196–204.
37. Zager RA. A focus of tissue necrosis increases renal susceptibility to gentamicin administration. *Kidney Int* 1988;33:84–90.
38. Zager RA. Gentamicin nephrotoxicity in the setting of acute renal hypoperfusion. *Am J Physiol* 1988; 254:F574–F581.
39. Houghton DC, Plamp CE, DeFehr JM, Bennett SM, Porter G, Gilbert D. Gentamicin and tobramycin nephrotoxicity. *Am J Pathol* 1978;93:137–152.
40. Venkatachalam MA, Bernard DB, Donohoe JF, Levinsky NG. Ischemic damage and repair in the rat proximal tubule. Differences among the S_1, S_2 and S_3 segments. *Kidney Int* 1978;14:31–49.
41. Jackson NM, Hsu CH, Visscher GE, Venkatachalam MA, Humes HD. Alterations in renal structure and function in a rat model of cyclosporine nephrotoxicity. *J Pharmacol Exp Ther* 1987;242:749–756.
42. Rosen S, Greenfeld Z, Brezis M. Chronic cyclosporine-induced nephropathy in the rat: a medullary ray and inner stripe injury. *Transplantation* 1990;49:445–452.
43. Epstein FH, Silva P, Spokes K, et al. Renal medullary Na-K-ATPase and hypoxic injury in perfused rat kidney. *Kidney Int* 1989;36:768–772.
44. Brezis M, Rosen S, Stoff JS, et al. Inhibition of prostaglandin synthesis in rat kidney perfused with and without erythrocytes: implication for analgesic nephropathy. *Miner Electrolyte Metab* 1986; 12:326–332.
45. Brezis M, Shina K, Kidroni G, et al. Calcium and hypoxic injury in the renal medulla of the perfused rat kidney. *Kidney Int* 1988;34:186–194.
46. Rosen S, Greenfeld Z, Bernheim J, Rathaus M, Podjarny E, Brezis M. Hypercalcemic nephropathy in the rat: chronic renal disease with predominent inner stripe injury. *Kidney Int* 1990;37:1067–1075.
47. Brezis M, Rosen S, Spokes K, Silva P, Epstein FH. Transport-dependent anoxic cell injury in the isolated perfused rat kidney. *Am J Pathol* 1984;116:327–341.
48. Brezis M, Rosen S, Silva P, Spokes K, Epstein FH. Mitochondrial activity: a possible determinant of anoxic injury in renal medulla. *Experientia* 1986;42:570–572.
49. Brezis M, Rosen S, Spokes K, Silva P, Epstein FH. Substrates induce hypoxic injury to medullary thick limbs of isolated kidneys. *Am J Physiol* 1986;251:F710–F717.
50. Epstein FH, Rosen S, Galicka-Piskorska G, et al. Relation of adenosine to medullary injury in the perfused rat kidney. *Miner Electrolyte Metab* 1990;16:185–190.
51. Dinour D, Brezis M. Effects of adenosine upon intrarenal oxygenation. *Am J Physiol* 1991; 261:F787–F791.
52. Gerkens JF, Branch RA. The influence of sodium status and furosemide on canine acute amphotericin B nephrotoxicity. *J Pharmacol Exp Ther* 1980;214:306.
53. The Canadian Multicentre Transplant Study Group. A randomized clinical trial of cyclosporine in cadaveric renal transplantation. *N Engl J Med* 1983;309:809.
54. Fisher MA, Talbot GH, Maislin G, McKeon BP, Tynan KP, Strom BL. Risk factors for amphotericin B-associated nephrotoxicity. *Am J Med* 1989;87:547–552.

55. Clive DM, Stoff JS. Renal syndromes associated with nonsteroidal anti-inflammatory drugs. *N Engl J Med* 1984;310:563.
56. Hricik DE, Browning PJ, Kopelman R, et al. Captopril-induced functional renal insufficiency in patients with bilateral renal-artery stenoses or renal-artery stenosis in a solitary kidney. *N Engl J Med* 1983;308:373.
57. Zager RA. *Escherichia coli* endotoxin infections potentiate experimental ischemic renal injury. *Am J Physiol* 1986;251:F988.
58. Hamilton RW, Gardner LB, Penn AS, Goldberg M. Acute tubular necrosis caused by exercise-induced myoglobinuria. *Ann Intern Med* 1982;77:77.
59. Jaenike JR. The renal lesion associated with hemoglobinemia. I. Its production and functional evolution in the rat. *J Exp Med* 1966;123:523.
60. DeFronzo RA, Humphrey RL, Wright JR, Cooke CR. Acute renal failure in multiple myeloma. *Medicine* 1975;54:209.
61. Benabe JE, Martinez-Maldonado M. Hypercalcemic nephropathy. *Arch Intern Med* 1978;138:777.
62. Shanley PF, Rosen MD, Brezis M, Silva P, Epstein FH, Rosen S. Topography of focal proximal tubular necrosis after ischemia with reflow in the rat kidney. *Am J Pathol* 1986;122:462.
63. Brezis M, Epstein FH. A closer look at radiocontrast nephropathy. *N Engl J Med* 1989;320:179.
64. Heyman SN, Brezis M, Epstein FH, Spokes K, Silva P, Rosen S. Early renal medullary hypoxic injury from radiocontrast and indomethacin. *Kidney Int* 1991;40:632–642.

Toxicology of the Kidney, Second Edition,
edited by Jerry B. Hook and Robin S. Goldstein.
Raven Press, Ltd., New York © 1993.

6

Mechanisms of Glomerular Injury

*Mauro Abbate, *Daniela Macconi, and *†Giuseppe Remuzzi

**Mario Negri Institute for Pharmacological Research, 24100 Bergamo, Italy; and †Division of Nephrology, Ospedali Riuniti di Bergamo, 24100 Bergamo, Italy*

The glomerulus is the target of toxic effects of a number of drugs and chemical agents that may cause changes in glomerular morphology and/or function both in humans and in experimental animals (Table 1) (1,2). Toxic agents can damage primarily selective glomerular components to which the structural changes are confined, at least initially. Evidence of a direct mechanism of glomerular injury has been derived from the Adriamycin and puromycin aminonucleoside models of nephrotic syndrome in the rat. A primary endothelial cell injury is likely responsible for the development of glomerular damage after mitomycin administration. However, more frequently extrarenal effects of nephrotoxic agents have been shown to set in motion a sequence of pathophysiological changes that indirectly cause the development of glomerular injury. Thus, disordered cell-mediated immunity and abnormal production of lymphokines are suspected to result in increased glomerular permeability in cases of drug-induced minimal change disease and focal segmental glomerulosclerosis in humans. Indirect mechanisms of glomerular injury act in forms of immune complex glomerulonephritis in which drugs or toxic substances are thought to interfere with the immune system, resulting in antibody formation. Experimental mercuric chloride–induced glomerulonephritis is associated with polyclonal B-cell activation and production of autoantibodies directed against components of the glomerular basement membrane, resulting in the formation of immune aggregates in the glomerular capillary wall with a linear and later granular distribution. The production of antinuclear and antihistone antibodies followed by the formation of circulating immune complexes and their deposition in the subendothelial and mesangial space have been proposed to promote the development of the glomerular disease observed with procainamide, hydralazine, and nifedipine.

Toxic effects of drugs in the glomerulus are not necessarily associated with glomerular structural changes. Cyclosporin A, gentamicin, and amphotericin B are examples of drugs that can affect functional properties of the glomerulus without loss of structural integrity, thereby leading to significant decline in glomerular filtration rate. In this chapter potential mechanisms of proteinuria and altered

TABLE 1. *Forms of glomerular injury caused by drugs and toxic substances in humans or experimental animals*

Toxic effect	Clinicopathologic picture	Agents
Epithelial cell disease	Minimal change disease, proteinuria	Puromycin aminonucleoside Adriamycin Hexadimethrine Cimetidine Gold Lithium Cadmium Fenoprofen Nonsteroidal anti-inflammatory drugs Heroin Antibiotics Leukocyte interferon-α
Endothelial cell disease	Hemolytic uremic syndrome/Thrombotic thrombocytopenic purpura	Mitomycin Cyclosporin A
Immune complex disease		
Subepithelial deposits	Membranous glomerulonephritis	Mercuric chloride Gold Cadmium Penicillamine Captopril Hydrocarbons Trimethadione Chlormethiazole
Antiglomerular basement membrane antibodies	Proliferative glomerulonephritis	Mercuric chloride Volatile hydrocarbons Solvents
Subendothelial, mesangial deposits	Systemic lupus erythematosus-like	Hydralazine Procainamide Nifedipine

glomerular filtration induced by toxic agents and drugs that directly interfere with the glomerular microcirculation will be reviewed. The relevance of oxygen free radicals as mediators of glomerular injury will be also discussed.

GLOMERULAR PERMSELECTIVE PROPERTIES

The normal glomerular capillary wall is endowed with both size- and charge-selective properties that modulate the filtration of circulating macromolecules to the Bowman's space (3), so that large molecular weight proteins are denied access to the urine. *In vivo* studies with macromolecular solutes have elucidated the basis of size and charge glomerular permselectivity (4–9). The fractional clearance of a molecule is the ratio of the clearance of the molecule relative to the clearance of a reference molecule such as insulin. Test molecules such as dextrans are neither secreted nor reabsorbed along the nephron. Thus, in the absence of demonstrable effects of dextrans on glomerular hemodynamic determinants, which also influence the filtration of macromolecules, their fractional clearance reflects permselective properties intrinsic to the glomerular capillary wall. Both in humans and rats no restriction to filtration is found for molecules <20 Å, with nearly complete restriction for molecules >42 Å (4–6). However, the filtration of albumin is restricted to a much greater extent than is that of neutral dextran having the same effective molecular radius of approximately 36 Å (7,8). Since albumin behaves as a polyanion, the charge-selective barrier has been analyzed by studying the sieving characteristics of dextrane sulfate, an anionic polymer of dextran (9). For any given size, the fractional clearance of dextran sulfate is lower than that of neutral dextran, indicating that native anionic residues of the glomerular capillary wall serve to retard the transcapillary passage of circulating polyanions.

Several histochemical and immunochemical studies have investigated the structural and biochemical basis of the glomerular permselectivity. The fenestrated endothelial cells may contribute to the charge selectivity by virtue of negative charges provided by their sialoglycoprotein coat (10-12). However, several experimental results have suggested that the principal barrier to albumin loss is the glomerular basement membrane, whose physiochemical and permselective properties might become altered even in the absence of ultrastructural changes (13–16). The lamina densa of the glomerular basement membrane with its network of fibrils containing type IV collagen (17) might offer a significant size-selective barrier to neutral plasma proteins (18). The laminae rarae interna and externa contain "fixed" anionic sites that, after staining with cationic ferritin or ruthenium red, appear spaced at regular intervals of approximately 60 nm and arranged in a lattice-like network (19). Kanwar and Farquhar (20,21) demonstrated that fixed anionic sites are enriched with heparan sulfate proteoglycan (HSPG), which is made up of heparan sulfate–rich glycosaminoglycan chains covalently bound to a core peptide. The surface coat of visceral glomerular epithelial cells could also play a role in the glomerular charge barrier, by virtue of its high content in negatively charged sialic acid–rich glycoproteins that constitute the so-called epithelial polyanion (22,23).

Sialic acid residues and podocalyxin, a 140-kd sialoprotein that is considered the major component of the epithelial polyanion (24), have been shown to be localized on the surface of the foot process above the slit diaphragm and the main cell body, as well as on the luminal surface of the endothelial cell (12,25). Of interest, it has been recently reported that besides sialic acid residues, sulfate residues contribute to the negative charge of the epithelial polyanion (26). That anionic charges influence the permselective properties has been also documented with digestion (27,28) and neutralization (29,30) experiments. However, the question of which is the most important site of the charge-dependent barrier remains unanswered. It should be emphasized that the sulfate, carboxyl, and sialic acid residues on structural (glyco)proteins that are considered to represent the biochemical basis for the charge-selective barrier have a complex distribution in the glomerular capillary wall (20–

23,26,31). Moreover, the size and charge barriers are likely intimately interrelated. Sulfate and carboxyl groups in the glomerular basement membrane may play a role both for charge and size selectivity, as suggested by the observation that in the rat the infusion of the polycation hexadimethrine induces an increase in the pore size (32). A defective charge density of the glomerular capillary wall might determine reorientation and defective interactions of basement membrane components leading to altered size selectivity (33). Conversely, an enlargement of the effective radius of the theoretical "pores" responsible for the size-selective barrier would prevent anionic charge–carrying moieties to restrict the passage of macromolecules through the capillary wall, thus producing the development of an apparent charge-selective defect (34).

Besides producing the development of proteinuria, the exposure of the rat kidney to polycations, such as protamine or polylysine which bind to anionic sites of the glomerular capillary wall, causes the foot processes to "efface," that is, to be replaced by a continuous cytoplasmic bond along the lamina rara externa (30,35). Perfusion of the rat kidney with neuraminidase, which removes sialic acid, causes detachment of both endothelial and epithelial cells from the glomerular basement membrane (29). Epithelial cell damage is the morphological hallmark of minimal change nephrotic syndrome and other proteinuric conditions in man (36). Studying the mechanisms by which drugs are directly toxic to structures of the glomerular capillary wall, and in particular the visceral epithelial cells, has contributed to a better understanding both of determinants of the glomerular permselective barrier and of pathogenetic mechanisms of altered glomerular permeability to proteins.

The Glomerular Capillary Wall as Target of the Toxic Effects of Drugs that Cause Abnormal Permeability to Proteins in Experimental Nephropathy

Puromycin aminonucleoside (PA) nephrosis and Adriamycin (ADR) nephrosis in the rat can be regarded as two well-defined experimental models of *epithelial cell disease* (37). This term has been used to identify diseases with ultrastructural damage selectively involving glomerular visceral epithelial cells (38). Both drugs induce nephrotic syndrome with selective proteinuria, anasarca, hypoalbuminemia, and high plasma cholesterol. During the early stages of disease, glomerular filtration rate is also depressed in PA and, to a lesser extent, in ADR nephrosis (39). These models share many clinical and morphological findings with human minimal change glomerulopathy and focal segmental glomerulosclerosis.

Puromycin aminonucleoside (6-dimethylaminopurine, 3-amino-d-ribose) is a purine antagonist with antibiotic activity. The drug inhibits protein synthesis by acting on the RNA synthesis at the level of the ribosome (40). Besides the rat, monkeys, but not mice, rabbits, guinea pigs, and dogs, have been reported to be sensitive to PA nephrotoxicity (41,42). The onset of nephrotic syndrome has also been observed in humans following PA administration (43). At least two different patterns of PA nephrotoxicity have been described. In a "single-shot" model selective proteinuria starts at 4 to 5 days after a single peripheral intravenous or intraperitoneal injection of 0.5 to 1.5 mg PA/kg, reaches peak values averaging 100 to 900 mg/24 hr after 7 to 14 days, and disappears within 4 weeks (44–46). At light microscopy examination no pathological abnormalities can be detected except for moderate swelling of glomerular visceral epithelial cells. Electron microscopy shows striking epithelial cell damage as early as 24 hr after the injection, consisting of effacement of foot processes, followed by the formation of cytoplasmic vacuoles, protein reabsorption droplets, and villous transformation (45). When proteinuria ensues, these changes are accompanied by focal loss of covering epithelium outside the glomerular basement membrane (47). All ultrastructural alterations disappear with the remission of proteinuria.

Subsequently, no remarkable glomerular changes are detectable up to 35 weeks after a single injection of PA; then segmental sclerosis becomes discernible in a minor proportion of glomeruli (44). Besides glomerular changes, the signs of acute tubulointerstitial nephritis with macrophage accumulation have been also described, starting as soon as 3 days after a single intraperitoneal injection of PA (48). In contrast to the reversible glomerular disease induced with a single dose of PA via the tail vein, recent studies have documented that when PA (5 mg/kg) is administered directly into the central venous circulation a chronic, progressive disease develops (49). The early appearance of proteinuria is associated with light microscopy findings of mesangial cell proliferation and matrix expansion, loss of glomerular capillary lumina, and occasional adhesions between the glomerular tuft and the Bowman's capsule (49,50). On electron microscopy, marked changes of glomerular epithelial cells are observed. Thereafter urinary protein excretion rate declines but persists above normal control levels. With continuing proteinuria, glomerular lesions markedly worsen and segmental glomerulosclerosis is detectable at 18 weeks after the injection (49). The higher severity of this variant as compared to that observed after a single peripheral intravenous injection (44) has been related to higher drug levels reached in the kidney after central venous injection. Previous studies have shown that a form of chronic PA nephrosis can be induced by repeated subcutaneous doses (51,52). In Sprague-Dawley rats, proteinuria reaches values of 200 to 400 mg/24 hr at 7 weeks and persists thereafter, associated with segmental glomerular sclerotic lesions starting from 3 months after drug administration (52).

Adriamycin (ADR), the trademark for doxorubicin, one of the most employed antineoplastic drugs for clinical use, is an anthracycline that inhibits RNA and DNA synthesis through intercalation into DNA double helyx (53), binds to the cell membrane (54), and induces the formation of free oxygen radicals (55). Unlike PA, a single peripheral intravenous injection of ADR at doses of 5 to 7.5 mg/kg induces persisting proteinuria in the rat that evolves to glomerulosclerosis (56,57). The rabbit is also sensitive to the nephrotoxic effects of ADR, which have been observed with doses of 8 to 19 mg/kg (58). In humans the use of ADR (cycles of 1 mg/kg daily for 2 to 6 days) is associated with a cumulative dose-related cardiac toxicity, which manifests at total doses higher than 800 mg (59,60), but not with renal toxicity. ADR nephrosis in the rat is characterized by early morphological changes of glomerular visceral epithelial cells associated with proteinuria that manifests a few days after the injection of the drug (Fig. 1). However, the renal function is relatively preserved (61–63). Chronic ADR nephrosis is marked by sustained proteinuria, with light microscopy changes consisting of tubular cast formation and tubulointerstitial inflammation. Glomerular sclerotic lesions are observed in a significant proportion of glomeruli several weeks after the drug administration and are associated with progressive decrease in glomerular filtration (57,64,65).

Several studies have tried to clarify structural targets of the abnormal glomerular permeability to proteins induced by PA and ADR in the rat. Transplant experiments have demonstrated that proteinuria is the result of a direct insult on the kidney (66). Moreover, perfusion of a single kidney with PA or ADR causes unilateral renal damage (37,52,67). At the glomerular level, the main target of these molecules is likely the glomerular visceral epithelial cell. Glomerular epithelial cells exposed *in vitro* to PA or ADR loose their capacity to adhere to the plastic substratum and become unable to proliferate (68,69). However, whether severe proteinuria induced by PA and ADR is secondary to changes in the glomerular basement membrane or the podocyte remains largely unknown. One reason is that, as outlined before, both components of the capillary wall may serve to restrict the passage of proteins to the Bowman's space. Further, the effacement of foot processes, which is likely associated with epithelial cell dysfunction, can be regarded both as primary toxic effect of the drug and as consequence of proteinuria (70,71).

The glomerular epithelial cell is able to take up macromolecules such as albumin from the glomerular basement membrane by an endocytic process and to concentrate them in lysosomes (70). By measuring the disappearance rate of electron-dense protamine-heparin aggregates in the lamina rara externa after intravenous injection of protamine and heparin to PA nephrotic rats, Schwartz et al. (70) have evaluated whether PA may directly inhibit glomerular visceral epithelial cell endocytosis. Prior to the onset of PA-induced proteinuria the endocytic function of the podocyte was active, at a time when diffuse intracellular droplets of albumin were detectable along with the presence of focal loss of foot processes. Therefore, the glomerular basement membrane may represent the early site of altered permselectivity to proteins in this model. However, during the proteinuric phase of PA nephrosis, but not in a protein overload model with comparable degrees of proteinuria, the endocytic function was decreased in parallel with the disappearance of albumin droplets from the glomerular basement membrane, suggesting that PA directly causes defective endocytosis by inhibiting uptake of albumin and formation of lysosomes in the podocyte (72). Thus, toxic agents and drugs such as PA might induce early changes in the sieving characteristics of the different structural components of the glomerular capillary wall, possibly by inducing complex biochemical defects in the glomerular visceral epithelial cell.

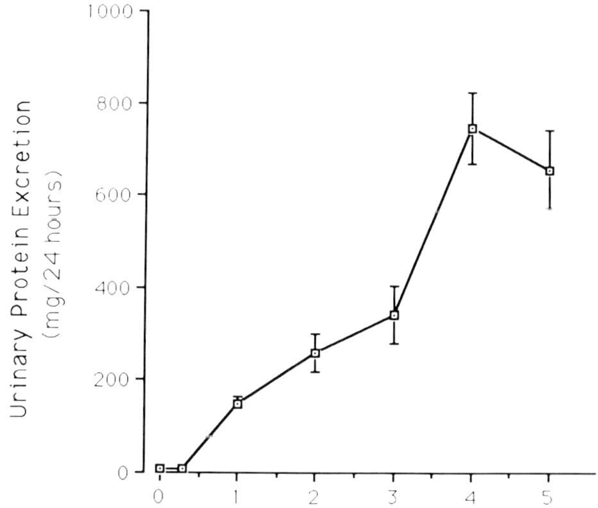

A

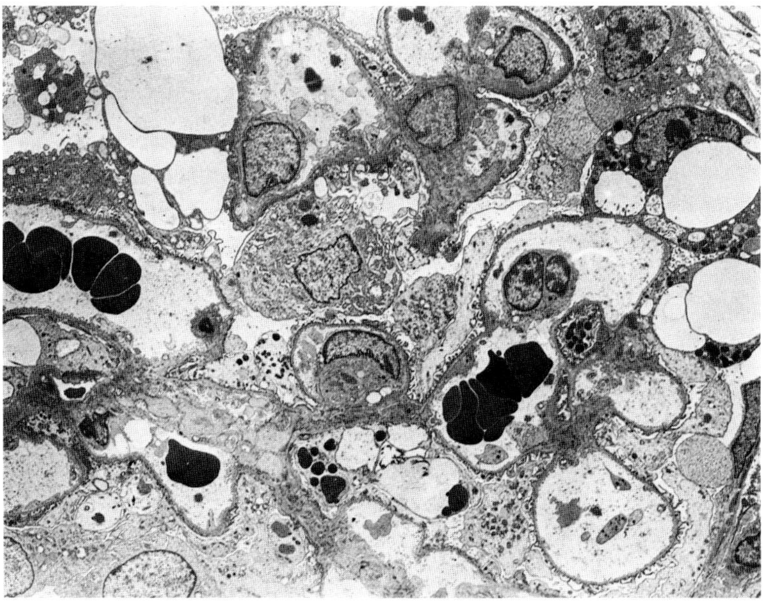

B

FIG. 1. A: Urinary protein excretion in rats following a single intravenous injection of Adriamycin (7.5 mg/kg/body weight). **B:** Electron micrograph of glomerular capillaries in nephrotic rat 28 days after injection of Adriamycin (7.5 mg/kg/body weight). Note the replacement of epithelial foot processes by expanses of epithelial cytoplasm, numerous vacuoles, and protein inclusion droplets. (×1,430.)

Drugs that are Toxic to the Glomerular Capillary Structures and Cause Abnormal Glomerular Permeability to Proteins by Altering Size and Charge Selectivity

Studies with macromolecular tracers have shown that in PA nephrosis both the size and the charge-selective properties of the glomerular capillary wall are impaired (39,47). Olson et al. (47) found that the fractional clearance of neutral dextrans and native horseradish peroxidase was significantly higher than normal, indicating a size-selective defect. However, the increased fractional clearance of anionic dextran sulfate and anionic horseradish peroxidase dextran sulfate indicated the coexistence of a charge-selective defect. In ADR nephrosis, Weening and Rennke (62), by measuring fractional clearances of anionic, native, and cationic horseradish peroxidases, found that the charge barrier was preserved. That ADR-induced proteinuria can result from a size-selective defect has been documented by the increased clearance of neutral dextran with molecular radius greater than 50 Å (62,73) and by the increased glomerular sieving coefficient of neutral IgG (74). However, the glomerular sieving coefficient for native anionic but not neutral bovine serum albumin was higher in ADR-treated rats than in control rats, indicating that charge barrier to albumin is also impaired (74). By fractional clearances of neutral and charged dextrans of different molecular radius it has been recently documented that both size- and charge-dependent permselective properties are altered in ADR nephrosis as previously found in PA nephrosis (75).

The defect in charge selectivity both in PA and ADR nephrosis has been attributed to the loss of anionic sites on the glomerular capillary wall. However, data from studies with cationic probes and autoradiographic techniques are not conclusive. With lysozyme and alcian blue staining the anionic sites of the glomerular capillary wall appeared significantly reduced (72,76), whereas data with cationic ferritin and ruthenium red in PA nephrosis failed to document the loss of polyanions, at least in the glomerular basement membrane (77). A loss of charge selectivity has been suggested by binding studies with protamine-heparin aggregates (78), showing an almost complete failure of these molecules to bind to the glomerular capillary wall in PA-nephrotic rats. Decreased binding of cuprolinic blue has also been reported in PA-treated rats, indicating a decrease of anionic charge, particularly of that endowed by sulfated groups and perhaps carboxyl groups present on structural proteins of the glomerular basement membrane (79). Kanwar and Jakubowski (80), employing a quantitative ultrastructural autoradiographic technique, were unable to find differences between normal and nephrotic rats in the binding of ^{125}I cationic ferritin to the glomerular basement membrane (80). In ADR nephrosis, Weening and Rennke (62), using the cationic probe polyethylenimine also failed to document a reduction of fixed anionic sites in the glomerular basement membrane. By contrast, Mahan et al. (81) and more recently Whiteside et al. (82), using a quantitative method with the same probe, found significantly fewer anionic sites in the basement membrane both of PA- (81,82) and ADR-treated rats (82) than in control animals. The charge defect was observed within 1 and 5 days from PA and

ADR injection, respectively, and preceded foot process effacement and nephrotic proteinuria (81,82).

Mechanisms and Mediators of Drug-Induced Changes in Glomerular Size and Charge Selectivity

Detachment of Epithelial Foot Processes

The loss of the size-selective barrier in epithelial cell disease has been related to focal detachment of podocytes from the glomerular basement membrane, at sites where increased passage of macromolecular tracers such as ferritin and peroxidase is visualized (47,83). Actually, the development of heavy proteinuria appears strictly associated with the detachment of the podocyte in this model. Results of early studies with peroxidase and catalase in PA-treated rats documented the penetration of exogenous tracers into basal pockets and vacuoles of epithelial cytoplasm overlying the glomerular basement membrane, thus suggesting that plasma proteins that penetrate the abnormally leaky glomerular basement membrane are then transferred across the epithelial layer of the capillary wall to the Bowman's space through a system of cytoplasmic vacuoles (83,84). That this may represent a major pathway for the passage of plasma proteins across the epithelial layer of the glomerular capillary wall is also indicated by recent findings obtained with ultrastructural analysis of serially sectioned glomeruli at different, timely closed stages in acute PA nephrosis (85). Before the onset of proteinuria the podocyte showed foot process effacement and cytoplasmic vacuoles. Coinciding with the sudden onset of proteinuria, large balloon-like spaces were found associated with a sevenfold increase in the number of sites of epithelial detachment from the glomerular basement membrane. Notably, a direct continuity was documented between sites of denuded glomerular basement membrane and the lumens of many large vacuoles, which now appeared to have ruptured into the urinary space. It was proposed that after the formation of small basal pockets of flattened epithelium over the glomerular basement membrane, a slow insudation of plasma across the denuded sites into the pockets may cause them to expand with formation and eventual rupture of large vacuoles. A similar sequence of events has been recently described in both PA and ADR nephrosis (82). The possibility that the vacuolar pathway may be responsible for proteinuria is intriguing. However, the incidence of transepithelial ruptures on transmission electron microscopy appears much less than that of focal detachments (82). Since the latter may directly allow increased bulk flow of plasma proteins to the Bowman's space through the defects, accurate morphometric analysis of detachment sites and ruptures is required to better define the contribution of the vacuolar pathway to the passage of proteins to the Bowman's space.

Altered Metabolism of Heparan Sulfate Proteoglycan and Sialoglycoproteins

Changes of the content of heparan sulfate proteoglycan in the capillary wall, as presumably reflected by reduced binding of polyethylenimine (37), may represent a major determinant of altered charge selectivity. By immunocytochemical detection of HSPG, a loss of the antigen has been observed after multiple PA injections (86). It has been recently reported that both renal and glomerular mRNA levels for HSPG markedly decrease in PA-nephrotic rats (87,88) and that they are improved by treatment with glucocorticosteroids, which are known to ameliorate proteinuria in PA nephrosis (88). Remarkably, dexamethasone has been shown recently to cause a dose- and time-dependent selective increase in the transcription and content of HSPG core protein in cultured glomerular epithelial cells (89). In this regard, Fishman and Karnovsky (68) studied the effects of PA on cultured visceral epithelial cells and demonstrated direct effects on cell membrane characteristics possibly through protein-lipid disorganization, and changes in the glucosamine and sulfated glycoprotein metabolic pathway.

Before the discovery of HSPG within the glomerular basement membrane, epithelial sialoproteins were considered the most important anionic components of the glomerulus. Both in PA (90) and ADR nephrosis (56,62), glomerular sialoproteins were markedly reduced by light microscopy examination after colloidal iron staining but unchanged by ultrastructural studies of the binding of cationic molecules (91). Thus, the light microscopy finding of reduced colloidal iron staining could have been due to a reduction of visceral epithelial cell surface consequent to obliteration of foot processes. This interpretation was challenged by Kerjaschki et al. (24), who found in PA nephrosis a markedly reduced sialylation of podocalyxin of the glomerular epithelial cell together with loss of foot processes and slit organization. Similar results have been obtained with a lectin-gold technique (25) and with the measurement of the total membrane-bound sialic acid content of isolated glomeruli obtained from PA-treated rats before the onset of nephrotic proteinuria (82). Conversely, measurements of the activity of neuraminidase, a lysosomal enzyme that cleaves sialic acid from sialoglycoproteins and sialoglycolipids, failed to show significant changes in glomeruli of rats with PA nephrosis both at the onset and peak proteinuria (46). That abnormal sialylation may occur also in ADR nephrosis is indicated by reduced labeling of sialic acid residues within the capillary wall with a biotinylation procedure (31). However, the functional significance of this finding in ADR nephrosis needs to be clarified, since a reduction in the glomerular sialic acid content may follow rather than precede the onset of nephrotic proteinuria (82). Sialoglycoproteins appear crucial to the attachment of epithelial cell foot processes to the basement membrane, so that their loss might favor focal detachment of the podocyte and altered size permselectivity of the glomerular barrier (17,24, 28,77).

Altered Metabolism of Laminin, Collagen, and Fibronectin

Besides proteoglycans and sialoglycoproteins, PA may interfere with the synthesis and degradation of other structural proteins and enzymes in the glomerulus that might be relevant to the glomerular permeability. Thus, during the acute phase of PA nephrosis mRNA levels for laminin, collagen, and fibronectin are abnormal in the kidney. Actually, the renal content of mRNA for type IV collagen and laminin decreased (92) followed by a marked increase of glomerular mRNAs for these molecules (87,92) and for fibronectin (88) in the nephrotic stage of the disease. Findings that the neutral proteinase metalloendopeptidase and the tissue inhibitor of metalloproteinases can be released by cultured glomerular mesangial cells and that metalloendopeptidase extensively degrades the glomerular basement membrane and type IV collagen suggest that these enzymes play a role in the turnover of glomerular basement membrane glycoproteins *in vivo* (93). Imbalances in the glomerular content of metalloendopeptidase and the tissue inhibitor of metalloendopeptidase may result in altered production of type IV collagen and changes in the permselective properties of the glomerular capillary wall. In this regard, Davin et al. (94) found in acute PA nephrosis a significant increase in urinary excretion of neutral proteinases, which correlated both with proteinuria and urinary excretion of type IV collagen and laminin, suggesting that neutral proteinases may be involved in the altered glomerular permeability. That changes in these enzymatic pathway occur in PA nephrosis is further indicated by the finding of higher renal mRNA levels for tissue inhibitor of metalloproteinases at 1 week after PA injection (92).

The effects of these metabolic changes on the glomerular permselectivity are presently unknown. Altered macromolecular assemblage of the glomerular basement membrane might directly cause abnormal permselectivity of the capillary wall (33) (Fig. 2). Further, matrix proteins can modify cell shape (95) and function (96). In this respect, since β_1-integrins, which bind components of the basement membrane, are present on the soles of foot processes (24,97), one can speculate that both altered matrix composition and changes in glomerular synthesis and distribution of molecules that anchor the cell membrane to the glomerular basement membrane contribute to detachment of podocytes from the basement membrane.

Lipid Mediators, Oxygen Free Radicals, and Cytokines

Altered arachidonic acid metabolism seems to be involved in the pathogenesis of proteinuria in epithelial cell disease. Conflicting results have emerged on the role of thromboxane (TX) A_2 in PA nephrosis, since some authors have found that urinary excretion and glomerular production of TXA_2, measured as immunoreactive TXB_2, did not increase (98,99), whereas others have shown that inhibiting TXA_2 synthesis is of value (100). In rats with ADR nephrosis a significant increase both of glomerular synthesis and urinary excretion of TXB_2 has been documented. The increase of TXB_2 was concomitant with the appearance of proteinuria and reached its maximum at the time of peak proteinuria. Administration of UK-38485, a selective thromboxane synthase inhibitor, significantly reduced the exaggerated renal TXB_2 production and lowered proteinuria in ADR nephrotic rats (101). Experiments with isolated perfused kidneys of rats given ADR have documented that the exaggerated TXB_2 excretion in ADR nephrosis originates from resident renal cells (102). The mecha-

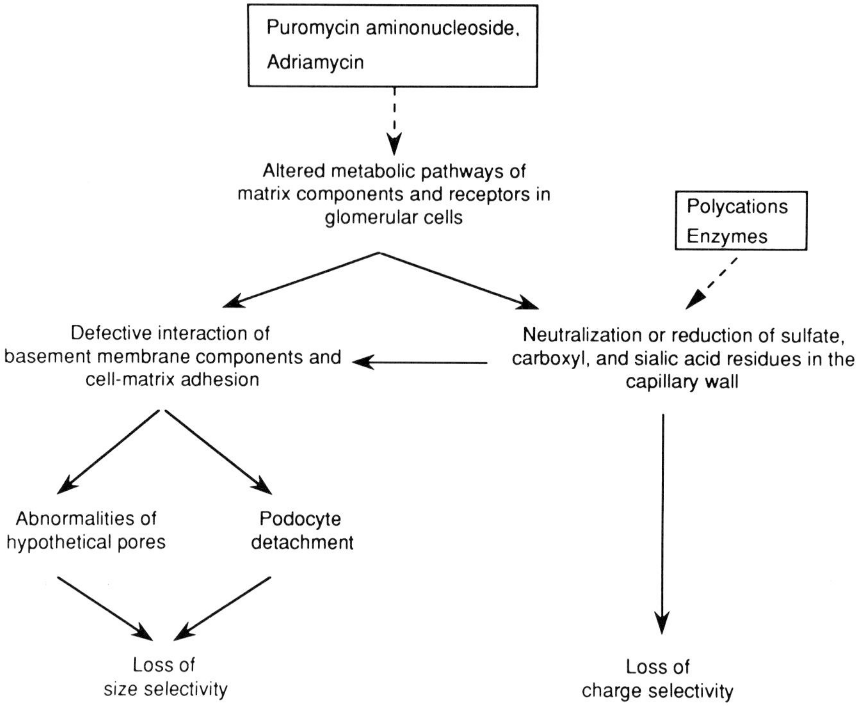

FIG. 2. Potential mechanisms of altered glomerular size and charge selective properties induced by drugs and toxic substances.

nism by which TXB_2 might induce abnormal permeability to proteins is largely unknown. Inhibiting TXA_2 synthesis is likely to interfere directly with TXA_2-dependent changes in permselective properties of the glomerular barrier (103).

Platelet activating factor (PAF) released by resident glomerular cells might cooperate with TXA_2 in inducing proteinuria in toxic models of epithelial cell disease. Recently it has been documented that a specific PAF receptor antagonist is able to ameliorate proteinuria and glomerular injury in ADR nephrosis (104). PAF directly causes proteinuria without inducing altered distribution of polyethylenimine stainable anionic sites when perfused in isolated rat kidney preparations (105). That PAF modifies glomerular size-selective properties is indicated by findings of increased fractional clearance of large dextrans (radius >50 Å) but not small neutral dextrans (24 to 48 Å) during PAF infusion (106).

Studies with pharmacological manipulations have suggested that reactive oxygen species, in particular superoxide anion and hydroxyl radical, may mediate effects of PA and ADR on the glomerular permselectivity (50,104,107,108). Cellular mechanisms by which oxygen metabolites damage the glomerular capillary wall are discussed below. However, it should be emphasized that in these models reactive oxygen species may induce proteinuria through perturbations in the epithelial synthesis of proteoglycans and sialoproteins (109).

As sources of eicosanoids, PAF, and reactive oxygen species, the mesangial cell may play a role in the development and evolution of toxic glomerular injury. In this respect it is possible that ADR and PA damage the glomerulus through effects on mesangial cells. Schreiner et al. (110) showed that 10 to 14 days after injection of PA there is an increase both in the number of glomerular macrophages and in their Ia expression accompanying peak proteinuria. Essential fatty acid deficiency prevents the increases both in glomerular macrophage number in glomerular TXB_2 production during the peak albuminuric phase, 2 weeks after injection of PA (99). The relationship between mesangial cell dysfunction and proteinuria in acute PA nephrosis is unclear. In a recent report by Harris et al. (98), essential fatty acid deficiency was associated with amelioration both of proteinuria and hypoalbuminemia at 14 to 21 days after PA administration. In rats with acute ADR nephrosis an increase of Ia-bearing glomerular macrophages has been found to correlate with proteinuria (111). In addition, increased secretion of tumor necrosis factor (TNF) has been found (112) both from glomeruli of rats with ADR nephrosis and from glomeruli, glomerular macrophages, and mesangial cells stimulated *in vitro* with ADR, suggesting a role for macrophages and mesangial cell-derived cytokines in this model. Of interest, TNF might mediate glomerular effects of PAF after ADR administration, as indicated by the finding that ADR nephrotic rats given a PAF receptor antagonist, BN 52021, had a decrease both in proteinuria (104,112) and glomerular production of TNF as compared to untreated rats with ADR nephrosis (112). Further studies are needed to clarify possible effects of cytokines on the glomerular permselective properties and their significance as mediators of toxic-induced glomerular damage.

Is Altered Glomerular Permeability that Results from a Toxic Insult to the Capillary Wall Responsible for the Progression of the Disease?

In analogy to various human diseases of the kidney and other rat models of chronic proteinuria, ADR and PA nephrosis progress to glomerulosclerosis and end-stage renal failure. Some human diseases, such as the nephropathy of acquired immune deficiency syndrome and heroin-associated nephropathy, are suspected to result from a primary insult to the glomerular visceral epithelial cells (36). The precise biochemical and molecular mechanisms of glomerulosclerosis after epithelial cell damage are still largely unknown. Glomerulosclerosis is considered the consequence of the interaction of diverse pathophysiological processes common to a wide spectrum of diseases (36,71). According to Brenner et al.'s (113) group hypothesis, sustained elevation of glomerular pressures and flows in remnant glomeruli is responsible for progressive renal insufficiency after loss of a critical number of functioning nephrons. In rat models, such as remnant kidney and streptozotocin-induced diabetes, protein restriction protects animals against proteinuria and renal disease progression.

The beneficial effects of low protein feeding are associated with prevention of glomerular capillary hypertension and hyperperfusion. The crucial role of altered glomerular hemodynamics in the development of glomerular injury in these models has been documented by the finding that angiotensin-converting enzyme inhibitors reduce urinary protein excretion rate by preventing glomerular capillary hypertension (114,115). Since both in PA and ADR nephrosis low protein diet is also of benefit (63,116), the question arises of whether altered glomerular hemodynamics play a role in the abnormal permeability to proteins in these settings. However, no conclusive data are available so far. In PA nephrosis, Fogo et al. (65) found normal intraglomerular capillary pressure in the early phase of the disease. This is challenged by the work of Anderson et al. (117), who found that glomerular capillary pressure in the early phase of PA nephrosis was normal but increased later in the course of the disease. In the latter phase, angiotensin-converting enzyme inhibition lessened both abnormal urinary protein excretion and glomerulosclerosis (117). In ADR nephrosis Fogo et al. measured normal glomerular capillary hydraulic pressure (65), whereas others found a significant increase (61,118). In the same model Scholey et al. (118) demonstrated that enalapril preserves glomerular filtration rate compared to untreated animals, without beneficial effects on proteinuria and glomerulosclerosis (118). Other recent studies have confirmed that angiotensin-converting enzyme inhibition is unable to decrease proteinuria in ADR nephrosis (119,120).

Although these data are conflicting as to the role of altered glomerular hemodynamics in PA and ADR nephrosis, they lend support to the hypothesis that abnormal transit of plasma proteins through the glomerular capillary wall may be the key factor in glomerulosclerosis (71). Glomerular obsolescence induced by nephrotoxic drugs, extensive renal ablation, or aging shares a sustained abnormality in glomerular permeability to macromolecules that can be regarded as the common determinant of glomerulosclerosis (71). Increased flux of macromolecules may induce dysfunction of mesangial, epithelial, and tubular cells in such a way as to favor the process of glomerulosclerosis. Thus, enhanced mesangial traffic of macromolecules may stimulate mesangial cells to proliferate and produce mesangial matrix components. This is suggested by the observation that in rats with PA nephrosis (121) sclerotic lesions develop in areas of increased accumulation of colloidal carbon tracer, so that glomeruli with focal sclerosis contain significantly more carbon than normal. Visceral glomerular epithelial cells react to filtered proteins with the development of functional and structural abnormalities (71), such as reduced release of heparin-like factor(s) that control the proliferation of mesangial cells (68,71), and focal detachment from basement membrane. The latter further favors the passage of macromolecules across the glomerular capillaries (36). This results in an increased amount of proteins in the ultrafiltrate that overwhelms proximal tubular epithelial cell reabsorption capacity (122). Thus, in ADR nephrosis the abnormal amount of proteins delivered to distal tubuli leads to the formation of casts breaking off the tubular basement membrane and to an interstitial inflammatory reaction (122). Inflammatory cells surrounding the glomeruli release factors that directly or through activation of resident glomerular cells may stimulate mesangial cells to proliferate and generate abnormal mesangial matrix. Inflammatory mediators such as TXA_2, interleukin-1, platelet-derived growth factor, and transforming growth factor-β are likely involved in this process (71). Findings that the TXA_2 mimetic U-46619 stimulates [^{3}H]-thymidine uptake in quiescent human mesangial cells in culture (123) suggest that TXA_2 could contribute to the process of glomerulosclerosis by inducing mesangial cells proliferation. Further, U-46619 increases the expression of genes for type IV collagen (α_1 and α_2) via activation of DNA regulatory regions in mesangial cells (124). The role of TXA_2 in regulating the expression of extracellular matrix components *in vivo* is suggested by the observation that in mice with non-insulin-dependent diabetes the TXA_2 synthase inhibitor U-63557 prevented the increase in type IV collagen mRNA levels of basement membrane of kidney cortex (125).

GLOMERULAR HEMODYNAMICS AND ULTRAFILTRATION

In recent years, the knowledge of potential mechanisms of regulation of determinants of glomerular filtration rate (GFR) has been considerably expanded (126,127). Alterations in afferent and/or efferent arteriolar tone result in changes in renal blood flow (RBF) and glomerular plasma flow rate. Evidence is now accumulating that the contraction of glomerular mesangial cells in response to vasoactive agents can regulate the glomerular capillary surface area and therefore the glomerular ultrafiltration coefficient (K_f) (126). Actually, the glomerular mesangial cells are endowed with numerous cytoplasmic contractile myofilaments and express on the plasma membrane specific receptors for several vasoactive substances, such as angiotensin II, TXA_2, PAF, and endothelin (128–130), all of which stimulate the contraction of mesangial cells *in vitro*. In addition, the mesangial cells synthesize vasoactive substances, including TXA_2, PAF, and endothelin (128,131), that may act by an autocrine pattern on the glomerular filtration. More in detail, neurohormonal mediators subserve renal microvascular responses that are responsible for changes in determinants of GFR *in vivo*. Afferent and efferent arteriolar resistances are increased by direct and reflex increases in *renal nerve activity* (132,133). The enhancement of adrenergic tone also determines a fall in K_f, likely through reduction in available filtering surface area (134).

The *renin-angiotensin system* is well known to contribute to the control of GFR. Intravenous infusion of angiotensin II induces increase in afferent and efferent arteriolar resistances (132) as well as a significant reduction in K_f (135). Angiotensin II is thought to mediate the so-called tubuloglomerular feedback mechanism (136). This is a reflex that reduces both glomerular plasma flow rate and K_f in response to increased chloride uptake by the macula densa subsequent to increase in the flow rate in the loop of Henle (126,137), thus contributing to the control of single nephron-GFR. *Arachidonate metabolites* are also known to influence GFR. Among metabolites derived from the cyclooxygenase pathway, TXA_2 is a potent vasoconstrictor that reduces GFR in normal rats by increasing glomerular afferent and efferent arteriolar resistances (138). TXA_2 also stimulates contraction of cultured rat mesangial cells through an elevation of free cytosolic calcium (130). In contrast, prostaglandins E_2 (PGE_2) and I_2 (PGI_2) act as vasodilators in the kidney, reduce renal vascular resistance, and antagonize angiotensin II–induced and TXA_2-induced mesangial contraction (139). Sulfidopeptide leukotrienes LTC_4 and LTD_4, arachidonate metabolites formed via the 5-lipoxygenase pathway, increase renal vascular resistance and reduce GFR when infused in the intact animal (140) as well as in the isolated perfused rat kidney (141). The infusion of *endothelin*, a novel constrictor peptide derived from vascular endothelial cells (142), elicits in the rat a concentration-dependent increase in renal vascular resistance and reduction in GFR (127). Similarly, in isolated perfused rat kidneys, proportional changes in GFR and renal plasma flow (RPF) have been reported over a wide range of endothelin doses (143). Further, endothelin contracts mesangial cells *in vitro* and lowers K_f through stimulation of inositol 1,4,5-triphosphate generation associated with elevation of intracellular calcium (144,145).

Mechanisms and Mediators by which Drugs Cause Acute Impairment of Glomerular Filtration

The above-mentioned vasoactive mediators have potential pathophysiological relevance in models of renal injury in which RBF and K_f are low. For instance, in experimental congestive heart failure and acute water deprivation renal denervation attenuates renal vasoconstriction and increases K_f (146), suggesting that reductions in both RBF and K_f in these settings may be caused by increased renal nerve activity. The renin-angiotensin system has also been implicated in the impaired glomerular filtration in models of renal disease (147,148). Activation of the renin angiotensin system may be associated with stimulation of the tubuloglomerular feedback. This may occur as an indirect consequence of damage to the proximal convoluted tubule (137) and perhaps as a direct functional effect of toxic molecules, thus leading to impaired glomerular filtration. Recent experimental evidence indicates that arachidonate metabolites are critical in volume-depleted animals and in disease conditions (149,150). Thus, a marked increase in TXA_2 synthesis not counterbalanced by a parallel increase in PGE_2 and PGI_2 is expected to decrease GFR and renal plasma flow. This mechanism likely plays a role in renal function impairment during glomerular diseases, such as in the autologous phase of rabbit nephrotoxic nephritis (150). Endothelin has recently been found to have a pivotal role in the renal vasoconstriction characteristic of postischemic renal failure (151).

There are examples of how mechanisms and mediators of altered glomerular hemodynamics may variably contribute to impaired glomerular filtration in drug nephrotoxicity. Thus, acute renal vasoconstriction seems to play a major role both in cyclosporin A and amphotericin B nephrotoxicity; in the latter setting, evidence has been provided that the decreased K_f also significantly contributes to reduction of GFR. Reduction in K_f has been shown to account for the hemodynamic component of gentamicin nephrotoxicity, even in the absence of significant changes in the rate of renal perfusion.

Cyclosporin A

The clinical use of cyclosporin A (CyA) is often associated with acute dose-related decrease in renal function (152,153). The episodes of acute renal insufficiency are usually rapidly reversible after the daily dose of CyA is reduced (154). The acute effect of CyA on renal function in animal models varies with respect to species or strain of animal as well as dose, mode of administration, and duration of treatment (155). Initial studies aimed at identifying the structural targets of acute CyA nephrotoxicity in the rat have documented proximal tubule epithelial cell damage (156) and leakage into the urine of lysosome-associated enzymes, such as *N*-acetyl-*p*-glucosaminidase (157). Tubular morphological changes have been also described in patients with CyA-induced acute renal failure (158,159). The tubular toxicity may be the result of deposition of CyA or its metabolites in tubular cells when high concentrations of the drug are reached in the blood. It has been proposed that the toxic effect to the tubular epithelium leads to increased back pressure along nephrons blocked by damaged tubules, and activation of tubuloglomerular feedback that lowers glomerular flow (160). However, findings of enhanced proximal tubular reabsorption and decreased distal delivery of sodium in CyA-treated rats (161) make such possibility unlikely. Moreover, several studies in the rat have documented elevated renovascular resistance, diminished RBF, and decline in GFR (155,162, 163) after CyA administration, without evidence of tubular cell injury or even before tubular damage develops (161). These data suggest that CyA induces impairment of renal function by primarily affecting renal vessels rather than proximal tubules. In order to divorce direct acute effects on renal function from indirect effects caused by systemic CyA toxicity, experiments have been performed with the model of isolated perfused rat kidney, a preparation in which systemic influences on renal function can be eliminated (164,165). With this technique it has been shown that CyA causes a dose-dependent fall in renal perfusate flow associated with a concomitant increase in renal vascular resistance (164). Accordingly, a concentration-dependent increase in perfusion pressure has been found in isolated rat kidneys perfused at constant flow and exposed to CyA (165). The morphological correlate to these functional changes has been recently provided by a study with scanning electron microscopy, showing progressive narrowing in afferent arteriolar diameter that paralleled the decrease in inulin clearance (166).

Several mechanisms have been proposed to mediate CyA-induced renal vasoconstriction. No definitive evidence has been provided of activation of the renin-angiotensin system and sympathetic nervous system. CyA stimulates *in vitro* renin release both in renal cortical slices (167) and isolated juxtaglomerular cells (168). However, although plasma renin is increased in CyA-treated animals, improvements in renal hemodynamics have not been uniformly observed following converting enzyme inhibition in rats given CyA (163,169,170). Recent studies have shown that CyA increases the activity of the renal sympathetic nerves (171). Findings that denervated kidneys fail to constrict in response to CyA *in vivo* (163) and that α-adrenergic inhibitors antagonize CyA-induced renal vasoconstriction in innervated kidneys (163), support the contention that the renal sympathetic nerves mediate CyA-induced renal vasoconstriction, at least in part. However, acute CyA toxicity with a decrease in GFR and RPF is seen in denervated human renal transplants (172). α-Adrenergic antagonism also fails to affect significantly renal function in CyA-treated transplant recipients (173).

Arachidonic acid metabolites likely play a role in CyA-induced renal vasoconstriction. Although effects on vasodilatory prostaglandins are controversial (163, 174–176), CyA consistently augments the generation of TXA_2. Incubation of cultured bovine endothelial cells with CyA causes cell injury associated with dose and time-dependent increase in TXA_2 production (176). *In vivo* studies have shown increased urinary excretion of immunoreactive TXB_2 in rats given short-term CyA (177–179). Further, specific inhibition of endogenous TXA_2 activity with a receptor antagonist, GR 32191, partially prevents the decline in GFR and RPF induced by acute CyA administration to rats, pointing out a major role for TXA_2 as hemodynamic mediator of renal toxicity (180,181). The administration of a specific TXA_2 synthase inhibitor also enhances GFR and RPF in patients with a recent renal transplant treated with CyA (181). Additional support is garnered by the finding that the use of fish oil vehicle rich in eicosapentaenoic acid, which inhibits renal eicosanoids synthesis, increases GFR, and reduces renal TXA_2 content in rats with experimentally induced CyA toxicity (182). The fact that inhibiting TXA_2 synthesis or biological activity ameliorates but does not normalize renal function suggests that in addition to TXA_2 other factors are involved in the acute reduction of GFR induced by CyA. Among arachidonate metabolites, LTC_4 and LTD_4 may play a role in mediating this effect of CyA. This has been suggested by the demonstration that a specific LTC_4/LTD_4 receptor antagonist, L-649,923, also partially prevents the fall in GFR and RPF caused by acute CyA administration to rats (180). Remarkably, TXA_2 and LTC_4/LTD_4 may act in concert to mediate acute renal vasoconstriction caused by CyA, as indicated by the observation that the combined administration of a specific TXA_2 receptor antagonist and a LTC_4/LTD_4 receptor antagonist completely abolishes CyA-induced fall in GFR and RPF (180).

An interrelationship between arachidonate metabolites and other vasoactive substances may also occur in the course of increasing renal vascular resistance following CyA administration. In this regard, the exposure of umbilical vein endothelial cells in culture to the TXA_2 mimetic U-46619 enhances the expression of preproendothelin mRNA associated with synthesis and release of the corresponding peptide in the cell supernatant (131). U-46619 stimulates endothelin gene expression and production also in human glomerular mesangial cells in culture (131). That CyA induces alterations in endothelin synthesis and/or metabolism is indicated by data showing that human aortic and glomerular endothelial cells in culture exposed to CyA released endothelin in a dose-dependent manner (183) and that in rats serum endothelin levels, 20 min after acute CyA infusion, were remarkably higher than in rats given vehicle (184). The possibility that the increased renal vascular resistance caused by CyA can be attributed at least in part to actions of endothelin at the glomerular level is consistent with the fact that the effects of CyA and endothelin on glomerular hemodynamics are very similar (145). Evidence for the role of endothelin in acute CyA nephrotoxicity has been recently provided in isolated perfused rat kidney preparations in which preexposure to a specific antiendothelin antibody markedly prevented CyA-induced reduction in GFR and renal perfusate flow and increased renal vascular resistance (164) (Fig. 3). Additional support comes from *in vivo* experiments, showing that an antiendothelin antibody prevented the decline in GFR induced by giving CyA to normal rats (164). In line with these findings, recent micropuncture studies of Kon et al. (184) also documented a protective effect of an antiendothelin antibody on CyA-induced acute glomerular vasoconstriction. Of note, the recent finding that, as compared to coronary, bronchial, and femoral, the renal vascular bed is most sensitive to the vasoconstrictory effect of endothelin (185) provides an explanation for the clinical observation that CyA has a peculiar toxic effect on the kidney.

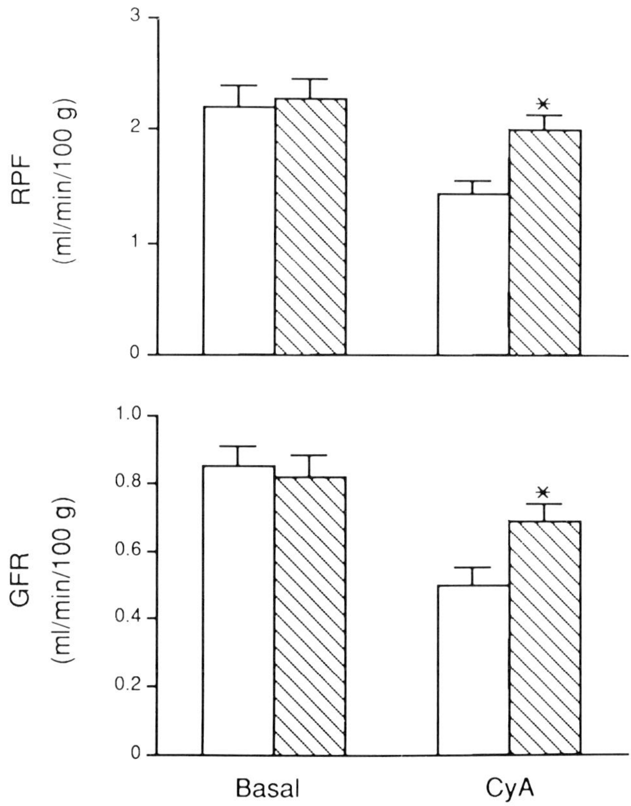

FIG. 3. Effect of nonimmune serum (□) or antibody antiendothelin (▧) infusion on renal plasma flow (RPF) and glomerular filtration rate (GFR) in the baseline period and after cyclosporin A intravenous administration in rats. *$p < .01$ vs. nonimmune serum after cyclosporin A infusion.

Gentamicin

At variance with CyA, a form of toxic injury to the proximal tubule cell is considered the predominant process responsible for impaired renal function in gentamicin nephrotoxicity (186). However, micropuncture studies have documented changes in hemodynamic determinants of glomerular filtration (148,187,188), thus raising the possibility that primary disturbances in the glomerular filtration contribute to the reduction of GFR that occurs with the administration of gentamicin. In the study of Baylis et al. (187), Munich-Wistar rats treated with gentamicin for 10 days at the dose of 4 or 40 mg/kg/day exhibited decreases in the mean values of both total and single-nephron GFR. A small reduction in the mean value of glomerular plasma flow was also found only in animals given 40 mg/kg. The primary cause for the reduction in single-nephron GFR was a marked decrease in the average value of K_f. In spite of extensive tubular damage, there was no evidence of altered tubular permeability to inulin (187). Electron microscopy examination revealed no obvious glomerular abnormalities (187), despite dose-dependent decrements in glomerular endothelial fenestral size, density, and area documented by some authors in rats given gentamicin (189). Although the specificity of glomerular endothelial abnormalities in this as well as other forms of acute renal failure is uncertain (190), their presence would suggest that glomerular endothelial cell dysfunction may contribute to impaired glomerular filtration in these settings.

Relatively few studies have investigated mechanisms underlying the defect in glomerular ultrafiltration associated with gentamicin. Schor et al. (148) examined the effects of angiotensin II blockade or long-term high salt intake on gentamicin nephrotoxicity in male Munich-Wistar rats. Inhibiting angiotensin II generation almost completely prevented gentamicin-induced changes in single-nephron GFR, K_f, and glomerular plasma flow. That angiotensin-converting enzyme inhibition protects from the K_f-lowering action of gentamicin has been confirmed recently in female Munich-Wistar rats (188). However, in other experiments angiotensin-converting enzyme inhibition with captopril did not prevent the decrease in GFR and the development of tubular and glomerular morphological changes in male Sprague-Dawley rats given gentamicin at the dose of 80 mg/kg/day for 10 days (191). Further when gentamicin was administered to rats with chronic potassium depletion, captopril worsened renal function, morphology, and glomerular ultrafiltration (192). In addition to differences in doses and rat strains, these apparently conflicting results may be reconciled by the observation that captopril, besides inhibiting angiotensin II formation, exerts other actions including stimulation of the renal release of TXB_2 and kinins, which may have adversely influenced renal function in potassium depleted rats given gentamicin (193). Actually, *ex vivo* perfused kidneys from potassium depleted rats that received both gentamicin and captopril produced significantly greater amounts of TXA_2, measured as immunoreactive TXB_2 in the venous effluent, than did kidneys from potassium-depleted rats given gentamicin alone (192). In rats given gentamicin and captopril, RBF and the clearance of inulin increased during intrarenal infusion of imidazole, a thromboxane synthase inhibitor, or aprotinin, a kallikrein antagonist (192). Thus, although the glomerular toxicity of gentamicin is likely mediated by mechanisms that are sensitive to converting enzyme inhibition, hemodynamic mediators other than angiotensin II, such as TXB_2 and kinins, may also be involved in the decreased GFR observed in this setting.

Amphotericin B

The use of amphotericin B is frequently complicated by renal dysfunction. Signs of renal toxicity, including azotemia associated with depressed GFR, have been reported in more than 80% of treated patients (194). The renal functional changes induced by amphotericin B are dose related and usually reversible after the withdrawal of the drug (194). Pathological examination in humans shows acute tubular necrosis, with tubular dilatation and calcifications (195). Glomerular and vascular morphological changes have also been reported including thickening of the glomerular basement membrane, glomerular hypercellularity and hyalinization (196, 197), and vacuolization of the media of small arteries and arterioles (195).

Altered renal hemodynamics contribute to impaired glomerular function in amphotericin B nephrotoxicity (198–201). Butler et al. (199) reported that a single intravenous bolus of amphotericin B in dogs produces a decrease in RBF and GFR. Renal angiograms showed decreased accumulation of contrast in the renal cortex, suggesting that acute infusion of amphotericin B induces preglomerular vessel constriction. In rats, the calculated whole renal vascular resistance was more than doubled and the calculated glomerular capillary hydrostatic pressure was decreased after the intravenous infusion of the drug, consistent with afferent arteriolar constriction (202). RPF rose to control levels immediately after the end of the infusion. However, it was decreased significantly 3 hr later. At this time the decrease in the clearance of inulin was much greater than the decrease in RPF (68% vs. 33%), suggesting that beside depressed RPF and GFR increased tubular permeability with increased "backleak" of tubule fluid may also contribute to the decreased clearance of inulin in this model. Renal dysfunction and hemodynamic changes were reversible within 24 hr. The absence of obvious histological abnormalities, in particular tubular cell necrosis, in this study favors a functional nature of the hemodynamic and tubular changes in amphotericin B nephrotoxicity (202). A biphasic response to acute infusion of amphotericin B in rats has been also described more recently by Tolins and Raij (203). Further, they found a marked increase in renal vascular resistance and a fall in RPF and GFR in rats treated for 21 days with amphotericin B, suggesting that renal vasoconstriction also operates in a chronic model of amphotericin B nephrotoxicity (203).

In addition to increased afferent arteriolar resistance with reduction of RPF, a decrease in K_f may mediate the depressant action of amphotericin B on GFR. Calcium channel blockade with verapamil inhibited completely the renal vasoconstriction induced by the intravenous infusion of amphotericin B in rats (203). This effect was associated with a delayed and blunted decline in GFR during the infusion of amphotericin B. However, in the early postinfusion period GFR fell to a similar extent to that in rats not pretreated with verapamil. Therefore, the renal vasoconstrictive effect, preventable by calcium channel blockade, does not fully account for the decline in GFR, which in this model may result in part from a decrease in K_f (203). Actually, a micropuncture study from the group of Badr has recently documented that intrarenal infusion of amphotericin B in rats induces both significant increases in pre- and postglomerular resistances and a significant (25%) decrease in K_f (204). These changes were associated with decreases in single-nephron RPF and GFR in the absence of effects on the mean arterial pressure and the net hydrostatic pressure difference across the glomerular capillary, thereby indicating that amphotericin B causes reduction in single-nephron GFR both through afferent and efferent arterial vasoconstriction-induced fall in RPF and through a reduction in K_f (204).

The mechanisms by which amphotericin B is able to elicit renal microvascular responses have not been identified so far. It seems unlikely that amphotericin B is directly toxic to renal microcirculation by the same mechanisms that are thought responsible for its cytotoxic effects on tubular cells. Rather, the observation that amphotericin B is able to induce contraction of mesangial cells *in vitro* would suggest that the drug may directly elicit renal microvascular responses (204). The ability of amphotericin B to induce contraction of smooth muscle–like cells *in vivo* may be linked also to interference with the local release of vasoactive agents. This could occur via activation of the tubuloglomerular feedback, a mechanism that is suspected to be involved in amphotericin B nephrotoxicity. Salt loading, furosemide, or theophylline administration, maneuvers that inhibit tubuloglomerular feedback, have been shown to inhibit the decrease in RBF and GFR induced by amphotericin in experimental animals (200,205). Likewise, increasing sodium intake improved renal function in patients in whom amphotericin B nephrotoxicity developed (201). Since angiotensin II is considered an important mediator of the tubuloglomerular feedback, as suggested by the fact that angiotensin-converting enzyme inhibition is associated with attenuation of the feedback response (136), the role of the renin-angiotensin system in the renal hemodynamic effects of amphotericin B has been examined. The pretreatment with sar-gly angiotensin II, an angiotensin II receptor blocker, failed to prevent the decreases in GFR and RBF induced in the rat by the infusion of a vasoconstrictive dose of amphotericin B (203). Therefore, the roles both of tubuloglomerular feedback and the renin-angiotensin system in amphotericin B–induced renal vasoconstriction and impaired renal function remain uncertain. Similarly, adrenergic and ganglion blocking agents (199) and unilateral renal denervation (203) failed to protect animals against hemodynamic changes induced by amphotericin B, indicating that the sympathetic nervous system does not directly mediate these effects of the drug. The beneficial effects of verapamil on renal perfusion in amphotericin B nephrotoxicity (203) may be related to a direct vasodilatory action of calcium channel blocking. However, changes in cytoplasmic calcium concentration may also act to attenuate the generation of vasoactive mediators, such as arachidonic acid metabolites and PAF (206), that might contribute to impaired renal function in this setting. Further studies are needed to clarify the role of these vasoactive substances in amphotericin B nephrotoxicity.

Persistent Renal Vasoconstriction and Progressive Renal Damage in Chronic Drug Nephrotoxicity

Hormonally mediated mechanisms may contribute to acute decrease in glomerular filtration induced by nephrotoxic drugs in the absence of renal structural changes. In the case of gentamicin and amphotericin B, clinical nephrotoxicity is observed with acute and short-term administration and is usually reversible after cessation of therapy or reduction in dose. Little is known about potential effects of prolonged treatment with these drugs on renal morphology and glomerular filtration. Conversely, the use of CyA has recently provided evidence that long-term administration of a drug that causes acute reversible renal dysfunction may promote progressive decrease in GFR and eventual loss of renal function associated with the development of irreversible anatomical changes at the level of the renal microcirculation. Actually, the form of renal injury that develops after long-term exposure to the drug is the main clinical problem related to CyA administration in humans (207–209). Clinical trials have demonstrated a sustained increase in serum creatinine in CyA-treated patients versus patients on conventional immunosuppression (210–214), indicating that CyA causes a chronic form of renal injury. Evidence is available that liver (215) and pancreas (173) allograft recipients or patients with autoimmune diseases (216,217) have low GFR. In heart transplant recipients with healthy native kidneys, both high (218,219) and low (219) doses of CyA, if given for more than 12 months, were associated with a marked decline in GFR and RPF. Chronic renal injury, once established, was not reversed either by substantial reduction of CyA dose or by its complete withdrawal (218). Further, end-stage renal failure developed in a proportion of these patients (218,219). Progressive deterioration in renal function has been documented also in CyA-treated cadaveric renal transplant recipients (220).

The pattern of pathological changes that are associated with chronic CyA nephrotoxicity includes vascular damage, the so-called CyA-associated arteriolopathy, tubular atrophy, and interstitial fibrosis (156,159,221). These lesions have been described in transplant recipients (159,215,219,221) as well as in patients with autoimmune diseases (217), indicating that CyA therapy leads to chronic renal damage irrespective of the underlying disease. The renal vascular lesions are almost exclusively located in the arterioles (afferent vessels) and small arteries (156,159). The most frequent form consists of circular nodular protein deposits in the arteriolar wall, resulting in narrowing or even occlusion of the vascular lumen. The deposits contain IgM and/or C_3/C_{1q} complement as well as fibrin in up to 20% of the cases. Another form of vascular lesion is characterized by a mucoid thickening of the intima, which also contributes to narrow or occlude the vascular lumen. Minor changes of endothelial and smooth muscle cells, including vacuolization and single cell necrosis, have been also reported (158).

Associated with vascular lesions are variable tubular atrophy, interstitial fibrosis and chronic inflammation (156,159,218,222,223). These changes may be nearly diffuse, but usually exhibit narrow stripes of atrophy and fibrosis, apparently corresponding to areas of cortex associated with afferent arteriolar lesions (158). In addition, lesions have been described in the glomeruli including juxtaglomerular apparatus hyperplasia, focal and segmental sclerosis, and thickening and wrinkling of capillary basement membrane (207,208,215,218,219,224,225).

Recent studies performed in heart transplant patients showed that the glomerular hypofiltration associated with chronic CyA therapy was due in large part to a reduction in RPF combined with a depressed K_f (207,218,219) that could not be attributed to impaired performance of cardiac graft. Renal vascular resistance was elevated in cardiac transplant recipients treated with CyA for more than 1 year (219). However, after 12 months of continuous therapy, it appears unlikely that elevated renal vascular resistance remains purely functional. The occlusive arteriolopathy that is observed at this time (219) or later (226) contributes to maintain the renal vascular resistance permanently elevated later on in the course of CyA therapy. In these patients renal artery to peritubular capillary pressure gradient increased between 1 and 12 months of CyA therapy, indicating a predilection for preglomerular sites of elevated renovascular resistance (219). Findings of striking elevation in transglomerular dextran transport both after 1 to 4 weeks and 12 months of therapy suggest that the afferent arteriole is the predominant site of increased renovascular resistance in CyA-treated heart transplant recipients (219).

Notably, the estimated K_f in these patients apparently failed to decline further after 12 months of CyA therapy, which is consistent with the relative constancy of GFR despite progressive obliteration of cortical microvessels (219). A possible interpretation for this finding is that the single nephron GFR of remnant glomeruli that remained perfused was adaptively increased, thereby compensating for the declining number of functional nephrons (219). To address this issue, Myers et al. (219) performed morphometric analysis of the glomerular cross sections on CyA recipients, in whom biopsies were done at 12 months, and compared it to that of healthy kidney donors (219). The pattern of distribution of glomerular capillary tuft cross-sectional area, which was bell-shaped in normal kidneys, was lost in CyA-treated patients, with a shift to both smaller and larger size glomeruli, presumably reflecting collapse and sclerosis of some glomeruli and the appearance of a subset of spared remnant glomeruli that became enlarged (219). Thus, in these patients the relative stability of GFR despite progressive pathological changes was ascribed to hypertrophy of the remaining glomeruli, which compensated for the loss of surface area in damaged glomeruli. Like remnant glomeruli of the rat following extensive ablation of renal mass (227), adaptive hemodynamic changes may occur with subsequent glomerular hypertension, which might result in expansion of the mesangial matrix, increase in glomerular permeability, and ultimately glomerular sclerosis (218,219). Actually, this evolution occurs in humans with a more prolonged CyA treatment. In the study of Myers et al. (219), CyA-treated heart transplant recipients who developed end-stage renal failure had 36% to 92% of glomeruli involved by sclerosis or ischemic collapse, and a yet more prominent shift to glomeruli of smaller size, whereas only a few glomeruli were enlarged. These observations have been recently extended with a three-dimensional morphometric analysis of individual glomeruli in renal biopsies taken from cardiac transplant patients on CyA for more than 2 years (130). Forty percent of glomeruli had global or segmental sclerotic changes. Moreover, in keeping with the findings of Myers et al., smaller (42%) and larger (24%) than normal glomeruli were found, the majority of glomeruli with global or segmental sclerosis belonging to the subset of small glomeruli.

The majority of initial animal studies focused on renal effects of short-term CyA administration; thus, the form of chronic CyA nephrotoxicity has not been evaluated carefully in an animal model. However, it has been documented that rats given orally CyA for 5 months at the dose of 40 mg/kg on alternate days had a marked decrease in GFR with pathological changes consisting of mild glomerular endothelial damage, glomerular hypercellularity, and mesangial matrix expansion (228). Isometric vacuolization in the proximal tubules, together with limited areas of interstitial fibrosis with perivascular distribution in the absence of vascular lesions, were also found in these animals. Similarly, the development of renal insufficiency associated with tubular atrophy and interstitial fibrosis has been reported in rats given CyA at the dose of 10 and 20 mg/kg/24 hr for up to 84 days (229). In addition to these morphological changes, a marked juxtaglomerular apparatus hypertrophy and hyperplasia has been described in rats treated with CyA (25 mg/kg/24 hr intraperitoneally) for 28 days (230). Striped interstitial fibrosis with no vascular changes has been observed also after oral chronic administration of CyA (12.5 or 25 mg/kg/24 hr) to normal rats for 16 weeks (231).

Persistent renal vasoconstriction likely plays a central role in the pathogenesis of chronic CyA nephropathy. In allograft recipients given long-term CyA the fall in GFR is accompanied by a parallel reduction in RPF after several weeks of treatment. It has been proposed that persistent afferent arteriolar vasospasm associated to CyA administration leads to structural alteration and eventual obliteration of a portion of these preglomerular vessels. The resulting impediment to glomerular perfusion, in turn, could result in downstream glomerular damage that is irreversible. When extensive, this process could lead to a loss of ultrafiltration pressure and filtration surface area sufficient to explain the development of end-stage renal failure in heart transplant patients given long-term CyA. The recent availability of experimental models resembling the chronic form of CyA nephrotoxicity (228–230) has offered the opportunity to investigate mechanisms of chronic CyA nephrotoxicity. In this regard, the lack of correlation between the reduction in GFR and proximal tubular abnormalities in rats chronically treated with CyA (228) gives further support to the notion that renal vasoconstriction, rather than tubular injury, is a major factor in chronic experimental CyA nephrotoxicity, as it is in humans. Further, a complete reconstruction of the glomerular corpuscule has been observed in rats given long-term CyA to evaluate the consequence of CyA-induced renal ischemia on capillary tuft volume (232). In accord with the results obtained in human studies, in rats given CyA for 3 months glomerular volume distribution was shifted toward small glomeruli in parallel with a significant reduction in GFR. Prolongation of CyA administration for up to 5 months did not result in a further decrease in GFR, and was associated with the appearance of a subset of glomeruli that became larger than normal (232).

Vasoactive substances previously recognized as participating in the acute form of CyA nephrotoxicity may also play a role in chronic renal vasoconstriction and progressive impairment of glomerular filtration. Given the notion that CyA is a potential stimulus for endothelin release (183), it has been recently evaluated whether synthesis of endothelin occurs in a rat model of chronic CyA nephrotoxicity (233). In contrast to results obtained with vehicle, 30 days' CyA administration resulted in a significant elevation in the urinary excretion of endothelin as compared with pretreatment values. The enhanced urinary excretion rate of endothelin in CyA-treated rats can be taken as to reflect an increased renal production of the peptide (234). This is consistent with the finding that, at variance with the urinary excretion rate, plasma levels of endothelin were unchanged in rats on chronic CyA therapy (233). Since in these animals a significant correlation was found between the urinary excretion of endothelin and the serum creatinine levels, a possible contribution of this vasoactive peptide, also, to the chronic CyA nephrotoxicity has been postulated.

In addition to directly eliciting renal vasoconstriction, other actions of endothelin may be involved in chronic CyA nephrotoxicity. For example, endothelin stimulates 15-lipoxygenase activity leading to 15-hydroxyeicosatetraenoic acid (15-HETE) formation (235). 15-HETE is chemotactic for inflammatory cells (236), and may represent a signal for circulating inflammatory cells and platelets to accumulate within the glomerular capillaries, a typical feature of rats chronically given CyA (228,237). Activation of inflammatory cells and platelets entrapped within the glomerular tuft during long-term CyA administration might result in the generation of vasoactive substances. Among them TXA_2 has been postulated to play a role in rats chronically treated with CyA, on the basis of increased urinary levels of i-TXB_2, its stable breakdown product, that correlated negatively with GFR values (238). Further, a selective TXA_2 synthase inhibitor ameliorated GFR in these animals (238). The effect of chronic CyA administration to rats on urinary excretion of TXB_2 has been confirmed by Coffman et al. (239), who found in a postischemic, denervated rat model a decline in renal function associated with an increase in urinary excretion of 2,3-dinor-TXB_2 and TXB_2. Additional evidence is that in a model of renal isograft the combination of GR 32191, a specific TXA_2 receptor antagonist, with CyA treatment partially prevented the deterioration in renal function found in rats given CyA alone for 30 days (240). That chronic CyA administration is associated with exaggerated synthesis of TXA_2 has also been documented in humans. Kuhn et al. (241), studying 40 patients with multiple sclerosis who received a 2-year treatment with CyA (5 mg/kg/24 hr), found an increased urinary excretion of 2,3-dinor-TXB_2, accompanied by significant increase in serum creatinine. Of note, withdrawal of CyA was followed by a return to normal of renal function and by a reduction in 2,3-dinor-TXB_2 excretion. Moreover, in accordance with animal studies (182), it has been recently shown that in renal transplant patients on CyA a period of dietary supplementation with fish oil, that prevented TXA_2 production, significantly increased GFR and RPF and reduced total renal vascular resistance as compared with pretreatment values (242). As for the cellular origin of TXA_2 in CyA-treated animals, results of biochemical measurements and morphological evidence of intracapillary hypercellularity *in vivo* but not in isolated perfused rat kidney prepared from animals previously treated for 30 days with CyA suggest that besides inflammatory cells, resident renal cells possibly contribute to the exaggerated urinary excretion of i-TXB_2 in CyA-treated animals (237).

Vasoconstrictors such as endothelin and TXA_2 may participate in the chronic renal ischemia in CyA-treated animals and humans, thus favoring the development of glomerular ischemia and subsequent sclerosis. Moreover, TXA_2 may promote glomerulosclerosis by stimulating an excessive formation of extracellular matrix components (124,243). In this regard, experiments have shown that renal fibroblasts from mice given CyA for 4 weeks have a dose-dependent increase in mRNA expression for protocollagen types I and IV (244), indicating that during chronic CyA administration spatial and temporal expression of specific proteins of extracellular matrix are modified, as occurs in other conditions of excessive renal formation of TXA_2 (125).

EFFECT OF REACTIVE OXYGEN SPECIES ON GLOMERULAR FUNCTION

The process of reduction of oxygen to water normally takes place by single electron transfers. When the reduction is incomplete reactive intermediates are generated that ultimately cause oxygen toxicity (245,246) (Fig. 4). Such species are the univalent and divalent reduction oxygen products, i.e., free radical superoxide anion ($O_2^{\cdot-}$) and hydrogen peroxide (H_2O_2). The latter is formed by spontaneous or enzymatically catalyzed dismutation of $O_2^{\cdot-}$ (247,248). More reactive oxidants that include the hydroxyl radical (OH·) and halide oxidation products can also be generated by the former species. Thus OH· formation is the likely result of the interaction of $O_2^{\cdot-}$ and H_2O_2 in the metal-catalyzed Haber-Weiss reaction, that is catalyzed by iron (249,250) (Fig. 4). Superoxide anion first reacts to reduce Fe^{3+} and H_2O_2 then interacts with the reduced Fe^{2+} in a Fenton reaction to form OH· or species with similar reactivity. Additional reactive metabolites can be formed as the result of the metabolism of H_2O_2 by cellular enzymatic systems. Leukocyte-derived myeloperoxidase reacting with H_2O_2 forms an enzyme substrate complex that can catalyze oxidation of the halides, chloride (Cl^-), iodide (I^-), or bromide (Br^-), producing highly reactive toxic products (251,252). Because of the wide distribution of chloride ion in biological systems, hypochlorous acid (HOCl) formed by the myeloperoxidase-H_2O_2 complex is probably the most significant reactant (Fig. 4). This oxidant reacts rapidly with amines, amino acids, sulfhydryl compounds, thioethers, aromatics, and other unsaturated carbon groups (253–255). Of interest is the fact that HOCl reacts with $O_2^{\cdot-}$ to form OH· (256).

Under physiological conditions $O_2^{\cdot-}$ is a minor product of the cellular metabolism. It is formed by autooxidation of a wide variety of small molecules or membrane-bound cytochromes and by numerous enzymes, localized in the cytosol, mitochondria, peroxisomes, and plasma membranes (246). A soluble cytosolic en-

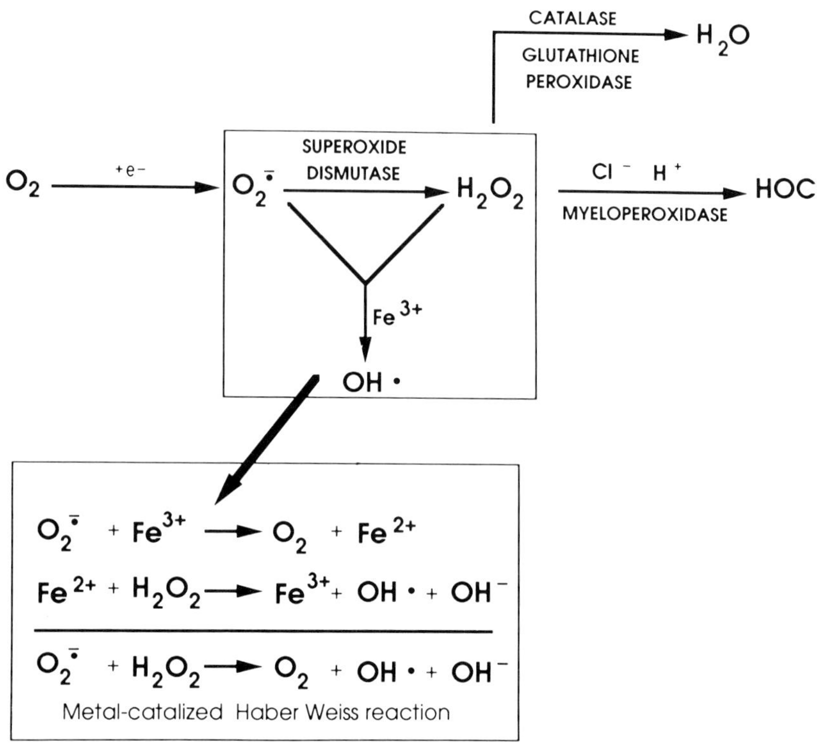

FIG. 4. Reactive oxygen species generation.

zyme, xanthine oxidase, generates $O_2^{\cdot -}$ during the reduction of oxygen to H_2O_2. *In vivo*, the enzyme is synthesized as NAD^+-dependent dehydrogenase (type D) which catalyzes uric acid formation by xanthine (257). Proteolysis, acidosis, sulfhydryl reagents, and ischemic conditions convert the enzyme from type D to $O_2^{\cdot -}$ and H_2O_2 producing oxidase form type O (258).

Besides xanthine oxidase, the cell membrane-associated NADPH oxidase is one of the major enzymes involved in reactive oxygen species (ROS) production (259). Cells appear to protect themselves against oxidative stress by low molecular weight free radical scavengers as well as by various enzyme systems (246). Superoxide dismutases, which dismute $O_2^{\cdot -}$ to H_2O_2 (247), and the enzymes that remove H_2O_2, catalase (260), and glutathione peroxidase (261), are major intracellular antioxidants. Reactive oxygen species may mediate ischemic, toxic, and possibly immune injury (262–266). It is well documented that ROS plays an active role in the acute immune complex-induced lung injury (267,268) as well as in the myocardial cellular damage due to ischemia and reperfusion (269). More recently several lines of evidence have indicated that ROS mediates glomerular injury induced by immune complexes or nephrotoxic drugs (270,271). Rehan et al. (272) provided the first evidence that ROS participates in the acute (heterologous) phase of a complement and neutrophil-dependent model of antiglomerular basement membrane nephritis. Catalase significantly reduced urinary protein excretion and preserved glomerular endothelial and epithelial cell structure in nephritic rats (272). By contrast treatment with superoxide dismutase resulted in a non–statistically significant reduction of proteinuria, and a scavenger of OH·, dimethyl sulfoxide, was ineffective (272). These data suggest that glomerular injury was due to H_2O_2 production from activated neutrophils.

In vitro studies have demonstrated that neutrophils incubated with immune complexes undergo a burst in O_2 consumption coincident with the generation of $O_2^{-\cdot}$ and H_2O_2 (273,274). Of interest is the observation that neutrophils adherent to a nonphagocytosable surface, such as glomerular basement membrane, containing immune globulin G aggregates, produce oxidants only at the site of attachment which may be inaccessible to circulating scavengers, such as superoxide dismutase or catalase, and therefore may be more exposed to the toxic effect of oxygen metabolites (275).

A recent study has shown that the injection into the renal artery of phorbol myristate acetate, a potent stimulus of leukocyte "respiratory burst" (276), resulted in the development of proteinuria associated with the morphological evidence of glomerular injury (277). Both neutrophil depletion and catalase treatment significantly reduced proteinuria and minimized glomerular endothelial cell damage, suggesting that neutrophil-derived H_2O_2 and/or its conversion products were responsible for such an effect. Boyce and Holdsworth (278) have demonstrated that an iron chelator deferoxamine prevented the development of proteinuria in rabbits with antiglomerular basement membrane glomerulonephritis and inhibited OH· generation by immunologically activated neutrophils *in vitro*. Similarly, a potent OH· scavenger dimethylthiourea was highly effective in blocking renal injury. The protective effect of both the compounds implies a role for OH· in neutrophil-dependent immune renal injury.

Direct evidence for a role of ROS in altering glomerular permeability has been recently provided by Yoshioka et al. (279), who showed that infusion of H_2O_2 into the renal artery in Munich-Wistar rats was associated with a transient massive proteinuria as well as with an increased fractional clearance of neutral dextran of effective molecular radii ranging from 42 to 60 Å. Both catalase and colloid-conjugated deferoxamine significantly reduced proteinuria, suggesting that iron-mediated metabolites of H_2O_2, including OH·, may be responsible for the altered glomerular basement membrane size-selective properties (279). Previous studies have suggested that leukocytes may induce proteinuria in glomerulonephritis by releasing lysosomal enzymes that may degrade the glomerular basement membrane (280–282). Several *in vitro* studies indicated that various species of oxygen free radicals can have a direct destructive effect on extracellular matrix macromolecules. Actually oxygen radicals generated by xanthine oxidase and hypoxanthine or by stimulated neutrophils can degrade collagen and cause depolymerization of hyaluronic acid (283–285). It has been shown that ROS may render proteins more susceptible to proteolysis (283,286). In this context a study by Fligiel et al. (287) has demonstrated that pretreament of preparation of rat glomerular basement membrane or fibronectin with H_2O_2 increased their sensitivity to subsequent proteolytic attack.

Recent studies have also documented that ROS generated by either myeloperoxidase-halide system (288) or by immune-complex–stimulated neutrophils (289) inactivated α_1-proteinase inhibitor, the primary regulator of neutrophil elastase, thus allowing the released elastase to degrade extracellular matrix more readily. A more recent study has shown that neutrophils stimulated with phorbol myristate acetate, along with elastase, generated an HOCl-like oxygen metabolite that potentiated elastase in its effect of solubilizing subendothelial basement membrane in the presence of α_1-proteinase inhibitor (290). In addition, ROS may be involved in the regulation of latent metalloproteinase activity (291–293).

Recent studies have documented that neutrophils stimulated with phorbol myristate acetate release their latent collagenase or gelatinase, which are activated by an oxidative process dependent on the HOCl or a similar oxidant generated by the H_2O_2-myeloperoxidase-halide system (291–293). Johnson et al. (294) reported that the infusion of myeloperoxidase followed by H_2O_2 in a chloride-containing solution into the renal artery of rats caused significant proteinuria and glomerular injury characterized by endothelial cell swelling and epithelial cell foot process effacement. That myeloperoxidase, H_2O_2, and a halide can interact in the glomeruli was documented by autoradiographic studies revealing the oxidant-dependent iodination of glomerular structures in myeloperoxidase-H_2O_2–perfused rats. The basement membrane was the major site of iodination and therefore the primary target of the halogenation reaction catalyzed by myeloperoxidase in the capillary wall (294). These observations were extended by a subsequent study (295) that provided a detailed sequential analysis of the morphological consequences of myeloperoxidase-H_2O_2-halide–induced glomerular injury. Within 10 min from the infusion of myeloperoxidase followed by H_2O_2, an acute injury occurred characterized by extensive swelling and necrosis of endothelial cells and possibly mesangial cells associated with marked influx of platelets in the glomerular capillary loops and activation at areas of denuded glomerular basement membrane. A recent finding of glomerular iodination in rats with concanavalin A–anticoncanavalin A glomerulonephritis (an *in situ* model of immune-complex glomerulonephritis) supports the hypothesis that the myeloperoxidase system participates in mediating neutrophil-dependent glomerulonephritis (296). In this context, of interest is the observation that myeloperoxidase-derived oxidants may directly induce *in vitro* covalent cross-linking of various natural antibodies to their respective antigens bound to a solid phase (297).

As mentioned above, the earliest morphological changes that accompany ROS-mediated glomerular injury in neutrophil-dependent glomerulonephritis consist of glomerular endothelial cell swelling and necrosis. Several *in vitro* studies indicate that ROS released from activated leukocytes may be directly cytotoxic to vascular endothelial cells. Indeed, phorbol myristate acetate–stimulated neutrophils have been shown to cause endothelial cell lysis by a process that was catalase inhibitable

(298). Sacks et al. (299) showed that granulocytes, when exposed to activated complement, induced ^{51}Cr release from human umbilical vein endothelial cells in culture. ^{51}Cr leak could be effectively inhibited by the simultaneous addition of superoxide dismutase and catalase. Consistent with these data is the observation that intravascular activation of complement in the rat causes proteinuria and glomerular injury characterized by blebbing of endothelial cells associated with epithelial cell foot process fusion. Both neutrophil depletion and catalase significantly reduced proteinuria and glomerular lesions (300).

Altogether, these observations suggest that H_2O_2 and/or its conversion products are the main determinant of neutrophil-mediated endothelial destruction. Recent studies confirm previous findings and provide suggestive evidence for a role of hydroxyl radicals and intracellular iron in leukocyte-induced endothelial cell damage (301,302). It appears that neutrophil-generated H_2O_2 may readily diffuse into endothelial cells and reacts with free iron in its transition redox state Fe^{2+} to produce the cytotoxic OH· (303). The most likely source of the intracellular iron seems to be the low molecular weight iron chelates and/or heme-associated iron rather than ferritin-bound iron (303).

Recent studies have contributed to expand our knowledge on the cellular events resulting from an oxidant injury to endothelial cells. Shasby et al. (304) have documented that xanthine/xanthine oxidase induced a reversible increase in albumin transfer across cultured endothelium that was associated with changes in cell shape and increase in calcium efflux from endothelial cells. These effects were reversed by the calcium antagonist lanthanum chloride and mimicked by calcium ionophore A23187. Moreover, chelation of extracellular calcium was shown to inhibit lysis of endothelium. These data suggest that oxygen radicals can alter vascular permeability through changes in endothelial cell shape and cytoskeleton that are related to altered calcium homeostasis. Increased vascular permeability can also be a consequence of a perturbation of the organization of vascular endothelial cell membrane as suggested by Freeman et al. (305). Vascular endothelial cells exposed to a superoxide-generating system showed an increase in membrane fluidity as assessed by electron paramagnetic resonance spectrometry. Superoxide anion increased the degree of disorder of the cellular membrane without destroying the mode of protein attachment.

Recently, it has been shown that endothelial cells undergo alterations in adenylate metabolism after exposure to H_2O_2 (306,307) or xanthine-xanthine oxidase (308). Ager and Gordon (306) reported increased release of ^3H-purines from cells preincubated with ^3H-adenosine and then exposed to H_2O_2. Separation of labeled purines by thin layer chromatography showed that H_2O_2 stimulated the release of nucleosides including inosine and hypoxanthine. Spragg et al. (307) documented a rapid and substantial loss of intracellular adenosine triphosphate (ATP) after exposure of endothelial cells to increasing concentrations of H_2O_2. This loss persisted for 3 hr without evidence of recovery. Finally, a recent study (308) has demonstrated that endothelial cells when exposed to xanthine/xanthine oxidase respond to the oxidant injury with an early decline in ATP levels and efflux in ^3H-adenine metabolites and later with cell detachment. Hydrogen peroxide seems responsible for ATP depletion and efflux of ^{3}H-adenine, whereas cell detachment is mediated both by H_2O_2 and OH·. Since adenosine nucleotides participate in many metabolic reactions and are major factors in maintaining homeostasis, impaired adenylate metabolism might contribute to cell dysfunction and death observed after exposure to oxidants. Moreover, the oxidative breakdown of ATP into nucleoside could provide additional substrate for xanthine oxidase. This enzyme has been found in endothelial cells (309,310) and may be activated by stimulated neutrophils (311). A rapid conversion of xanthine dehydrogenase to xanthine oxidase also occurs when endothelial cells are exposed to several chemotactic mediators such as the human recombinants C5a and TNF and the peptide *N*-formyl-*L*-methionyl-*L*-leucyl-*L*- phenylalanine (312).

In addition to being a target of injury, endothelial cells may represent a potential source of ROS (313), thus contributing to their own oxidant injury initiated by activated neutrophils. On the other hand, endothelial cells can protect themselves from H_2O_2 induced injury by endogenous antioxidant defense mechanisms mainly related to the glutathione redox cycle and catalase (314,315). Thus, for an oxidant injury to occur, it is necessary that the amount of ROS produced exceeds enzymatic and nonenzymatic antioxidant defenses of a given cell. Antioxidant enzymes may be modulated by drugs. Glucocorticoids, which are widely used in the treatment of human glomerulonephritis, have been shown recently to increase antioxidant enzyme activity in glomerular endothelial cells in culture, and this was associated with a significant reduction in H_2O_2 generation (316). Moreover, in PA nephrosis methylprednisolone was able to raise renal manganese-superoxide dismutase and catalase activities, and significantly reduced proteinuria and renal cortical malondialdehyde levels with a marked attenuation of epithelial cell foot process fusion and cell vacuolization (317). By contrast diethyldithiocarbamate, an inhibitor of superoxide dismutase, as well as diethyl maleate, a glutathione-depleting drug, contributed to worsen PA-induced nephrosis (318,319).

A significant reduction in urinary protein excretion together with a less severe damage of glomerular epithelial cells was also documented in nephrotic rats treated with superoxide dismutase or allopurinol, an inhibitor of xanthine oxidase (50). It has been suggested that the nephrotoxic effect of PA is related to the formation of its metabolic by-product hypoxanthine, which can serve as a substrate for $O_2^{\overline{\cdot}}$ production via the xanthine oxidase system (50). PA might also indirectly provide the intracellular compartment with ample precursor for hypoxanthine by virtue of its ability to induce increase in the membrane permeability for the intracellular flux of adenosine in glomerular epithelial cells (68). The enhanced generation of $O_2^{\overline{\cdot}}$ can be accompanied by generation of other reactive oxygen metabolites, mainly OH·. Actually, recent experiments have documented that both OH· scavengers and the iron chelator deferoxamine are protective against PA-induced proteinuria, indicating that OH·, likely generated from the interaction of $O_2^{\overline{\cdot}}$ and H_2O_2 in the presence of iron, may be partially responsible for altered glomerular permeability in this model (107).

As in PA nephrosis and ADR cardiotoxicity (60), oxygen free radicals may contribute to ADR nephrotoxicity *in vivo*. This is suggested by the observed beneficial effects of a free radical scavenger, dimethylthiourea, against glomerular injury in this model, possibly through stimulatory effects on glutathione metabolism (320). Additional evidence comes from findings of a marked activation of renal xanthine oxidase observed as early as 24 hr after ADR injection. Moreover, allopurinol, which inhibits renal xanthine oxidase, effectively reduces proteinuria in this model (108). A mechanism by which ADR can initiate free radical formation is its reduction to the semiquinone radical that reacts with oxygen to generate $O_2^{\cdot -}$, H_2O_2, OH· (55). Results from micropuncture studies have suggested that cortical nephrons of Munich-Wistar rats are less sensitive to the toxic effects of ADR than are juxtamedullary nephrons (321). Since in kidneys of rabbits treated with ADR morphological changes have been described almost exclusively in the inner cortex (58), it has been proposed that the higher oxygen supply in juxtamedullary nephrons may enhance oxidative stress, which is possibly mediated by ADR semiquinone radical (321).

Reactive oxygen species may damage glomerular epithelial cells in both PA and ADR nephrosis by causing oxidative injury to the cell membrane via lipid peroxidation (322). Actually, ROS alters the synthesis of proteoglycans and sialoproteins, as documented in isolated rat kidney preparations (109). Other potential negative effects of free radicals in such models involve the possible inhibition of membrane-associated enzymes. This has been recently suggested by findings that adenosine triphosphatase (ATPase) activity is decreased in kidney sections incubated either with ADR or a superoxide generating system, and that such an effect is inhibited by superoxide dismutase (323). Reactive oxygen species may mediate glomerular damage in other models. Thus, Shah (324) has reported that in passive Heymann nephritis, a complement-dependent rat model of membranous nephropathy, either scavengers of OH· (dimethylthiourea and sodium benzoate) or an iron chelator (deferoxamine) significantly reduced proteinuria. These results would suggest that OH· played a role in the altered glomerular permeability to proteins in Heymann nephritis. A potential role for OH· as mediator of proteinuria has been also documented in cationized bovine gamma globulin–induced glomerulonephritis, a model of immune-complex glomerular disease with subepithelial as well as mesangial immune-complex deposition, which is independent of glomerular complement deposition and intraglomerular infiltration of leukocytes (325).

Besides proteinuria, glomerular diseases are also characterized by a fall in GFR. Pharmacological maneuvers aimed at preventing the formation of ROS both in immune-mediated glomerulonephritis (272) and PA-induced nephropathy (50,107) were ineffective in preventing renal function impairment. However, other studies suggest that ROS may cause changes in hemodynamic determinants of GFR. Both neutrophil depletion and catalase largely prevented the fall in single nephron GFR and K_f and the increase in renal arteriolar resistance induced by the unilateral infusion of phorbol myristate acetate into the renal artery in Munich-Wistar rats (326). In this model, activated neutrophils infiltrating the glomerulus likely are the source of ROS, which may induce a vasoconstrictive response in the glomerular and post-glomerular microcirculation, leading to a fall in glomerular filtration.

Beside neutrophil-derived oxidants, enzymatically generated ROS may also determine glomerular hemodynamic changes. In this respect, recently ROS generated via the xanthine/xanthine oxidase system, namely H_2O_2, has been shown to contract isolated glomeruli and cultured mesangial cells by reducing the glomerular cross-sectional area and planar cell surface, respectively, effects that were completely inhibited by catalase (327). Therefore, ROS, by inducing a fall in K_f secondary to mesangial cell contraction, could contribute to the reduction in GFR observed in glomerular diseases, whether associated or not with glomerular neutrophil infiltration. ROS may act to alter renal vascular resistance and K_f by interfering with the synthesis and/or the action of vasoactive molecules.

It has been documented that vascular and glomerular endothelial cells produce potent vasoactive factors such as nitric oxide among vasodilators (328,329) and endothelin as vasoconstrictor (142,183), which also influence mesangial cell contraction and K_f (144,145,330). On the other hand, *in vitro* data are available that indicate that ROS impairs vascular endothelial cell function (298,299,304–308). Thus, oxidants might alter the rate of production of vasoactive substances by endothelial cells, which in turn may result in glomerular hemodynamic changes. Oxidant-induced glomerular dysfunction may also occur through altered synthesis of cyclic nucleotides and secondary mediators of inflammation at the glomerular level.

Enzymatically generated ROS increases glomerular adenosine 3′, 5′-cyclic monophosphate (cAMP) levels, an effect that was selectively inhibited by catalase (331). Since infusion of dibutyl cAMP or hormones, which stimulate glomerular cAMP, cause a decrease in K_f (332), one can speculate that the fall in K_f induced by neutrophil-derived oxidants may be mediated by an increase in glomerular cyclic nucleotide content. This possibility is consistent with the finding that cell-free supernatants from stimulated neutrophils caused an increase in cAMP content in isolated glomeruli which was significantly reduced by catalase and scavengers of HOC1 (333). Experiments using prostaglandin synthesis inhibitors suggested that ROS increases the cAMP content in glomeruli by enhancing prostaglandin synthesis (331,333). Platelet activating factor may be regarded as an additional mediator of ROS-induced fall in K_f as documented by the fact that a PAF receptor antagonist inhibited the contraction of isolated glomeruli and cultured mesangial cells exposed to xanthine/xanthine oxidase or H_2O_2 (327).

There is increasing evidence that glomerular mesangial cells play an active role in acute and chronic renal diseases (128). A preliminary report has documented that both xanthine/xanthine oxidase and H_2O_2 stimulated the proliferation of cultured rat mesangial cells associated with an increase in intracellular calcium concentration (334). That a similar mechanism could occur *in vivo* is indirectly suggested by the beneficial effects of allopurinol and superoxide dismutase against the mesangial cell proliferation and matrix expansion observed in rats with PA nephrosis (50). Mesangial cells may also contribute to glomerular injury by virtue of their ability to generate ROS in response to various stimuli. When exposed to serum-treated zymosan, rat cultured mesangial cells exhibited phagocytic activity resulting in $O_2^{\cdot -}$ and H_2O_2 generation associated with the release of arachidonic acid and its conversion into lipoxygenase products (335). Soluble stimuli such as phorbol myristate acetate

(336), calcium ionophore (336), and PAF (336,337), also stimulate ROS release from rat mesangial cells, although to a lesser extent. Further, human mesangial cells generated ROS in response to TNF and interleukin-1α (IL/1α) (338). These findings, together with the observation that the glomerular production of PAF, TNF, or IL-1 is increased in experimental immune-mediated renal diseases (339,340), suggest that ROS generated by mesangial cells in response to inflammatory mediators may contribute to glomerular injury. Recently, it has been shown that immune-complexes (341) and C5b-9 membrane attack complex (342) stimulate $O_2^{\cdot -}$ production by rat mesangial cells *in vitro*. These findings raise the possibility that the glomerular localization of immune-complexes and complement in glomerulonephritis may promote mesangial cell release of ROS. Interestingly, the glomerulonephritis characterized by mesangial immune deposits containing C5b-9 (343) is also characterized by mesangial cell proliferation and matrix expansion.

REFERENCES

1. Hoedemaker PhJ. Drug induced immune complex glomerulonephritis in man. In: Bertani T, Remuzzi G, Garattini S, eds. *Drugs and kidney*. New York: Raven Press, 1986;75–94.
2. Cattell V. Endothelial cell diseases in experimental models: mitomycin. In: Bertani T, Remuzzi G, Garattini S, eds. *Drugs and kidney*. New York: Raven Press, 1986;26–35.
3. Brenner BM, Bohrer MP, Baylis C, Deen WM. Determinants of glomerular permselectivity: insights derived from observations in vivo. *Kidney Int* 1977;12:229–237.
4. Arturson G, Groth T, Grotte G. Human glomerular membrane porosity and filtration pressure: dextran clearance data analyzed by theoretical models. *Clin Sci* 1971;40:137–158.
5. Hardwicke J, Cameron JS, Harrison JF, Hulme G, Soothill JF. Proteinuria, studied by clearances of individual macromolecules. In: Manuel Y, Revillard JP, Betuel H, eds. *Proteins in normal and pathological urine*. Baltimore: University Park Press, 1970;111–152.
6. Verniory A, DuBois R, DeCoodt P, Gassée JP, Lambert PP. Measurement of the permeability of biological membranes: application to the glomerular wall. *J Gen Physiol* 1973;62:489–507.
7. Eisenbach GM, Van Liew JB, Boylan JW. Effect of angiotensin on the filtration of protein in the rat kidney: a micropuncture study. *Kidney Int* 1975;8:80–87.
8. Gaizutis M, Pesce AJ, Lewy JE. Determination of nanogram amounts of albumin by radioimmunoassay. *Microchem J* 1972;17:327–337.
9. Chang RLS, Deen WM, Robertson CR, Brenner BM. Permselectivity of the glomerular capillary wall. III. Restricted transport of polyanions. *Kidney Int* 1975;8:212–218.
10. Kerjaschki D, Sharkey DJ, Farquhar MG. Identification and characterization of podocalyxin—the major sialoprotein of the renal glomerular epithelial cell. *J Cell Biol* 1984;98:1591–1596.
11. Horvat R, Hovoka A, Dekan G, Poczewski H, Kerjaschki D. Endothelial cell membranes contain podocalyxin—the major sialoprotein of visceral glomerular epithelial cells. *J Cell Biol* 1986; 102:484–491.
12. Sawada H, Stukenbrok H, Kerjaschki D, Farquhar MG. Epithelial polyanion (podocalyxin) is found on the sides but not the soles of the foot processes of the glomerular epithelium. *Am J Pathol* 1986;125:309–318.
13. Brenner BM, Hostetter TH, Humes MD. Glomerular permselectivity: barrier function based on discrimination of molecular size and charge. *Am J Physiol* 1978;234:F455–F460.
14. Bray J, Robinson GB. Influence of charge on filtration across renal basement membrane films in vitro. *Kidney Int* 1984;25:527–533.
15. Kaysen GA, Myers BD, Couser WG, Rabkin R, Felts JM. Mechanisms and consequence of proteinuria. *Lab Invest* 1986;54:479–498.
16. Latta H, Johnston WH. The glycoprotein inner layer of glomerular capillary basement membrane as a filtration barrier. *J Ultrastruct Res* 1976;57:65–67.
17. Kanwar YS. Biophysiology of glomerular filtration and proteinuria. *Lab Invest* 1984;51:7–21.

18. Batsford SR, Rohrbach R, Vogt A. Size restriction in the glomerular capillary wall: importance of lamina densa. *Kidney Int* 1987;31:710–717.
19. Kanwar YS, Farquhar MG. Anionic sites in the glomerular basement membrane. In vivo and in vitro localization to the lamina rarae by cationic probes. *J Cell Biol* 1981;81:137–153.
20. Kanwar YS, Farquhar MG. Presence of heparan sulfate in the glomerular basement membrane. *Proc Natl Acad Sci USA* 1979;76:1303–1307.
21. Kanwar YS, Farquhar MG. Isolation of glycosaminoglycans (heparan sulfate) from glomerular basement membranes. *Proc Natl Acad Sci USA* 1979;76:4493–4497.
22. Jones DB. Mucosubstances of the glomerulus. *Lab Invest* 1969;21:119–125.
23. Latta H, Johnston WH, Stanley TM. Sialoglycoproteins and filtration barriers in the glomerular capillary wall. *J Ultrastruct Res* 1975;51:354–376.
24. Kerjaschki D, Vernillo AT, Farquhar MG. Reduced sialylation of podocalyxin—the major sialoprotein of the rat kidney glomerulus—in aminonucleoside nephrosis. *Am J Pathol* 1985; 118:343–349.
25. Charest MP, Roth J. Localization of sialic acid in kidney glomeruli: regionalization in the podocyte plasma membrane and loss in experimental nephrosis. *Proc Natl Acad Sci USA* 1985;82:8508–8512.
26. Dekan G, Gabel C, Farquhar MG. Sulfate contributes to the negative charge of podocalyxin, the major sialoglycoprotein of the glomerular filtration slits. *Proc Natl Acad Sci USA* 1991;88: 5398–5402.
27. Kanwar YS, Linker A, Farquhar MG. Increased permeability of the glomerular basement membrane to ferritin after removal of glycosaminoglycans (heparan sulfate) by enzyme digestion. *J Cell Biol* 1980;86:688–693.
28. Rosenzweig LJ, Kanwar YS. Removal of sulfated (heparan sulfate) or nonsulfated (hyaluronic acid) glycosaminoglycans results in increased permeability of the glomerular basement membrane to ^{125}I-bovine serum albumin. *Lab Invest* 1982;47:177–185.
29. Kanwar YS, Farquhar MG. Detachment of endothelium and epithelium from the glomerular basement membrane produced by kidney perfusion with neuraminidase. *Lab Invest* 1980;42:375–384.
30. Seiler MW, Venkatachalam MA, Cotran RS. Glomerular epithelium: structural alterations induced by polycations. *Science* 1975;189:390–393.
31. Bertolatus JA. Affinity cytochemical labeling of glomerular basement membrane anionic sites using specific biotinylation and colloidal gold probes. *J Histochem Cytochem* 1990;38:377–384.
32. Bertolatus JA, Abuyousef M, Hunsicker LG. Glomerular sieving of high molecular weight proteins in proteinuric rats. *Kidney Int* 1987;31:1257–1266.
33. Lelongt B, Makino H, Kanwar YS. Status of glomerular proteoglycans in aminonucleoside nephrosis. *Kidney Int* 1987;31:1299–1310.
34. Glassock RJ. Normal physiology and pathophysiology of proteinuria. In: Cameron JS, Glassock RJ, eds. *The nephrotic syndrome*. New York: Marcel Dekker, 1988;219–249.
35. Barnes JL, Radnik RA, Gilchrist EP, Venkatachalam MA. Size and charge selective permeability defects induced in glomerular basement membrane by polycation. *Kidney Int* 1984;25:11–19.
36. Rennke HG, Klein PS. Pathogenesis and significance of nonprimary focal and segmental glomerulosclerosis. *Am J Kidney Dis* 1989;13:443–456.
37. Bertani T, Remuzzi G. Epithelial cell damage. In: Bertani T, Remuzzi G, eds. *Glomerular injury 300 years after Morgagni*. Milano: Wichtig, 1983;163–177.
38. Spargo BH, Seymour AE, Ordonez NG. Epithelial cell disease. In: Spargo BH, Seymour AE, Ordonez NG, eds. *Renal biopsy pathology with diagnostic and therapeutic implications*. New York: Wiley, 1983;34.
39. Bohrer MP, Baylis C, Robertson CR, Brenner BM, et al. Mechanisms of the puromycin-induced defects in the transglomerular passage of water and macromolecules. *J Clin Invest* 1977;60: 152–161.
40. Siegrist S, Velitchkovitch S, Moreau N, Le Goffic F. Effect of P and A site substrates on the binding of a macrolide to ribosomes: analysis of the puromycin-induced stimulation. *Eur J Biochem* 1984;143:23–26.
41. Michael AF, Venters HD, Worthen HG, Good RA. Experimental renal disease in monkeys. *Lab Invest* 1962;11:1266–1278.
42. Wilson SGF, Hackel DB, Harwood S, Nash G, Heymann W. Aminonucleoside nephrosis in rats. *Pediatrics* 1985;21:963–973.
43. Nussenzveig I, Vilela de Faria C, Lopez de Faria J, Magaldi BJ. Aminonucleoside induced ne-

phrotic syndrome in human beings: report of five cases. *Proc 2nd Int Congr Nephrol Prague* 1963;78:506–510.
44. Lannigan R. The production of chronic renal disease in rats by single intravenous injection of aminonucleoside of puromycin and effect of low dosage continuous hydrocortisone. *Br J Exp Pathol* 1962;326.
45. Ryan GB, Karnovsky MJ. An ultrastructural study of the mechanisms of proteinuria in aminonucleoside nephrosis. *Kidney Int* 1975;8:219–232.
46. Baricos WH, Cortez-Schwartz S, Shah SV. Renal neuraminidase: characterization in normal rat kidney and measurement in experimentally induced nephrotic syndrome. *Biochem J* 1986; 239:705–710.
47. Olson JL, Rennke HG, Venkatachalam MA. Alterations in the charge and size selectivity barrier of the glomerular filter in aminonucleoside nephrosis in rats. *Lab Invest* 1981;44:271–279.
48. Eddy AA, Michael AF. Acute tubulointerstitial nephritis associated with aminonucleoside nephrosis. *Kidney Int* 1988;33:14–23.
49. Diamond JR, Karnovsky MJ. Focal and segmental glomerulosclerosis following a single intravenous dose of puromycin aminonucleoside. *Am J Pathol* 1986;122:481–487.
50. Diamond JR, Bonventre JV, Karnovsky MJ. A role for oxygen free radicals in aminonucleoside nephrosis. *Kidney Int* 1986;29:478–483.
51. Velosa JA, Glasser RJ, Nevins TE, Michael AF. Experimental model of focal sclerosis. II. Correlation with immunopathologic changes, macromolecular kinetics, and polyanion loss. *Lab Invest* 1977;36:527–534.
52. Grond J, Weening JJ, Elema JD. Glomerular sclerosis in nephrotic rats. Comparison of the long term effects of Adriamycin and aminonucleoside. *Lab Invest* 1984;51:277–285.
53. Painter RB. Inhibition of DNA replicon initiation by 4-nitroquinoline 1-oxide, Adriamycin and ethyleneimine. *Cancer Res* 1978;38:4445–4449.
54. Young RC, Ozols RF, Myers CE. The anthracycline antineoplastic drugs. *N Engl J Med* 1981; 305:139–153.
55. Bachur N, Gordon GL, Gee MV. Anthracyclin antibiotic augmentation of microsomal electron transport and free radical formation. *Mol Pharmacol* 1977;13:901–910.
56. Bertani T, Poggi A, Pozzoni R, et al. Adriamycin-induced nephrotic syndrome in rats. Sequence of pathologic events. *Lab Invest* 1982;46:16–23.
57. Bertani T, Rocchi G, Sacchi G, Mecca G, Remuzzi G. Adriamycin-induced glomerulosclerosis in the rat. *Am J Kidney Dis* 1986;7:12–19.
58. Fajardo LF, Eltringham JR, Stewart JR, Klauber MR. Adriamycin nephrotoxicity. *Lab Invest* 1980;43:242–253.
59. Calabresi P, Parks RE Jr. Chemotherapy of neoplastic diseases. In: Goodman Gilman A, Goodman LS, Rall TW, Murad F, eds. *The pharmacological basis of therapeutics*. New York: Macmillan, 1985;1283–1285.
60. Speyer JL, Green MD, Kramer E, et al. Protective effect of the bispiperazinedione ICRF-187 against doxorubicin-induced cardiac toxicity in women with advanced breast cancer. *N Engl J Med* 1988;319:745–752.
61. O'Donnell MP, Michels L, Kasiske B, Raij L, Keane WF. Adriamycin induced chronic proteinuria: a structural and functional study. *J Lab Clin Med* 1985;106:62–67.
62. Weening JJ, Rennke HG. Glomerular permeability and polyanion in Adriamycin nephrosis in the rat. *Kidney Int* 1983;24:152–159.
63. Remuzzi G, Zoja C, Remuzzi A, et al. Low-protein diet prevents glomerular damage in Adriamycin-treated rats. *Kidney Int* 1985;28:21–27.
64. Okuda S, Oh Y, Tsruda H, Onoyama K, Fujimi S, Fujishima M. Adriamycin-induced nephropathy as a model of chronic progressive glomerular disease. *Kidney Int* 1986;29:502–510.
65. Fogo A, Yoshida Y, Glick AD, Homma T, Ichikawa I. Serial micropuncture analysis of glomerular function in two rat models of glomerular sclerosis. *J Clin Invest* 1988;82:322–330.
66. Hoyer JR, Ratte J, Potter AH, Mauser SM, Michael AF. Transfer of aminonucleoside nephrosis by renal trasplantation. *J Clin Invest* 1972;51:277–280.
67. Hoyer JR, Mauer SM, Michael AF. Unilateral renal disease in the rat. I. Clinical morphologic and glomerular mesangial functional features of the experimental model produced by renal perfusion with the aminonucleoside of puromycin. *J Lab Clin Med* 1975;85:756.
68. Fishman JA, Karnovsky MJ. Effects of aminonucleoside of puromycin on glomerular epithelial cells in vitro. *Am J Pathol* 1985;118:398–407.

69. Bertelli R, Ginevri F, Gusmano R, Ghiggeri GM. Cytotoxic effect of adriamycin and agarose-coupled on glomerular epithelial cells: role of free radicals. *In Vitro Cell Dev Biol* 1991; 27A: 799–804.
70. Schwartz MM, Sharon Z, Pauli BU, Lewis DJ. Inhibition of glomerular visceral epithelial cell endocytosis during nephrosis induced by puromycin aminonucleoside. *Lab Invest* 1984;51:690–696.
71. Remuzzi G, Bertani T. Is glomerulosclerosis a consequence of altered glomerular permeability to macromolecules? *Kidney Int* 1990;38:384–394.
72. Caufield JP, Farquhar MG. Loss of anionic sites from the glomerular basement membrane in aminonucleoside nephrosis. *Lab Invest* 1978;39:505–512.
73. Remuzzi A, Battaglia C, Rossi L, Zoja C, Remuzzi G. Glomerular size selectivity in nephrotic rats exposed to diets with different protein content. *Am J Physiol* 1987;253:F318–F327.
74. Bertolatus JA, Hunsicker LG. Glomerular sieving of anionic and neutral bovine albumins in proteinuria rats. *Kidney Int* 1985;28:467–476.
75. Remuzzi A, Perticucci E, Battaglia C, D'amico G, Gentile MG, Remuzzi G. Low-protein diet and glomerular size-selective function in membranous glomerulopathy *AM J Kidney Dis* 1991; 17:317–322.
76. Caufield JP. Alterations in the distribution of alcian blue staining fibrillar anionic sites in the glomerular basement membrane in aminonucleoside nephrosis. *Lab Invest* 1979;40:503–511.
77. Kanwar YS, Rosenzweig LJ. Altered glomerular permeability as a result of focal detachment of the visceral epithelium. *Kidney Int* 1982;21:565–575.
78. Seiler MW, Hoyer JR, Krueger TE. Altered localization of protamine-heparin complexes in aminonucleoside nephrosis. *Lab Invest* 1980;43:9–17.
79. Kobayashi S, Nagase M, Honda N, Adachi K, Ichinose N, Hishida A. Analysis of anionic charge of the glomerular basement membrane in aminonucleoside nephrosis. *Kidney Int* 1989;35:1405–1408.
80. Kanwar JS, Jakubowski ML. Unaltered anionic sties of glomerular basement membrane in aminonucleoside nephrosis. *Kidney Int* 1984;25:613–618.
81. Mahan JD, Sisson-Ross S, Vernier RL. Glomerular basement membrane anionic charge site changes early in aminonucleoside nephrosis. *Am J Pathol* 1986;125:393–401.
82. Whiteside C, Prutis K, Cameron R, Thompson J. Glomerular epithelial detachment, not reduced charge density, correlates with proteinuria in Adriamycin and puromycin nephrosis. *Lab Invest* 1989;61:650–660.
83. Venkatachalam MA, Karnovsky MJ, Cotran RS. Glomerular permeability. Ultrastructural studies in experimental nephrosis using horseradish peroxidase as a tracer. *J Exp Med* 1969;130:381–399.
84. Venckatakalam MA, Cotran RS, Karnovsky MJ. An ultrastructure study of glomerular permeability in aminonucleoside nephrosis using catalase as tracer protein. *J Exp Med* 1970;132:1168–1180.
85. Messina A, Davies DJ, Dillane PC, Ryan GB. Glomerular epithelial abnormalities associated with the onset of proteinuria in aminonucleoside nephrosis. *Am J Pathol* 1987;126:220–229.
86. Mynderse LA, Hassel JR, Kleinman HK, Martin GR, Martinez-Hernandez A. Loss of heparan sulfate proteoglycan from glomerular basement membrane of nephrotic rats. *Lab Invest* 1983; 48:292–302.
87. Ebihara I, Nakamura T, Suzuki S, Tomino Y, Koide H. Altered mRNA expression of basement membrane components in focal glomurular sclerosis. *Contrib Nephrol* 1991;95:102–106.
88. Nakamura T, Ebihara I, Fukui M, Tomino Y, Koide H. Effects of Methylprednisone on glomerular and medullary mRNA levels for extracellular matrices in puromycin aminonucleoside nephrosis. *Kidney Int* 1991;40:874–881.
89. Kasinath BS, Singh AK, Kanwar YS, Lewis EJ. Dexamethasone increases heparan sulfate proteoglycan core protein content of glomerular epithelial cells. *J Lab Clin Med* 1990;115:196–202.
90. Michael AF, Blau E, Vernier RL. Glomerular polyanion. Alteration in aminonucleoside nephrosis. *Lab Invest* 1970;23:649–657.
91. Faraggiana T, Grishman E. The podocyte cell coat in experimental nephrosis. *J Ultrastruct Res* 1981;74:296–306.
92. Jones C, Buch S, Post M, Eddy A. Production of extracellular matrix in purine aminonucleoside (PAN) nephrosis. *J Am Soc Nephrol* 1990;1:550.
93. Martin J, Davies M, Thomas G, Lovett DH. Human mesangial cells secrete a GBM-degrading neutral proteinase and a specific inhibitor. *Kidney Int* 1989;36:790–801.

94. Davin JC, Davies M, Foidart JM, Foidart JB, Dechene CA, Mahieu PR. Urinary excretion of neutral proteinases in nephrotic rats with a glomerular disease. *Kidney Int* 1987;31:32–40.
95. Grinnel F, Head JR, Hopepauir J. Fibronectin and cell shape in vivo: studies on the endometrium during pregnancy. *J Cell Biol* 1982;94:579–606.
96. Hedin U, Bottger BA, Forsberg E, Johansson S, Thyberg J. Diverse effects of fibronectin and laminin on fenotypic properties of cultured arterial smooth muscle cells. *J Cell Biol* 1988;107:307–319.
97. Cosio FG, Sedmak DD, Nahman SN Jr. Cellular receptors for matrix proteins in normal human kidney and human mesangial cells. *Kidney Int* 1990;38:886–895.
98. Harris KPG, Lefkowith JB, Klahr S, Schreiner GF. Essential fatty acid deficiency ameliorates acute renal dysfunction in the rat after the administration of the aminonucleoside of puromycin. *J Clin Invest* 1990;86:1115–1123.
99. Diamond JR, Pesek I, Ruggieri S, Karnovsky MJ. Essential fatty acid deficiency during acute puromycin nephrosis ameliorates late renal injury. *Am J Physiol* 1989;257:F798–F807.
100. Goto T, Mune M, Mayoba K, Yukawa S, Nomoto H. Effects of selective thromboxane A2 synthetase inhibitor on aminonucleoside induced nephrotic rat. *Proc Int Congr Nephrol 10th* 1987; 227(abstract).
101. Remuzzi G, Imberti O, Rossini M, et al. Increased glomerular thromboxane synthesis as a possible cause of proteinuria in experimental nephrosis. *J Clin Invest* 1985;75:94–101.
102. Benigni A, Perico N, Dadan J, Valoti N, Piccinelli A, Remuzzi G. The increased thromboxane B2 (TxB2) urinary excretion in experimental nephrosis originates from resident renal cells. *Kidney Int* 1990;37:345(abstract).
103. Imberti O, Remuzzi A, Benigni A, Puntorieri S, Perico N, Remuzzi G. Thromboxane (TX) A2 synthase inhibitor reduces urinary protein excretion in experimental nephrosis by a mechanism independent by changes in glomerular hemodynamics. *J Am Soc Nephrol* 1990;1:632.
104. Egido J, Robles A, Ortiz A, et al. Role of platelet-activating factor in Adriamycin-induced nephropathy in rats. *Eur J Pharmacol* 1987;138:119–123.
105. Perico N, Delaini F, Tagliaferri M, et al. The effect of platelet-activating factor and its specific receptor antagonist on glomerular permeability to proteins in isolated perfused rat kidney. *Lab Invest* 1988;58:163–171.
106. Perico N, Remuzzi A, Dadan J, Battaglia C, Remuzzi G. Platelet-activating factor alters glomerular barrier size selectivity for macromolecules in the rat. *Am J Physiol* 1991; 261:F85–F90.
107. Thakur V, Walker PD, Shah SV. Evidence suggesting a role for hydroxyl radical in puromycin aminonucleoside-induced proteinuria. *Kidney Int* 1988;34:494–499.
108. Ginevri F, Ghiggeri GM, Oleggini R, et al. Renal xanthine oxidase in the pathogenesis of experimental Adriamycin nephrosis in rats. *VIII Congress of the International Pediatric Nephrology Association August 27-September 1 1989*; (abstract).
109. Kashihara N, Dalecki T, Watanabe Y, Liu Z, Makino H, Kanwar Y. Effect of reactive oxygen species on glomerular extracellular matrix proteoglycans. *J Am Soc Nephrol* 1990;1:527.
110. Schreiner GF, Cotran RS, Unanue ER. Modulation of IA and leukocyte common antigen expression in rat glomeruli during the course of glomerulonephritis and aminonucleoside nephrosis. *Lab Invest* 1984;51:524–533.
111. Bricio TR, Mampaso F, Egido J, Molina A, Gonzales E. Interleukin-1 cytokine production in Adriamycin induced nephrosis. *Cancer Chemother Rep* 1990;1:517(abstract).
112. Gomez-Chiarri M, Lerma JL, Gonzalez E, Ortiz A, Hernando L, Egido J. Involvement of tumor necrosis factor (TNF) in the pathogenesis of experimental nephrotic syndrome. *J Am Soc Nephrol* 1990;1:522(abstract).
113. Brenner BM, Meyer TW, Hostetter TH. Dietary protein intake and the progressive nature of kidney disease: the role of hemodynamically mediated glomerular injury in the pathogenesis of progressive glomerular sclerosis in aging, renal ablation, and intrinsic renal disease. *N Engl J Med* 1982; 307:652–659.
114. Anderson S, Meyer TW, Rennke HG, Brenner BM. Control of glomerular hypertension limits glomerular injury in rats with reduced renal mass. *J Clin Invest* 1985;76:612–619.
115. Zatz R, Dunn BR, Meyer TW, Anderson S, Rennke HG, Brenner BM. Prevention of diabetic glomerulopathy by pharmacological amelioration of glomerular capillary hypertension. *J Clin Invest* 1986;77:1925–1930.
116. Diamond JR, Karnovsky MJ. Ameliorative effects of dietary protein restriction in chronic aminonucleoside nephrosis. *J Lab Clin Med* 1987;109:538–544.

117. Anderson S, Diamond JR, Karnovsky MJ, et al. Mechanisms underlying transition from acute glomerular injury to late glomerular sclerosis in a rat model of nephrotic syndrome. *J Clin Invest* 1988;82:1757–1768.
118. Scholey JW, Miller PL, Rennke HG, Meyer TW. Effect of converting enzyme inhibition on the course of Adriamycin-induced nephropathy. *Kidney Int* 1989;36:816–822.
119. Hall RL, Wilke WL, Fettman MJ. The progression of Adriamycin-induced nephrotic syndrome in rats and the effect of captopril. *Toxicol Appl Pharmacol* 1986;82:164–174.
120. Beukers JJB, Hoedemaeker PJ, Weening JJ. A comparison of the effects of converting-enzyme inhibition and protein restriction in experimental nephrosis. *Lab Invest* 1988;59:631–640.
121. Grond J, Koudstaal J, Elema JD. Mesangial function and glomerular sclerosis in rats with aminonucleoside nephrosis. *Kidney Int* 1985;27:405–410.
122. Bertani T, Cutillo F, Zoja C, Broggini M, Remuzzi G. Tubulo-interstitial lesions mediate renal damage in Adriamycin glomerulopathy. *Kidney Int* 1986;30:488–496.
123. Mené P, Abboud HE, Dunn MJ. Regulation of human mesangial cell growth in culture by thromboxane A2 and prostacyclin. *Kidney Int* 1990;38:232–239.
124. Bruggeman LA, Burbelo PD, Yamada Y, et al. Regulation of renal transcriptional factors for type IV collagen gene expression by thromboxane. *XI International Congress of Nephrology Tokyo, 15–20 July 1990*;30A(abstract).
125. Ledbetter S, Copeland EJ, Noonan D, et al. Altered steady-state mRNA levels of basement membrane proteins in diabetic mouse kidneys and thromboxane synthase inhibition. *Diabetes* 1990;39:196–203.
126. Dworkin JD, Brenner BM. Biophysical basis of glomerular filtration. In: Seldin DW, Giebisch G, eds. *The kidney, physiology and pathophysiology*. New York: Raven Press, 1985;397–426.
127. King AJ, Brenner BM, Anderson S. Endothelin: a potent renal and systemic vasoconstrictor peptide. *Am J Physiol* 1989;256:F1051–F1058.
128. Schlondorff D. The glomerular mesangial cell: an expanding role for a specialized pericyte. *FASEB J* 1987;1:272–281.
129. Badr KF, Munger KA, Sugiura M, Snajdar RM, Schwartzberg M, Inagami T. High and low affinity bindings sites for endothelin on cultured rat glomerular mesangial cells. *Biochem Biophys Res Commun* 1989;161:776–781.
130. Mené P, Dunn MJ. Contractile effects of TxA2 and endoperoxide analogues on cultured rat glomerular mesangial cells. *Am J Physiol* 1986;251:F1029–F1035.
131. Zoja C, Orisio S, Perico N, et al. Constitutive expression of endothelin gene in cultured human mesangial cells and its modulation by transforming growth factor-b, thrombin, and a thromboxane A2 analogue. *Lab Invest* 1991;64:16–20.
132. Myers BD, Deen WM, Brenner BM. Effects of norepinephrine and angiotensin II on the determinants of glomerular ultrafiltration and proximal tubule fluid reabsorption in the rat. *Circ Res* 1975;37:101–110.
133. DiBona G. The function of the renal nerves. *Rev Physiol Biochem Pharmacol* 1982;94:75–171.
134. Kon V. Karnovsky MJ. Morphologic demonstration of adrenergic influences on the glomerulus. *Am J Pathol* 1989;134:1039–1046.
135. Blantz RC, Konnen KS, Tucker BJ. Angiotensin II effects upon the glomerular microcirculation and ultrafiltration coefficient in the rat. *J Clin Invest* 1976;57:419–434.
136. Ploth DW, Rudolph J, LaGrange R, Navar LG. Tubuloglomerular feedback and single nephron function after converting enzyme inhibition in the rat. *J Clin Invest* 1979;64:1325–1335.
137. Blantz RC, Pelayo JC. A functional role for the tubuloglomerular feedback mechanism. *Kidney Int* 1984;25:739–746.
138. Baylis C. Effects of administered thromboxanes on the intact, normal rat kidney. *Renal Physiol* 1987;10:110–121.
139. Schor N, Ichikawa U, Brenner BM. Mechanisms of action of various hormones and vasoactive substances on glomerular ultrafiltration in the rat. *Kidney Int* 1981;20:442–451.
140. Badr KF, Baylis C, Pfeffer JM, et al. Renal and systemic hemodynamic responses to intravenous infusion of leukotriene C4 in the rat. *Circ Res* 1984;54:492–499.
141. Rosenthal A, Pace-Asciak CR. Potent vasoconstrictor of the isolated perfused rat kidney by leukotrienes C4 and D4. *Can J Physiol Pharmacol* 1983;61:325–328.
142. Yanagisawa M, Kurihara H, Kimura S, et al. A novel potent vasoconstrictor peptide produced by vascular endothelial cells. *Nature* 1988;332:411–415.
143. Perico N, Dadan J, Gabanelli M, Remuzzi G. Cyclooxygenase products and atrial natriuretic peptide modulate renal response to endothelin. *J Pharmacol Exp Ther* 1990;252:1213–1220.

144. Simonson MS, Wann S, Mené P, et al. Endothelin stimulates phospholipase C, Na^+/H^+ exchange, c-fos expression and mitogenesis in rat mesangial cells. *J Clin Invest* 1989;83:708.
145. Badr KF, Murray JJ, Breyer MD, Takahashi K, Inagami T, Harris RC. Mesangial cell, glomerular and renal vascular responses to endothelin in the rat kidney. *J Clin Invest* 1989;83:336–342.
146. Kon V, Yared A, Ichikawa I. Role of renal sympathetic nerves in mediating hypoperfusion of renal cortical microcirculation in experimental congestive heart failure and acute extravascular fluid volume depletion. *J Clin Invest* 1985;76:1913–1920.
147. Blantz RC, Pelayo JC, Gushwa LC, et al. Functional basis for the glomerular alteration in uranyl nitrate acute renal failure. *Kidney Int* 1985;28:733–743.
148. Schor N, Ichikawa I, Rennke HG, Troy JL, Brenner BM. Pathophysiology of altered glomerular function in aminoglycoside-treated rats. *Kidney Int* 1981;19:288–296.
149. Clive DM, Stoff JS. Renal syndromes associated with nonsteroidal antiinflammatory drugs. *N Engl J Med* 1984;310:563–572.
150. Macconi D, Benigni A, Morigi M, et al. Enhanced glomerular thromboxane A2 mediates some pathophysiologic effect of platelet-activating factor in rabbit nephrotoxic nephritis: evidence from biochemical measurements and inhibitor trials. *J Lab Clin Med* 1989;113:549–560.
151. Kon V, Yoshioka T, Fogo A, et al. Glomerular actions of endothelin in vivo. *J Clin Invest* 1989; 83:1762.
152. Salaman JR. Cyclosporine in a renal trasplantation: a guide to management. *Lancet* 1984;2:269–271.
153. Powell-Jackson PR, Young B, Calne RY, Williams R. Nephrotoxicity of parenterally administered cyclosporine after orthotopic liver transplantation. *Transplantation* 1983;36:505–508.
154. Flechner SM, van Buren C, Kerman RH, Kahan DB. The nephrotoxicity of cyclosporine in renal transplant recipients. *Transplant Proc* 1983;15(suppl 1):2689–2694.
155. Sullivan BA, Hak LJ, Finn WF. Cyclosporine nephrotoxicity: studies in laboratory animals. *Transplant Proc* 1985;17(suppl 1):145–154.
156. Mihatsch MJ, Thiel G, Basler V, et al. Morphological patterns in cyclosporine-treated renal transplant recipients. *Transplant Proc* 1985;17:101–116.
157. Whiting PH, Thomson AW, Blair JT, Simpson JG. Experimental cyclosporin A nephrotoxicity. *Br J Exp Pathol* 1982;63:88–94.
158. Mihatsch MJ, Thiel G, Ryffel B. Histopathology of cyclosporine nephrotoxicity. *Transplant Proc* 1988;20(suppl 3):759–771.
159. Mihatsch MJ, Thiel G, Spicktin MP, et al. Morphological findings in kidney transplants after treatment with cyclosporine. *Transplant Proc* 1983;15(suppl 1):2821.
160. Ryffel B. Experimental toxicological studies with cyclosporin A nephrotoxicity. In: White DJG, ed. *Cyclosporin A*. Amsterdam: Elsevier, 1982;45–75.
161. Dieperink H, Starklint H, Leyssac PP. Nephrotoxicity of cyclosporine—an animal model: study of the nephrotoxic effect of cyclosporine on overall and renal tubular function in conscious rats. *Transplant Proc* 1983;15:2736.
162. Humes HD, Jackson NM, O'Connor RP, Hunt DA, White MD. Pathogenetic mechanisms of nephrotoxicity: insights into cyclosporine nephrotoxicity. *Transplant Proc* 1985;17(suppl 1):51–62.
163. Murray BM, Paller MS, Ferris TF. Effect of cyclosporine administration on renal hemodynamics in conscious rat. *Kidney Int* 1985;28:767–774.
164. Perico N, Dadan J, Remuzzi G. Endothelin mediates in the renal vasoconstriction induced by cyclosporine in the rat. *J Am Soc Nephrol* 1990;1:76–83.
165. Rossi NF, Churchill PC, McDonald FD, Ellis VR. Mechanism of cyclosporine A–induced renal vasoconstriction in the rat. *J Pharmacol Exp Ther* 1989;250:896–901.
166. English J, Evan A, Houghton DC, Bennett WM. Cyclosporine-induced acute renal dysfunction in the rat. Evidence of arteriolar vasoconstriction with perservation of tubular function. *Transplantation* 1987;44:135–141.
167. Baxter CR, Duggin GG, Hall BM, Horvath JS, Tiller DJ. Stimulation of renin release from rat renal cortical slices by cyclosporin A. *Res Commun Chem Pathol Pharmacol* 1984;43:417–423.
168. Kurtz A, Della Bruna R, Kuhn K. Cyclosporine A enhances renin secretion and production in isolated juxtaglomerular cells. *Kidney Int* 1988;33:947–953.
169. Barros EJG, Boim MA, Ajzen H, Ramos OL, Schor N. Glomerular hemodynamics and hormonal participation in cyclosporine nephrotoxicity. *Kidney Int* 1987;3:219–225.
170. Jao S, Waltzer W, Arbeit LA. Acute cyclosporine induced decrease in GFR is mediated by changes in renal blood flow and renal vascular resistance. *Kidney Int* 1986;29:431.

171. Moss NG, Powell SL, Falk RJ. Intravenous cyclosporine activates afferent and efferent renal nerves and causes sodium retention in innervated kidneys in rats. *Proc Natl Acad Sci USA* 1985;82:8222–8226.
172. Curtis JJ, Luke RG, Dubovsky E. Cyclosporin in therapeutic doses increases renal allograft vascular resistance. *Lancet* 1986;2:477–479.
173. Bantle JP, Paller MS, Boudreau RJ. Long-term effects of cyclosporine on renal function in organ transplant recipients. *J Lab Clin Med* 1990;115:233–240.
174. Lau DCW, Wong KL, Hwang WS. Cyclosporine toxicity on cultured rat microvascular endothelial cells. *Kidney Int* 1989;35:604–613.
175. Adu D, Lote CJ, Michael J, Turney JH, McMaster P. Does cyclosporine inhibit renal prostaglandin synthesis? *Proc Eur Dial Transpl Assoc* 1985;21:969–972.
176. Zoja C, Furci L, Ghilardi F, Zilio P, Benigni A, Remuzzi G. Cyclosporin-induced endothelial cell injury. *Lab Invest* 1986;55:455–462.
177. Perico N, Zoja C, Benigni A, Ghilardi F, Gualandris L, Remuzzi G. Effect of short-term cyclosporine administration in rats on renin-angiotensin and thromboxane A2: possible relevance to the reduction in glomerular filtration rate. *J Pharmacol Exp Ther* 1986;239:229–235.
178. Kawaguchi A, Goldman MH, Shapiro R, Foegh ML, Ramwell PW, Lower RR. Increase in urinary thromboxane B2 in rats caused by cyclosporine. *Transplantation* 1985;40:214–216.
179. Smeesters C, Chaland P, Giroux L, et al. Prevention of acute cyclosporine A nephrotoxicity by thromboxane synthetase inhibitor. *Transplant Proc* 1988;20(suppl 3):658–664.
180. Perico N, Pasini M, Gaspari F, Abbate M, Remuzzi G. Co-participation of thromboxane A_2 and leukotriene C_4 and D_4 in mediating cyclosporine-induced acute renal failure. *Transplatation* 1991;52:873–878.
181. Coffman TM, Smith SR, Creech EA, et al. The thromboxane (Tx) synthetase inhibitor CSG 13080 improves renal allograft function in patients taking cyclosporine (CyA). *Kidney Int* 1990; 37: 604(abstract).
182. Elzinga L, Kelley VE, Houghton DC, Barrett LV, Bennett WM, Strom TB. Modification of experimental nephrotoxicity with fish oil as the vehicle of cyclosporine. *Transplantation* 1987; 43:271–281.
183. Bunchman TE, Brookshire CA. Cyclosporine stimulated synthesis of endothelin by human endothelial cells in tissue culture. *Kidney Int* 1990;37:365.
184. Kon V, Sugiura M, Inagami T, et al. Role of endothelin in cyclosporine-induced glomerular dysfunction. *Kidney Int* 1990;37:1487.
185. Pernow J, Boutier J-F, Franco-Cereceda A, et al. Potent selective vasoconstrictor effects of endothelin in the pig kidney in vivo. *Acta Physiol Scand* 1988;134:573.
186. Humes DH. Aminoglycoside nephrotoxicity. *Kidney Int* 1988;33:900–911.
187. Baylis C, Rennke HR, Brenner BM. Mechanisms of the defect in glomerular ultrafiltration associated with gentamicin administration. *Kidney Int* 1977;12:344–353.
188. Baylis C. Gentamicin-induced glomerulotoxicity in the pregnant rat. *Am J Kidney Dis* 1989; 13:108–113.
189. Luft FC, Evan AP. Glomerular filtration barrier in aminoglycoside induced nephrotoxic acute renal failure. *Renal Physiol* 1980;3:265–271.
190. Bulger RE, Eknoyan G, Purcell DJ, Dobyan DC. Endothelial characteristics of glomerular capillaries in normal, mercuric chloride-induced, and gentamicin-induced acute renal failure in the rat. *J Clin Invest* 1983;72:128–141.
191. Luft FC, Aronoff GR, Evan AP, Connors BA, Weinberger MH, Kleit SA. The renin-angiotensin system in aminoglycoside-induced acute renal failure. *J Pharmacol Exp Ther* 1982;220:433–439.
192. Klotman PE, Boatman JE, Volpp BD, Baker JD, Yarger WE. Captopril enhances aminoglycoside nephrotoxicity in potassium-depleted rats. *Kidney Int* 1985;28:118–127.
193. Gotoh S, Ogihara T, Nakamaru M, et al. Effect of captopril on renal vascular resistance, renin, prostaglandins and kinin in the isolated perfused kidney. *Life Sci* 1983;33:2409–2425.
194. Sande MA, Mandell GL. Antimicrobial agent. Antifungal antiviral agents. In: Goodman Gilman A, Goodman LS, Rall TW, Murad F, eds. *The pharmacological basis of therapeutics*. New York: Macmillan, 1980;453–464.
195. Wertlake PT, Butler WT, Hill GH, Utz JP. Nephrotoxic tubular damage and calcium deposition following amphotericin B therapy. *Am J Pathol* 1963;43:449–457.
196. McCurdy DK, Frederic M, Elkinton JR. Renal tubular acidosis due to amphotericin B. *N Engl J Med* 1968;278:124–131.
197. Douglas JB, Healy JK. Nephrotoxic effects of amphotericin B, including renal tubular acidosis. *Am J Med* 1969;46:154–162.

198. Utz JP, Bennett JE, Brandiss MD, Butler WT, Hill GJ. Amphotericin B toxicity. *Ann Intern Med* 1964;61:334–354.
199. Butler WT, Hill GJ, Szwed CF, Knight V. Amphotericin B renal toxicity in the dog. *J Pharmacol Exp Ther* 1964;143:47–56.
200. Gerkens JF, Branch RA. The influence of sodium status and furosemide on canine acute amphotericin B nephrotoxicity. *J Pharmacol Exp Ther* 1980;214:306–311.
201. Heidemann HT, Gerkens JF, Spickard WA, Jackson EK, Branch RA. Amphotericin B nephrotoxicity in human decreased by salt repletion. *Am J Med* 1983;75:476–481.
202. Cheng J-T, Witty RT, Robison RR, Yarger WE, Schrader NW, Kennedy BM. Amphotericin B nephrotoxicity: increased renal resistance and tubule permeability. *Kidney Int* 1982;22:626–633.
203. Tolins JP, Raij L. Adverse effect of amphotericin B administration on renal hemodynamics in the rat. Neurohumoral mechanisms and influence of calcium channel blockade. *J Pharmacol Exp Ther* 1990;245:594–599.
204. Sabra R, Takahashi K, Branch RA, Badr KF. Mechanisms of amphotericin B–induced reduction of the glomerular filtration rate: a micropuncture study. *J Pharmacol Exp Ther* 1990;253:34–37.
205. Gerkens JF, Heidemann HTh, Jackson EK, Branch RA. Aminophylline inhibits renal vasoconstriction induced by intrarenal hypertonic saline. *J Pharmacol Exp Ther* 1983;225:609–615.
206. Badr KF, DeBoer DK, Takahashi K, Harris RC, Fogo A, Jacobson HR. Glomerular responses to platelet activating factor in the rat: role of thromboxane A2. *Am J Physiol* 1989;256:F35–F43.
207. Myers BD, Ross J, Newton L, Leutscher J, Perlroth M. Cyclosporine-associated chronic nephropathy. *N Engl J Med* 1984;311:699–705.
208. Moran M, Tomlanovich S, Myers BD. Cyclosporine-induced chronic nephropathy in human recipients of cardiac allografts. *Transplant Proc* 1985;17(suppl 1):185–190.
209. Remuzzi G, Bertani T. Renal vascular and thrombotic effects of cyclosporine. *Am J Kidney Dis* 1989;13:261–272.
210. Starzl TE, Hakala TR, Rosenthal JT, et al. Colorado-Pittsburgh cadaveric renal transplantation study with cyclosporine. *Transplant Proc* 1983;15:2463–2468.
211. Flechner SM, Payne WD, van Buren, et al. The effect of cyclosporine on early graft function in human renal transplantation. *Transplantation* 1983;36:268.
212. Najarian JS, Ferguson RM, Sutherland DE, Rynasiewicz JJ, et al. A prospective trial of the efficacy of cyclosporine in renal transplantation at the University of Minnesota. *Transplant Proc* 1983;15:438.
213. Canadian Multicentre Transplant Study Group. A randomized clinical trial of cyclosporine in cadaveric renal transplants. *N Engl J Med* 1983;309:809–815.
214. European Multicenter Trial Group. Cyclosporine in cadaveric renal transplantation: one-year follow-up of multicenter trial. *Lancet* 1983;2:986–989.
215. Dische FE, Neuberger J, Keating J, et al. Kidney pathology in liver allograft recipients after long-term treatment with cyclosporin A. *Lab Invest* 1988;58:395–402.
216. Stiller CR, Keown PA, Heinrichs D, et al. The effect of cyclosporine on renal function in newly diagnosed diabetics. *Transplant Proc* 1985;17:202.
217. Von Graffenreid B, Harrison WB. Renal function in patients with autoimmune diseases treated with cyclosporine. *Transplant Proc* 1985;17:215.
218. Myers BD, Sibley R, Newton L, et al. The long-term course of cyclosporine-associated chronic nephropathy. *Kidney Int* 1988;33:590–600.
219. Myers BD, Newton L, Boshkos C, et al. Chronic injury of human renal microvessels with low-dose cyclosporine therapy. *Transplantation* 1988;46:694–702.
220. Sweny P, Lui SF, Scoble JE, et al. Conversion of stable renal allografts at one year from cyclosporin A to azathioprine: a randomized controlled study. *Transplant Int* 1990;3:19–22.
221. Nizze H, Mihatsch MJ, Zollinger HU, et al. Cyclosporine-associated nephropathy in patients with heart and bone marrow transplants. *Clin Nephrol* 1988;30:248–260.
222. Thiru S, Maher ER, Hamilton DV, et al. Tubular changes in renal transplant recipients on cyclosporin. *Transplant Proc* 1983;15:2846.
223. Klintmalm G, Bohman SO, Sundelin E, et al. Interstitial fibrosis in renal allografts after 12 to 40 months of cyclosporine treatment. Beneficial effects of lower doses early after transplantation. *Lancet* 1984;2:950–953.
224. Devinemi R, McKenzie N, Wall N, et al. Renal function in patients receiving cyclosporine for orthotopic cardiac transplantation. *Transplant Proc* 1985;17:1256.
225. Wallace AC. Histopathology of cyclosporine. *Transplant Proc* 1985;17 (4 suppl 1):117–122.
226. Bertani T, Ferrazzi P, Shieppa HA, et al. Nature and extent of glomerular injury induced by cyclosporine in heart transplant patients. *Kidney Int* 1991;40:243–250.

227. Olson JL, Hostetter TH, Rennke HG, Brenner BM, Venkatachalam MA. Altered glomerular permeability and progressive sclerosis following ablation of renal mass. *Kidney Int* 1982;22:112–126.
228. Bertani T, Perico N, Abbate M, Battaglia C, Remuzzi G. Renal injury induced by long-term administration of cyclosporin A to rats. *Am J Pathol* 1987;127:569–579.
229. Simpson JG, Saunders NJ, Thomson KJ, et al. Chronic renal damage caused by cyclosporine. *Transplant Proc* 1988;20:792–794.
230. Gillum DM, Truong L, Tasby J, et al. Chronic cyclosporine nephrotoxicity. A rodent model. *Transplantation* 1988;46:285–292.
231. Dieperink H, Leyssac PP, Starklint H, Kemp E. Long-term cyclosporin nephrotoxicity in the rat: effects on renal function and morphology. *Nephrol Dial Transplant* 1988;3:317–326.
232. Perico N, Remuzzi A, Imberti O, et al. Morphometrical analysis of glomerular changes induced by cyclosporine in the rat. *Am J Kidney Dis* 1991;17:537–543.
233. Benigni A, Perico N, Ladny JR, et al. Increased urinary excretion of endothelin-A and its precursor, big-endothelin-1 in rats chronically treated with cyclosporine. *Transplantation* 1991;52:175–177.
234. Benigni A, Perico N, Gaspari F, et al. Increased renal endothelin production in rats with reduced renal mass. *Am J Physiol* 1991;260:F331-F339.
235. Nagase T, Fukuchi Y, Jo C, et al. Endothelin-1 stimulates arachidonate 15-lipoxygenase activity and oxygen radical formation in the rat distal lung. *Biochem Biophys Res Commun* 1990;168:485–489.
236. Goetzl EJ, Pickett WC. The human PMN leukocyte chemotactic activity of complex hydroxyeicosatetraenoic acids (HETEs). *J Immunol* 1980;125:1789.
237. Benigni A, Chiabrando C, Piccinelli A, et al. Increased urinary excretion of thromboxane B2 and 2,3-dinor-TxB2 in cyclosporin A nephrotoxicity. *Kidney Int* 1988;34:164–174.
238. Perico N, Benigni A, Zoja C, Delaini F, Remuzzi G. Functional significance of exaggerated renal thromboxane A2 synthesis induced by cyclosporin A. *Am J Physiol* 1986;251:F581–F587.
239. Coffman TM, Carr DR, Yarger WE, Klotman PE. Evidence that renal prostaglandin and thromboxane production is stimulated in chronic cyclosporine nephrotoxicity. *Transplantation* 1987;43:282–285.
240. Rossini M, Belloni A, Remuzzi G, Perico N. Thromboxane receptor blockade attenuates the toxic effect of cyclosporine in experimental renal transplantation. *Circulation* 1990;81(suppl I):61–67.
241. Kuhn K, Forstermann U, Frolich JC, et al. Effect of cyclosporine A (CyA) on blood pressure and prostacyclin and thromboxane A2 production. *Xth International Congress of Nephrology London, 26–31 July 1987*; 231.
242. van der Heide JJH, Bilo HJG, Tegzess AM, Donker AJM. The effects of dietary supplementation with fish oil on renal function in cyclosporine-treated renal transplant recipients. *Transplantation* 1990;49:523–527.
243. Bruggeman LA, Horigan EA, Horikoshi S, et al. Thromboxane stimulates synthesis of extracellular matrix proteins in vitro. *Am J Physiol* 1991;261:F488–F494.
244. Wolf G, Killen PD, Neilson EG. Cyclosporin A stimulates transcription and procollagen secretion in tubulointerstitial fibroblasts and proximal tubular cells. *J Am Nephrol* 1990;1:918–922.
245. Fridovich I. Oxygen radicals, hydrogen peroxide and oxygen toxicity. In: Pryor WA, ed. *Free radicals in biology*. New York: Academic Press, 1976;239–277.
246. Freeman BA, Crapo JD. Biology of disease, free radicals and tissue injury. *Lab Invest* 1982;47:412–426.
247. Fridovich I. Superoxide dismutases. *Annu Rev Biochem* 1975;44:147.
248. Marklund SL. Extracellular superoxide dismutase and other superoxide dismutase isoenzymes in tissues from nine mammalian species. *Biochem J* 1984;222:649–655.
249. Halliwell B, Gutteridge JMC. Oxygen toxicity, oxygen radicals, transition metals and disease. *Biochem J* 1984;219:1–14.
250. Aust SD, Morehouse LA, Thomas CE. Role of metals in oxygen radical reactions. *J Free Radicals Biol Med* 1985;1:3–25.
251. Harrison JE, Schultz J. Studies on the chlorinating activity of myeloperoxidase. *J Biol Chem* 1976;251:1371–1374.
252. Weiss St, Test ST, Eckman CH, Roos D, Regiani S. Brominating oxidants generated by human eosinophils. *Science* 1986;234:200–203.
253. Agner K. Biological effects of hypochlorous acid formed by "MPO" peroxidation in the presence of chloride ions. In: Akeson A, Ehrenburg A, eds. *Structure and function of oxidation-reduction enzymes*. New York: Pergamon Press, 1972;329–335.
254. Albrich JM, McCarthy CA, Hurst JK. Biological reactivity of hypochlorous acid: implications for

microbicidal mechanisms of leukocytes myeloperoxidase. *Proc Natl Acad Sci USA* 1981;78:210–214.
255. Weiss SJ, Lampert MB, Test ST. Long-lived oxidants generated by human neutrophils: characterization and bioactivity. *Science* 1983;222:625–628.
256. Lang CA, Bielski BHJ. Rate of reaction of superoxide radicals with chloride containing species. *J Physiol Chem* 1980;84:555–557.
257. Battelli MG, Della Corte E, Stirpe F. Xanthine oxidase type D (dehydrogenase) in the intestine and other organs of the rat. *Biochem J* 1972;126:747–749.
258. Roy RS, McCord JM. Superoxide and ischemia: conversion of xanthine dehydrogenase to xanthine oxidase. In: Greenwald R, Cohen G, eds. *Oxygen radicals and their scavenger systems—cellular and molecular aspect*. New York: Elsevier Science, 1983;145–153.
259. Rossi F. The O_2^--forming NADPH oxidase of the phagocytes: nature, mechanisms of activation and function. *Biochim Biophys Acta* 1986;853:65–89.
260. Deisseroth A, Dounce AL. Catalase: physical and chemical properties, mechanism of catalysis, and physiological role. *Physiol Rev* 1970;50:319–375.
261. Mc Cay FPB, Gibson DD, Fong KC, Hornbrook KR. Effect of gluathione peroxidase activity on lipid peroxidation in biological membranes. *Biochim Biophys Acta* 1976;431:459.
262. McCord JM. Oxygen-derived free radicals in postischemic tissue injury. *N Engl J Med* 1985; 312:159–163.
263. Dormandy TL. An approach to free radicals. *Lancet* 1983;2:1010–1014.
264. Fantone JC, Ward PA. Role of oxygen-derived free radicals and metabolites in leukocyte-dependent inflammatory reactions. *Am J Pathol* 1982;107:397–418.
265. Johnson KJ, Ward PA. Biology of disease. Newer concepts in the pathogenesis of immune complex-induced tissue injury. *Lab Invest* 1982;47:218–226.
266. Marx JL. Oxygen free radicals linked to many diseases. *Science* 1987;235:529–531.
267. Johnson KJ, Ward PA. Role of oxygen metabolites in immune complex injury of lung. *J Immunol* 1981;126:2365–2369.
268. McCormick JR, Harkin MM, Johnson KJ, Ward PA. Suppression by superoxide dismutase of immune-complex induced pulmonary alveolitis and dermal inflammation. *Am J Pathol* 1981;102: 55–61.
269. Simpson PJ, Lucchesi BR. Free radicals and myocardial ischemia and reperfusion injury. *J Lab Clin Med* 1987;110:13–30.
270. Baud L, Ardaillau R. Reactive oxygen species: production and role in the kidney. *Am J Physiol* 1986;251:F765–F776.
271. Shah SV. Role of reactive oxygen metabolites in experimental glomerular disease. *Kidney Int* 1989;35:1093–1106.
272. Rehan A, Johnson KJ, Wiggins RC, Kunkel RG, Ward PA. Evidence for the role of oxygen radicals in acute nephrotoxic nephritis. *Lab Invest* 1984;51:396–403.
273. Weissman G, Smolen J, Korchak HM. Release of inflammatory mediators from stimulated neutrophils. *N Engl J Med* 1980;303:27.
274. Weiss SJ, Ward PA. Immune complex induced generation of oxygen metabolites by human neutrophils. *J Immunol* 1982;129:309–313.
275. Vissers MCM, Day WA, Winterbourn CC. Neutrophils adherent to a nonphagocytosable surface (glomerular basement membrane) produce oxidants only at the site of attachment. *Blood* 1985; 66:161–166.
276. DeChatelet LR, Shirley PS, Johnston RB. Effect of phorbol myristate acetate on the oxidative metabolism of human polymorphonuclear leukocytes. *Blood* 1976;47:545–554.
277. Rehan A, Johnson KJ, Kunkel RG, Wiggins RC. Role of oxygen radicals in phorbol myristate acetate–induced glomerular injury. *Kidney Int* 1985;27:503–511.
278. Boyce NW, Holdsworth SR. Hydroxyl radical mediation of immune renal injury by desferrioxamine. *Kidney Int* 1986;30:813–817.
279. Yoshioka T, Ichikawa I, Fogo A. Reactive oxygen metabolites cause massive, reversible proteinuria and glomerular sieving defect without apparent ultrastructural abnormality. *J Am Soc Nephrol* 1991;2:902–912.
280. Davies M, Barrett AJ, Travis J, Sanders E, Coles GA. The degradation of human glomerular basement membrane with purified lysosomal proteinases: evidence for the pathogenic role of the polymorphonuclear leucocyte in glomerulonephritis. *Clin Sci Mol Med* 1978;54:233–240.
281. Vissers MCM, Winterbourn CC, Hunt JS. Degradation of glomerular basement membrane by human neutrophils in vitro. *Biochim Biophys Acta* 1984;804:154–160.

282. Johnson RJ, Couser WG, Alpers CE, Vissers M, Schulze M, Klebanoff SJ. The human neutrophil serine proteinases, elastase and cathepsin G, can mediate glomerular injury in vivo. *J Exp Med* 1988;168:1169–1174.
283. Greenwald RA, Moy WW. Inhibition of collagen gelation by action of the superoxide radical. *Arthritis Rheum* 1979;22:251–259.
284. Curran SF, Amoruso MA, Goldstein BD, Berg RA. Degradation of soluble collagen by ozone or hydroxyl radicals. *FEBS Lett* 1984;176:155–160.
285. Greenwald RA, Moy WW. Effect of oxygen-derived free radicals on hyaluronic acid. *Arthritis Rheum* 1980;23:455–463.
286. Wolf SP, Dean RT. Fragmentation of proteins by free radicals and its effect on their susceptibility to enzymatic hydrolysis. *Biochem J* 1982;234:399–403.
287. Fligiel SEG, Lee EC, McCoy JP, Johnson KJ, Varani J. Protein degradation following treatment with hydrogen peroxide. *Am J Pathol* 1984;115:418–425.
288. Clark RA, Stone PT, El Hag A, Calore JD, Franzblan C. Myeloperoxidase-catalyzed inactivation of alpha 1-inhibitor by human neutrophils. *J Biol Chem* 1981;256:3348–3353.
289. Carp H, Janoff A. In vitro suppression of serum elastase-inhibitory capacity by reactive oxygen species generated by phagocytosing polymorphonuclear leukocytes. *J Clin Invest* 1979;63:793–797.
290. Weiss SJ, Regiani S. Neutrophils degrade subendothelial matrices in the presence of alpha-1-proteinase inhibitor. Cooperative use of lysosomal proteinases and oxygen metabolites. *J Clin Invest* 1984;73:1297–1303.
291. Weiss SJ, Peppin G, Ortiz X, Ragsdale C, Test ST. Oxidative autoactivation of latent collagenase by human neutrophils. *Science* 1985;227:747–749.
292. Peppin GJ, Weiss SJ. Activation of the endogenous metalloproteinase, gelatinase, by triggered human neutrophils. *Proc Natl Acad Sci USA* 1986;83:4322–4326.
293. Shah SV, Baricos WH, Basci A. Degradation of human glomerular basement membrane by stimulated neutrophils. Activation of a metalloproteinase(s) by reactive oxygen metabolites. *J Clin Invest* 1987;79:25–31.
294. Johnson RJ, Couser WG, Chi EY, Adler S, Klebanoff SJ. New mechanism for glomerular injury. Myeloperoxidase-hydrogen peroxide-halide system. *J Clin Invest* 1987;79:1379–1387.
295. Johnson RJ, Guggenheim SJ, Klebanoff SJ, et al. Morphologic correlates of glomerular oxidant injury induced by the myeloperoxidase-hydrogen peroxide-halide system of the neutrophil. *Lab Invest* 1988;58:294–301.
296. Johnson RJ, Klebanoff SJ, Ochi RF, et al. Participation of myeloperoxidase-H_2O_2-halide system in immune complex nephritis. *Kidney Int* 1987;32:342–349.
297. Jasin HE. Oxidative cross-linking of immune complexes by human polymorphonuclear leukocytes. *J Clin Invest* 1988;81:6–15.
298. Weiss SJ, Young J, LoBuglio AF, Slivka A Nimeh NF. Role of hydrogen peroxide in neutrophil-mediated destruction of cultured endothelial cells. *J Clin Invest* 1981;68:714–721.
299. Sacks T, Moldow CF, Craddock PR, Bowers TK, Jacob HS. Oxygen radicals mediate endothelial cell damage by complement-stimulated granulocytes. *J Clin Invest* 1978;61:1161–1167.
300. Rehan A, Wiggins RC, Kunkel RG, Till GO, Johnson KJ. Glomerular injury and proteinuria in rats after intrarenal injection of cobra venom factor. *Am J Pathol* 1986;123:57–66.
301. Varani J, Fligiel SEG, Till GO, Kunkel RG, Ryan US, Ward PA. Pulmonary endothelial cell killing by human neutrophils. Possible involvement of hydroxyl radical. *Lab Invest* 1985;53:656–663.
302. Gannon DE, Varani J, Phan SH, et al. Source of iron in neutrophil-mediated killing of endothelial cells. *Lab Invest* 1987;57:37–44.
303. Kvietys PR, Inauen W, Bacon BR, Grisham MB. Xanthine oxidase-induced injury to endothelium: role of intracellular iron and hydroxyl radical. *Am J Physiol* 1989;257:H1640–H1646.
304. Shasby DM, Lind SE, Shasby SS, Goldsmith JC, Hunninghake GW. Reversible oxidant-induced increases in albumin transfer across cultured endothelium: alterations in cell shape and calcium homeostasis. *Blood* 1985;65:605–614.
305. Freeman BA, Rosen GM, Barber MJ. Superoxide perturbation of the organization of vascular endothelial cell membranes. *J Biol Chem* 1986;261:6590–6593.
306. Ager A, Gordon JL. Differential effects of hydrogen peroxide on indices of endothelial cell function. *J Exp Med* 1984;159:592–603.
307. Spragg RG, Hinshaw DB, Hyslop PA, Schraufstatter IU, Cochrane CG. Alterations in adenosine

triphosphate and energy charge in cultured endothelial and P388D1 cells after oxidant injury. *J Clin Invest* 1985;76:1471–1476.
308. Andreoli SP, McAteer JA. Reactive oxygen molecule-mediated injury in endothelial and renal tubular epithelial cells in vitro. *Kidney Int* 1990;38:785–794.
309. Ratych RE, Chuknyske RS, Bulkley GB. The primary localization of free radical generation after anoxia/reoxygenation in isolated endothelial cells. *Surgery* 1987;102:122–131.
310. Jarasch E-D, Grund C, Bruder G, Heid HW, Kennan TW, Franke WW. Localization of xanthine oxidase in mammary gland epithelium and capillary endothelium. *Cell* 1981;25:67–82.
311. Phan SH, Gannon DE, Varani J, Ryan US, Ward PA. Xanthine oxidase activity in rat pulmonary artery endothelial cells and its alteration by activated neutrophils. *Am J Pathol* 1989;134:1201–1211.
312. Friedl HP, Till GO, Ryan US, Ward PA. Mediator-induced activation of xanthine oxidase in endothelial cells. *FASEB J* 1989;3:2512–2518.
313. Rosen GM, Freeman BA. Detection of superoxide generated by endothelial cells. *Proc Natl Acad Sci USA* 1984;81:7269–7273.
314. Harlan JM, Levine JD, Callahan KS, Schwartz BR, Harker LA. Glutathione redox cycle protects cultured endothelial cells against lysis by extracellularly generated hydrogen peroxide. *J Clin Invest* 1984;73:706–713.
315. Dobrina A, Patriarca P. Neutrophil-endothelial cell interaction. Evidence for and mechanisms of the self-protection of bovine microvascular endothelial cells from hydrogen peroxide-induced oxidative stress. *J Clin Invest* 1986;78:462–471.
316. Kawamura T, Yoshioka T, Moore-Jarrett T, Hoover RL, Ichikawa I. Glucocorticoid (G) raises antioxidant enzyme (AOE) activity and attenuates hydrogen peroxide (H_2O_2) generation in glomerular endothelial cells (GEC). *J Am Soc Nephrol* 1990;1:528.
317. Kawamura T, Yoshioka T, Bills T, Fogo A, Ichikawa I. Glucocorticoid activates glomular antioxidant enzymes and protects glomeruli from oxidant injuries. *Kidney Int* 1991;291–301.
318. Hara T, Miyai T, Iida T, Futenma A, Nakamura S, Kato K. Aggravation of puromycin aminonucleoside (PAN) nephrosis by the inhibition of endogenous superoxide dismutase (SOD). *XI International Congress of Nephrology Tokyo, 15–20 July 1990*;442(abstract).
319. Miyai H, Hara T, Yamada K, Nakamura S, Futenma A, Kato K. Aggravation of puromycin aminonucleoside (PAN) nephrosis by glutathione-depleting agent. *XIth International Congress of Nephrology Tokyo, 15–20 July 1990*;442.
320. Milner LS, Wei SH, Houser MT. Amelioration of glomerular injury in doxorubicin hydrochloride nephrosis by dimethylthiourea. *J Lab Clin Med* 1991;118:427–434.
321. Soose M, Haberstroh U, Rovira-Halbach G, Brunkhorst R, Stolte H. Heterogeneity of glomerular barrier function in early Adriamycin nephrosis of MWF rats. *Clin Physiol Biochem* 1988;6:310–315.
322. Halliwell B, Gutteridge JMC. *Free radicals in biology and medicine*, Oxford, UK: Clarendon, 1985;20–64.
323. Bakker WW, Kalicharan D, Donga J, Hulstaert CE, Hardonk MJ. Decreased ATPase activity in Adriamycin nephrosis is independent of proteinuria. *Kidney Int* 1987;31:704–709.
324. Shah SV. Evidence suggesting a role for hydroxyl radical in passive Heymann nephritis in rats. *Am J Physiol* 1988;254:F337–F344.
325. Rahman MA, Emancipator SS, Sedor JR. Hydroxyl radical scavengers ameliorate proteinuria in rat immune complex glomerulonephritis. *J Lab Clin Med* 1988;112:619–626.
326. Yoshioka T, Ichikawa I. Glomerular dysfunction induced by polymorphonuclear leukocyte-derived reactive oxygen species. *Am J Physiol* 1989;257:F53–F59.
327. Rodriguez-Puyol D, Duque I, Obregon L, Moliz MA, Hernando L. Reactive oxygen species (ROS) contract isolated glomeruli and cultured rat mesangial cells. *Kidney Int* 1989;35:219(abstract).
328. Palmer RMJ, Ashton DS, Moncada S. Vascular endothelial cells synthesize nitric oxide from L-arginine. *Nature* 1988;333:664–666.
329. Marsden PA, Brock TA, Ballerman BJ. Glomerular endothelial cells respond to calcium-mobilizing agonists with release of EDRF. *Am J Physiol* 1990;258:F1295–F1303.
330. Shultz PA, Schorer AE, Raij L. Effect of endothelium-derived relaxing factor and nitric oxide on rat mesangial cells. *Am J Physiol* 1990;258:F162–F167.
331. Shah SV. Effect of enzymatically generated reactive oxygen metabolites on the cyclic nucleotide content in isolated rat glomeruli. *J Clin Invest* 1984;74:393–401.

332. Dworkin LD, Ichikawa I, Brenner BM. Hormonal modulation of glomerular function. *Am J Physiol* 1983;244:F95–F104.
333. Basci A, Wallin JD, Shah SV. Effect of stimulated neutrophils on cyclic nucleotide content in isolated rat glomeruli. *Am J Physiol* 1987;252:F429–F436.
334. Rodriguez-Puyol D, Duque I, Gonzales-Rubio M, et al. Stimulation of cultured rat mesangial cell (CRMC) proliferation by reactive oxygen species (ROS). *J Am Soc Nephrol* 1990;1:448(abstract).
335. Baud L, Hagege J, Sraer J, Rondeau E, Perez J, Ardaillou R. Reactive oxygen production by cultured rat glomerular mesangial cells during phagocytosis is associated with stimulation of lipoxygenase activity. *J Exp Med* 1983;158:1836–1852.
336. Baud L, Perez J, Ardaillou R. Dexamethasone and hydrogen peroxide production by mesangial cells during phagocytosis. *Am J Physiol* 1983;250:F596–F604.
337. Sedor JR, Abboud HE. Platelet activating factor stimulates oxygen radical release by rat mesangial cells. *Kidney Int* 1985;27:222(abstract).
338. Radeke HH, Meier B, Topley N, Floge J, Habermehl GG, Resch K. Interleukin-1α and tumor necrosis factor-α induce oxygen radical production in mesangial cells. *Kidney Int* 1990;37:767–775.
339. Lianos EA, Zanglis A. Glomerular platelet-activating factor levels and origin in experimental glomerulonephritis. *Kidney Int* 1990;37:736–740.
340. Boswell JM, Yui MA, Burt DW, Kelley VE. Increased tumor necrosis factor and IL-1β gene expression in the kidneys of mice with lupus nephritis. *J Immunol* 1988;141:3050–3054.
341. Sedor JR, Carey SW, Emancipator SN. Immune complexes bind to cultured rat glomerular mesangial cells to stimulate superoxide release. *J Immunol* 1987;138:3751–3757.
342. Adler S, Baker PJ, Johnson RJ, Ochi RF, Pritzl P, Couser WG. Complement membrane attack complex stimulates production of reactive oxygen metabolites by cultured rat mesangial cells. *J Clin Invest* 1986;77:726–767.
343. Biesecker G, Katz S, Koffler D. Renal localization of the membrane attack complex in systemic lupus erythematosus nephritis. *J Exp Med* 1981;154:1779–1794.

Toxicology of the Kidney, Second Edition,
edited by Jerry B. Hook and Robin S. Goldstein.
Raven Press, Ltd., New York © 1993.

7

Biochemical Heterogeneity and Site-Specific Tubular Injury

Robin S. Goldstein

Department of Toxicology, SmithKline Beecham Pharmaceuticals, King of Prussia, Pennsylvania 19406

The majority of nephrotoxicants appear to have their primary effects on discrete segments or regions of the nephron. The proximal tubule, for example, is the primary target for many nephrotoxic antibiotics, antineoplastics, halogenated hydrocarbons, mycotoxins, and heavy metals, whereas the glomerulus is the primary target for immune complexes, the loop of Henle/collecting duct for fluoride ions, and the medulla/papilla for chronically consumed analgesic mixtures. The reasons underlying this site-selective injury in the kidney are complex but appear to be due in part to segmental differences in morphology, physiology, and biochemistry. Specifically, segmental differences in regional blood flow, transport and accumulation of chemicals, bioactivation and detoxicification capacity, cellular energetics, and tissue repair mechanisms may contribute individually or in concert to segmental differences in chemically induced injury.

The concept of site-selective nephrotoxic injury suggests that a chemical produces localized injury, targeting only a single segment/site within the nephron. Such a concept can be misleading since assessment of localized injury is biased to a large extent by our current state of technology. Although the majority of nephrotoxicants have their primary site of action in the proximal tubule, identification of more distal tubular segments as potential targets of injury has been hampered by limitations in assessing specialized functions and/or biochemical properties of these cell types. Clearly, our current state of knowledge and technology in assessing unique proximal tubular functions (i.e., organic ion transport, reabsorption of glucose, amino acids, etc.) far exceeds our ability to specifically assess the functional integrity of the more distal regions of the tubule where function(s) are very closely integrated with, and often inseparable from, other segments of the nephron. Structural damage to the more distal regions of the tubule also may be difficult to detect, particularly for cell types with thin and poorly characterized epithelium such as the thin ascending and descending limbs of the loop of Henle. Thus, detection of chemically induced damage to the distal segments of the nephron may be overlooked with routine functional and light microscopic evaluation, hindering recognition of these sites as potential targets. Detection of nephrotoxic damage to distal tubule segments therefore may require a rigorous evaluation of localized structural and functional damage, using techniques that are sensitive enough to detect subtle cell injury (i.e., cell proliferation assays or ultrastructural/morphometric analyses).

Detection of damage to multiple cell types also may require a thorough evaluation of dose-response and time-response relationships. Increasing dose or duration of treatment, for example, may result in recruitment of additional cellular targets as intrarenal exposure to the nephrotoxicant becomes more widespread or as other biochemical mechanisms of toxicity are triggered. Acute administration of large doses of acetaminophen, for example, is known to produce proximal tubule necrosis in rats, whereas chronic administration of smaller doses results in papillary necrosis. In such instances, identification of site-selective nephrotoxic injury may be a dose- and/or time-dependent phenomenon and thus, multiple cellular targets of nephrotoxic injury may be overlooked if dose-response and time-response curves are not fully explored.

The concept of site-selective injury in this chapter will refer to the occurrence of a predominant site, not necessarily an exclusive site, of nephrotoxic damage as assessed by our current state of technology. The focus of this chapter is twofold: (a) to review our current state of knowledge of the biochemical heterogeneity of the nephron, which may contribute to site-selective tubule injury, and (b) to provide specific examples of site-specific nephrotoxicants, emphasizing the intimate relationship between biochemical heterogeneity of the nephron and site-specific injury.

BIOCHEMICAL HETEROGENEITY

Blood flow to the cortex is disproportionately high compared to other regions of the kidney. Thus, blood-borne toxicants will be delivered preferentially to this region, rendering cortical structures, predominantly proximal tubules, more vulnerable to chemically induced injury. Although the relatively high systemic delivery of toxicants to cortical structures likely contributes to site-selective injury in this region, site-selective nephrotoxic injury does persist *in vitro* under conditions in which both cortical and medullary structures are exposed to equivalent extracellular concentrations of nephrotoxicants. For example, *in vitro* exposure of microdissected nephron segments to either ochratoxin A or cisplatin selectively targets the proximal tubule segments, and not the medullary thick ascending limbs or medullary collecting tubules (1,2), suggesting that site-selective injury to the proximal tubule *in vivo* cannot be attributed solely to regional differences in systemic delivery of these toxicants. Furthermore, *in vivo* and *in vitro* studies demonstrating selective injury to specific cell types within the renal cortex suggests that factors other than, or in addition to, regional blood flow contribute to site-selective injury. Using precision-cut renal cortical slices, equivalent extracellular exposure of different cell types to nephrotoxicants such as mercuric chloride, potassium dichromate, cisplatin, hexachlorbutadiene, or dichlorovinylcysteine produces the same pattern of selective cellular injury *in vitro* as reported by others following *in vivo* administration (3–6). Thus, although regional differences in blood flow may contribute to site-selective injury, these studies suggest that localized nephrotoxic injury is not due to systemic delivery of toxicants alone but rather may be attributed to the intrinsic biochemical properties of the cell types in question. These intrinsic biochemical properties of the renal tubule are reviewed below, highlighting the tubular heterogeneity in (a) cellular energetics and metabolism, (b) transport mechanisms, and (c) xenobiotic metabolism.

Cellular Energetics and Metabolism

Oxygen Tension and Consumption

Oxygen availability, like renal blood flow, is not uniform within the renal parenchyma, but rather exhibits a corticomedullary gradient. Cortical tissue P_{O_2} (approximately 70 to 90 mm Hg) is slightly less than arterial P_{O_2} and drops dramatically beyond the corticomedullary junction to approximately 10 to 20 mm Hg, a value that is close to the "critical P_{O_2}" at which mitochondrial cytochrome oxidase becomes reduced and respiration is decreased (7). The steep corticomedullary gradient for oxygen tension has been attributed to a large extent to the countercurrent microcirculatory arrangement in the medulla, allowing countercurrent diffusion or shunting of oxygen between the arterial and venous branches of the vasa recta, and thus reducing oxygen supply to the deeper portions of the medulla and papilla. Further, the decreased oxygen tension beyond the corticomedullary junction may be due to a relatively high extraction and consumption of oxygen by outer and/or inner medullary tissue. Recent studies have indicated that in the outer stripe of the outer medulla, the oxidative state of this cytochrome is governed primarily by changes in blood flow (and hence, oxygen delivery) whereas in the inner stripe of the outer medulla, the rate of oxygen consumption is the primary determinant (8). Thus, the intrarenal gradients in oxygen tension can be attributed to several factors including the countercurrent oxygen shunt, regional differences in blood flow (oxygen delivery), and oxygen consumption.

Oxygen consumption is unusually high in the kidney and is exceeded only by that of the heart. In fact, although the kidney represents less than 0.5% of total body mass, renal oxygen consumption constitutes approximately 8% of whole body oxygen consumption. Despite the high rates of oxygen consumption, the even higher rate of renal blood flow results in a very low arteriovenous difference, which is lower in kidney than in any other major organ. The relationship between renal blood flow and oxygen consumption in the kidney is rather unique in that the rate of oxygen consumption is directly related to renal blood flow; i.e., as renal blood flow increases, oxygen consumption increases and vice versa. The reasons underpinning this response relate to the intimate relationship between oxygen consumption and tubular work. As renal blood flow and glomerular filtration rate increase, solute delivery and the mitochondrial energy needed to support tubular reabsorption of solutes also increase. Indeed, if NaCl transport in the outer medullary region of the nephron is inhibited via furosemide or ouabain, tissue pO_2 increases and cytochrome oxidase becomes less reduced and more oxidized, substantiating the critical relationship between oxygen supply and demand and tubular reabsorptive work (9).

Marked intranephron heterogeneity in rates of oxygen consumption appear to parallel differences in mitochondrial density along the length of the nephron (Fig. 1). Specifically, *in vitro* rates of basal oxygen consumption are highest in the

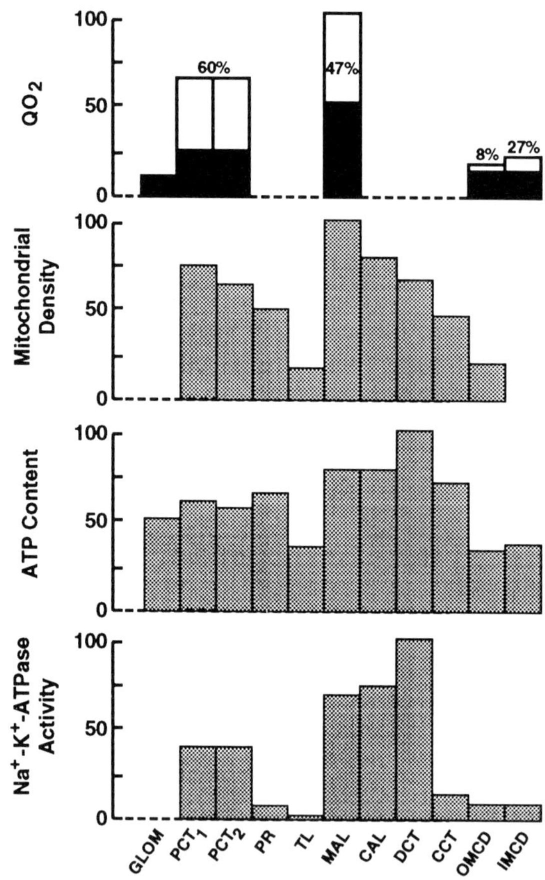

FIG. 1. Relative distribution of oxygen consumption (QO_2) (*open bars*, ouabain-inhibitable oxygen consumption, mitochondrial density, ATP content, and Na^+K^+–ATPase activity along the nephron. All data are expressed as percent of the maximal values observed. GLOM, glomerulus; PCT_1, S_1 segment of proximal convoluted tubule; PCT_2, S_2 segment of proximal convoluted tubule; PR, pars recta; TL, thin limb of the loop of Henle; MAL, medullary thick ascending limb; CAL, cortical thick ascending limb; DCT, distal convoluted tubule; CCT, cortical collecting tubule; OMCD, outer medullary collecting duct; IMCD, inner medullary collecting duct. (Reproduced from Gullans and Hebert, ref. 10, with permission.)

medullary thick ascending limb, intermediate in the proximal convoluted tubular segments, and least in the outer and inner medullary collecting duct (10). Similarly, mitochondrial density (mitochondrial volume/cytosolic volume) is greatest in the medullary and cortical thick ascending limbs and decreases progressively in the distal convoluted tubule, cortical collecting tubule, and medullary collecting tubule (Fig. 1). Both oxygen consumption and mitochondrial density of the S_1 segment of the proximal tubule is slightly less than that of the thick ascending limbs. Within the proximal tubular segments, mitochondrial density in the S_2 and S_3 segments are less than that of the S_1 (10). Despite segmental differences in basal oxygen consumption, both the proximal tubule and medullary thick ascending limb of the rabbit share in common a mitochondrial reserve capacity, suggested by the ability of the cationophore nystatin to increase oxygen consumption approximately two- to threefold over basal rates in both segments (11). In these studies, nystatin is used as a probe to assess respiratory capacity (or state 3 respiration) vis-a-vis the ability of nystatin to increase intracellular sodium and hence sodium-potassium–adenosine triphosphatase (Na-K–ATPase) activity; oxygen consumption, in turn, is increased to support the energetic requirements created by the large increase in Na-K–ATPase activity. Under these conditions, Na-K–ATPase activity is limited by the rate of oxidative phosphorylation. Although nystatin increases oxygen consumption by both proximal tubules and medullary thick ascending limbs of rabbits, absolute rates of nystatin-stimulated oxygen consumption in these segments are significantly different; i.e., that of the thick ascending limb is approximately twofold greater than that of the proximal tubule (12). Although these data suggest that both basal and nystatin-stimulated oxygen consumption are greater in the medullary thick ascending limb than in the proximal tubule, it must be borne in mind that these *in vitro* assessments do not take into account segmental differences in blood flow, substrate delivery, and oxygen tension, all of which significantly impact mitochondrial respiration. Further, segmental differences in respiratory capacity, as reflected by nystatin-stimulated oxygen consumption, may reflect segmental differences in Na-K–ATPase activities (see below) rather than intrinsic differences in respiratory capacity.

Adenine Nucleotides

Under steady-state conditions, the consumption of adenosine triphosphate (ATP) by endergonic processes in renal tubular cells is matched by the production of ATP, resulting in maintenance of a fairly constant intracellular concentration of ATP. Approximately 95% of the ATP in the kidney is supplied by oxidative metabolism (13) and thus, renal mitochondria play a crucial role in maintaining the ATP needed to support ATP-dependent processes of the kidney. Measurements of the relative distribution of ATP content along the length of the rat nephron, when expressed per milligram of dry weight or protein, suggest that ATP concentration is greater in the ascending limbs (14) or distal convoluted tubule (13) than in the S_1, S_2, or S_3 segments of the proximal tubule; differences in intracellular ATP concentration between the thick ascending limbs and the proximal tubular segments are modest (Fig. 1). However, the relative distribution of ATP along the nephron is remarkably different when data are normalized for tubule length. Specifically, ATP content/millimeter tubule in the rat nephron is greatest in the S_2, followed in descending order by the S_3, S_1, medullary thick ascending limb, distal tubule, and cortical thick ascending limb (14). This discrepancy in the relative distribution of ATP is likely related to the fact that the ratio of dry weight/tubule length can vary up to threefold for different nephron segments (15).

The rate of ATP production is equally (if not more) important than absolute concentrations of ATP when considering segmental differences in the capacity to support ATP-dependent functions. In the rat, the maximal rates of substrate-supported ATP formation *in vitro* in microdissected nephron segments averaged 1.5 to 2.0 pmol/mm tubule/15 min in the proximal tubular segments and medullary thick ascending limb and 0.5 to 1.0 pmol/mm tubule/15 min in the cortical ascending limb, distal convoluted tubule, and cortical collecting tubule (14). In the rabbit, estimates of the maximal rate of ATP production from empirical measurements of nystatin-stimulated oxygen consumption (assuming 6 mol of ATP formed/O_2 consumed), suggest that ATP production/milligram protein/min in thick ascending limbs is at least twofold greater than that in the proximal tubules (16).

Na-K–ATPases

Parallel alterations in oxygen consumption and sodium transport suggest that the rate of ATP production is tightly coupled to the rate of ATP utilization by Na-K–ATPase. Studies evaluating the heterogeneity of Na-K–ATPase activity along the rat, rabbit, and mouse nephron have indicated that enzymatic activity per millimeter tubule length is greatest in the distal convoluted tubule and thick ascending limbs, intermediate in the proximal tubule, and lowest in the collecting tubule (Fig. 2). Within the proximal tubule, enzyme activity is greatest in the proximal convoluted tubule and least in the pars recta (17). Theoretically, this distribution of Na-K–ATPase activity along the nephron may be related to segmental differences in the number or density of enzymatic units and/or in the specific activity of the enzyme. The number of pumps, estimated in microdissected nephron segments using [^{3}H]-ouabain binding techniques, correlates well with estimates of Na-K–ATPase activities and thus, contributes in part to segmental differences in enzymatic activity. Specifically, 40 to 50 million binding sites/cell were noted in the medullary ascending limb and distal convoluted tubule of rabbits, 25 million in the proximal convoluted tubule, and 8 to 10 million in the pars recta, cortical ascending limb, and cortical collecting tubule (18). These data must be interpreted carefully, however, since it has been demonstrated that the affinity of ouabain for Na-K–ATPase varies along the length of the nephron. For example, Na-K–ATPase is 10 to 30-fold more sensitive to ouabain in the collecting tubule than in more proximal segments of the nephron (19). In evaluating the nephron heterogeneity of Na-K–ATPase activity, it

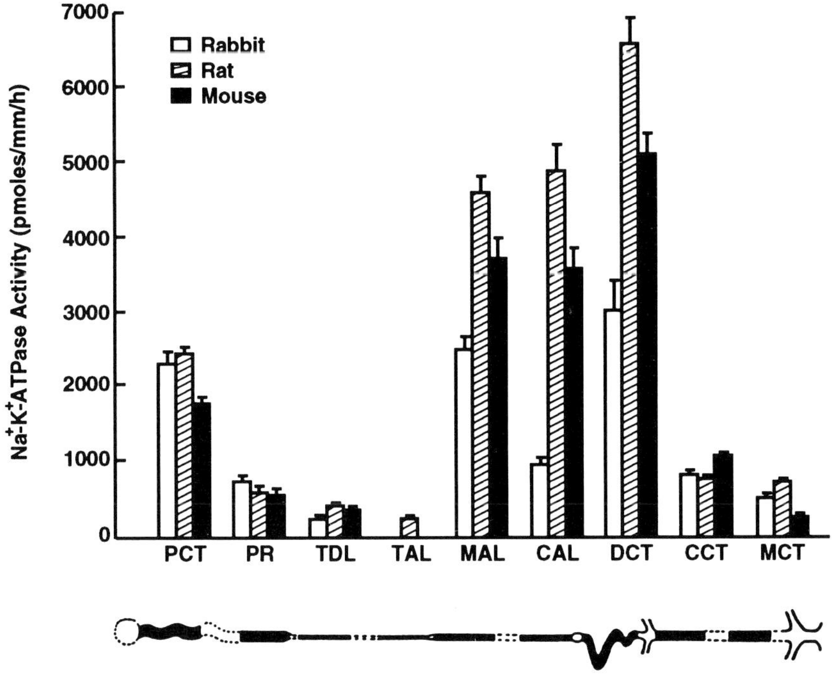

FIG. 2. Na^+K^+–ATPase activity in the rabbit, rat, and mouse nephron. PCT, proximal convoluted tubule; PR, pars recta; TDL, thin descending limb; TAL, thin ascending limb; MAL, medullary thick ascending limb; CAL, cortical thick ascending limb; DCT, distal convoluted tubule; CCT, cortical collecting tubule; MCT, outer medullary collecting tubule. (Reproduced from Katz, Doucet, and Morel, ref. 193, with permission.)

also must be borne in mind that enzymatic activity is assessed under conditions supporting V_{max}, thus providing an index of the enzymatic capacity of individual nephron segments rather than actual rates of Na-K–ATPase activity under normal physiological conditions *in vivo*.

In general, there is a fairly good correlation between segmental differences in oxygen consumption, mitochondrial density, and Na-K–ATPase activity; increased mitochondrial density and oxygen consumption in the thick ascending limb and proximal convoluted tubule are accompanied by relatively high rates of Na-K–ATPase activity (Fig. 1). Not surprisingly, ouabain-sensitive oxygen consumption, i.e., that portion of oxygen consumption utilized to support Na-K–ATPase activity, is greatest in those segments with the highest Na-K–ATPase activity, specifically thick ascending limbs and proximal convoluted tubules, and least in the outer and inner medullary collecting duct where enzyme activity is the lowest (Fig. 1). Sodium transport and oxygen consumption appear to be linearly related over a wide range of sodium transport rates (16). The metabolic efficiency of sodium transport (i.e., moles of oxygen consumed to support transport of 1 mEq of sodium), however, can vary considerably from one segment to another. This heterogeneity in metabolic efficiency can be attributed to the heterogeneity in the relative contribution of passive and active transepithelial transport of sodium and the relative contribution of nonoxidative ATP synthesis (i.e., anaerobic glycolysis) to support sodium reabsorption. For example, in the proximal tubule, approximately 30% of sodium transport is passive, whereas in the medullary thick ascending limb, there is negligible, if any, passive sodium transport. Thus, the number of calories required to transport 1 mEq of sodium by the proximal tubule is substantially less than that required by the thick ascending limb.

Further evaluation of the relationship between sodium transport and oxygen consumption *in vivo* suggests that there is a significant fraction of oxygen consumption that is independent of sodium transport; i.e., 3% to 18% of total oxygen consumption in the mammalian kidney is used to support sodium transport-independent processes (e.g., active transport processes not coupled to sodium transport, synthetic functions [gluconeogenesis, triglycerides], cell growth and repair, and other metabolic processes) (10). However, *in vitro* studies have suggested that oxidative support of these basal processes is considerably higher than 3% to 18% (15). Specifically, in the proximal convoluted tubule and medullary thick ascending limbs, 40% to 50% of oxygen consumption is ouabain-insensitive, i.e., the percentage of oxygen consumption supporting metabolic processes that are independent of sodium transport. In inner and outer medullary cortical collecting tubules, where Na-K–ATPase activity is relatively low, ouabain-insensitive oxygen consumption represents as much as 70% to 92% of total oxygen consumption. The reasons for the *in vivo* and *in vitro* discrepancy in estimating the relative percentage of oxygen consumption needed to support basal metabolism is not clear, but may relate to *in vivo–in vitro* differences in Na-K–ATPase activity and in the relative activities of multiple, and perhaps competing, sodium-dependent and -independent metabolic processes.

Substrate Utilization

There is marked regional and segmental heterogeneity in the metabolic fuels supporting cell respiration. Segmental differences in substrate utilization may reflect segmental differences in cellular uptake and/or mitochondrial transport of the substrate in question or, alternatively, segmental differences in activities of the enzymes needed for substrate oxidation. Although transporters for a variety of energy substrates (glucose, lactate, citric acid cycle intermediates, amino acids, glutamine) have been identified in the basolateral and/or luminal membranes of the proximal tubular segments, very little is known about substrate transport in the more distal segments. For the most part, it appears that at least in the proximal tubule, uptake of a substrate does not represent a rate-limiting step to its subsequent metabolism and oxidation. Since in the normal healthy kidney, proximal tubular reabsorption of metabolizable substrates (e.g., amino acids, glucose) is nearly complete, it is likely that luminal concentrations of these substrates is negligible downstream. Thus, transport of these substances into the distal tubular cells most likely does not occur from the luminal side but rather from the basolateral membrane. Equally important to substrate support for cell respiration is transport of the substrate in question across the mitochondrial membrane. Transport of substrates into mitochondria is mediated by a variety of mechanisms, including dicarboxylate and tricarboxylate exchangers, α-ketoglutarate/malate exchanger, glutamate/aspartate exchanger, glutamine uniporter, etc. All of these transporters mediate passive, reversible transport driven entirely by electrochemical gradients of the transported solutes across mitochondrial membranes. However, the nature and relative distribution of these specific transporters along the nephron is not known. Thus, the role of segmental differences in intracellular and/or intramitochondrial transport to segmental differences in substrate utilization remains unclear.

In general, metabolism in the renal cortex is characterized by aerobic oxidation of substrates and gluconeogenesis, whereas that in the renal medulla is via aerobic and anaerobic glycolysis (20). Furthermore, the respiratory quotient (CO_2 generated per O_2 consumed) is relatively low in the cortex, suggestive of fatty acid oxidation, whereas the renal medulla is characterized by a respiratory quotient of unity, suggestive of carbohydrate metabolism. More specific evaluation of the metabolic characteristics of the individual nephron segments within the cortex and medulla have relied on measuring $^{14}CO_2$ production from ^{14}C-labeled substrates *in vitro*. Early studies demonstrated that in renal cortical slices, fatty acids and acetoacetate are rapidly decarboxylated (21), consistent with *in vivo* studies indicating a low respiratory quotient in the cortex. Subsequent studies utilizing isolated nephron segments indicated that in proximal convoluted tubules of rats, marked $^{14}CO_2$ is generated from radiolabeled succinate, 2-oxoglutarate, glutamate, glutamine and malate, moderate $^{14}CO_2$ production from citrate, and negligible $^{14}CO_2$ production from glucose and lactate (22). In contrast, medullary and cortical thick ascending limb segments oxidize glucose, 2-oxoglutarate, lactate, glutamate, and glutamine, but not malate, succinate, and citrate. Unfortunately, interpretation of these data are confounded by potential segmental differences in isotopic dilution with endogenous metabolic pools. More recently, Jung et al. (14) evaluated substrate utilization in ATP-depleted microdissected nephron segments by measuring ATP synthesis following addition of a variety of substrates. In these studies, the rank order of preferred substrates in the proximal tubular segments of the rat has been reported to be pyruvate = glutamine > lactate > β-hydroxybutyrate > glucose. Within the proximal tubule, the relative increase in pyruvate or glutamine-supported ATP synthesis is greatest in the S_2 segment. In contrast, the preferred substrates in the distal tubular segments are glucose = pyruvate = lactate > β-hydroxybutyrate > glutamine. Of the distal tubular segments, the relative increase in glucose and pyruvate-supported ATP synthesis is greatest in the medullary thick ascending limb and the medullary collecting tubule.

To a large extent, our current understanding of substrate utilization by various nephron segments is based on studies evaluating the metabolism of single substrates in substrate-deprived renal slices, nephron segments, or cells *in vitro*. Clearly, in the *in vivo* state the milieu is quite different as a mixture of diverse, and perhaps, competing substrates are delivered to the tubular cell. Since substrate utilization is known to vary directly with systemic delivery and availability of substrates (23), it is unclear to what extent single substrate utilization *in vitro* reflects *in vivo* metabolism by discrete regions or segments of the nephron. Since the substrates utilized will vary with their plasma concentration, identification of the "preferred substrates" in *in vitro* studies using substrate-deprived tissue may not necessarily reflect metabolism *in vivo*. Thus, *in vivo* utilization and metabolism of substrates by the nephron is likely to be far more complex than suggested by *in vitro* work.

Carbohydrate Metabolism

In the kidney, the initial substrate for glycolysis is glucose since renal glycogen stores are very low. Segmental differences in glucose utilization are consistent with the known segmental differences in activities of enzymes mediating glycolysis. For example, in the rat nephron, activities of the rate-limiting kinases for glycolysis, i.e., hexokinase, phosphofructokinase, and pyruvate kinase, are higher in the more distal segments of the nephron than in the proximal tubular segments (Fig. 3) (15,24,25), consistent with the greater utilization of glucose in the more distal segments. Indeed, activity of hexokinase is often used as a marker for assessing the relative enrichment of distal tubular cells (26). Although the distribution of glycolytic enzymes strongly suggests that glycolysis plays an important role in energy metabolism in the distal tubular segments, enzymatic activity *in vitro* under V_{max} conditions may not reflect glycolytic fluxes *in vivo*. An alternative approach in assessing glycolytic flux in nephron segments has relied on the measurement of lactate production from glucose. Under aerobic conditions, lactate production from glucose has been observed in all segments beyond the proximal tubule (27). These data must not be overinterpreted to reflect aerobic glycolytic flux, however, since the terminal reaction in glycolysis, i.e., reductive metabolism of pyruvate to lactate, may not proceed under aerobic conditions. Rather, pyruvate may be further metabolized via the TCA cycle and thus, assessment of lactate production from glucose under these circumstances would underestimate glycolytic flux. Indeed, lactate oxidation has been reported to be substantial in the S_2 and S_3 segments of the rabbit proximal tubule (28). In contrast, under anaerobic conditions, i.e., anoxia or inhibition of oxidative phosphorylation with respiratory site II inhibitor (e.g., antimycin A), pyruvate is not further oxidized and lactate production can be used to estimate glycolytic flux. Indeed, incubation of nephron segments with antimycin A results in substantial lactate production in the medullary thick ascending limb, cortical collecting tubule, and outer medullary collecting duct, intermediate production in the cortical ascending limbs and distal convoluted tubules, and negligible lactate production by proximal tubular segments (27). Similarly, in the rabbit, antimycin A does not increase glucose-supported lactate production in proximal tubular suspensions (29). However, other inhibitors of the respiratory chain, i.e., rotenone (site I)

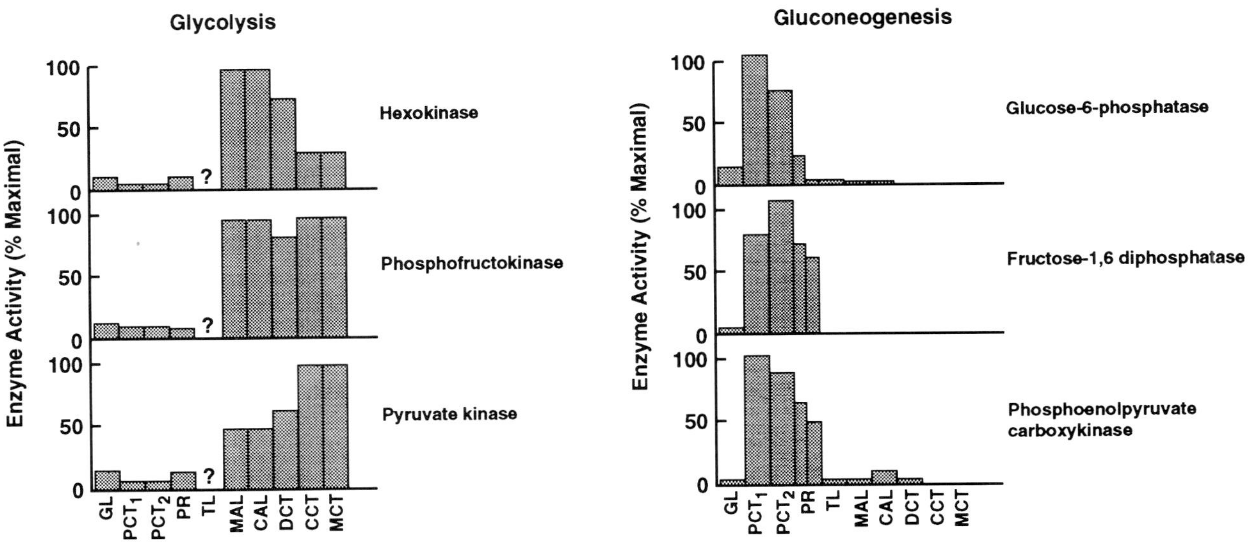

FIG. 3. Distribution of glycolytic and gluconeogenic enzymes along the rat nephron. Nephron segments were dissected from fed (glycolysis) and fasted (gluconeogenesis) rats. Enzyme activities are expressed as percent of the maximal value observed based on the activity per gram of dry weight. GL, glomerulus; PCT_1, early proximal convoluted tubule; PCT_2, late proximal convoluted tubule; PR, pars recta; TL, thin limb of loop of Henle; MAL, medullary thick ascending limb; CAL, cortical ascending limb; DCT, distal convoluted tubule; CCT, cortical collecting tubule; MCT, medullary collecting tubule. (Reproduced from Guder and Ross, ref. 25, with permission.)

and the uncoupler, carbonyl cyanide-*p*-trifluoromethoxyphenylhydrazone (FCCP), appear to be potent stimuli for lactate production by proximal tubular segments. Thus, rabbit proximal tubules do have an anaerobic glycolytic capability, but activation of glycolysis does not appear to be directly linked to mitochondrial inhibition since neither antimycin A nor incubation under anoxic conditions stimulated lactate production. Although both proximal and distal tubular structures have an anaerobic glycolytic capacity, this metabolic pathway may be more important for cell viability and function in medullary than in cortical structures, considering the low oxygen tension in the medulla.

Recent evidence further suggests marked differences in glucose oxidation between S_1/S_2 and S_3 rabbit proximal tubular segments. Ruegg and Mandel (30) reported that oxygen consumption and ATP concentrations are maintained by glucose (as the only metabolic substrate) in the S_3, but not S_1/S_2, suggesting that glucose supports oxidative metabolism in the S_3 but not S_1/S_2 segments. In these studies, the maximal glycolytic flux rate under aerobic conditions was estimated from nystatin-stimulated oxygen consumption in the presence and absence of glucose. In S_3 segments, the estimated aerobic glycolytic flux was 3 to 6 nmol glucose/mg protein/min, whereas no evidence of aerobic glycolytic flux was observed in the S_1/S_2 segments. Thus, this study demonstrates that within the proximal tubule, only the S_3 segment has the capacity for aerobic glycolysis. Lactate oxidation (the terminal glycolytic reaction in aerobic glycolysis) has been demonstrated in the S_2 and S_3, but not S_1, segments of rabbit nephrons (28). Thus, the absence of aerobic glycolysis in the S_1/S_2 population reported by Ruegg and Mandel might be due to a decrease in glycolytic reactions preceding lactate oxidation.

In contrast to the intranephron distribution of glycolytic enzymes, the distribution of rate-limiting enzymes mediating gluconeogenesis, i.e., glucose-6-phosphatase, fructose 1,6-disphosphatase, pyruvate carboxylase, and phosphoenolpyruvate carboxykinase, are localized almost exclusively in the proximal tubule; within the proximal tubule, enzymatic activities are higher in the S_1 and S_2 segments than in the S_3 (Fig. 3) (25). These differences in enzyme distribution essentially mirror segmental differences in gluconeogenic rates. Specifically, pyruvate or glutamine-supported glucose production in microdissected nephron segments was greatest in the S_1,intermediate in the S_2, and least in the S_3 segments in rats (31). The axial heterogeneity of glycolysis and gluconeogenesis has prompted the speculation that glucose synthesized in the proximal tubules contributes to and is used for glycolysis by the more distal segments and conversely, that lactate produced by the more distal structures supports gluconeogenesis or respiration in the proximal tubule (32,33).

Lipid Metabolism

Several studies have suggested that only a small percentage of radiolabeled free fatty acids removed by the kidney is oxidized to CO_2. The magnitude of free fatty acid uptake by the kidney varies from species to species, but in general, arteriovenous differences of 10% to 25% have been reported. The majority of radiolabel is incorporated into triglycerides, an observation reported both *in vivo* and *in vitro*.

The cortex appears to be the predominant, but certainly not the exclusive, site of free fatty acid oxidation (34). In proximal tubular suspensions, short-chain fatty acids, e.g., butyrate, valerate, and heptanoate, dramatically stimulate oxygen consumption (35). Indeed, butyrate supports mitochondrial oxidative phosphorylation to a greater degree than lactate, glucose, or alanine when Na-K–ATPase is maximally stimulated by addition of nystatin to suspensions of proximal tubules (11). In contrast to proximal tubule suspensions, medullary thick ascending limbs maintain viability and function in the absence of exogenous substrates, suggesting that endogenous fuels support respiration. Furthermore, inhibitors of fatty acid oxidation, e.g., bromooctanoate or tetradecyglycidic acid, inhibit oxygen consumption of the medullary thick ascending limb in substrate-free media, suggesting that endogenous lipids are used to meet the energy needs of these cells. These and other data suggest that the most effective endogenous substrates for rabbit medullary thick ascending limbs are fatty acids (12). Butyrate increases both ouabain-sensitive and ouabain-insensitive components of oxygen consumption, suggesting that this fatty acid stimulates energy-requiring processes associated with Na-K–ATPase activity as well as Na-K–ATPase–independent processes.

Oxidation of fatty acids to acetylcoenzyme A (acetyl-CoA) is mediated by β-oxidation, which in the kidney is localized within both the mitochondria and the peroxisomes. Enzymes mediating β-oxidation appear to be present in all segments of the nephron with the intranephron distribution paralleling segmental differences in mitochondrial density. Activity of 3-hydroxyacl-CoA dehydrogenase is highest in the distal convoluted tubule and also is relatively high in the proximal convoluted tubule and the thick ascending limbs; activity is low in the cortical collecting tubule (36).

Tubular Transport

Numerous studies suggest that segmental differences in transport of xenobiotics across the cell membrane contribute importantly to segmental differences in intracellular accumulation, and hence in toxicity, of these chemicals. In addition to segmental differences in the specific transport mechanisms discussed below, segmental differences in intracellular accumulation of chemicals may occur even for chemicals transported into the cell via passive diffusion. Although intraluminal concentrations of toxicants are likely to be higher in the distal regions of the renal tubule, providing a greater concentration gradient to drive passive diffusion from lumen to cell, the distal tubule is characterized by a relatively "tight" epithelium with high electrical resistance, a feature that may impede diffusion of solutes. In contrast, the proximal tubule is characterized by a "leaky" epithelium; thus, small lipophilic compounds are more likely to diffuse into the proximal tubular cells than into distal tubular cells.

Organic Ion Transport

Active transport processes, such as organic anion and cation transport, may raise the intracellular concentration of nephrotoxicants significantly by driving concentrative, uphill movement of these substances into tubular cells. Indeed, a large number of xenobiotics are transported by the organic anion and/or cation transport systems and such transport appears to be directly related to the onset and development of tubular injury induced by several nephrotoxicants including β-lactam antibiotics, cisplatin, ochratoxin A, and haloalkene-S-conjugates (37–39).

Recent studies have suggested the presence of at least three basolateral organic anion transport systems in rat proximal tubular cells: (a) a sulfate/oxalate system, (b) an Na^+-dicarboxylate cotransport system, and (c) a system for hydrophobic negatively charged molecules and long-chain fatty acids, the so-called *p*-aminohippuric acid (PAH) system (Fig. 4) (40,41). The seminal event in organic anion transport is the creation of a transmembrane electrochemical potential difference for sodium ions via Na-K–ATPase located in the basolateral membrane. ATP is not directly utilized by organic anion transporters but rather, the cellular mechanisms of anion transport appear to depend upon either a secondary or tertiary active process (40). Specifically, the normal operation of the sodium pump drives the steep gradient needed for the inward movement of dicarboxylic acids; Na^+ dicarboxylate transport systems are present in both the luminal and basolateral membrane, resulting in high intracellular concentration of these substances. Intracellularly accumulated dicarboxylates, most likely 2-oxoglutarate (40), then exchange with interstitial PAH or related hydrophobic anions using a distinct transporter (PAH transporter), resulting in efflux of dicarboxylic acids coupled to an influx of PAH into the proximal tubular cell (Fig. 4). Once inside the cell, PAH may be transported into the tubular lumen in exchange for another anion, e.g., urate, to complete the process of tubular secretion. In the course of tubular secretion, proximal tubular cells can concentrate PAH and related anions to levels several hundred times higher than that of interstitial fluid.

Substrates for the Na^+-dicarboxylate cotransporter include all citric acid cycle intermediates and aliphatic substrates carrying two or three negative ionic charges at a distance of two to five carbons. Shorter and longer dicarboxylates are not substrates for this system. Virtually all substrates of the dicarboxylate transporter are also substrates for the PAH transporter, although affinities for these transporters are different. The substrate specificity of the PAH system is broader; common to all substrates of this transporter is a hydrophobic moiety, such as a methylene chain or a benzene ring and at least one negatively charged ionic group (COO^-, SO_3^-, O^-) or two, partially negative charges. Thus, the PAH transport system handles fatty acids, steroid hormones, small peptides, and anionic xenobiotics. Similar to the dicarboxylate/PAH exchange, urate also may enter the proximal tubular cell following basolateral exchange with acids; however, it is not entirely clear whether urate transport utilizes a transporter distinct from PAH. Probenecid has been used as a classic inhibitor of organic anion transport. Importantly, probenecid inhibits not

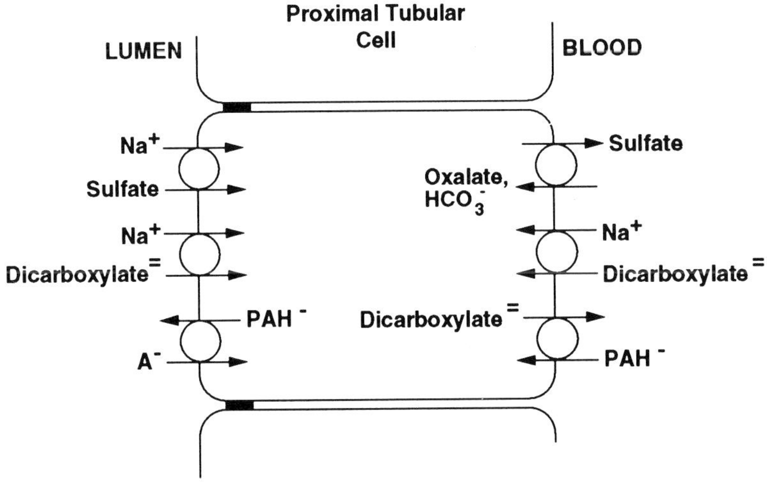

FIG. 4. Organic anion transport systems in the proximal tubular cell. (Modified from Ullrich and Rumrich, ref. 41, with permission.)

only PAH transport, but also sulfate and urate transport, and thus may not be a specific inhibitor of any one organic anion system. Furthermore, although probenecid competes with PAH and related anions for uptake by the basolateral exchanger, the presence of probenecid-sensitive luminal transport of PAH (and urate) has been suggested (42).

Sodium-coupled transport of sulfate in the luminal membrane results in accumulation of sulfate within the cell, providing a driving force for transport across the basolateral membrane into the peritubular blood. This basolateral transport of sulfate out of the proximal tubular cell involves exchange with anions such as oxalate, thiosulfate, and some of the phenylsulfonphthalein dyes.

Isolated perfused rabbit nephrons and *in situ* micropuncture studies have indicated remarkable heterogeneity of organic anion transport. In the rabbit, the highest rate of secretion of PAH, for example, is in the S_2 segments (43); secretion by the S_1 is comparable to that of the S_3 segments (Fig. 5). Secretory rates are comparable between superficial and juxtamedullary nephrons for any given segment. In a more detailed study of PAH secretion in rabbit superficial proximal tubules, Shimomura et al. (44) have reported that the K_m for PAH transport is not significantly different between the S_1, S_2, and S_3 segments of rabbit proximal tubules; however, maximal transport rates (V_{max}) are approximately six to sevenfold greater in the S_2 segment than in the S_1 or S_3, suggesting an increased density or number of PAH transporters in the S_2 segment. The segmental heterogeneity of PAH secretion by the proximal tubules does not pertain to all organic anions. For example, maximal rates of urate secretion are higher and of the same magnitude in rabbit superficial S_1 and S_2 than in S_3 segments (45). Unfortunately, the intranephron distribution of organic anion transport in species other than the rabbit has not been determined.

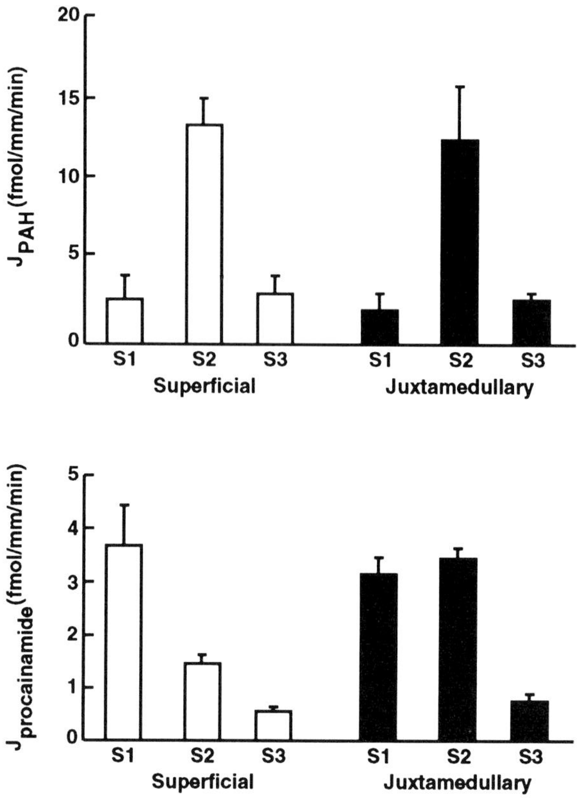

FIG. 5. Rates of p-aminohippuric acid (PAH) and procainamide secretion by different proximal tubular segments of superficial and juxtamedullary nephrons of rabbits. The rate of PAH or procainamide secretion was determined by adding radiolabeled PAH or procainamide to the perfusate and measuring radioactivity appearing in the tubular fluid. The rate of secretion (fmol/mm/min) was calculated as $C_L \times V_L/S \times L$, where C_L is concentration of radiolabel in the tubular fluid, V_L is the tubular fluid collection rate, S is the specific activity of radiolabel in the perfusate, and L is the tubular length. (Modified from McKinney, ref. 52, with permission.)

Organic cation transport has been studied less extensively than organic anion transport and consequently, the exact mechanisms of organic cation transport are less well understood. There is considerable debate, for example, as to the precise mechanisms mediating organic cation transport across the basolateral membrane. Holohan and Ross (46) proposed that uptake of organic cations across basolateral membrane vesicles occurs via facilitated diffusion, driven by the electronegative milieu of the interior of the renal tubular cell, and thus, unlike organic anion transport, does not involve active transport across the basolateral membrane. However, several studies have indicated that in isolated nonperfused proximal tubules, accumulation of organic cations is greater than could be accounted for by passive equilibration (47,48). Recent evidence suggests that in rabbit S_2 proximal tubule segments, uptake of a prototypical organic cation, tetraethylammonium (TEA), is mediated by both active and passive transport across the basolateral membrane (48). Further, TEA uptake of proximal tubular segments is significantly inhibited by ouabain, suggesting that transport is dependent on Na-K–ATPase activity.

The exact mechanisms by which organic cations enter the lumen of proximal tubules also is poorly understood. Mediated transport across the luminal membrane is suggested by the observation that ouabain inhibits transport of a prototype organic cation (e.g., procainamide) into the tubular fluid but does not reduce intracellular concentrations of the drug (49,50). Studies of organic cation transport in membrane vesicles prepared from dog renal cortex have led to the hypothesis that organic cations are actively extruded from the proximal tubular cell into the tubular fluid, a process believed to be secondary to an organic cation-proton exchange in the luminal membrane, driven by a lumen-to-cell proton gradient (51). The proton gradient needed for operation of the exchanger has been suggested to be established by proton secretion via a Na/H exchange mechanism and by the concentration of intracellular organic cations. Thus, these investigators further proposed that the rate-limiting step for organic cation secretion is at the luminal membrane, not the basolateral membrane, and is driven by countertransport with protons secondary to Na/H exchange.

In general, molecules secreted by the organic cation system contain a nitrogen atom and carry a net positive charge at physiological pH; this positive charge appears to be a requisite for transport. Molecules transported by this system include endogenous compounds such as choline, dopamine, serotonin, norepinephrine, and histamine, and xenobiotics such as cimetidine, morphine, procainamide, paraquat, and quinine. Studies in rabbit tubules indicated that procainamide and TEA are secreted by superficial proximal tubules in a sequential pattern of $S_1 > S_2 > S_3$; in contrast, in juxtamedullary tubules secretion is greatest in the S_1 and S_2 segments and lowest in S_3 segments (Fig. 5) (47,52).

Low Molecular Weight Proteins

Many biologically important low molecular weight proteins (LMWPs) (<50,000 d) are filtered and subsequently reabsorbed and degraded by the renal tubules. Indeed, renal tubular uptake and degradation of LMWP appears to be an early biochemical target for injury produced by nephrotoxicants such as the aminoglycoside antibiotics (53). These LMWPs include most if not all circulating peptide hormones (e.g., insulin, glucagon, growth hormone, parathyroid hormone), enzymes (e.g., lysozyme, ribonuclease), immunoprotein fragments (e.g., Bence Jones protein) and membrane antigens (β_2-microglobulin). The role of filtration in the uptake of LMWPs has been suggested by the marked decreases in renal uptake of proteins by the nonfiltering, isolated perfused kidney when compared with the filtering perfused kidney (54). In general, the most important determinants of filtration of LMWPs is molecular weight and size; net electrical charge has little or no influence on the glomerular sieving coefficient for small proteins with a molecular radius of 20 Å or less. The glomerular sieving coefficient of anionic β_2-microglobulin (MW = 11,600; radius = 16 Å), for example, is comparable to that of cationic cytochrome c(MW = 12,400; radius = 15 Å). Net electrical charge, however, does become critical as proteins reach 30 Å in size, reflected by significant differences in the glomerular sieving coefficients for neutral, anionic, and cationic horseradish peroxidase.

Despite the significant filtration of LMWPs, only minimal amounts of these proteins are detected in the urine, suggesting substantial tubular reabsorption at the luminal membrane. The transport of LMWPs into and across the tubular cell has been studied extensively by ultrastructural and autoradiographic techniques (54–56). Tubular reabsorption of proteins is believed to be high capacity and low affinity, and is initiated by binding of substances to endocytotic sites at the surface of the cell membrane and ultimately, by segregation and internalization of endosomes (Fig. 6) (57). Endocytotic sites comprise only a small fraction of the total luminal cell membrane and are situated at the bases of long and narrowly separated microvilli. The luminal membrane is covered with a thick external coat and, in addition, a cytoplasmic coat containing clathrin, which corresponds to the endocytotic invaginations. The negative surface charges of the endocytotic site facilitate access/binding of cationic proteins and hinder access to anionic proteins. Thus, electrostatic interactions between the positively charged groups of the protein in question and anionic sites at the luminal membrane appear to be an important determinant for tubular reabsorption. However, other factors likely are involved since net electrical charge does not always influence reabsorption, suggested by the observation that reabsorption of anionic and cationic horseradish peroxidase is comparable. Thus, other physicochemical parameters may impact accessibility of proteins to endocytotic sites, e.g., rigidity of protein, type of anionic/cationic residue, and molecular size and shape.

Following binding, the protein migrates to the base of the microvilli and invagination of the surface membrane and formation of small endocytotic vesicles begins, a process commonly referred to as adsorptive endocytosis. Alternatively, fluid-phase endocytosis may occur, involving internalization of tubular fluid (and

FIG. 6. Renal tubular uptake and metabolism of low molecular weight proteins. The endocytotic pathway is illustrated on the *right* of the schematic beginning with the initial binding of the ligand to its binding site at the brush border or at the plasma membrane. The invaginations have a cytoplasmic clathrin coat (represented by *dots*). The proteins bound or taken up are represented by *crosses* (smaller peptides and proteins) or *asterisks* (larger proteins). Small endocytotic vesicles are formed from the coated invaginations; the vesicles fuse with larger endocytotic vacuoles, which transfer the protein to the lysosomes for degradation. Membrane constituents recycle back to the luminal plasma membrane, most likely mediated by dense apical tubules. Proteins are degraded in the lysosomes to constituent amino acids, which probably diffuse through the lysosome membrane into the cytoplasm and from there to the peritubular capillaries. The *left* side of the schematic depicts the autophagic components of the vacuolar apparatus. (Reproduced from Christensen and Nielsen, ref. 55, with permission.)

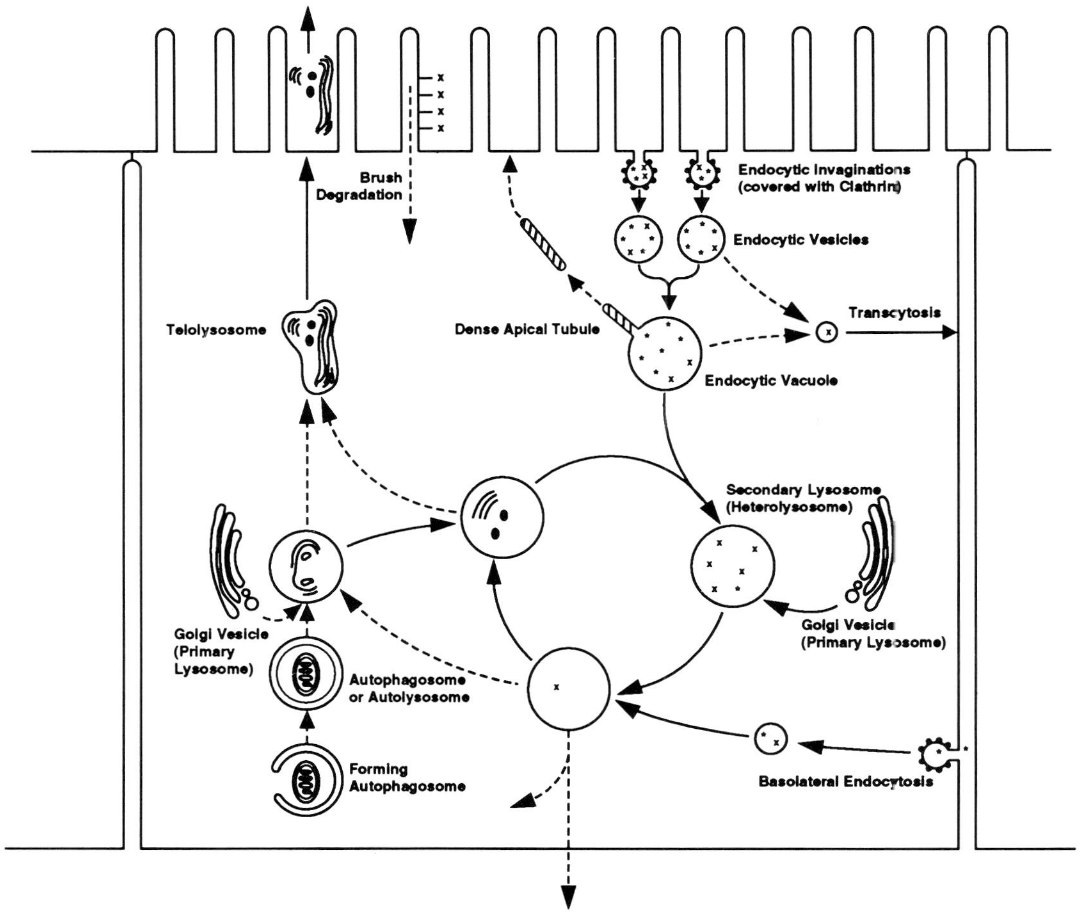
Endocytic Invaginations
(covered with Clathrin)
Endocytic Vesicles
Transcytosis
Dense Apical Tubule
Endocytic Vacuole
Brush
Degradation
Telolysosome
Secondary Lysosome
(Heterolysosome)
Golgi Vesicle
(Primary Lysosome)
Golgi Vesicle
(Primary
Lysosome)
Autophagosome
or Autolysosome
Forming
Autophagosome
Basolateral Endocytosis

proteins), which appears to be slow and relatively nonspecific. Formation and internalization of endocytotic vesicles appears to be (directly or indirectly) dependent upon cell energy inasmuch as metabolic inhibitors, anoxia and/or cytochalasin B, inhibit this process. Once formed and internalized, the endocytotic vesicles migrate to and subsequently fuse with lysosomes where proteins are catabolized to their constituent amino acids by hydrolytic enzymes, e.g., acid phosphatase, β-glucuronidase, the cysteine proteinases (cathepsins B, H, and L), and the aspartic acid proteinase (cathepsin D) (Fig. 6). The rate of hydrolysis appears to depend on the nature of the protein in question. For example, albumin and cytochrome c are rapidly degraded, whereas degradation of lysozyme is much slower (58,59). In general, lysosomal hydrolysis is not saturated over a wide range of filtered loads; thus, increased filtered loads of LMWP generally are associated with a proportional increase in tubular uptake and metabolism (60). Exceptions to this rule include circulating proteins that appear to be relatively resistant to hydrolytic enzymes, such as lysozyme, light chains, and α-$_{2u}$-globulin. An imbalance between the rate of absorption and the rate of intralysosomal hydrolysis of protein may result in the intralysosomal or intracellular accumulation of protein absorption droplets (60). Since tubular uptake of LMWPs is high capacity, accumulation of proteins in lysosomes in general is dependent on the rate of hydrolysis. Intracellular defects in lysosomal catabolism thus may lead to lysosomal accumulation of proteins. For example, it is well documented that the acid milieu within the lysosomes is essential for normal hydrolysis inasmuch as alkalinization of lysosomal pH inhibits catabolism of absorbed proteins; alkalinization may result from inhibition of the lysosomal proton pump or from increased permeability of the lysosomal membrane to hydrogen ions. Thus, alkalinization of intralysosomal pH, by inhibiting catabolism of absorbed proteins and thereby creating an imbalance between protein uptake and catabolism, may lead to intracellular accumulation of protein droplets.

The tubular handling of larger molecular weight proteins that escape the glomerular capillary wall, however, appears to be somewhat different than that for LMWPs. Park and Maack (61) demonstrated a dual transport system for albumin in isolated proximal tubules from normal rabbits characterized by (a) a low-capacity system that becomes saturated at physiological protein concentrations in the tubular fluid, and (b) a high-capacity, low-affinity system that is operative at high tubular fluid concentrations of albumin. The low affinity, high capacity for albumin uptake suggests that an increase in the filtered load of albumin may lead to albuminuria before the system becomes saturated. Thus, in protein-overload situations, the low-affinity, high-capacity system will result in a proportionality between filtered loads and urinary excretion of albumin, resulting in albuminuria. Nonetheless, several lines of evidence suggest that in response to glomerular proteinuria, tubular uptake of proteins is increased as reflected by the increased number of apical vacuoles and lysosomes (62), and lysosomal enzyme activity (cathepsins B and L) (63,64). These latter observations further substantiate the high-capacity nature of both uptake and lysosomal degradation of filtered proteins.

In rats, sex-related differences in the proximal tubular reabsorption of exogenous cytochrome c or ovalbumin (fluorescein-isothiocyanate labeled) have been reported. Tubular uptake and reabsorption of cytochrome c and ovalbumin appear to be greater in females than in males (65,66), suggesting sex-related differences in both adsorptive and fluid-phase endocytosis, respectively. Further, both proximal tubular uptake of ovalbumin and lysosomal peptidase activity are greater in females than in males and increase significantly in males following castration (65), suggesting that sex hormones play a significant role in proximal tubular uptake and catabolism of proteins.

The intranephron site of renal accumulation of proteins has been shown to reside principally in the S_1 segment of the proximal tubules where under normal circumstances exposure to protein load is the greatest (67). Cortney et al. (68) reported significant reabsorption when proteins were infused in the initial parts of the proximal convoluted tubule, and little uptake when the more distal regions of the tubule were infused. Morphometric analysis revealed that in the normal rabbit kidney, the volume of lysosomes and endocytotic vacuoles per millimeter of tubule are greater in the S_1 segment than in the S_2 or S_3 segment (69). Indeed, activities of lysosomal enzymes, cathepsins B, H, and L, are greatest in the S_1 and less in the S_2 and S_3 in proximal tubules from young adult rabbits or rats, reflected by differences in enzymatic activity (63,64,69) or by immunocytochemical techniques (70,71). In contrast, acid phosphatase activity was significant in S_1, S_2, and S_3 segments of the rabbit proximal tubule (72), suggesting heterogeneity in lysosomal populations; i.e., large lysosomes with high cathepsin activity are prominent in the S_1, whereas smaller lysosomes with low cathepsin but high acid phosphatase activity are prominent in the S_3. In proteinuric states, activity of cathepsins B and L is significantly increased in the S_2 and S_3, but not S_1, segments (63,64), suggesting compensatory response of the S_2 and S_3 segments to an increased filtered load of protein.

Small, linear peptides (e.g., bradykinin, angiotensin) may be hydrolyzed at the luminal membrane by brush border proteases; the resulting amino acids are then transported via an energy-dependent transport process (73). Peptides that contain a disulfide linkage, such as vasopressin and insulin, or peptides containing β-alanine, proline, or sarcosine residues, appear to be resistant to luminal hydrolysis. In addition to luminal uptake and metabolism of proteins, several hormones (parathyroid hormone [PTH], glucagon, growth hormone, insulin) may be taken up and/or metabolized at the basolateral membrane. The renal extraction of proglucagon, for example, is significantly greater than can be accounted for by filtration and cannot be completely blocked by rendering the kidney nonfiltering (74), suggesting significant peritubular extraction and/or metabolism of this prohormone. Significant basolateral extraction of insulin and PTH also occurs; however, metabolism at this site does not result in complete catabolism to constituent amino acids, but rather results in the formation of large peptides.

Glutathione and Glutathione Conjugates

Several mechanisms appear to be involved in the renal handling and uptake of glutathione (GSH) and thus may mediate uptake of GSH S- (or related) conjugates

(Fig. 7). Greater than 80% of plasma GSH is extracted in a single pass by the kidney (75). Plasma GSH is filtered in proportion to the filtration fraction (i.e., 20% to 30%) and is degraded in a stepwise fashion by enzymes mediating mercapturate synthesis, specifically, γ-glutamyl transpeptidase (γ-GT), cysteinylglycine dipeptidase, and *N*-acetyltransferase. However, renal extraction of GSH is significant despite inhibition of total renal γ-GT (76,77) or cessation of glomerular filtration (78), suggesting that mechanisms other than filtration and γ-GT metabolism must contribute to the renal extraction of GSH. Indeed, renal extraction of GSH is significantly inhibited by probenecid, a competitive inhibitor of organic anion transport. Studies using basolateral membrane vesicles indicated that *in vitro* basolateral transport of GSH is electrogenic, Na^+-coupled, has a broad substrate specificity for γ-glutamyl compounds, and is probenecid-sensitive (79), consistent with transport of GSH via a basolateral organic anion transporter. The renal extraction of GSH therefore is mediated by a sodium-coupled, probenecid-sensitive transporter as well as via γ-GT metabolism and uptake; the relative contribution of these mechanisms to total renal GSH clearance/extraction is not known.

The exact mechanisms mediating the tubular uptake of nonfiltered GSH S-conjugates, or metabolites thereof, have been studied fairly extensively. Circulating GSH S-conjugates may be transported intact across the basolateral membrane by a sodium-dependent, electrogenic, and probenecid-sensitive transporter (Fig. 7) (79, 80). Intracellular GSH conjugates may then enter tubular fluid via a membrane potential–sensitive transporter (81) and be metabolized via γ-GT and peptidases. Alternatively, nonfiltered GSH S-conjugates may be cleaved by γ-GT and dipeptidases located in the basolateral membrane (82); the resulting cysteine conjugate may then be transported into the proximal tubule via an amino acid transporter.

The majority of GSH conjugates are likely formed in the liver, are excreted in the bile, and degraded to cysteine conjugates in canaliculi and/or biliary or intestinal epithelium (83). Cysteine conjugates undergo enterohepatic reabsorption and are taken up by the liver, perhaps via an amino acid transporter. Following hepatic *N*-acetylation, the *N*-acetylcysteine conjugate is returned to the systemic circulation and is an excellent substrate for the renal organic anion transporter. Recent studies on the mechanism of cysteine conjugate transport have revealed that in the isolated perfused kidney, clearance of a cysteine conjugate, S-pentachlorobutadienyl-L-cysteine (PCBC), was sixfold higher than inulin clearance; in the presence of probenecid, the fractional clearance approximates unity (84), suggesting that this conjugate is excreted principally via probenecid-sensitive tubular secretion. However, others have suggested that renal transport of cysteine conjugates is not mediated via an organic anion transporter (6,85), but mediated principally via a probenecid-insensitive amino acid transport system (85,86). Transport of the cysteine conjugate, S-(1,2- dichlorovinyl)-L-cysteine (DCVC), for example, is sodium dependent in brush border membrane vesicles and is inhibited by a variety of neutral amino acids and other cysteine conjugates (87). In contrast, transport of *N*-acetylcysteine conjugates occurs via a probenecid-sensitive organic anion transporter (85,88,89). Multiple mechanisms have been suggested to mediate the tubular uptake of GSH

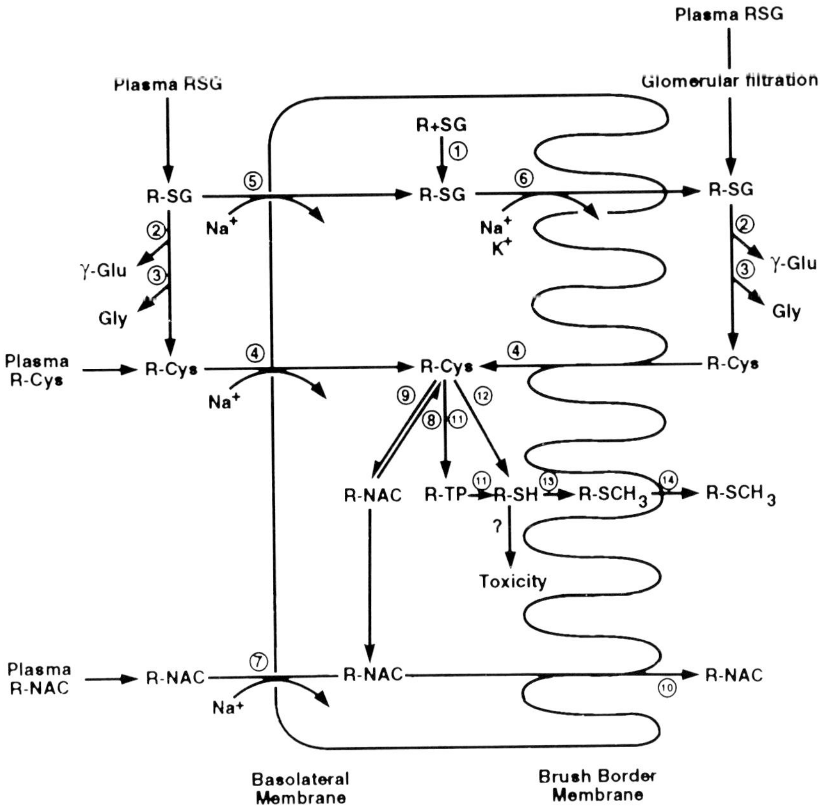

FIG. 7. Renal tubular uptake and metabolism of GSH conjugates. (*1*) Intracellular formation of GSH conjugates catalyzed by renal GSH S-transferase(s); (2) GGT-mediated catabolism of RGSH and formation of the corresponding S-cysteinylglycine conjugate (*3*) and of the corresponding cysteine (R-Cys) conjugate; (*4*) Na^+ coupled transport of R-Cys into the renal proximal tubular cell; (*5*) Na^+ coupled transport of RSG across the basolateral membrane; (*6*) translocation of RSG and excretion across the brush border membrane into the tubular lumen; (*7*) Na^+ coupled and probenecid-sensitive transport of the mercapturate (R-NAC) across the basolateral membrane; (*8*) deacetylation of R-NAC to R-Cys and (*9*) acetylation of R-Cys to R-NAC; (*10*) excretion of the mercapturate into the tubular lumen; (*11*) thiol formation (R-SH) via the intermediate formation of the thiopyruvic acid conjugate (R-TP) or (*12*) via β-lyase; (*13*) methylation of the reactive thiol and (*14*) excretion of reactive thiol into the urine. (Modified from Monks and Lau, ref. 39, with permission.)

S-conjugates and cysteine S-conjugates; however, the exact nature, number, and tubular distribution of these transporter(s) are not known with certainty.

Xenobiotic Metabolism

In general, xenobiotic metabolism is not a one-step event but rather occurs via multiple competing and sequential pathways. The relative balance between bioactivation and detoxification activities may be a critical determinant to the onset and development of toxicant-induced damage. Thus, intrarenal and intranephron heterogeneity in bioactivation and detoxification pathways may contribute significantly to site-selective nephrotoxic injury.

Mixed-Function Oxidases

The specific activities of renal mixed-function oxidases vary widely across species, strain, and sex. In general, however, renal cytochrome P-450 concentration is approximately 10% of hepatic cytochrome P-450; in rabbits, for example, hepatocytes contain approximately 1.3 nmol cytochrome P-450/mg protein (90), whereas renal proximal tubules contain 0.15 nmol cytochrome P-450/mg protein (91). Similarly, renal NADPH cytochrome P-450 reductase also is about 10% of hepatic activity in rabbits (90,91). Low cytochrome P-450 concentration in the kidney compared to that of the liver has led to the suggestion that the kidney has a limited capacity for P-450 metabolism. However, with certain substrates, the metabolic activity of the renal cytochrome P-450 may exceed that of the liver. For example, chloroform metabolism, reflected as CO_2 evolution, by renal cortical microsomes from male mice is approximately 50% of that observed in hepatic microsomes when expressed as total protein. However, when metabolic activity is expressed as a function of cytochrome P-450 content, renal activity is twofold higher than hepatic activity (92).

Mixed-function oxidase activity is not distributed uniformly throughout the kidney. Cytochrome P-450 and NADPH–cytochrome P-450–reductase concentrations exhibit a corticomedullary gradient in rats (93) and rabbits (90); concentrations are highest in the renal cortex and progressively decrease in the outer and inner medulla (Fig. 8). Within the renal cortex, the greatest activity of cytochrome P-450 is localized within the proximal tubules; distal tubules have negligible activity (26,91). Further, within the proximal tubule of the rabbit, cytochrome P-450 concentration is two to threefold greater in the S_2 segment than in the S_1 or S_3 segments, whereas cytochrome P-450 has not been detected in either the distal or cortical collecting tubules (Fig. 8). NADPH–cytochrome P-450–reductase activity in rabbits is highest in the S_2 and S_3 segments. However, in contrast to the intrarenal distribution of cytochrome P-450, NADPH–cytochrome P-450–reductase activity also is present in detectable amounts in the distal tubule and collecting tubule, exhibiting about half the activity as that observed in the S_2 and S_3 segments (Fig. 8).

Multiple forms of cytochrome P-450 have been identified in the mammalian kidney. In rat kidneys, at least five isozymes have been identified, corresponding to hepatic cytochromes P-450IA1, P-450IIC2, P-450IID1, P-450IID2, P-450IIE1, and P-450IVA1 (94). In mice, at least six renal isozymes have been detected, corresponding to P-450IIA1, P-450IIB1, P-450IIC6, P-450IIE1, P-450IIIA1, and P-450IVA1 (95). In rabbit kidney at least four isozymes of cytochromes P-450 have been identified: forms 2 (phenobarbital inducible; P-450IIB1), 3 (ethanol-inducible;

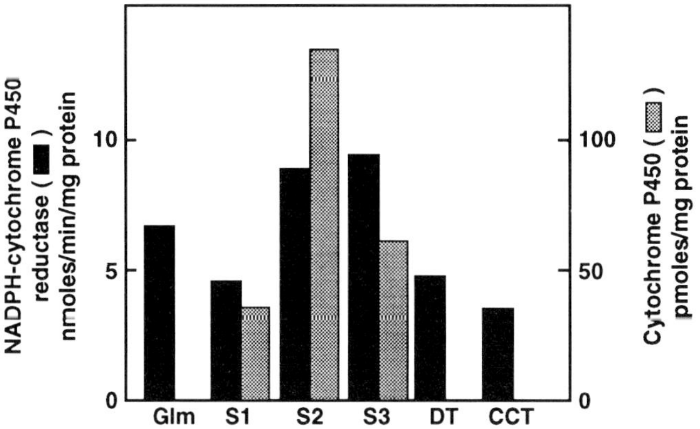

FIG. 8. Segmental distribution of cytochrome P-450 and NADPH–cytochrome P-450 reductase in rabbit kidney. Glm, glomerulus; S_1, S_1 segment of proximal tubule; S_2, S_2 segment of proximal tubule, S_3, S_3 segment of proximal tubule; DT, distal tubule; CCT, cortical collecting tubule. (Reproduced from Tarloff et al., ref. 194, with permission.)

P-450IIE1), 4 (polycyclic aromatic compound-inducible; P-450IA2), and 6 (polycyclic aromatic compound-inducible; P-450IA1) (94). Low concentrations of these isozymes in the kidney, coupled with inherent technological difficulties in obtaining pure preparations for production of monoclonal antibodies, has hindered complete classification of renal cytochrome P-450s; thus, definition of intrarenal and intranephron distribution of these isozymes is still evolving.

Several studies have suggested sex-related differences in renal cytochrome P-450 activity/content in mice. Renal cytochrome P-450 activity/content in males is greater than that of females and may contribute in part to sex-related differences in nephrotoxicity requiring P-450 bioactivation (95,96). Using immunoblotting techniques, Henderson et al. (95) have reported similar sex-related differences in the expression of six gene families or subfamilies of P-450 isozymes. Northern blot analysis indicated that these sex-related differences in P-450 isozymes are mirrored by changes in mRNA content (95), suggesting that sexual differentiation of P-450s from the gene families studied may be regulated at the transcriptional level. Furthermore, castration of male mice results in a pattern of cytochrome P-450 expression that is similar to that observed in females; the male pattern of P-450 expression is restored following treatment of castrated mice with testosterone. In contrast, ovariectomy of female mice does not affect the pattern of renal P-450 isoenzyme expression, suggesting that the expression of renal cytochrome P-450 genes is inducible or repressible by testosterone.

Although total P-450 content is greater in the renal cortex than in the medulla, the intranephron distribution of specific isozymes may not necessarily follow such a corticomedullary gradient. For example, microsomal NADPH-dependent P-450 metabolism of arachidonic acid has been identified in both cortical and medullary renal tissue of pigs, rabbits, and rats, and P-450–mediated arachidonic acid metabolites have been detected in human urine (97–100). This renal P-450 system catalyzes the transformation of arachidonic acid via either an epoxygenase system yielding 5,6-, 8,9-, 11,12- and 14,15-epoxides (epoxyeicosatrienoic acid [EET], which can be hydrolyzed to their respective vicinal diols, or a monooxygenase system yielding ω and ω-1 oxidation products (e.g., 19-hydroxyeicosatetraenoic acid [HETE], 20-HETE). The formation of these metabolites is dependent on NADPH, is inhibited by carbon monoxide or SK&F 525-A, and is not affected by indomethacin (97,98). Induction of P-450 content increases the formation of NADPH-dependent metabolites of arachidonic acid to the same extent as aryl hydrocarbon hydroxylase activity, whereas inhibition of P-450 content causes a corresponding decrease in arachidonic acid metabolites (98). Recent data suggest that these novel arachidonic acid metabolites may influence Na^+-K^+–ATPase activity, renal tubular sodium handling, and control of systemic blood pressure (98–102). Schwartzman et al. (98) have demonstrated that the specific activity for formation of arachidonate metabolites (expressed per nanomole cytochrome P-450) in outer medulla of rabbit kidney is significantly greater (threefold increase) than that of the renal cortex or liver. Moreover, the highest activity of this isozyme is in the inner stripe of the outer medulla, in the region of the medullary thick ascending limb (98,100,101). Thus, the intranephron distribution of this specific isozyme of cytochrome P-450 does not follow that of total P-450 content.

Uridine Diphosphate Glucuronyltransferase (UDPGT)

Although in general renal UDPGT activity is less than that of the liver, tissue differences in UDPGT activity appear to be substrate-dependent. For example, glucuronidation of acetaminophen in isolated renal cells is only 5% of that produced by hepatocytes (103), whereas glucuronidation of 7-hydroxycoumarin is comparable between isolated hepatocytes and renal cells (104). Similarly, although glucuronidation of *o*-aminophenol by rat renal homogenates is only 30% of that by liver, glucuronidation of *p*-nitrophenol is 2 to 2.5 times greater in renal homogenates than in hepatic tissue (105).

Similar to the regional distribution of mixed function oxidases (MFOs), renal UDPGT activity and its cofactor, UDP-glucuronic acid, is not uniformly distributed but follows a corticomedullary gradient; i.e., highest activity is in the cortex and lowest in the medulla (106). In rat kidney, UDPGT activity is observed in both proximal and distal tubules; glucuronidation capacity of the distal tubule is approximately 50% that of proximal tubules (28). Although multiple isozymes of UDPGT are present in the kidney, the intranephron distribution of these isozymes is not known.

Sulfotransferases

Sulfation represents an important detoxification step inasmuch as sulfate conjugates are highly polar and rapidly excreted in urine. However, because of the limited pool of available sulfate in the body, sulfate conjugation generally is quantitatively less than that of glucuronide conjugation. Comparison of maximal rates of sulfation measured in isolated liver and kidney cell suspensions from rats indicates that renal sulfotransferase activity is significantly less than that of liver (104). In rabbits, the activity of sulfotransferase is fairly comparable in cortical and outer medullary homogenates; however, its cofactor, adenosine 3′-phosphate 5′-phosphosulfate (PAPS) is approximately twofold greater in cortical than in medullary tissue (106).

GSH Transferases

Total renal GSH transferase activity, expressed per gram of wet tissue, is markedly less than that of hepatic activity; the relative differences are dependent upon the substrate in question. For example, in male and female rats, renal GSH aryl transferase activity is approximately 3% to 5% of hepatic activity, whereas renal GSH S–alkyl transferase activity is 90% to 120% of hepatic activity (96). In rats, GSH S-transferase is localized primarily in the proximal tubule (107); intracellular GSH concentrations, however, are not appreciably different between proximal and distal tubular cells (25,108). In the rabbit nephron, GSH transferase activity toward 1-chloro-2,4-dinitrobenzene is present exclusively and to an equal extent in the S_2 and S_3 segments of the proximal tubule and not detected in the thin descending and ascending limbs, the thick ascending limb, or cortical and medullary collecting tubules (109).

Mercapturic Acid Formation

Although GSH S-transferase activity in the kidney generally is lower than that of the liver, enzymatic activities catalyzing mercapturic acid formation (e.g., γ-glutamyl transpeptidase (γ-GT), cysteinylglycine dipeptidase, and cysteine conjugate *N*-acetyltransferase) are considerably greater in the kidney than in the liver. All three enzymes are predominantly localized to the outer stripe of the renal medulla (110). γ-GT catalyzes the first step in the metabolism of GSH S-conjugates by cleaving the γ-glutamyl linkage, yielding the corresponding cysteinylglycine conjugate. γ-GT activity, although ubiquitous, is highest in the kidney; most tissues have only 1% of the activity found in the kidney. γ-GT is concentrated primarily in the brush border of proximal tubular cells, specifically in the early and late proximal tubule of rats and rabbits (111,112); γ-GT activity has also been detected in the basolateral membranes (82). Its active site is oriented on the outer surface of the cell membrane, thus hydrolyzing substrates within the tubular lumen or peritubular capillary. The cysteinylglycine conjugate formed is a substrate for numerous peptidases, including aminopeptidase M and a dipeptidase, both located within the brush border. These peptidases catalyze the removal of the glycine residues of the GSH S-conjugates to yield the corresponding cysteine S-conjugate. The resulting cysteine S-conjugate may be excreted or, more likely, taken up by the proximal tubule cell and metabolized further by the microsomal cysteine-thioether *N*-acetyltransferase to produce *N*-acetylcysteine conjugate (mercapturic acid) (113) which is readily excreted in the urine.

Cysteine Conjugate β-Lyase

Although GSH conjugation generally functions as a detoxification pathway, the kidney contains an enzyme, cysteine conjugate β-lyase, which is a pyridoxal-phosphate–dependent enzyme capable of cleaving the β-carbon bond between cysteine and sulfur, forming ammonia, pyruvate, and a reactive thiol intermediate (114). Cysteine conjugate β-lyase is inactive with aliphatic cysteine conjugates and requires compounds that bear a good leaving group on the β-carbon of cysteine (115). Cysteine conjugate β-lyase activity is present in rat liver, kidney, and gut microflora. β-Lyase is present in outer mitochondrial membrane and cytosol (114) and is virtually absent from brush border membranes (86). Liver and kidney cytosolic enzymes are distinct proteins insofar as the antibody to the liver enzyme does not cross-react with the kidney cytosolic enzyme (116). The major cytosolic β-lyase has been purified from rat kidneys and is identical to rat kidney cytosolic glutamine transaminase K (117). In the kidney, cytosolic enzyme is localized specifically in the proximal tubule; no β-lyase has been detected in glomeruli, distal tubules, or collecting tubules (118). There appears to be some controversy over the distribution of cytosolic β-lyase within the proximal tubule of rats, with some investigators reporting a fairly uniform distribution between the S_1, S_2, and S_3 segments (119), whereas others have indicated a higher concentration in the S_3 segment (118).

Prostaglandin H Synthase

Prostaglandin (PG) H synthase is a hemoprotein involved in the biosynthesis of prostaglandins, thromboxanes, and prostacyclins, and is composed of two enzymes, fatty acid cyclooxygenase and prostaglandin hydroperoxidase. Fatty acid cyclooxygenase catalyzes the initial bis-oxidation of unsaturated fatty acids, converting arachidonic acid to the hydroperoxide, PGG_2. Prostaglandin hydroperoxidase catalyzes the reduction of PGG_2 to PGH_2. Several xenobiotics have been demonstrated to serve as electron donors in the catalysis of PGG_2 to PGH_2, resulting in co-oxidation of the xenobiotic. Indeed, intrarenal prostaglandin H synthase has been implicated in the co-oxidation of the xenobiotic. Indeed, intrarenal prostaglandin H synthase has been implicated in the co-oxidation, and bioactivation, of several xenobiotics, including acetaminophen, *p*-aminophenol, *p*-phenetidine, benzidine, and *N*-[4-(5-nitro-2-furyl)-2-thiazolyl] formamide (FANFT) (120).

In rabbit kidney, prostaglandin H synthase is not distributed uniformly but is highest in inner medulla, intermediate in outer medulla, and is barely detectable in the cortex, a concentration gradient opposite to that of mixed-function oxidases

(120). Intracellular prostaglandin H synthetase is localized in the endoplasmic reticulum and nuclear membrane.

SITE-SPECIFIC TUBULAR INJURY

Proximal Convoluted Tubule (S_1/S_2 Segment)

Cephalosporin Antibiotics

Of the nephrotoxic cephalosporin antibiotics, cephaloridine has been studied the most extensively. In laboratory animals, cephaloridine nephrotoxicity is characterized by widespread areas of necrosis and hydropic changes confined to the subcapsular proximal convoluted tubules, specifically the S_2 segments (121). Several studies have suggested that the varying incidence and severity of cephaloridine nephrotoxicity observed in different species, strains, and age groups is directly related to differences in renal cortical concentrations and accumulation of this drug. For example, renal cortical concentrations and nephrotoxicity of cephaloridine are greatest in rabbits, intermediate in guinea pigs, and least in rats (122). Furthermore, within a given species, such as the mouse, the susceptibility of males and females of different strains varies and appears to be dependent upon similar strain and sex-related differences in renal cortical accumulation of cephaloridine. C57BI female mice, for example, exhibit greater renal cortical concentrations of cephaloridine and are more susceptible to cephaloridine nephrotoxicity than C57BI male mice or female mice of other strains (123). Age also significantly affects both renal cortical concentrations and, hence, nephrotoxicity of cephaloridine. Neonatal rabbits, for example, do not significantly accumulate cephaloridine and are not susceptible to the nephrotoxic effects of this antibiotic (124). On the other hand, aging rats are more susceptible to cephaloridine nephrotoxicity than young adult rats, reflected by more profound drug-related changes in blood urea nitrogen (BUN) concentration, kidney weight, and renal cortical slice accumulation of PAH and TEA in aging rats (125). The enhanced susceptibility of older rats is accompanied by an increase in renal cortical concentrations of cephaloridine, which, in turn, may be secondary to age-dependent changes in the pharmacokinetics of this drug.

The mechanisms mediating the renal cortical accumulation of cephaloridine have been studied in detail in the rabbit. Pretreatment of rabbits with inhibitors of renal organic anion transport, such as probenecid, decreases the cortex/serum concentration ratio of cephaloridine (122,126), suggesting that cephaloridine is actively transported into proximal tubular cells by an organic anion transporter. Unlike other cephalosporins, however, cephaloridine is a zwitterion containing a positive charge at the 3 positions of the cephem ring, and organic cation transport also appears to be important to the renal tubular handling of cephaloridine. Efflux of cephaloridine from renal cortical slices is significantly decreased in the presence of organic cation inhibitors such as cyanine 863 or mepiperphenidol (127), suggesting that transport of cephaloridine from cell to lumen is mediated by an organic cation transporter. Indeed, these inhibitors of organic cation transport enhance cephaloridine nephrotoxicity in rabbits (128), presumably by decreasing efflux and, hence, increasing intracellular concentrations and nephrotoxicity of cephaloridine. Cephaloridine transport from proximal tubular cell to tubular fluid is restricted, compared with other cephalosporins, resulting in little or no net tubular secretion into the tubular fluid.

These studies of cephaloridine transport in rabbit kidney collectively suggest that in the rabbit, net intracellular accumulation of cephaloridine is dependent upon at least two components: active basolateral transport via an organic anion transporter and limited efflux across the luminal membrane via an organic cation transporter. The role of tubular transport to the nephrotoxicity of cephaloridine in rabbits has been suggested by the observation that inhibitors of organic anion transport, such as probenecid, *p*-aminohippurate, and benzylpenicillin, reduce both the renal cortical concentration and nephrotoxicity of cephaloridine (126,129). Furthermore, the S_2 segment of the proximal tubule represents the site of greatest activity of organic anion transport in the rabbit nephron and is the primary target of cephaloridine-induced injury, suggesting a relationship between transport and nephrotoxic injury.

Although the mechanisms of the tubular transport of cephaloridine in the rabbit are well characterized, recent studies have called into question the exact mechanisms of transport in the rat kidney. Using stop-flow capillary perfusion methods, Ullrich et al. (130) recently reported that unlike monocarboxylic penicillins (benzylpenicillin, phenoxymethylpenicillin), monocarboxylic cephalosporins (6315 S Shionogi, cefotaxime, ceftriaxone, cefodizime) or aminocephalosporins (cephalexin, defadroxil), cephaloridine does not inhibit the basolateral influx of the prototype organic anion, PAH, into rat cortical tubular cells. Further, cephaloridine does not inhibit basolateral influx of other prototype organic anions, e.g., succinate or sulfate, suggesting that in the rat, cephaloridine may not be transported by these basolateral organic anion transporters. The absence of interaction of cephaloridine with a basolateral organic anion transporter in rat kidneys in these studies is consistent with the observation that cephaloridine does not inhibit PAH transport by rat basolateral membrane vesicles, but does inhibit PAH transport by rabbit basolateral membrane vesicles (131). Although these *in vitro* studies call into question the mechanisms mediating the tubular transport of cephaloridine in the rat, the organic anion transport inhibitor probenecid is known to reduce the renal cortical accumulation and nephrotoxicity of cephaloridine in rats (132,133).

Although renal tubular transport and accumulation of cephaloridine likely contributes to some extent to its site-selective injury to the S_2 segment of the rabbit proximal tubule, the relationship between renal cortical uptake and the nephrotoxic potential of other β-lactam antibiotics does not appear to be precise or predictive. For example, similar to cephaloridine, cephaloglycin is transported across the basolateral membrane via an organic anion transporter in rabbits and probenecid decreases both the renal cortical concentrations and nephrotoxicity of cephaloglycin

(134). Thus, qualitatively, the relationship between transport, accumulation, and toxicity appears to be similar for both cephaloridine and cephaloglycin. However, the rank order of intracellular concentration does not correlate with the rank order of nephrotoxic potential of these two cephalosporins; that is, renal cortical concentrations of cephaloglycin are significantly lower than those of cephaloridine, yet, cephaloglycin is significantly more nephrotoxic (135). Similarly, although renal cortical concentrations of cephaloglycin and cephalexin are similar, there are dramatic differences in nephrotoxic potential between these two antibiotics; cephaloglycin is nephrotoxic whereas cephalexin is not (135). Taken collectively, these data suggest that although transport and accumulation of β-lactams may be important to the incidence and severity of site-selective nephrotoxic injury, other mechanisms ultimately determine the nephrotoxic potential of the cephalosporin in question. Thus, once transported and sequestered into the targeted cell, the incidence/severity of nephrotoxic injury may be dependent upon the reactivity of the cephalosporin (or metabolite) with subcellular or molecular targets. Furthermore, recent *in vitro* data suggest that in rats site-selective injury is not solely due to segmental differences in cephalosporin transport. *In vitro* exposure of suspensions of rat proximal tubular versus distal tubular cells to cephaloridine results in a selective cytotoxicity to proximal tubular cells, despite comparable intracellular concentrations of cephaloridine in both cell populations (136,137). Similarly, cephaloridine is not cytotoxic to suspensions of rat hepatocytes under conditions in which hepatocellular concentrations of cephaloridine exceed those associated with cytotoxicity to rat renal cortical slices (137). Thus, intracellular accumulation of cephaloridine does not appear to be the sole determinant of site-selective injury to the proximal tubular cell. Collectively, these data suggest that intracellular accumulation is a necessary but not sufficient event in the site-selective nephrotoxicity of cephaloridine. Rather, other segmental features of the proximal tubular cell are likely to be important in rendering this segment of the nephron susceptible to cephalosporin nephrotoxicity.

Aminoglycoside Antibiotics

The clinical utility of aminoglycoside antibiotics is frequently limited by a dose-related nephrotoxicity as suggested by an 8% to 26% incidence of acute renal failure in patients receiving aminoglycosides (138). Hallmarks of aminoglycoside-induced renal dysfunction include tubular proteinuria (β_2-microglobulin), enzymuria (brush border membrane– and lysosomal-associated enzymes), glycosuria, aminoaciduria, nephrogenic diabetes insipidus, magnesium and potassium wasting, and decreased glomerular filtration rate (139). The predominant sites of aminoglycoside nephrotoxicity are the S_1 and S_2 segments of the proximal tubule; the distal tubule and glomerulus are also affected albeit to a lesser extent (140–143). The earliest morphological changes of aminoglycoside nephrotoxicity include an increase in the number and size of secondary lysosomes containing myeloid bodies, electron-dense lamellar structures of concentrically arranged and densely packed membranes (143–

145). Following these lysosomal changes, there is a decrease in the density and height of brush border microvilli, dilatation of the cisternae of rough endoplasmic reticulum, and cytoplasmic vacuolization in the tubular epithelium. As injury progresses, mitochondrial swelling, tubular necrosis, and desquamation occur.

Aminoglycosides accumulate within the renal cortex of laboratory animals and humans, and it is generally thought that the susceptibility of the kidney to aminoglycosides toxicity is related to the ability of the kidney to transport/accumulate these molecules. Indeed, for any given aminoglycoside, the incidence and severity of nephrotoxicity appears to be directly related to renal cortical concentrations of drug. Variables such as dose, dosing frequency, and duration of treatment each influence the renal cortical concentrations of drug and, hence, similarly influence the incidence and severity of nephrotoxicity.

The renal handling of aminoglycosides has been studied in detail and the relative contribution of reabsorptive and secretive processes has been somewhat controversial. In Sprague-Dawley rats, gentamicin clearance is comparable to that of inulin clearance (146), suggesting that gentamicin is freely filtered at the glomerulus and does not undergo net reabsorption or secretion. Microinjection studies, however, have indicated that gentamicin does undergo significant reabsorption in the early and late proximal tubular segments, reflected by decreased urinary recovery of radiolabeled gentamicin compared with that of inulin at these sites (146). Similarly, the aminoglycoside netilmicin undergoes reabsorption along the early proximal convoluted tubule (147). At relatively low doses, fractional urinary excretion of gentamicin exceeds the fractional delivery of drug to the superficial distal tubule (148,149), suggesting net secretion of gentamicin by the deeper juxtamedullary nephrons (148). In contrast, at relatively high doses of netilmicin, the fractional delivery to the early proximal tubule exceeds the filtered load, suggestive of proximal tubular secretion (147). Thus, aminoglycosides appear to undergo proximal tubular reabsorptive and secretory processes; the latter may occur in the early proximal tubule (high-dose netilmicin) and/or in the late proximal tubule of juxtamedullary nephrons (low-dose gentamicin).

The exact mechanisms of renal tubular uptake and accumulation of aminoglycosides likely involve both luminal and basolateral transport mechanisms. The polycationic aminoglycosides bind to anionic phospholipids, such as the polyphosphinositides, in the brush border of the proximal tubule (150). Indeed, the affinity for the brush border membrane binding site correlates with the number of free amino groups and hence the cationic charge of the aminoglycoside molecule, suggesting the importance of electrostatic binding (150). Although the precise structural features of aminoglycosides required for brush border membrane binding have not been clearly defined, net charge per se does not appear to be the sole determinant of binding as suggested by the observation that gentamicin binding to brush border membrane vesicles is inhibited by polymers of cationic (lysine, ornithine, arginine, and histidine), neutral (asparagine), and acidic (asparate and glutamate) amino acids (151). Thus, the number of amino groups, regardless of net charge, may be important to binding affinity. The bound aminoglycoside is taken up via a high-capacity, adsorptive endocytotic mechanism, analogous to that mediating uptake of low molecular weight proteins. Indeed, aminoglycosides appear to competitively inhibit the tubular uptake of low molecular weight proteins such as lysozyme (152). Following pinocytosis, aminoglycosides are sequestered and stored in secondary lysosomes. The relative contribution of these luminal transport processes to the nephrotoxic effects of aminoglycosides has been suggested by the observation that the early deleterious effects of gentamicin, i.e., inhibition of Na- K–ATPase, occurs only in the filtering, and not nonfiltering, isolated perfused kidney (153). Furthermore, renal cortical accumulation of radiolabeled gentamicin is decreased by as much as 75% when isolated perfused kidneys are rendered nonfiltering (154), suggesting that luminal transport represents the predominant mode of aminoglycoside uptake and accumulation. Thus, basolateral membrane binding and uptake appears to represent a quantitatively minor mechanism for total renal cortical accumulation of aminoglycosides.

The relationship between the renal tubular handling and nephrotoxicity of aminoglycosides is suggested by several lines of evidence. First, earlier comparative studies of aminoglycosides have suggested a direct relationship between membrane binding and nephrotoxic potential (150). For example, among the older aminoglycosides the rank order of clinical nephrotoxic potential is neomycin>gentamicin>kanamycin, which is similar to that observed for brush border membrane binding affinity (150). Second, the S_1 and S_2 segments of the proximal tubule exhibit the greatest endocytotic activity in the nephron and are the primary sites of aminoglycoside nephrotoxicity, suggesting (a) a relationship between segmental differences in endocytotic reabsorption and site-selective injury, and (b) a relationship between luminal binding/uptake and aminoglycoside nephrotoxicity. Third, aminoglycosides accumulate within the lysosome, which is an early target of injury, suggesting a relationship between luminal uptake, accumulation, and nephrotoxic injury. Finally, several studies have indicated that sex and age-related differences in the nephrotoxic potential of aminoglycosides parallel differences in the renal cortical accumulation of drug, suggesting the possibility of a cause-effect relationship. Specifically, neonatal male rats (155,156) or young adult female rats (157) are less susceptible than young adult male rats to gentamicin nephrotoxicity, a phenomenon associated with decreased renal cortical accumulation of gentamicin. Similarly, in diabetic rats decreased renal cortical accumulation of gentamicin is believed to contribute to the reported decreased incidence and severity of gentamicin nephrotoxicity (158).

Although these studies suggest a relationship between renal uptake, accumulation, and nephrotoxicity of aminoglycosides, these variables are not inextricably linked. For example, neomycin is the most potent nephrotoxic aminoglycoside; yet, renal cortical accumulation of drug is less than that of gentamicin and comparable to that of the relatively nontoxic tobramycin (Table 1) (159), suggesting that factors other than, or in addition to, cortical accumulation are important to aminoglycoside nephrotoxicity. Also, the binding affinity to rat brush border membranes does not correlate well with the extent of intracellular uptake or the nephrotoxic potential in

TABLE 1. *Relationship between renal cortical concentrations and nephrotoxic potential of aminoglycosides*

	Renal cortical (μg/g)	Serum creatinine (mg/dl)
Saline	—	0.34 ± .02
Streptomycin (100 mg/kg/day)	76 ± 10	0.33 ± .02
Tobramycin (100 mg/kg/day)	833 ± 61	0.32 ± .02
Neomycin (100 mg/kg/day)	940 ± 171	7.19 ± .58
Kanamycin (500 mg/kg/day)	1,156 ± 53	2.18 ± .24
Amikacin (500 mg/kg/day)	1,759 ± 111	0.96 ± .15
Netilmicin (100 mg/kg/day)	2,142 ± 222	0.34 ± .01
Gentamicin (100 mg/kg/day)	2,230 ± 275	4.73 ± .60

Data are expressed as means ± SEM. Rats were administered vehicle or drug once daily for 4 consecutive days and renal cortical concentrations of drug and serum creatinine concentrations measured. (Modified from Kalyonadies and Pastoriza-Munoz, ref. 159.)

rats. Gentamicin, tobramycin, and netilmicin have five ionizable amino groups and have roughly the same affinity for rat brush border membrane sites (150). Yet, there are substantial differences between the renal cortical accumulation of these aminoglycosides (Table 1), e.g., gentamicin≈netilmicin>tobramycin (159,160) and in nephrotoxic potential, e.g., gentamicin>netilmicin≈tobramycin (159). Thus, brush border membrane binding affinity does not correlate precisely with renal cortical accumulation and accumulation does not correlate precisely with nephrotoxic potential. Williams et al. (161) have observed that polyamino acids decrease both the renal brush border membrane binding and nephrotoxicity of aminoglycosides, but do not decrease total cortical accumulation of drug, suggesting that membrane binding may be a better correlate and predictor of nephrotoxicity than tissue accumulation per se. Indeed, the rank order of brush border membrane binding of various aminoglycosides parallels that of nephrotoxic potential (162). Also, polyamino acids such as polyaspartate confer significant protection against gentamicin nephrotoxicity despite a tenfold increase in renal cortical accumulation of gentamicin (163,164), further suggesting a dissociation between renal cortical accumulation and nephrotoxicity of gentamicin.

Despite the poor correlation between net renal cortical accumulation and nephrotoxicity of aminoglycosides, the site-selective injury of aminoglycosides to the S_1 and S_2 proximal tubular cells is likely to be related, at least in part, to the accumulation of drug within these cell types. Combined immunofluorescence microscopy and section freeze-dry autoradiography studies have indicated rapid localization of labeled gentamicin in S_1 and S_2 segments, whereas no significant uptake of gentamicin by S_3 cells has been observed (165); thus, cell-specific uptake likely contributes to some extent to cell-specific injury. The renal tubular uptake of aminoglycosides is likely to represent a necessary but not sufficient factor for inducing nephrotoxic injury. Once sequestered within the S_1 and S_2 cells, the nephrotoxic potential of aminoglycosides may be dependent upon residence time within the cells and/or intrinsic reactivity of the aminoglycoside with subcellular or molecular targets.

Pars Recta (S_3 Segment)

Haloalkene S-Conjugates

Several halogenated alkenes, e.g., hexachlorobutadiene (HCBD), perfluoropropene, and trichloroethylene (TCE), produce injury to the proximal tubule, predominantly the pars recta or S_3 segment. These nephrotoxic haloalkenes are metabolized to glutathione S-conjugates, which are believed to be key intermediates in haloalkene nephrotoxicity. Although kidney microsomal and cytosolic fractions contain glutathione S-transferases capable of conjugating haloalkenes with glutathione, hepatic GSH conjugation plays a more predominant role. Indeed, a number of GSH-related metabolites have been identified in bile of HCBD-treated rats; the principal metabolites identified are S-(1,2,3,4,4-pentachloro-1,3-butadienyl) glutathione (PCBDG) and S-(1,2,3,4,4-pentachloro-1,3-butadienyl)cysteinylglycine (166). *In vitro* studies have indicated that rat hepatic microsomal and cytosolic fractions catalyze the formation of PCBDG from HCBD (167). The involvement of these hepatobiliary GSH conjugates in HCBD nephrotoxicity has been suggested by the observation that (a) administration of lyophilized bile, collected from HCBD-treated rats, to naive rats produces necrosis of the pars recta, a lesion that is similar in nature to that following HCBD administration; and (b) interruption of the enterohepatic circulation, by cannulation and exteriorization of the bile duct, prevents HCBD nephrotoxicity (166). Furthermore, chemically synthesized PCBDG causes a renal lesion identical to that seen with HCBD (168). Glutathione conjugates of other haloalkenes also have been reported; biliary glutathione or cysteine conjugates have been identified in tetrafluoroethylene (TFE)- and in TCE-treated rats (169).

The mechanism of nephrotoxicity of these chlorinated and fluorinated olfins appears to involve complex sequential interorgan metabolism and translocation. Once formed, glutathione conjugates may be excreted in the bile and metabolized by hepatobiliary γ-glutamyl transpeptidase (γ-GT) and dipeptidase to yield the corresponding cysteine S-conjugates. Following enterohepatic circulation, the cysteine conjugates may be delivered and taken up by the kidney or may be *N*-acetylated to mercapturic acid within the liver prior to renal tubular uptake. The cysteine conjugates and mercapturic acids are then delivered to the kidney where they are transported into tubular cells by different transport mechanisms. Alternatively, glutathione conjugates formed in the liver may be transported across the hepatic sinusoidal membrane, enter the systemic circulation, and are delivered to the kidneys. Metabolism of these GSH conjugates to the corresponding cysteine conjugates may occur via γ-GT and dipeptidases associated with the brush border of proximal tubular cells. Thus, haloalkene metabolites reaching the kidney may include GSH S-conjugates, cysteine conjugates, and *N*-acetylated (NAC; mercapturate) conjugates.

The exact reasons for the selective injury of haloalkenes to the pars recta are not known but likely involve any one or a combination of contributing factors, e.g., cell-specific tubular transport, and metabolism and/or intrinisic susceptibility to the biochemical effects of the proximate nephrotoxicant(s). The role of renal transport/accumulation in the nephrotoxicity of haloalkene–GSH conjugates is suggested by the observation that renal accumulation of radiolabeled HCBD is localized to the outer stripe of the outer medulla (166), coinciding with the site of renal necrosis (170–172). However, the exact mechanisms of transport and the relative contribution of cysteine conjugate transport versus mercapturate transport leading to renal accumulation of HCBD-related material are not known. Mercapturates are substrates for the renal tubular organic anion transporter; the *N*-acetylcysteine conjugate of HCBD, PCBD-NAC, accumulates in renal cortical slices via an energy-dependent transport system and uptake is significantly reduced by substrates of the organic anion transport system (172). Furthermore, probenecid blocks the renal cortical accumulation and nephrotoxicity of HCBD and PCBD-NAC (173), suggesting that accumulation of *N*-acetylcysteine conjugate plays an important role in HCBD nephrotoxicity. These data further suggest that HCBD nephrotoxicity is not dependent upon the renal tubular transport of the cysteine S-conjugate, since the renal tubular uptake of the cysteine conjugate appears to be mediated by a probenecid-insensitive transporter (86,87). Probenecid also inhibits proximal tubular accumulation of the mercapturate of TCE, *N*-acetylcysteine dichlorovinylcysteine (NAC-DCVC), but not DCVC, in rabbit renal slices *in vitro* (6). Although probenecid blocks the nephrotoxicity of NAC-DCVC, organic anion transport is not the sole determinant of site-specific nephrotoxic injury since the S_2 segment, and not the S_3 segment (site of injury), has the highest organic anion transport activity in rabbits. Thus, factors other than or in addition to organic anion transport of haloalkene S-conjugates must contribute to the site-selective injury to the pars recta.

The role of cell-specific metabolism in the site-selective injury of haloalkenes also has been investigated. Once accumulated within the cell, the NAC-conjugate may be deacetylated to the corresponding cysteine conjugate. The cysteine conjugates, in turn, are excellent substrates for the cysteine conjugate β-lyase, resulting in the formation of pyruvate, ammonia, chloride, and a reactive mercaptan moiety. The latter is believed to be the ultimate nephrotoxicant, capable of reacting with intracellular proteins, nucleic acids, and/or thiols to produce cytotoxicity (174–176). Cysteine conjugates rapidly impair succinate dependent state 3 respiration, mitochondrial calcium sequestration, membrane potential, and metabolism *in vitro*, indicating that mitochondria are important cellular targets (175). Thus, site-selective injury may be due to segmental differences in deacetylase/acetylase activity, β-lyase activity, and/or segmental differences in the intrinsic susceptibility of mitochondria to toxicant damage. Studies evaluating the segmental distribution of β-lyase activity have been inconsistent with some reports indicating a uniform distribution of β-lyase between S_1, S_2, and S_3 cells (119), whereas others have suggested that β-lyase is specifically localized in the S_3 segment (118). Wolfgang et al. (6) have suggested the possibility that the lower number and size of mitochondria in the S_3 segment may render this segment of the nephron more susceptible to mitochondrial effects of haloalkenes. Although an attractive hypothesis, this is unlikely to be the sole explanation for haloalkene-induced site-selective nephrotoxic injury, since the S_1/S_2 segments appear to be more susceptible to hypoxia, anoxia, or mitochondrial toxicants than the S_3 segments (3,176). Thus, segmental differences in any one variable alone is unlikely to adequately explain the site-selective injury of haloalkene S-conjugate nephrotoxicity. Rather, site-selective injury of haloalkene nephrotoxicity may be due to segmental differences in transport/accumulation of haloalkene S-conjugates coupled with the net effect of segmental differences in acetylase/deacetylase activity, β-lyase activity, and/or intrinsic susceptibility of the mitochondria.

Loop of Henle/Distal Tubule/Collecting Duct

Methoxyflurane

The general anesthetic, methyoxyflurane, produces renal failure characterized by vasopressin-resistant polyuria and increases in serum sodium, osmolality, and BUN. Methoxyflurane is metabolized to two major metabolites, inorganic fluoride and oxalic acid, detected in serum and urine of methoxyflurane-treated patients and animals. Patients with clinically evident nephrotoxicity exhibit greater serum and urine concentrations of these metabolites than do patients with subclinical abnormalities (177), suggesting that these metabolites may mediate methoxyflurane nephrotoxicity. The role of metabolism in methoxyflurane nephrotoxicity is suggested by the observation that induction of hepatic mixed-function oxidases in F-344 rats by phenobarbital treatment increases defluorination and nephrotoxicity of methoxyflurane, whereas administration of SK&F 525-A, an inhibitor of mixed-function oxidases, results in decreased defluorination and decreased nephrotoxicity (178). Importantly, phenobarbital alters rat hepatic, but not renal, mixed-function oxidase activity, suggesting that hepatic metabolism of methoxyflurane is important to its nephrotoxicity. Furthermore, strain-related differences in methoxyflurane metabolism in rats correlates fairly well with strain-related differences in the incidence/severity of methoxyflurane nephrotoxicity. For example, F-344 rats metabolize methoxyflurane to the greatest extent and also develop the greatest degree of renal damage (179). However, the Buffalo rat, which metabolizes methoxyflurane to a similar extent as the F-334 rat, is not susceptible to methoxyflurane nephrotoxicity, suggesting that factors other than or in addition to strain-related differences in metabolism account for differences in susceptibility to methoxyflurane nephrotoxicity.

Fluoride appears to be the proximate nephrotoxicant inasmuch as administration of sodium fluoride produces vasopressin-resistant polyuria and morphological abnormalities similar to that observed with methoxyflurane, whereas administration of another metabolite of methoxyflurane, oxalic acid, causes anuria, not polyuria (178,180). The observation that methoxyflurane produces a vasopressin-resistant polyuria suggests that fluoride may be interfering with the action of vasopressin in the medullary thick ascending limb and/or the collecting duct. However, histological damage associated with methoxyflurane has been noted in the proximal convoluted tubule and not in the more distal segments (180). Thus, several mechanisms of fluoride-induced polyuria have been proposed: inhibition of salt and water reabsorption in the proximal tubule or in the thick ascending limb of the loop of Henle and/or decreased responsiveness of the collecting duct to vasopressin. Rush and Willis (181) reported that fluoride administration decreases free water excretion, suggesting that polyuria is not secondary to increased proximal tubular delivery of solutes to the distal tubule. Furthermore, fluoride was shown to diminish the solute gradient in renal medullary tissue and to increase the fractional excretion of sodium (181), suggesting that fluoride dissipates the concentration gradient in the renal medulla largely by inhibiting sodium chloride reabsorption by the thick ascending limb. In addition to these effects, fluoride inhibits vasopressin-induced increases in medullary adenosine 3′,5′-cyclic monophosphate (cAMP) content, suggesting that fluoride exerts an inhibitory effect on vasopressin action on the medullary collecting duct (181). Taken together, these studies suggest that methoxyflurane-induced polyuria is mediated by the ability of fluoride to inhibit sodium chloride reabsorption by the thick ascending limb and to inhibit the effects of vasopressin on water and urea reabsorption by the collecting duct. Since cAMP is known to play a crucial role in both of these functions, it is tempting to postulate that the inhibitory effects of fluoride may relate to its effects on adenine nucleotide metabolism. In both the medullary thick ascending limb and the medullary collecting duct, glucose is the primary substrate supporting ATP synthesis (2); in contrast, pyruvate and glutamine are the preferred substrates in the proximal tubular segments. Fluoride is known to inhibit glycolysis, the resulting inhibition of glycolysis theoretically would decrease availability of ATP for cAMP generation via adenylate cyclase, an effect that would lead to decreased responsivity of the medullary thick ascending limb (mTAL) and collecting duct to vasopressin and hence, resulting in polyuria. Although the exact molecular mechanisms of fluoride nephrotoxicity are not known, an effect on glycolysis and hence, on adenine nucleotide metabolism and vasopressin activity, would be consistent with the site-selective effects on the mTAL and collecting duct.

Amphotericin B

Amphotericin B nephrotoxicity is manifested as azotemia associated with decreased renal plasma flow and glomerular filtration rate, renal tubular acidosis, impaired concentrating ability, and electrolyte abnormalities, e.g., potassium wasting and hypokalemia (182-184). Two distinct mechanisms are involved in amphotericin B nephrotoxicity: renal arteriolar vasoconstriction and increased tubular permeability. Histologically, tubular changes are characterized by fragmentation and thickening of the basement membranes, necrosis of the distal tubular epithelium, nephrocalcinosis, and vacuolization of distal tubular cells (182).

Although multiple sites of the nephron are affected by amphotericin, the primary effects of this drug appear to involve the distal tubule. Both renal tubular acidosis and impaired concentrating ability occur early in the course of amphotericin nephrotoxicity and are hallmarks of the distal tubular effects of amphotericin B (182–184).

Impaired concentrating ability is not ameliorated by exogenous vasopressin, suggesting that the concentrating defect occurs at the level of the mTAL and/or collecting duct. Amphotericin treatment has been associated with a decreased ability to maintain medullary urea gradients (185), an effect consistent with impaired vasopressin activity in the collecting duct. Renal tubular acidosis is characterized by a defect in distal tubular acidification; specifically, amphotericin decreases net acid excretion and reduces acidification of the urine following an acid load. This drug-related acidification defect has been demonstrated to be related to increased back-diffusion of hydrogen ions in the form of carbonic acid, dissolved carbon dioxide, or a weak acid or proton (184).

The mechanisms of amphotericin-induced distal tubular/collecting duct effects are likely related to drug-induced alterations in membrane permeability. Amphotericin B is a polyene antibiotic containing a hydrophilic region and a sequence of conjugated double bonds that is lipophilic. This unique structure facilitates the incorporation of the drug into cellular membranes. Indeed, administration of amphotericin B *in vivo* results in binding to sterols in most tissues, with the highest binding occurring in the kidney (186). Amphotericin B has been demonstrated to increase the permeability of both artificial and natural membranes (187), an effect that is likely related to its interactions with sterol moieties (e.g., cholesterol, ergosterol) of cell membranes leading to the formation of aqueous pores. The relationship of membrane interactions to toxicity of amphotericin B has been suggested by early studies indicating that amphotericin is without effects in cell-free systems. Furthermore, bacteria and bluegreen algae, which have no membrane sterols, are resistant to the effects of amphotericin (188). Studies in toad and turtle urinary bladders indicated that amphotericin increases membrane permeability to a variety of small molecules, including urea, potassium, and chloride (189–190). Thus, interaction of amphotericin with membrane sterols is likely to result in formation of transmembrane channels or pores, increasing membrane permeability to ions and leading to membrane dysfunction. Consequently, amphotericin B can transform a relatively tight epithelium such as the distal tubule into one that is relatively leaky to water, hydrogen ions, and potassium. The exact reasons for the predominant distal tubular effects of amphotericin B are not known but it has been postulated that the distal tubular membrane may be richer in cholesterol, resulting in greater amphotericin-membrane interactions (191).

CONCLUDING REMARKS

In addition to segmental differences in transport and metabolism, the intrinsic susceptibility of each of the cell types to chemically induced injury also is a critical determinant of site-selective injury. The intrinsic susceptibility of tubular cells to injury can be assessed using a toxicant that does not require transport/metabolism to exert its toxic effects and using *in vitro* techniques in which variables such as blood flow and substrate delivery are eliminated. For example, the intrinsic susceptibility of proximal versus distal tubular cells to chemically induced oxidative injury has been evaluated by assessing the effects of peroxides and quinones on the viability of suspensions of proximal or distal tubular cells *in vitro*. Such studies have indicated that distal tubular cells are more susceptible to oxidative injury than proximal tubular cells, an effect that was attributed in part to the comparatively lower activities of enzymes involved in the detoxification of oxygen radicals or peroxides, specifically glutathione (GSSG) reductase, GSH peroxidase, and catalase, in the distal versus proximal tubular cell (192). Thus, in the absence of segmental differences in blood flow, oxygen tension, tubular transport, and bioactivation mechanisms, distal tubular cells appear to be more susceptible to oxidative stress and injury than proximal tubular cells. The intrinsic susceptibility of tubular cells to hypoxia/anoxia also has been evaluated *in vitro* using either renal cortical slices or suspensions of isolated tubular segments. These *in vitro* data suggest that the S_1/S_2 cells are more susceptible to oxygen deprivation than S_3 cells (6,176), a finding that contrasts to *in vivo* observations indicating that the S_3 segment is the primary site of injury following renal ischemia. Ruegg and Mandel (176) have suggested that *in vivo*, the nonuniform oxygen gradient renders the S_3 segments located in the distal capillary beds anoxic, whereas other nephron segments, perfused by the proximal capillary beds, extract the available oxygen under reduced oxygen delivery conditions. Thus, transient or sustained hypotension *in vivo* results in poor perfusion of the outer medullary stripe, leaving S_3 segments anoxic. In contrast, uniform oxygen deprivation (*in vitro* hypoxia/anoxia) results in S_1/S_2 injury, suggesting that in the absence of regional differences in oxygen delivery and regional blood flow, S_1/S_2 cells are intrinsically more susceptible to the effects of oxygen deprivation. Taken together, these apparent *in vitro/in vivo* discrepancies suggest that the intrinsic biochemical properties and susceptibility of different cell populations of the nephron (reflected *in vitro*) represent only one of many variables influencing site-selective nephrotoxic injury *in vivo*. Site-selective nephrotoxic injury, then, cannot be attributed to any one single factor, but rather must be viewed as the net balance of a variety of physiological, biochemical, and molecular determinants influencing cell survival/damage.

REFERENCES

1. Nakada J, Machida T, Endou H. Nephrotoxicity of cisplatin in rats. In: Tanabe T, Hook JB, Endou H, eds. *Nephrotoxicity of antibiotics and immunosuppressants*. New York: Elsevier, 1986; 179–182.
2. Jung KY, Endou H. Nephrotoxicity assessment by measuring cellular ATP content. II. Intranephron site of ochratoxin A nephrotoxicity. *Toxicol Appl Pharmacol* 1989;100:383–390.
3. Ruegg CE, Gandolfi AJ, Brendel K. Differential patterns of injury to the proximal tubule of renal cortical slices following in vitro exposure to mercuric chloride, potassium dichromate or hypoxic conditions. *Toxicol Appl Pharmacol* 1987;90:261–273.
4. Phelps JS, Gandolfi AJ, Brendel K, Dorr RT. Cisplatin nephrotoxicity: in vitro studies with precision-cut rabbit renal cortical slices. *Toxicol Appl Pharmacol* 1987;90:501–512.
5. Wolfgang GHI, Gandolfi AJ, Krumdieck CL, Brendel K. Evaluation of organic nephrotoxins in rabbit renal cortical slices. *Toxicol In Vitro* 1989;3:341–350.

6. Wolfgang GHI, Gandolfi AJ, Stevens JL, Brendel K. N-acetyl S-(1,2-dichlorovinyl)-L-cysteine produces a similar toxicity to S-(1,2-dichlorovinyl)-L-cysteine in rabbit renal slices: differential transport and metabolism. *Toxicol Appl Pharmacol* 1989;101:205–219.
7. Balaban RS, Silvia AL. Spectrophotometric monitoring of oxygen delivery to the exposed rat kidney. *Am J Physiol* 1981;241:F257–262.
8. Atkins JL, Lankford SP. Changes in cytochrome oxidation in outer and inner stripes of outer medulla. *Am J Physiol* 1991;261:F849–F857.
9. Brezis M, Rosen S, Silva P, Epstein FH. Transport activity modified thick ascending limb damage in the isolated perfused kidney. *Kidney Int* 1984;25:65–72.
10. Gullans SR, Hebert SC. Metabolic basis of ion transport. In: Brenner BM, Rector FC, eds. *The kidney*, 4th ed, vol 1. Philadelphia: WB Saunders, 1991;76–109.
11. Harris SI, Balaban RS, Barrett L, Mandel LJ. Mitochondrial respiratory capacity and Na^+ and K^+-dependent adenosine trisphosphatase-mediated ion transport in the intact renal cell. *J Biol Chem* 1981;256:10319–10328.
12. Chamberlain ME, Mandel LJ. Substrate support of medullary thick ascending limb oxygen consumption. *Am J Physiol* 1986;251:F758–763.
13. Soltoff SP. ATP and the regulation of renal cell function. *Annu Rev Physiol* 1986;48:9–31.
14. Jung KY, Uchida S, Endou H. Nephrotoxicity assessment by measuring cellular ATP content. I. Substrate specificities in the maintenance of ATP content in isolated rat nephron segments. *Toxicol Appl Pharmacol* 1989;100:369–382.
15. Vanderwalle A, Wirthensohn G, Heidrich HG, Guder WG. Distribution of hexokinase and phosphoenolcarboxykinase along the rabbit nephron. *Am J Physiol* 1981;240:F492–500.
16. Soltoff SP. Coupling renal metabolism to ion transport in renal epithelia. *Semin Nephrol* 1987; 7:20–28.
17. Katz AI. Distribution and function of classes of ATPases along the nephron. *Kidney Int* 1986; 29:21–31.
18. Jorgensen PL. Structure, function and regulation of Na,K-ATPase in the kidney. *Kidney Int* 1986;29:10–20.
19. Doucet A, Barlet C. Evidence for differences in the sensitivity to ouabain binding and turnover of Na-K-ATPase along the nephrons of rabbit kidney. *J Biol Chem* 1986;261:993–995.
20. Klahr S, Hammerman M. Renal metabolism. In: Seldin DW, Giebisch G, eds. *The Kidney: Physiology and Pathophysiology*, vol 1. New York: Raven Press, 1985;699–715.
21. Weidermann MJ, Krebs HA. The fuel of respiration of rat kidney cortex. *Biochem J* 1969; 112:149–166.
22. Klein KL, Wang MS, Torikai S, Davodson WD, Lirplawa L. Substrate oxidation by isolated single nephron segments of the rat. *Kidney Int* 1981;20:29–35.
23. Mandel LJ. Metabolic substrates, cellular energy production and the regulation of proximal tubular transport. *Annu Rev Physiol* 1985;47:85–101.
24. Schmidt U, Guder WG. Sites of enzyme activity along the nephron. *Kidney Int* 1976;9:233–242.
25. Guder WG, Ross BD. Enzyme distribution along the nephron. *Kidney Int* 1984;26:101–111.
26. Cojocel C, Maita K, Pasino DA, Kuo C-H, Hook JB. Metabolic heterogeneity of the proximal and distal kidney tubules. *Life Sci* 1983;33:855–861.
27. Bagnasco S, Good D, Balaban R, Burg M. Lactate production in isolated segments of the rat nephron. *Am J Physiol* 1985;248:F522–526.
28. Brand PH, Taylor BB. Lactate oxidation by three segments of the rabbit proximal tubule. *Proc Soc Exp Biol Med* 1986;182:454–460.
29. Dickman KG, Mandel LJ. Differential effects of respiratory inhibitors on glycolysis in proximal tubules. *Am J Physiol* 1990;258:F1608–1615.
30. Ruegg CE, Mandel LJ. Bulk isolation of renal PCT and PST I. Glucose-dependent metabolic differences. *Am J Physiol* 1990;259:F164–175.
31. Yamada H, Nakada J, Aizawa C, Endou H. Intra- and inter-nephron heterogeneity of gluconeogenesis in the rat: effects of chronic metabolic acidosis and potassium depletion. *Pflugers Arch* 1986;407:1–7.
32. Wang M-S, Kurokawa K. Renal gluconeogenesis: axial and internephron heterogeneity and the effect of parathyroid hormone. *Am J Physiol* 1984;246:F59–F66.
33. Ross BD, Espinal J, Silva P. Glucose metabolism in renal tubular function. *Kidney Int* 1986; 29:54–67.
34. Hohenegger M, Wittmann G, Dahlheim H. Oxidation of fatty acid by different zones of the rat kidney. *Pflugers Arch* 1973;341:105–112.

35. Balaban RS, Mandel LJ. Metabolic substrate utilization by rabbit proximal tubule. An NADH fluorescence study. *Am J Physiol* 1988;254:F407–F416.
36. Le Hir M, Dubach UC. Distribution of two enzymes of beta oxidation of fatty acid along the rat nephron. In: Morelm F, ed. *Biochemistry of Kidney Function*, INSERM Symposia No. 21. New York: Elsevier Biomedical, 1982;87–94.
37. Goldstein RS, Smith PF, Tarloff JB, Contardi L, Rush GF, Hook JB. Minireview: Biochemical mechanisms of cephalrodine nephrotoxicity. *Life Sci* 1988;42:1809–1816.
38. Sokol PP, Ripich G, Holohan PD, Ross CD. Mechanism of ochratoxin A transport in kidney. *J Pharmacol Exp Ther* 1988;246:460–465.
39. Monks TJ, Lau SS. Commentary: Renal transport processes and glutathione conjugate-mediated nephrotoxicity. *Drug Metab Dispos* 1987;15:437–441.
40. Burckhardt G, Ullrich KJ. Organic anion transport across the contraluminal membrane—dependence on sodium. *Kidney Int* 1989;36:370–377.
41. Ullrich KJ, Rumrich G. Contraluminal transport systems in the proximal renal tubule involved in secretion of organic anions. *Am J Physiol* 1988;254:F453–F462.
42. Moller JV, Sheikh MI. Renal organic anion transport system: pharmacological, physiological and biochemical aspects. *Pharmacol Rev* 1983;34:315–357.
43. Woodhall PB, Tisher CC, Simonton CA, Robinson RR. Relationship between para-aminohippurate secretion and cellular morphology in rabbit proximal tubules. *J Clin Invest* 1978;61: 1320–1329.
44. Shimomura A, Chonko AM, Grantham JJ. Basis for heterogeneity of para-aminohippurate secretion in rabbit proximal tubules. *Am J Physiol* 1981;240:F430–436.
45. Shimomura A, Chonko A, Tanner R, Edwards R, Grantham J. Nature of urate transport in isolated rabbit proximal tubules. *Am J Physiol* 1981;241:F565–F578.
46. Holohan PD, Ross CR. Mechanisms of organic cation transport in kidney plasma membrane vesicles: 1. Countertransport studies. *J Pharmacol Exp Ther* 1980;215:191–197.
47. Schali C, Schild L, Overney J, Roch-Ramel F. Secretion of tetraethylammonium by proximal tubules of rabbit kidneys. *Am J Physiol* 1983;245:F238–246.
48. Tarloff JB, Brand PH. Active tetraethylammonium uptake across the basolateral membrane of rabbit proximal tubule. *Am J Physiol* 1986;251:F141–149.
49. McKinney TD. Procainamide uptake by rabbit proximal tubules. *J Pharmacol Exp Ther* 1983; 224:302–306.
50. McKinney TD, Speeg KV Jr. Cimetidine and procainamide secretion by proximal tubules in vitro. *Am J Physiol* 1982;242:F672–680.
51. Holohan PD, Ross CR. Mechanisms of organic cation transport in kidney plasma membrane vesicles. 2. Delta-pH studies. *J Pharmacol Exp Ther* 1981;216:294–298.
52. McKinney TD. Heterogeneity of organic base secretion by proximal tubules. *Am J Physiol* 1982; 243:F404–407.
53. Cojocel C, Smith JH, Maita K, Sleight SD, Hook JB. Renal protein degradation: a biochemical target of specific nephrotoxicants. *Fundam Appl Toxicol* 1983;3:278–284.
54. Maack T, Johnson V, Kau ST, Figueiredo J, Sigulem D. Renal filtration, transport, and metabolism of low-molecular-weight proteins: a review. *Kidney Int* 1979;16:251–270.
55. Christensen EI, Nielsen S. Structural and functional features of protein handling in the kidney proximal tubule. *Semin Nephrol* 1991;11:414– 439.
56. Maack T, Park CH, Camargo MJF. Renal filtration, transport and metabolism of proteins. In: Seldin DW, Geibisch G, eds. *The Kidney: Physiology and Pathophysiology*. New York: Raven Press, 1985;1773–1803.
57. Sumpio BE, Maack T. Kinetics, competition, and selectivity of tubular absorption of proteins. *Am J Physiol* 1982;243:F379–392.
58. Christensen EI. Rapid protein uptake and digestion in proximal tubule lysosomes. *Kidney Int* 1976;10:301–310.
59. Christensen EI, Maunsbach AB. Intralysosomal digestion of lysozyme in renal proximal tubule cells. *Kidney Int* 1974;6:396–407.
60. Camargo MJF, Sumpio BE, Maack T. Renal hydrolysis of absorbed protein: influence of load and lysosomal pH. *Am J Physiol* 1984;247:F656–F664.
61. Park CH, Maack T. Albumin absorption and catabolism by isolated perfused proximal convoluted tubules of the rabbit. *J Clin Invest* 1984;73:767–777.
62. Ryan GB, Karnovsky MJ. An ultrastructural study of the mechanisms of proteinuria in aminonuceloside nephrosis. *Kidney Int* 1975;8:219–232.

63. Olbricht CJ, Cannon JK, Garg LC, Tisher CC. Activities of cathepsins B and L in isolated nephron segments from proteinuric and nonproteinuric rats. *Am J Physiol* 1986;250:F1055–F1062.
64. Olbricht CJ, Cannon JK, Tisher CC. Cathepsin B and L in nephron segments of rats with puromycin aminonucleoside nephrosis. *Kidney Int* 1987;32:354–361.
65. Sievers L, Kugler P. Reabsorption of fluorescein-isothiocyanate-labelled-ovalbumin in the kidney of normal and castrated male and female rats. *Histochemistry* 1986;86:215–220.
66. Kiesewetter F, Kugler P. Sex different cytochrome-c uptake in the proximal tubule of the rat kidney. *Histochemistry* 1985;82:557–564.
67. Bordeau JE, Carone FA, Ganote CE. Serum albumin uptake in isolated perfused renal tubules. *J Cell Biol* 1972;54:382–398.
68. Cortney MA, Sawin LL, Weiss DD. Renal tubular protein absorption in the rat. *J Clin Invest* 1970;49:1–4.
69. Madsen KM, Park CH. Lysosome distribution and cathepsin B and L activity along the rabbit proximal tubule. *Am J Physiol* 1987;253:F1290–1301.
70. Yokota S, Tsuji H, Kato K. Immunocytochemical localization of cathepsin B in rat kidney. I. Light microscopic study using the indirect immunoenzyme technique. *J Histochem Cytochem* 1986; 34:891–897.
71. Yokota S, Tsuji H, Kato K. Immunocytochemical localization of cathepsin B in rat kidney. II. Electron microscopic study using the protein A-gold technique. *J Histochem Cytochem* 1986; 34:899–907.
72. Olbricht CJ, Garg LC, Cannon JK, Tisher CC. Acid phosphatase activity in the mammalian nephron. *Am J Physiol* 1984;247:F252–259.
73. Carone FA, Peterson DR, Flouret G. Renal tubular processing of small peptide hormones. *J Lab Clin Med* 1982;100:1–14.
74. Emmanouel DS, Jaspan JB, Kuku SF, Rubinstein AH, Katz AI. Pathogenesis and characterization of hyperglucagonemia in the uremic rat. *J Clin Invest* 1976;58:1266–1272.
75. Haberle D, Wahllander A, Sies H. Assessment of kidney function in maintenance of plasma glutathione concentration and redox state in anesthetized rats. *FEBS Lett* 1979;108:335–340.
76. Rankin BB, Curthoys NP. Evidence for the renal paratubular transport of glutathione. *FEBS Lett* 1982;147:193–196.
77. Scott RD, Curthoys NP. Renal clearance of glutathione measured in rats pretreated with inhibitors of glutathione metabolism. *Am J Physiol* 1987;252:F877–F882.
78. Ormstad K. Metabolism of glutathione in the kidney. In: Bach PH, Lock EA, eds. *Nephrotoxicity in the Experimental and Clinical Situation*. Boston: Martinus Nijhoff, 1987;405–428.
79. Lash LH, Jones DP. Renal glutathione transport. Characteristics of the sodium-dependent system in the basal-lateral membrane. *J Biol Chem* 1984;259:14508–14514.
80. Lash LH, Jones DP. Transport of glutathione by renal basal-lateral membrane vesicles. *Biochem Biophys Res Commun* 1983;112:55–60.
81. Inoue M, Morino Y. Direct evidence for the role of membrane potential in glutathione transport by renal brush-border membranes. *J Biol Chem* 1985;260:326–331.
82. Spater HW, Poruchynsky MS, Quintana N, Inoue M, Novikoff AB. Immunocytochemical localization of γ-glutamyltransferase in rat kidney with protein A-horseradish peroxidase. *Proc Natl Acad Sci USA* 1982;79:3547–3550.
83. Inoue M, Okajima K, Morino Y. Hepato-renal cooperation in biotransformation, membrane transport and elimination of cysteine S-conjugates of xenobiotics. *J Biochem (Tokyo)* 1984;95:247–254.
84. Schrenk P, Dekant W, Henschler D. Metabolism and excretion of S-conjugates derived from hexachlorobutadiene in the isolated perfused rat kidney. *Mol Pharmacol* 1988;34:407–412.
85. Zhang G, Stevens JL. Transport and activation of S-(1,2-dichlorovinyl)-L-cysteine and N-acetyl-S-(1,2-dichlorovinyl)-L-cysteine in rat kidney proximal tubules. *Toxicol Appl Pharmacol* 1989; 100:51–61.
86. Schaeffer VH, Stevens JL. The transport of S-cysteine conjugates in LLC-PK1 cells and its role in toxicity. *Mol Pharmacol* 1987;31:506–512.
87. Schaeffer VH, Stevens JL. Mechanism of transport for toxic cysteine conjugates in rat kidney cortex membrane vesicles. *Mol Pharmacol* 1987;32:293–298.
88. Lock EA, Odum J, Ormond P. Transport of N-acetyl-S-pentachloro-1,3-butadienylcysteine by rat renal cortex. *Arch Toxicol* 1986;59:12–15.
89. Lock EA, Ishmael J. Effect of the organic acid transport inhibitor probenecid on renal cortical uptake and proximal tubular toxicity of hexachloro-1,3-butadiene and its conjugates. *Toxicol Appl Pharmacol* 1985;81:32–42.

90. Zenser TV, Mattammal MB, Davis BB. Differential distribution of the mixed function oxidase in rabbit kidney. *J Pharmacol Exp Ther* 1978;207:719–725.
91. Endou H. Cytochrome P450 monooxygenase system in the kidney: its intranephron localization and its induction. *Jpn J Pharmacol* 1983;33:423–433.
92. Smith J, Hook JB. Mechanism of chloroform nephrotoxicity. II. Renal and hepatic microsomal metabolism of chloroform in mice. *Toxicol Appl Pharmacol* 1984;73:511–524.
93. Fowler BA, Hook GER, Lucier GW. 2,3,7,8-Tetrachlorodibenzo-p-dioxin induction of renal microsomal enzyme systems: ultrastructural effects on pars recta (S3) proximal tubule cells of rat kidney. *J Pharmacol Exp Ther* 1977;203:712–721.
94. Tarloff JB, Goldstein RS, Hook JB. Xenobiotic biotransformation by the kidney: pharmacological and toxicological aspects. In: Gibson GG, ed. *Progress in Drug Metabolism*, vol 12. London: Taylor & Francis, 1990;1–40.
95. Henderson CJ, Scott AR, Yang CS, Wolf CR. Testosterone-mediated regulation of mouse renal cytochrome P-450 isoenzymes. *Biochem J* 1990;266:675–681.
96. Smith JH, Maita K, Sleight SD, Hook JB. Effect of sex hormone status on chloroform nephrotoxicity and renal mixed function oxidases in mice. *Toxicology* 1984;30:305–316.
97. Oliw EH, Lawson JA, Brash AR, Oates JA. Arachidonic acid metabolism in rabbit renal cortex. *J Biol Chem* 1981;256:9924–9931.
98. Schwartzman M, Abraham N, Carroll M, et al. Regulation of arachidonic acid metabolism by cytochrome P450 in rabbit kidney. *Biochem J* 1986;238:283–290.
99. Tot R, Siddhanta A, Mann S, et al. Arachidonic acid epoxygenase: detection of epoxyeicosatrienoic acids (EETs) in human urine. *Biochim Biophys Acta* 1987;919:132–139.
100. Carroll MA, Schwartzman M, Abraham NG, Pinto A, McGiff JC. Cytochrome P450-dependent arachidonate metabolism in renomedullary cells: formation of Na-K-ATPase inhibitor. *J Hypertension* 1986;4(Suppl):S33–42.
101. Carroll MA, Schwartzman M, Baba M, Abraham NG, McGiff JC. Formation of biologically active cytochrome P450-arachidonate metabolites in renomedullary cells. *Adv Prostaglandin Thromboxane Leukotriene Res* 1987;17:714–718.
102. McGiff JC, Carroll MA. Cytochrome P450-dependent arachidonate metabolites, renal function and blood pressure regulation. *Adv Prostaglandin Thromboxane Leukotriene Res* 1990;21:675–682.
103. Jones DP, Sundby GB, Ormstad K, Orrenius S. Use of isolated kidney cells for study of drug metabolism. *Biochem Pharmacol* 1979;28:929–935.
104. Fry JR, Perry NK. The effect of Aroclor 1254 pretreatment on the phase I and phase II metabolism of 7-ethoxycoumarin in isolated viable rat kidney cells. *Biochem Pharmacol* 1981;30:1197–1201.
105. Aitio A, Vainio H, Hanninen O. Enhancement of drug oxidation and conjugation by carcinogens in different rat tissues. *FEBS Lett* 1972;24:237.
106. Hjelle JT, Hazelton GA, Klaassen CD, Hjelle JJ. Glucuronidation and sulphation in rabbit kidney. *J Pharmacol Exp Ther* 1986;236:150–156.
107. Fleischner G, Mishkin D, Reyes H, Robbins J, Levy AJ, Gatmaitan A, Arias IM. *J Clin Invest* 1971;50:31a (abstract).
108. Lash LH, Tokarz JJ. Isolation of two distinct populations of cells from rat kidney cortex and their use in the study of chemical-induced cytotoxicity. *Anal Biochem* 1989;182:271–279.
109. Fine LG, Goldstein EJ, Trizna W, Rozmaryn L, Arias IM. Glutathione-S-transferase activity in the rabbit nephron: segmental localization in isolated tubules and formation of thiol adducts of ethacrynic acid (40018). *Proc Soc Exp Biol Med* 1978;157:189–193.
110. Hughey R, Rankin B, Elce J, Curthoys N. Specificity of a particulate rat renal peptidase and its localization along with other enzymes of mercapturic acid synthesis. *Arch Biochem Biophys* 1978;186:211–217.
111. Endou HH, Shimada H, Koseki C, Yokokura Y, Sakai Y. Distribution and possible functions of γ-glutamytranspeptidase in the kidney. *Jpn J Nephrol* 1981;23:981–988.
112. Heinle H, Wendel A, Schmidt U. The activities of the key enzymes of the γ-glutamyl cycle in microdissected segments of the rat nephron. *FEBS Lett* 1977;73:220–224.
113. Duffel MW, Jakoby WB. Cysteine S-conjugate N-acetyltransferase from rat kidney microsomes. *Mol Pharmacol* 1982;21:444–448.
114. Lash LH, Elfarra AA, Anders MW. Renal cysteine conjugate β-lyase. Bioactivation of nephrotoxic cysteine S-conjugates in mitochondrial outer membrane. *J Biol Chem* 1986;261:5930–5935.
115. Stevens JL. Cysteine conjugate β-lyase activity in rat kidney cortex: subcellular localization and relationship to the hepatic enzyme. *Biochem Biophys Res Commun* 1985;261:15529–15537.

116. Stevens J, Jakoby WB. Cysteine conjugate β-lyase. *Mol Pharmacol* 1983;23:761–765.
117. Stevens JL, Robbins JD, Byrd RA. A purified cysteine conjugate β-lyase from rat kidney cytosol. Requirement for an α-keto acid or an amino acid oxidase for activity and identity with soluble glutamine transaminase K. *J Biol Chem* 1986;261:15529–15537.
118. MacFarlane M, Foster JR, Gibson GG, Kind LJ, Lock EA. Cysteine conjugate β-lyase of rat kidney cytosol: characterization, immunocytochemical localization and correlation with hexachlorobutadiene nephrotoxicity. *Toxicol Appl Pharmacol* 1989;98:185–197.
119. Jones TW, Qin C, Schaeffer VH, Stevens JL. Immunohistochemical localization of glutamine transaminase K, a rat kidney cysteine conjugate β-lyase, and the relationship to the segment specificity of cysteine conjugate nephrotoxicity. *Mol Pharmacol* 1988;34:621–627.
120. Zenser TV, Davis BB. Oxidation of xenobiotics by prostaglandin H synthase. In: Goldstein RS, Hewitt WH, Hook JB, eds. *Toxic Interactions*. San Diego: Academic Press, 1990;62–86.
121. Silverblatt F, Turck M, Bulger R. Nephrotoxicity due to cephaloridine: a light and electron microscopic study in rabbits. *J Infect Dis* 1970;122:33–44.
122. Tune B. Relationship between the transport and toxicity of cephalosporins in the kidney. *J Infect Dis* 1975;132:189–194.
123. Pasino DA, Miura K, Goldstein RS, Hook JB. Cephaloridine nephrotoxicity: strain and sex differences in mice. *Fundam Appl Toxicol* 1985;5:1153–1160.
124. Wold JS, Joost RR, Owen NV. Nephrotoxicity of cephaloridine in newborn rabbits: role of the renal anionic transport system. *J Pharmacol Exp Ther* 1977;201:778–785.
125. Goldstein RS, Pasino DA, Hook JB. Cephaloridine nephrotoxicity in aging male Fischer-344 rats. *Toxicology* 1986;38:43–53.
126. Tune BM. Effect of organic acid transport inhibitors on renal cortical uptake and proximal tubular toxicity of cephaloridine. *J Pharmacol Exp Ther* 1972;181:250–256.
127. Wold JS, Turnipseed SA. The effect of renal cation transport inhibitors on the in vivo and in vitro accumulation and efflux of cephaloridine. *Life Sci* 1980;27:2559–2564.
128. Wold JS, Turnipseed SA, Miller BL. The effect of renal cation transport on cephaloridine nephrotoxicity. *Toxicol Appl Pharmacol* 1979;45:115–122.
129. Tune BM, Wu KY, Kempson RL. Inhibition of transport and prevention of toxicity of cephaloridine in the kidney. Dose-responsiveness of the rabbit and the guinea pig to probenecid. *J Pharmacol Exp Ther* 1977;202:466–471.
130. Ullrich KJ, Rumrich G, Kloss S. Contraluminal organic anion and cation transport in the proximal renal tubule: V. Interaction with sulfamoy- and phenoxy diuretics, and with β-lactam antibiotics. *Kidney Int* 1989;36:78–88.
131. Williams PD, Hitchcock MJM, Hottendorf GH. Effect of cephalosporins on organic ion transport in renal membrane vesicles from rat and rabbit kidney cortex. *Res Commun Chem Pathol Pharmacol* 1985;47:357–371.
132. Hori R, Ishikawa Y, Takano M, Okano T, Shikifumi K, Inui K-I. The interaction of cephalosporin antibiotics with renal cortex of rats: accumulation to cortical slices and binding to purified plasma membranes. *Biochem Pharmacol* 1982;31:2267–2272.
133. Cojocel C, Laeschke KH, Inselmann G, Baumann K. Inhibition of cephaloridine-induced lipid peroxidation. *Toxicology* 1985;35:295–305.
134. Tune BM, Fravert D. Cephalosporin nephrotoxicity. Transport, cytotoxicity and mitochondrial toxicity of cephaloglycin. *J Pharmacol Exp Ther* 1980;215:186–190.
135. Tune BM. The nephrotoxicity of cephalosporin antibiotics—structure activity relationships. *Comments Toxicol* 1986;1:145–170.
136. Lash LH. Personal communication.
137. Goldstein RS, Smith PF, Tarloff JB, Rush GF, Hook JB. Comparative susceptibility of kidney and liver cells to cephaloridine toxicity in vitro. *Toxicologist* 1987;7:28.
138. Leitman PS, Smith CR. Aminoglycoside nephrotoxicity in humans. *J Infect Dis* 1983;5(Suppl 2):S284–S293.
139. Humes HD, O'Connor RP. Aminoglycoside nephrotoxicity. In: Schrier RW, Gottschalk CW, eds. *Diseases of the Kidney*, vol 2, 4th ed. Boston: Little, Brown, 1988;1229–1273.
140. Kosek JC, Mazze RI, Cousins MJ. Nephrotoxicity of gentamicin. *Lab Invest* 1974;30:48–57.
141. Wellwood JM, Lovell D, Thompson AE, Tighe JR. Renal damage caused by gentamicin: a study of the effects on renal morphology and urinary enzyme excretion. *J Pathol* 1976;118:171–182.
142. Maita K, Cojocel C, Dociu N, Sleight SD, Hook JB. Effects of aminoglycosides on glomerular ultrastructure. *Pharmacology* 1984;29:292–300.

143. Houghton DC, Hartnett M, Campbell-Biswell M, Portrer G, Bennett W. A light and electron microscopic analysis of gentamicin nephrotoxicity in rat. *Am J Pathol* 1976;82:589–612.
144. Humes HD. Aminoglycoside nephrotoxicity. *Kidney Int* 1988;33:900–911.
145. Tulkens PM. Nephrotoxicity of aminoglycoside antibiotics. *Toxicol Lett* 1989;46:107–123.
146. Pastoriza-Munoz E, Bowman RL, Kaloyanides GL. Renal tubular transport of gentamicin in the rat. *Kidney Int* 1979;16:440–450.
147. Pastoriza-Munoz E, Timmerman D, Kaloyanides GJ. Renal transport of netilmicin in the rat. *J Pharmacol Exp Ther* 1984;228:65–72.
148. Sheth AU, Senekjian HO, Babino H, Knight TF, Weinman EJ. Renal handling of gentamicin by the Munich-Wistar rat. *Am J Physiol* 1981;241:F645–F648.
149. Senekjian HO, Knight TF, Weinman EJ. Micropuncture study of the handling of gentamicin by the rat kidney. *Kidney Int* 1981;19:416–423.
150. Sastrasinh M, Knauss TC, Weinberg JM, Humes HD. Identification of the aminoglycoside binding site in rat renal brush border membranes. *J Pharmacol Exp Ther* 1982;222:350–358.
151. Williams PD, Hottendorf GH, Bennett DB. Inhibition of renal membrane binding and nephrotoxicity of aminoglycosides. *J Pharmacol Exp Ther* 1986;237:919–925.
152. Cojocel CC, Docius N, Maita K, Smith JH, Hook JB. Renal ultrastructural and biochemical injuries induced by aminoglycosides. *Environ Health Perspect* 1984;57:293–299.
153. Williams PD, Trimble ME, Crespo L, Holohan PD, Freedman JC, Ross CR. Inhibition of renal Na+, K+-adenosine triphosphatase by gentamicin. *J Pharmacol Exp Ther* 1984;231:248–253.
154. Collier V, Lietman P, Mitch W. Evidence for luminal uptake of gentamicin in the perfused rat kidney. *J Pharmacol Exp Ther* 1979;210:247–251.
155. Marre R, Tarara N, Louton, Sack K. Age-dependent nephrotoxicity and the pharmacokinetics of gentamicin in rats. *Eur J Pediatr* 1980;133:25.
156. Cowan RH, Jukkola AF, Arant BS, Jr. Pathophysiologic evidence of gentomicin nephrotoxicity in neonatal puppies. *Ped Res* 1980;14:1204–1211.
157. Bennett WM, Parker RA, Elliot WC, Gilbert DN, Houghton DC. Sex-related differences in the susceptibility of rats to gentamicin nephrotoxicity. *J Infect Dis* 1982;145:370–373.
158. Ramsammy LS, Josepovitz C, Jones D, Ling K-Y, Lane BP, Kaloyanides GJ. Induction of nephrotoxicity by high doses of gentamicin in diabetic rats. *Proc Soc Exp Biol Med* 1987;186:306–312.
159. Kalyonadies GJ, Pastoriza-Munoz E. Aminoglycoside nephrotoxicity. *Kidney Int* 1980;18:571–582.
160. Soberon L, Bowman RL, Pastoriza-Munoz E, Kaloyanides GJ. Comparative nephrotoxicities of gentamicin, netilmicin and tobramycin in the rat. *J Pharmacol Exp Ther* 1979;210:334–343.
161. Williams PD, Hottendorf GH, Bennett DB. Inhibition of renal membrane binding and nephrotoxicity of aminoglycosides. *J Pharmacol Exp Ther* 1986;237:919–925.
162. Williams PD, Bennett DB, Gleason CR, Hottendorf GH. Correlation between renal membrane binding and nephrotoxicity of aminoglycosides. *Antimicrob Agents Chemother* 1987;31:570–574.
163. Gilbert DN, Wood CA, Kohlepp SJ, Kohnen PW, Houghton DC, Finkbeiner HC, Lindsley J, Bennett WM. Polyaspartic acid prevents experimental aminoglycoside nephrotoxicity. *J Infect Dis* 1989;159:945–953.
164. Ramsammy LS, Josepovitz C, Lane BP, Kaloyanides GJ. Polyaspartic acid protects against gentamicin nephrotoxicity in the rat. *J Pharmacol Exp Ther* 1989;250:149–153.
165. Wedeen RP, Batuman V, Cheeks C, Marquet E, Sobel H. Transport of gentamicin in rat proximal tubule. *Lab Invest* 1983;48:212–223.
166. Lock EA, Ishmael J. The acute toxic effects of hexachloro-1,3-butadiene in the rat kidney. *Arch Toxicol* 1979;43:47–57.
167. Ishamael J, Pratt IS, Lock EA. Necrosis of the pars recta (S3 segment) of the rat kidney produced by hexachloro-1,3-butadiene. *J Pathol* 1982;138:99–113.
168. Nash JA, King LJ, Lock EA, Green T. The metabolism and disposition of hexachloro-1:3-butadiene in the rat and its relevance to nephrotoxicity. *Toxicol Appl Pharmacol* 1984;73:124–137.
169. Wolf CR, Berry PN, Nash JA, Green T, Lock EA. Role of microsomal and cytosolic glutathione S-transferases in the conjugation of hexachloro-1:3-butadiene and its possible relevance to toxicity. *J Pharmacol Exp Ther* 1984;228:202–208.
170. Ishmael J, Lock EA. Nephrotoxicity of hexachlorobutadiene and its glutathione-derived conjugates. *Toxicol Pathol* 1986;14:258–262.
171. Lock EA. Studies on the mechanisms of nephrotoxicity and nephrocarcinogenicity of halogenated alkenes. *CRC Crit Rev Toxicol* 1988;19:23–42.

172. Lock EA, Odum J, Ormond P. Transport of N-acetyl-S-pentachloro-1,3-butadienylcysteine by rat renal cortex. *Arch Toxicol* 1986;59:12.
173. Koob M, Dekant W. Bioactivation of xenobiotics by formation of toxic glutathione conjugates. *Chem Biol Interact* 1991;77:107–136.
174. Anders MW, Banki K, Dohn DR, Lash LH. Biosynthesis and bioactivation of toxic glutathione S-conjugates. *Fed Proc* 1987;46:2434–2436.
175. Anders MW, Lash LH, Dekant W, Elfarra AA, Dohn DR. Biosynthesis and biotransformation of glutathione S-conjugates to toxic metabolites. *CRC Crit Rev Toxicol* 1988;18:311–342.
176. Ruegg CE, Mandel LJ. Bulk isolation of renal PCT and PST II. Differential responses to anoxia and hypoxia. *Am J Physiol* 1990;259:F176–F185.
177. Mazze RI, Shue GL, Jackson SH. Renal dysfunction associated with methoxyflurane anesthesia. A randomized prospective clinical evaluation. *JAMA* 1971;216:278–288.
178. Cousins MJ, Mazze RI, Kosek JC, Hitt BA, Love FV. The etiology of methoxyflurane nephrotoxicity. *J Pharmacol Exp Ther* 1974;190:530–541.
179. Mazze RI, Cousins MJ, Kosek JC. Strain differences in metabolism and susceptibility to the nephrotoxic effects of methoxyflurane in rats. *J Pharmacol Exp Ther* 1973;184:481–488.
180. Mazze RI, Cousins MJ, Kosek JC. Dose-related methoxyflurane nephrotoxicity in rats: a biochemical and pathologic correlation. *Anesthesiology* 1972;36:571–587.
181. Rush GF, Willis LR. Renal tubular effects of sodium fluoride. *J Pharmacol Exp Ther* 1982; 223:275–279.
182. Sabra R, Branch RA. Amphotericin B nephrotoxicity. *Drug Safety* 1990;5:94–108.
183. Gouge TH, Andriole VT. An experimental model of amphotericin B nephrotoxicity with renal tubular acidosis. *J Lab Clin Med* 1971;78:713–724.
184. Julka NK, Arruda JAL, Kurtzman NA. The mechanism of amphotericin-induced distal acidification defect in rats. *Clin Sci* 1979;56:555–562.
185. Kavlock RJ, Rehnberg BF, Rogers EH. Amphotericin B- and folic acid-induced nephropathies in developing rats. *Toxciol Appl Pharmacol* 1985;81:407–415.
186. Hoeprich PD. Chemotherapy of systemic fungal diseases. *Annu Rev Pharmacol Toxicol* 1978; 18:205–231.
187. Andriole VT. On the anatomy of amphotericin-B cholesterol pores in lipid bilayer membranes. *Kidney Int* 1973;4:337–345.
188. Kinsky SC. Polyene antibiotics. In: Gottlieb D, Shaw PD, eds. *Antibiotics I*. New York: Springer-Verlag, 1967;123–141.
189. Gatzy JT, Reuss L, Finn A. Amphotericin B and K^+ transport across excised toad urinary bladder. *Am J Physiol* 1979;237:F145–F156.
190. Lichtenstein NS, Leaf A. Effect of amphotericin B on the permeability of the toad bladder. *J Clin Invest* 1965;44:1328–1342.
191. Humes HD, Weinberg JM. Toxic nephropathies. In: Brenner BM, Rector FC, eds. *The Kidney*, vol 3. Philadelphia: WB Saunders, 1986;1491–1532.
192. Lash LH, Tokarz JJ. Oxidative stress in isolated rat renal proximal and distal tubular cells. *Am J Physiol* 1990;259:F338–F347.
193. Katz AI, Doucet A, Morel F. Na-K-ATPase activity along the rabbit, rat, and mouse nephron. *Am J Physiol* 1979;237:F114–F120.
194. Tarloff JB, Goldstein RS, Hook JB. In: Boch PH, Lock EA, eds. *Nephrotoxicity in the experimental and clinical situation*. Lancaster: Martinus Nijhoff, 1987;371–405.

Toxicology of the Kidney, Second Edition,
edited by Jerry B. Hook and Robin S. Goldstein.
Raven Press, Ltd., New York © 1993.

8

Nephrotoxicity of Protein Overloading

Jan J. Weening

Department of Pathology, University of Amsterdam, Academic Medical Center, 1105 AZ Amsterdam, The Netherlands

Under normal conditions only very small amounts of proteins can pass the glomerular capillary wall (GCW) and reach the urinary space. Its physicochemical properties based on the fenestrated endothelium, the tight epithelium, the basement membrane, and the highly negative charge of cell-associated mucopolysaccharides and extracellular heparan sulfate moieties, render the GCW into an efficient size- and charge-selective filter to circulating macromolecules (1,2). Glomerular filtration is more restricted for molecules with a relatively high molecular radius and negative isoelectric point (3–5). Molecular configuration also contributes to the filtration characteristics of a given substance. Globular proteins are less easily filtered than dextrans of the same molecular radius (6). Low molecular weight proteins that reach the outer side of the GCW are either endocytosed by the glomerular epithelial cells or enter the urinary space. Most of the filtered proteins are then taken up by the tubular epithelial cells in the normal process of reabsorption and are subsequently catabolized by intracellular lysosomal enzymes.

Under pathological conditions, such as an excessive increase in the concentration of circulating proteins in dysproteinemias or a leaky glomerular filter in certain forms of glomerulonephritis, the load of filtered proteins may increase and may lead to functional and structural alterations of the glomerulus and tubules (7–9).

In this chapter, I shall review some of these conditions of proteinuria-related nephrotoxicity in man and in experimental models and discuss the pathogenetic mechanisms that lead to renal cell damage.

PROTEIN-OVERLOAD PROTEINURIA

In man, the most frequent cause of protein-overload proteinuria is a group of hematologic disorders referred to as plasma-cell dyscrasias or dysproteinemias. These diseases are characterized by a monoclonal proliferation of plasma cells, producing large amounts of one type of immunoglobulin or its subunits. These plasma-cell dyscrasias include as the most frequent form multiple myeloma, and, in addition, Waldenström's macroglobulinemia and the cryoglobulinemias. Renal involvement is frequent in patients with multiple myeloma, often presenting with proteinuria with or without renal insufficiency. Renal involvement is less frequent in the other forms of dysproteinemias in which alterations are usually confined to the glomerulus (10).

Glomerular pathology in dysproteinemias includes mesangial accumulation of proteins associated with hypercellularity and increased matrix production. Deposition of immunoglobulins along the GCW may lead to light-chain nephropathy, membranous glomerulopathy, or membranoproliferative glomerulonephritis. A well-known complication of plasma cell dyscrasias is amyloidosis, which often involves the glomerulus and leads to massive proteinuria.

More frequent in multiple myeloma is tubulointerstitial involvement based on light-chain proteinuria and associated with varying degrees of renal insufficiency. Several factors such as dehydration, hypercalcemia, and tubular cell injury due to contrast media, antibiotics, or infection may lead to acute renal insufficiency in these patients through precipitation of light chains in the tubular lumina.

Pathology

At light microscopy, the usually enlarged kidneys of patients with multiple myeloma and massive light-chain proteinuria show extensive tubular cast formation, most commonly in the distal tubules, associated with chronic inflammation and interstitial fibrosis (Fig. 1). The casts usually contain, in addition to the light chains, other serum proteins such as albumin, immunoglobulins, complement components, and large amounts of Tamm-Horsfall protein that coprecipitates with the serum proteins. The inflammatory changes in the interstitium include accumulation of polymorphonuclear leukocytes and mononuclear cells. Frequently multinucleated giant cells derived from the tubular epithelium surround the casts. In the relatively recently recognized entity "light-chain disease," deposits of light chains are found in the outer part of the tubular basement membrane.

Pathophysiology

Protein-overload nephrotoxicity in multiple myeloma is related to the filtration and tubular accumulation of light-chain proteins (LCPs). Under normal conditions, LCPs can be detected in minute amounts in the circulation. LCPs are filtered freely in the glomerulus and reabsorbed in cells of the proximal convoluted tubule, similarly to other low molecular weight proteins (9,11,12). The LCPs are then catabolized by lysosomal enzymes. Since the kidney is the principal site of catabolism of LCPs, glomerular filtration and tubular cell function determine the clearance rate of LCPs.

Renal insufficiency in patients with multiple myeloma and light-chain proteinuria

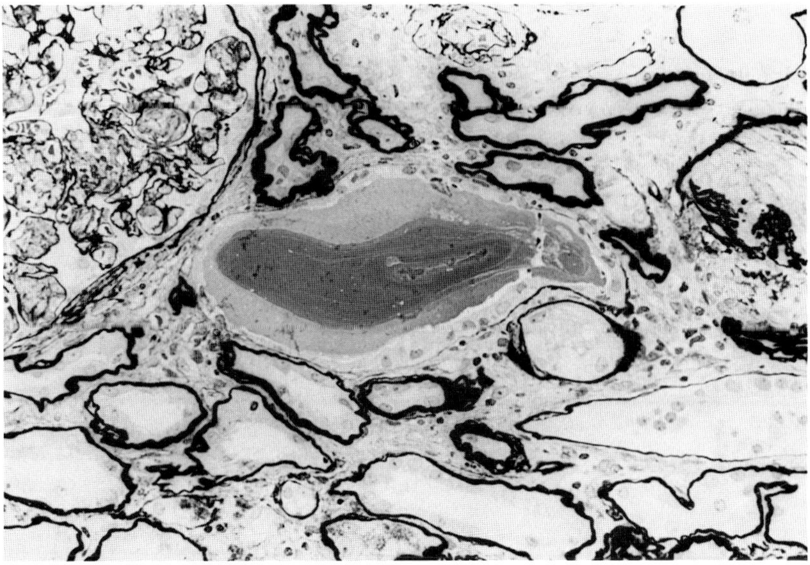

FIG. 1. Light micrograph showing a tubular cast surrounded by interstitial mononuclear infiltrate in the renal cortex of a patient with multiple myeloma, amyloidosis, and heavy proteinuria due to the loss of light-chain proteins and high molecular weight serum proteins (H&E, ×202.)

("myeloma kidney") is based upon tubular cell damage either due to overloading the catabolic capacity of tubular epithelial cells or to cellular toxicity of specific LCPs. Both hypotheses have been tested and proven to be true. The degree of tubulointerstitial lesions is dependent upon the serum concentration of LCPs and is increased under conditions of hydropenia (13,14). Experimental studies have revealed that some LCPs are more nephrotoxic than others, based upon their physicochemical properties (13). The isoelectric point (14), molecular size, polymerization (15), and degree of glycosylation (16) all influence the degree of filtration, reabsorption (17), and catabolization. A high isoelectric point facilitates the filtration and reabsorption, whereas LCPs with a low isoelectric tend to precipitate more easily (14,18).

LCPs were found to inhibit Na-K–ATPase activity in plasma membranes isolated from rat renal cortex (10). Functional studies have shown that LCPs have a toxic effect on proximal and distal tubular cells leading to symptoms of Fanconi's syndrome, polyuria, and concentration defects (19).

In summary, increased concentration of circulating intact and fragmented immunoglobulins in plasma cell dyscrasias may lead to glomerular and tubular abnormalities due to overloading, hyperfiltration, saturation of catabolic capacity, precipitation, and obstruction, as well as to epithelial cell toxicity. Some of these phenomena can also be seen in conditions of proteinuria due to a leaky glomerular filter in conditions of glomerulonephritis, discussed in the next paragraph.

GLOMERULAR PROTEINURIA

Hemodynamic, metabolic, toxic, immunologic, and inflammatory factors (4) may all damage the glomerular filter and cause an increased flux of serum proteins across the GCW. Urinary protein loss, usually less than 80 mg/24 hr, may exceed 10 g per day. As a result, the glomerular epithelial cells lose their highly differentiated foot processes, and show condensation of microtubules along the basal membrane, increased pinocytotic vesicles, and intracellular reabsorption droplets containing serum proteins. Large amounts of serum proteins are present extracellularly in Bowman's space and in tubular lumina. Proximal tubular epithelial cells are loaded with protein reabsorption droplets in the lysosomal compartment. Condensation in the tubular lumina leads to cast formation. When excreted, these casts are seen as waxy cylinders.

Laboratory animal models have been developed to study the pathogenetic mechanisms underlying the glomerular alterations in these diseases (9,20). Long-standing glomerular injury in many of the glomerulopathies in man and in these experimental models eventually leads to progressive glomerulosclerosis and renal insufficiency. Pathogenetic factors involved in this progression are intraglomerular hypertension and coagulation, hyperlipidemia, mesangial cell proliferation and mesangial influx of macrophages, and proteinuria per se (reviewed in 21–23).

Dietary protein and lipid and pharmacological intervention aimed at reducing glomerular and systemic blood pressure have been shown to modulate progression of renal insufficiency (21–23). The contribution of glomerular proteinuria in progressive glomerulosclerosis, tubular cell damage, and renal insufficiency has been recently reviewed by Remuzzi and Bertani (24). A central role is attributed to glomerular epithelial cell damage with formation of adhesions to Bowman's capsule and subsequent capillary collapse and to tubulointerstitial damage due to cast formation and inflammatory reactions (see Pathophysiology, above).

In addition to models of glomerular injury, conditions of protein-overload proteinuria have been studied in laboratory animals in order to distinguish between the effect of increased protein flux per se on renal cell damage and the primary underlying injurious factors caused by metabolic, toxic, immunologic, inflammatory, and other stimuli.

EXPERIMENTAL MODELS OF PROTEIN-OVERLOAD PROTEINURIA

Experimental models of protein-overload proteinuria include a rare genetic disorder in Wistar rats bearing a growth hormone producing pituitary tumor (25). This tumor causes liver cell hyperplasia and excessive albumin production, which in turn results in massive albuminuria (26). The rats bearing these tumors develop extensive glomerular cell damage characterized by dedifferentiation and loss of foot processes, accumulation of protein droplets, adhesions to Bowman's capsule, and formation of fibrous crescents. Tubules show extensive cast formation and tubular cell proliferation accompanied by interstitial inflammatory changes. These changes only partially disappear upon removal of the pituitary tumor (26).

Similar changes can be found in rats given high amounts of homologous or heterologous serum proteins by parenteral injection (27–31). Increased filtration of the exogenous proteins is accompanied by glomerular epithelial cell injury (Fig. 2). This leads to sieving defects of the glomerular filter to endogenous proteins as well (Fig. 3) (31–33). Charge-selective properties and endocytotic capacity of the glomerular epithelial cells remain intact (Fig. 4) (30,31). The administration of large amounts of exogenous or homologous proteins has no overt effect on glomerular filtration rate or renal plasma flow (31).

Tubulointerstitial changes have been documented extensively by Eddy et al. (34) in rats given daily injections of bovine serum albumin. At 1 week, interstitial influx of macrophages was noted, subsequently followed by helper and cytotoxic T cells. Tubular epithelial cells showed increased expression of vimentin and deposition of complement component C3 and neoantigen.The degree of tissue injury was directly related to the level of proteinuria (34).

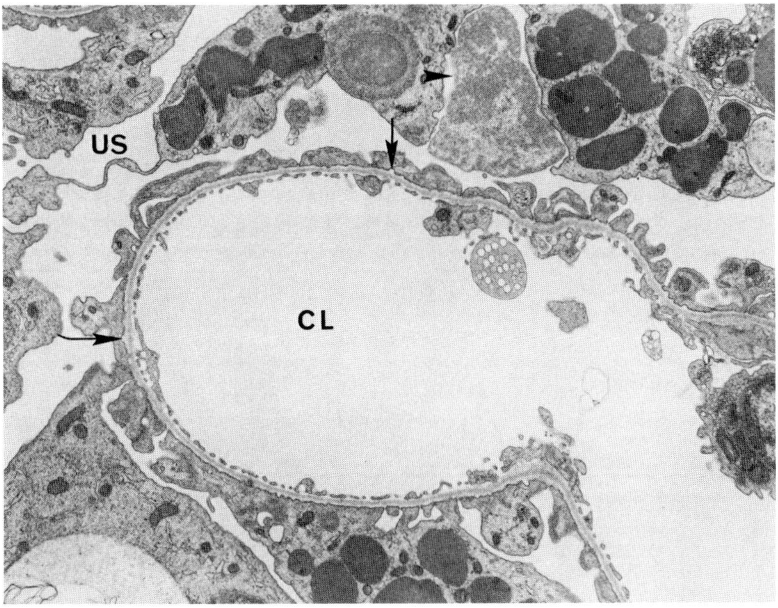

FIG. 2. Electron micrograph of a glomerular capillary loop from a proteinuric rat after two doses of 1.25 g bovine serum albumin (BSA), showing areas of foot process obliteration, a high number of developing pinocytic vesicles (*arrows*), protein reabsorption droplets in the epithelial cells, and accumulation of flocculent proteinaceous material (*arrowhead*) in the urinary space. CL, capillary lumen. (Uranyl acetate and lead citrate, ×6,825.) (Reproduced from Weening et al., ref. 31 with permission.)

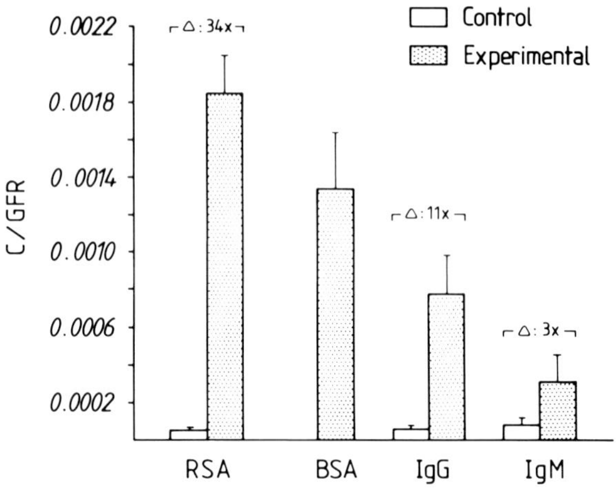

FIG. 3. Fractional clearances of rat serum albumin (RSA), bovine serum albumin (BSA), IgG and IgM in proteinuric and control rats, determined after two doses of 1.25 g BSA, when proteinuria was maximal (281 ± 64 mg per 24 hr). Values are the mean of five animals in each group ± SD of the mean. (Reproduced from Weening et al., ref. 31 with permission.)

Reviewing the literature, it becomes apparent that protein-overload proteinuria, induced by one or more daily injections of heterologous proteins, may result at a later stage in progressive glomerulosclerosis in some laboratory rats, but not in all (32,33,35). This discrepancy may be due to genetic factors governing vascular, inflammatory and epithelial cell reactivity (36). Sex and strain have been shown to influence the glomerular response to high parenteral doses of protein (37).

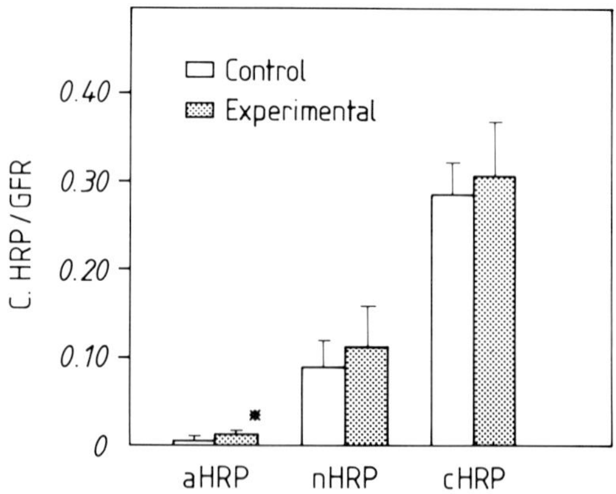

FIG. 4. Fractional clearance of anionic (a), native (n), and cationic (c) horseradish peroxidase (HRP) in proteinuric and control rats, determined after two doses of 1.25 g BSA, when proteinuria was maximal (281 ± 64 mg per 24 hr). Values are the mean of five animals in each group ± SD or the mean. (Reproduced from Weening et al., ref. 31 with permission.)

In summary, increased filtration of exogenous or endogenous proteins due to a high serum concentration or a leaky glomerular filter results in glomerular and tubular epithelial cell injury, which can become chronic and may lead to progressive renal insufficiency. Physicochemical properties of the filtered proteins determine their tendency to precipitation and their interaction with the epithelial cells. Tubular epithelial cell injury is related to saturation and excess of catabolic capacity and specific toxicity.

REFERENCES

1. Rennke HG, Venkatachalam MA. Structural determinants of glomerular permselectivity. *Fed Proc* 1977;36:2619–2926.
2. Brenner BM, Hostetter TH, Humes HD. Glomerular permselectivity: barrier function based on discrimination of molecular size and charge. *Am J Physiol* 1978;F455–F460.
3. Rennke HG, Cotran RS, Venkatachalam MA. Role of molecular charge in glomerular permeability: tracer studies with cationized ferritins. *J Cell Biol* 1975;67:638.
4. Chang RLS, Deen WM, Robertson CR, Brenner BM. Permselectivity of the glomerular capillary wall. III. Restricted transport of polyanions. *Kidney Int* 1975;8:212.
5. Rennke HG, Patel Y, Venkatachalam MA. Glomerular filtration of proteins: clearance of anionic, neutral and cationic horseradish peroxidase in the rat. *Kidney Int* 1978;13:278.
6. Rennke HG, Venkatachalam MA. Glomerular permeability of macromolecules: effect of molecular configuration on the fractional clearance of uncharged dextran and neutral horseradish peroxidase in the rat. *J Clin Invest* 1979;63:713.
7. Brenner BM, Hostetter TH, Humes HD. Molecular basis of proteinuria of glomerular origin. *N Engl J Med* 1978;298:826–833.
8. Kanwar YS. Biophysiology of glomerular filtration and proteinuria. *Lab Invest* 1984;51:7–21.
9. Kaysen GA, Myers BD, Couser WG, Rabkin R, Felts JM. Mechanisms and consequences of proteinuria. *Lab Invest* 1986;54:479–498.
10. Pirani CL, Silva FG, Appel GB. Tubulo-interstitial disease in multiple myeloma and other nonrenal neoplasias. In: Cotran RS, Brenner BM, Stein JH, eds. *Tubulo-interstitial nephropathies*. New York: Churchill Livingstone, 1983;288–309.
11. Maack T, Johnson V, Kau ST, Figueiredo J, Sigulem D. Renal filtration, transport and metabolism of low molecular weight proteins. A review. *Kidney Int* 1979;16:251–270.
12. Carone FA, Peterson DR. Hydrolysis and transport of small peptides by the proximal tubules. *Am J Physiol* 1980;238:F151–F158.
13. Koss MN, Pirani CL, Osserman FF. Experimental Bence Jones cast nephropathy. *Lab Invest* 1976; 34:579–591.
14. Clyne DH, Brendstrup L, First MD, Pesce AJ, Finkel PN, Pollak VE, Pirani CL. Renal effects of intraperitoneal kappa chain injection: induction of crystals in renal tubular cells. *Lab Invest* 1974;31: 131–142.
15. Ganeval D, Jungers P, Noel LH, Droz D. La nephropathie du myelome. *Actualites Nephrol Hôpital Necker* 1977;7:309–347.
16. Preud'Homme JL, Morel-Maroger L, Brouet JC, Cerf M, Mignon F, Guglielmi P, Seligmann M. Synthesis of abnormal immunoglobulins in lymphoplasmacytic disorders with visceral light chain deposition. *Am J Med* 1980;69:703–710.
17. Christensen EI, Rennke HG, Carone FA. Renal tubular uptake of protein: effect of molecular charge. *Am J Physiol* 1983;13:F436–F441.
18. Kant KS, Pesce AJ, Clyne DH, Pollak VE. Urinary cast formation: pH dependence and interaction of Tamm-Horsfall mucoprotein (TH) with myoglobin (Myo), hemoglobin (Hb), Bence Jones (BJ) protein and albumin. *Kidney Int* 1976;10:559.
19. McGeoch J, Ledingham J, Smith JF, Ross B. Inhibition of active-transport sodium-potassium-ATPase by myeloma protein. *Lancet* 1978;1:17.
20. Hoedemaeker PhJ, Weening JJ. Relevance of experimental models for human nephropathology. *Kidney Int* 1989;35:1015–1025.

21. Klahr S, Schreiner G, Ichikawa I. The progression of renal disease. *N Engl J Med* 1988;318: 1657–1666.
22. Weening JJ, Westenend PJ, Beukers JJB, Grond J. Experimental models of glomerulosclerosis. *Contrib Nephrol* 1990;77:65–76.
23. Grond J, Weening JJ. Mesangial cell injury, glomerulosclerosis and therapeutic intervention. *Contrib Nephrol* 1990;81:229–239.
24. Remuzzi G, Bertani T. Is glomerulosclerosis a consequence of altered glomerular permeability to macromolecules? *Kidney Int* 1990;38:384–394.
25. Makino S, Mori H, Koizumi K, Yamashita H, Hayashi Y, Aono T, Matsumoto K. Functional and morphological characteristics of transplantable rat pituitary tumors established in nude mice. *Cancer Res* 1984;44:487.
26. Mori H, Yamashita H, Nakanishi C, Koizumi K, Makino S, Kishimoto Y, Hayashi Y. Proteinuria induced by transplantable rat pituitary tumor MtT SA5. *Lab Invest* 1986;54:636.
27. Anderson MS, Recant L. Fine structural alterations in the rat kidney following intraperitoneal bovine albumin. *Am J Pathol* 1962;40:555–569.
28. Rollason TP, Brewer DB. A scanning and transmission electron microscopic study of glomerular damage in the rat following heterologous serum albumin overload. *J Pathol* 1981;134:39–56.
29. Davies DJ, Messina A, Thumwood CM, Ryan GB. Glomerular podocytic injury in protein overload proteinuria. *Pathology* 1985;17:412–419.
30. Schwartz MM, Bidani AK, Lewis EJ. Glomerular epithelial cell structure and function in chronic proteinuria induced by homologous protein-load. *Lab Invest* 1986;55:673.
31. Weening JJ, Guldener Cv, Daha MR, Klar N, Wal Avd, Prins FA. The pathophysiology of protein-overload proteinuria. *Am J Pathol* 1987;129:64–73.
32. Lippman RW. Mechanism of proteinuria: effect of parenteral bovine albumin injections on hemoglobin excretion in rats. *Am J Physiol* 1948;154:532–536.
33. Lippman RW. Mechanism of proteinuria: II. Identity of urinary protein in the rat following parenteral protein injection. *Proc Soc Exp Biol Med* 1949;71:546–549.
34. Eddy AA, McCulloch L, Adams J, Liu E. Interstitial nephritis induced by protein-overload proteinuria. *Am J Pathol* 1989;135:719–733.
35. Marks MI, Drummond KN. Nephropathy and persistent proteinuria after albumin administration in the rat. *Lab Invest* 1970;23:416–420.
36. Weening JJ, Beukers JJB, Grond J, Elema JD. Genetic factors in focal segmental glomerulosclerosis. *Kidney Int* 1986;29:789–798.
37. Lawrence GM, Brewer DB. Effect of strain and sex on the induction of hyperalbuminaemic proteinuria in the rat. *Clin Sci* 1981;61:751–756.

Toxicology of the Kidney, Second Edition,
edited by Jerry B. Hook and Robin S. Goldstein.
Raven Press, Ltd., New York © 1993.

9

The Nephrotoxicity of β-Lactam Antibiotics

Bruce M. Tune

Laboratory of Renal Pharmacology, Division of Nephrology, Department of Pediatrics, Stanford University School of Medicine, Stanford, California 94305-5119

The β-lactam antibiotics (penicillins, cephalosporins, carbapenems, and several structurally related compounds) are the largest and most rapidly expanding group of antimicrobial agents (Fig. 1). None of the penicillins released for clinical use has proved to be directly nephrotoxic. In contrast, several of the cephalosporins are toxic to the proximal renal tubule, with a spectrum of nephrotoxic/therapeutic ratios much broader than that of the aminoglycosides. Only a few carbapenems have been developed and evaluated for toxicity, but there is already evidence that this group of β-lactams may have a spectrum of renal toxicity similar to that of the cephalosporins.

This chapter will consider the following aspects of the nephrotoxicity of the β-lactams: (a) clinical toxicity; (b) studies of potentiating or risk factors in the laboratory and in human use; and (c) laboratory studies of the mechanisms of toxicity, with emphasis on the roles of tubular cell transport, molecular mechanisms of attack, and the molecular targets of injury. The cephalosporins have been available for study for over 25 years and will therefore be discussed in greatest detail. Where data are available, the carbapenems will be considered within each section.

CLINICAL TOXICITY

The extremes of β-lactam nephrotoxicity are illustrated by the first two ($R_1 =$ 2-thienylacetyl) cephalosporins (see Fig. 1) released for human use: cephalothin ($R_2 =$ acetoxy) and cephaloridine ($R_2 =$ pyridinium). When cephalothin was introduced in the mid-1960s, testing in laboratory animals showed minimal renal toxicity (1,2). It was therefore anticipated that the cephalosporins would have the negligible organ toxicity of the several penicillins already in use. This expectation was largely borne out by clinical experience with cephalothin (3).

However, cephaloridine, released shortly after cephalothin, was nephrotoxic in several laboratory species—with an intravenous ND-50 (50%-nephrotoxic single dose = mk/kg body weight producing tubular necrosis in half of the animals) as

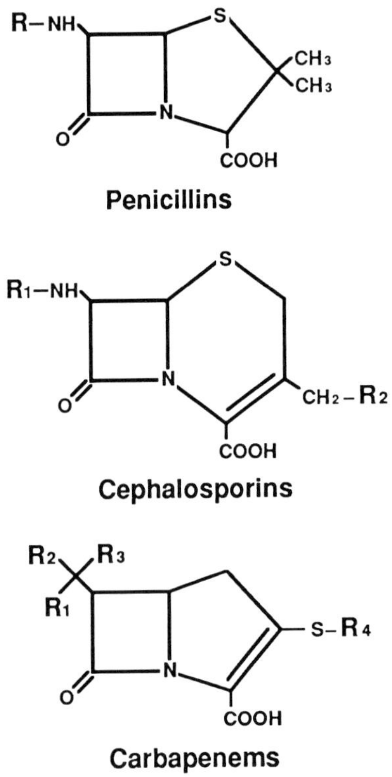

FIG. 1. Basic structures of the penicillins, cephalosporins, and carbapenems.

follows (4,5): rabbit, 90 to 140; monkey, 300; guinea pig, 400 to 700; rat, 1,000 to 1,400; mouse, 600 to 3,000. Early clinical experience showed cephaloridine toxicity in a number of patients (3). Nephrotoxicity in humans, presenting as acute renal failure due to acute tubular necrosis, usually followed doses in excess of 6 g per day, suggesting toxicity comparable to that in monkeys. Clinical nephrotoxicity due to cephaloridine was limited by restricting its dosage, avoiding its use in elderly patients or those with renal insufficiency, and, most importantly, through its later replacement by safer cephalosporins.

POTENTIATING FACTORS

Pharmacologic studies of newly developed antibiotics are done in healthy laboratory animals and human subjects. Toxicologic screening and subsequent clinical trials do not generally test potential toxic interactions. Thus, although acute renal failure is relatively common during serious bacterial infections, a single cause is not usually identified, leaving uncertainty about the contributory role of toxic antibiotics.

Table 1 shows data available for the three most nephrotoxic β-lactams, cephaloridine, cephaloglycin, and the carbapenem imipenem, listed as doses (mg/kg) that

TABLE 1. *Nephrotoxicity of three β-lactam antibiotics in several animal species*[a]

	Rat	Rabbit	Monkey	Human
Cephaloridine	1,200 (4)[b]	100 (4)	300 (4)	≥100 (3)
Cephaloglycin	700 (6)	60 (7)	—	—
Imipenem	≥1,250 (8)	100 (8)	180 (8)	—

[a]Parenteral dosage (mg/kg body weight × 1 in laboratory animals, mg/kg per day in humans) causing acute tubular necrosis.

[b]References given in parentheses.

produce tubular necrosis in rats, rabbits, monkeys, and humans. Cephaloridine produced enough renal injury in otherwise uncomplicated cases to provide a body of data regarding its toxicity to humans. Cephaloglycin, it appears, was not even tested in monkeys, but proved to be extremely toxic to the rabbit and was released only for oral use. Thus, cephaloglycin failed to produce the blood levels necessary to test its potential clinical toxicity. Imipenem has toxicity in rabbits and monkeys comparable to that of cephaloridine; it is marketed in combination with cilastatin, an inhibitor of its enzymatic breakdown in the kidney that also inhibits its nephrotoxicity.

These data show potentially severe nephrotoxicity of three clinically released β-lactams, and suggest that the rabbit provides a suitable model for the study of their toxicology. Several cephalosporins in common use, such as cefaclor, cefazolin, cefamandole, and to some extent cephalothin, are mildly to moderately toxic to the rabbit (9). Their potential for producing renal damage in this species is increased, through interactions at the subcellular or molecular level, by several clinical risk factors: combined use with aminoglycosides (7), renal ischemia (10), and endotoxemia (11,12).

The best-described state of potentiated toxicity in human use is the cephalosporin-aminoglycoside synergy. The three prospective, controlled series summarized in Table 2 documented significantly more renal functional impairment (shown as percent of patients with increased serum creatinine concentrations) with com-

TABLE 2. *Additive toxicity of aminoglycosides and cephalothin in the human kidney*[a]

	A[b]	C[b]	A + C[b]
Klastersky et al. (13)[c]	6%	2%	21%
Wade et al. (14)[d]	7%	—	26%
EORTC (15)[e]	2%	4%	12%

[a]Data given as percent of patients in each treatment group who developed elevations of serum creatinine (Cr_S, as defined below for each study).

[b]Aminoglycoside (A) or cephalothin (C) combined with methicillin or ticarcillin, or combined with one another (A + C). References given in parentheses.

[c]Aminoglycoside = tobramycin. Cr_S increased to > 2.0.

[d]Aminoglycoside = gentamicin or tobramycin. Cr_S increased by ≥0.4.

[e]Aminoglycoside = gentamicin. Cr_S increased to ≥2.5.

TABLE 3. *Impact of multiple risk factors on antibiotic nephrotoxicity (rabbit)*[a]

	Aminoglycoside[b] Cr_s[d]	Endotoxemia[c] Cr_s[d]	Cr_s >1.1[e]
C	0.74 ± 0.05	1.08 ± 0.12	2/12
A	0.95 ± 0.07	0.83 ± 0.03	0/12
E	—	0.76 ± 0.07	0/12
C + A	7.30 ± 2.24	0.77 ± 0.04	0/12
C + E	—	2.72 ± 1.12	4/12
A + E	—	3.04 ± 1.24	4/12
C + A + E	—	4.17 ± 1.20	11/12

[a]Cephalosporin (C), aminoglycoside (A), endotoxin (E) (*Escherichia coli* 0111:B4 lipopolysaccharide) given alone or in combination, as indicated.
[b]Cefaclor (C), 300 mg/kg, gentamicin (A), 100 mg/kg, or both (A + C) injected subcutaneously daily for 5 days. Animals killed on day 7. (From ref. 7.)
[c]Cephaloglycin (C), 60 mg/kg, neomycin (A), 60 mg/kg, endotoxin (E), 0.5 mg/kg, or combinations of these, given as single intravenous doses. Animals killed 2 days later. (From ref. 11.)
[d]Serum creatinine (Cr_s, mg/dl), mean ± SE. Normal = 0.79 ± 0.03 (24).
[e]Numbers of rabbits with serum creatinine concentrations >1.1.

bined compared to separate use of cephalothin and an aminoglycoside. Similar studies in rabbits (7) suggest an even greater risk with more toxic cephalosporins like cefaclor and cefazolin.

Studies of the cephalosporin-aminoglycoside interaction in humans have been challenged because broad-spectrum penicillins may have reduced cephalosporin or aminoglycoside toxicity in the control groups (16–18). Table 3 demonstrates the cephalosporin-aminoglycoside synergy in rabbits in the absence of this variable. On the left are shown serum creatinine concentrations in animals given 5 days of a cefaclor-plus-gentamicin combination in doses that caused little or no renal injury when given alone. In combination, the two antibiotics were nephrotoxic to every animal treated. On the right are the results of separate and combined administration of single, minimally toxic doses of cephaloglycin and neomycin too small to produce a toxic synergy by themselves, but strongly toxic in combination with a single dose of bacterial cell wall lipopolysaccharide (endotoxin). The combination of all three insults produced elevations of serum creatinine in more animals (11/12) than did the combination of any two of them (0 to 4/12). Although endotoxic shock is commonly blamed for the acute renal failure of bacterial septicemia, the dose of lipopolysaccharide, when given alone, caused no tubular necrosis or increase of serum creatinine at the 48-hr time of sacrifice.

MECHANISMS OF TOXICITY

The nephrotoxic β-lactams produce a selective necrosis of the proximal renal tubule (4,8,19,20). Because of their greater availability, the cephalosporins have been studied most extensively. Most studies have used cephaloridine (ND-50 = 90 mg/kg in the female rabbit) or cephaloglycin (60 mg/kg), which reproducibly cause acute tubular necrosis after single dosage. More limited studies with cefaclor (~500–800 mg/kg) and cefazolin (~1,500 mg/kg) support the conclusions reached with the more toxic cephalosporins (7,21). Imipenem, the first carbapenem released for clinical use and the one with the best-described toxic potential, is nephrotoxic to rabbits and monkeys in about the same dosage as cephaloridine (8,22).

Several mechanisms of nephrotoxicity have been proposed. (I) *Tubular transport*: concentrative uptake through a secretory carrier, based on the consistent correlation between transport and toxicity (23). (II) *Molecular mechanisms*: (a) production of a highly reactive acylating metabolite by a cytochrome P-450–dependent mixed-function oxidase (MFO) (24); (b) production of cell membrane lipid peroxidation (25); and (c) spontaneous acylation by the cephalosporins of their molecular targets through the intrinsic reactivity of their β-lactam ring (26). (III) *Molecular targets*: (a) inhibition of gluconeogenesis (27); (b) depletion of cytochrome P-450 (28); and (c) production of mitochondrial respiratory toxicity (29–31), recently shown to be mediated by (d) inactivation of the mitochondrial transporters of anionic metabolites such as succinate (32).

Tubular Transport

Like benzylpenicillin, many of the cephalosporins are secreted across the proximal tubule by the *p*-aminohippurate carrier on the antiluminal side (33–35), reaching intracellular concentrations orders of magnitude greater than in any other cell type. Evidence of the toxicologic importance of this transport is as follows (9): (a) the occurrence of toxic injury only with those β-lactams that undergo tubular secretion; (b) its restriction to the proximal tubule; (c) a correlation of cortical antibiotic concentrations with the toxic threshold; (d) the prevention of toxicity by different inhibitors of secretory transport; and (e) augmentation of toxicity by manipulations that increase cellular concentrations.

The degree and duration of concentrative uptake, or the area under the curve (AUC) of tubular cell concentration and time, varies greatly between individual β-lactams (Table 4). The net effects of differing antiluminal-side transport into the cell and luminal-side efflux into the tubular fluid (Fig. 2) result in (a) low levels for cefaclor and cephalothin, (b) an extremely high AUC for cephaloridine, (c) intermediate levels for cephaloglycin and cephalexin, and (d) no measurable uptake for ceftazidime (9).

Cephaloridine

Cephaloridine has two highly unusual properties: (a) it carries a fixed quarternary nitrogen in the pyridinium side-ring on its 3-methylene (R_2) position (Fig. 1); and (b) although cephaloridine is rapidly transported into the tubular cell at the basolateral side, its movement from cell to tubular fluid is greatly restricted compared to normally secreted organic anions (38). Because of this luminal membrane

TABLE 4. *Concentrative uptake of several cephalosporins by the in situ rabbit renal cortex*

	Concentrations[a,b]		Cortex-to-serum ratios[b,c]	Cortical half-lives (hr)[b]	Cortical AUCs[b,d]
	Cortex	Serum			
CLD	2,576 ± 267	167 ± 12	15.1 ± 0.8	1.30 ± 0.21	5023 ± 881
CGL	1088 ± 56	176 ± 25	6.9 ± 1.1	0.65 ± 0.06	1015 ± 93
CLX	1323 ± 258	180 ± 26	7.7 ± 1.6	0.42	798
CCL	499 ± 48	77 ± 9	6.8 ± 1.0	0.52	374
CTZ	406 ± 42	293 ± 33	1.4 ± 0.1	0.68	396
CPT	431 ± 122	127 ± 16	3.2 ± 0.4	[e]	[e]

[a]Peak or steady-state concentrations measured in cortex (μg/g wet tissue) or serum (μg/ml) after infusion of 100 mg/kg BW of each cephalosporin into female NZW rabbits. Values (means ± SEM) for cephaloridine (CLD) and cephaloglycin (CGL) derived from pooled data of several previously published studies (using 7 and 6 means, respectively), and values for cephalexin (CLX), cefaclor (CCL), ceftazidime (CTZ), and cephalothin (CPT) from single studies (n = 5–6 animals in each group), from the following sources: CLD: (9,11,17,36). CGL: (7,10,11,21,26,31). CLX: (9). CCL: (37). CTZ: (9). CPT: (26).

[b]The following comparisons are statistically significant (>95% by ANOVA): Cortical concentrations: CLD > CGL and CLX > CCL, CTZ, and CPT. Cortex-to-serum ratios (C/S): CLD > all others; CGL, CLX, and CCL > CPT > CTZ. Cortical half-lives: CLD > CGL and all other cephalosporins collectively. Cortical AUCs: CLD > CGL > all other cephalosporins collectively.

[c]C/S inulin = 1.4 ± 0.1 (from 7 means), not significantly different from C/S CTZ.

[d]Areas under the curves of cortical concentration and time, calculated as peak or steady-state cortical concentrations × cortical half-lives/0.693.

[e]Measurements made at one time only.

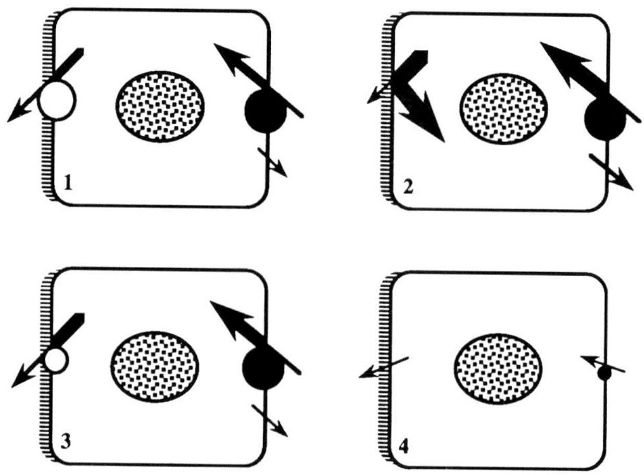

FIG. 2. Secretion of cephalosporin antibiotics across the proximal renal tubule. Differences in active transport from blood to tubular cell (shown on the *right side* in each example) and movement from cell to luminal fluid (*left side*) result in wide variations of intracellular AUCs of concentration and time. Specific examples of each pattern of transport are given in the text.

block, which is probably a result of its cationic charge (39,40), cephaloridine reaches tubular cell concentrations after mildly toxic dosage (100 mg/kg in the rabbit → peak renal cortical concentrations ~2,600 μg/g wet tissue) substantially higher than found after equivalent dosage of any other cephalosporin (≤1,300 μg/g) (31,37). The magnitude of this intracellular sequestration is best illustrated by the cortical AUCs (Table 4). Note here that ceftazidime, which also has an R_2 pyridinium, undergoes little or no concentrative uptake in renal cortex, possibly because a second carboxyl (in the R_1 side-group) restricts its transport into the tubule cell.

The importance of the transport-toxicity relationship of cephaloridine has been demonstrated in several ways: (I) large interspecies, intersex, and interstrain differences of cortical uptake, which correlate with proportionate variations of nephrotoxicity (41,42); (II) the maturation of concentrative uptake in the newborn rabbit, which also correlates with increasing toxicity (41,43); and (III) manipulations of toxicity with different inhibitors of transport: (a) Pretreatment with the organic anions probenecid or *p*-aminohippurate prevents cephaloridine nephrotoxicity only when enough of the inhibitor is given to produce a sustained reduction of cortical antibiotic concentration (36,44). (b) Pretreatment with cyanine 863, an inhibitor of organic cation transport, decreases cephaloridine efflux from the tubular cell, increasing both its intracellular concentrations and its nephrotoxicity (39,45).

Cephaloridine, therefore, has unique properties of high and prolonged intracellular concentrations, which have an almost certain pathogenic role in its nephrotoxicity. However, the discovery of cephaloglycin's greater toxicity in the presence of significantly lower AUCs (20,31) called for closer examination of the molecular properties of the toxic and nontoxic cephalosporins (9).

Cephaloglycin, Cephalexin, and Cefaclor

These R_1 = phenylglycyl cephalosporins were developed for their acid-stability and absorption across the gastrointestinal tract (46). Analysis of the widely different nephrotoxic potentials, cellular uptakes, and molecular properties of these closely related compounds provided the basis for the model of β-lactam–induced molecular injury to be developed later in this discussion.

Cephaloglycin (R_2 = acetoxy) is the most nephrotoxic of the commercially available cephalosporins. It is secreted across the tubular cell with a cortical AUC one-fifth of that of cephaloridine and about 2.5 times those of cephalothin and cefaclor (Table 4). Although cephaloglycin has an AUC much lower than cephaloridine, there is a close relationship between its uptake and toxicity in the tubular cell. Nephrotoxicity is prevented by decreasing intracellular concentrations with probenecid (31) and augmented by increasing cellular concentrations through transient ureteral occlusion (21).

Cephalexin (R_2 = hydrogen), which is virtually nontoxic to the kidney, is secreted across the tubular cell with an AUC almost the same as that of cephaloglycin (Table 4). Cefaclor (3-CH_2-R_2 = Cl), which is mildly nephrotoxic, is efficiently secreted

TABLE 5. *Side-group substituents of several cephalosporins*[a]

Cephalosporin[b]	R_1 side-group	R_2 side-group
Cephaloglycin	Phenylglycyl	Acetoxy
Cephaloridine	2-Thienylacetyl	Pyridinium
Cefaclor	Phenylglycyl	Chlorine[c]
Cephalothin	2-Thienylacetyl	Acetoxy
Cephalexin	Phenylglycyl	Hydrogen

[a]See Fig. 1 for core structure (46).
[b]Listed from top to bottom in decreasing order of nephrotoxicity to the rabbit (9).
[c]CH_2-R_2 replaced by Cl.

across the tubular cell. The very low degree of intracellular sequestration of cefaclor (Table 4) could be sufficient to account for its limited toxicity compared to that of cephaloglycin. In support of this interpretation is the large increase of nephrotoxicity when tubular cell cefaclor concentrations are increased by a brief period of ureteral obstruction (21). However, the virtual absence of toxicity with cephalexin cannot be explained by similar analysis.

The following can be concluded from experience with these four cephalosporins: (a) concentrative uptake is necessary, but not sufficient for the production of cytotoxic injury; (b) simple comparison of the R_1 and R_2 side-groups of the toxic and nontoxic cephalosporins (Table 5) does not reveal the basis of their toxic potentials; and (c) the very similar AUCs and very different toxicities of cephaloglycin and cephalexin must nevertheless be related to the only structural difference between the two, their R_2 side-groups. This apparent paradox will be further explored later in the discussion of the molecular mechanisms of toxicity.

Molecular Mechanisms

MFO-Metabolite Hypothesis

Cobaltous chloride and piperonyl butoxide, which block and compete, respectively, for cytochrome P-450–dependent MFO activity, reduce the nephrotoxicity of cephaloridine in the mouse and the rat (24). It was therefore proposed that MFO activity produces a toxic metabolite, through epoxidation of the thiophene ring on the thienylacetyl R_1 side-group common to cephaloridine and cephalothin. Because cephalothin secretion involves very little intracellular sequestration (Table 4), it need not have major MFO-mediated nephrotoxicity.

The validity of this hypothesis came into early question for several reasons: (a) There was no demonstration of energy-dependent, MFO-mediated binding of cephaloridine to renal microsomes, as shown with other MFO-activated cytotoxins (24). (b) Most nephrotoxic cephalosporins (cephaloglycin, cefaclor, cefazolin, cefamandole, and others) do not have a thiophene or similar side-ring (9). (c) None of the different side-groups on the nephrotoxic cephalosporins is consistently associated with toxicity.

The metabolite hypothesis has been further refuted by the following lines of evidence: (a) Studies with cephaloglycin showed no protection by piperonyl butoxide (47). (b) Although piperonyl butoxide protects against cephaloridine in the rabbit, cobaltous chloride does not (47). (c) Piperonyl butoxide reduces the cortical concentrations of cephaloridine by 50% in the rabbit (47); this reduction of net uptake, which is sufficient to account for the protective effect, appears to be the result of an increased efflux of cephaloridine (48). (d) Although cephaloglycin binds to renal cortical microsomes *in vitro* and *in vivo*, this binding appears to be unrelated to MFO activity (26); unlike binding resulting from MFO activation, cephaloglycin binding is decreased—not increased—by nicotinamide-adenine dinucleotide phosphate, reduced (NADPH), and is not decreased by piperonyl butoxide.

Lipid Peroxidation

Kuo and associates (25) first observed that cephaloridine induces lipid peroxidation in rat and rabbit kidneys. Pursuing their earlier observation (49,50) that cephaloridine depleted renal cortical glutathione (GSH) without forming a GSH conjugate, these investigators found that the cephalosporin produces a rise in cortical oxidized glutathione (GSSG). They went on to demonstrate that the antibiotic causes the formation of conjugated dienes, as evidence of cell membrane lipid peroxidation, and that selenium deficiency and vitamin E deficiency, both of which enhance lipid peroxidation, potentiate the production of tubular necrosis and renal failure by cephaloridine. The authors suggested that redox cycling of cephaloridine's pyridinium ring is the vehicle of electron transfer causing peroxidation.

These observations have been generally confirmed and extended by the following findings: (a) Cephaloridine and NADPH undergo reduction and oxidation, respectively, in an *in vitro* system containing each in the presence of active renal cortical microsomes (51). (b) Cephaloridine generates the production of superoxide anion and hydrogen peroxide in a similar *in vitro* system (51). (c) Cephaloridine induces malondialdehyde (MDA) production, another indicator of lipid peroxidation, in cortical microsomes and mitochondria (12,51) and in renal cortical slices (52,53), and this effect is prevented by various antioxidants and radical scavengers (52,53). Cefotaxime and cephalexin, which are not nephrotoxic, cause little or no similar reaction (12,51). (d) Cephaloridine-induced MDA or conjugated diene production is concentration- and dose-dependent (increasing over the range of 400 to 4,000 μg/ml *in vitro* or 100 to 300 mg/kg body weight *in vivo*) and time-dependent (commencing at 0.25 to 1.5 hr) and precedes the nephrotoxic reduction of cortical uptake of *p*-aminohippurate and tetraethylammonium in renal cortical slices (52–54). (e) Cephaloridine-induced MDA production is decreased by the cytochrome P-450 inhibitor cobaltous chloride, suggesting a role of a P-450–dependent reductase in the generation of lipid peroxides (52).

Several observations are difficult to reconcile with lipid peroxidation being a primary mechanism of cephalosporin nephrotoxicity. (a) Cephalothin, which lacks a pyridinium ring, induces malondialdehyde generation in cortical slices as well as cephaloridine does (55). (b) GSH depletion by cephaloridine is not prevented by antioxidants (53). (c) The other highly toxic β-lactams do not have pyridinium in their side-groups (Table 5) and do not cause significant peroxidative injury (22,54).

Spontaneous β-Lactam Reactivity

The β-lactam antibiotics are modified cyclic dipeptides with three-dimensional configurations closely resembling the D-alanyl-D-alanine (D-ala-D-ala) carboxyterminal sequence of bacterial cell wall precursor peptidoglycans (56). The β-lactams are accepted as the precursor substrates of a number of bacterial membrane-bound 40 to 50 kd peptidoglycan carboxypeptidases (CPases) essential for cell wall formation. Once in place, they form a covalent complex with the CPases, blocking their ability to cross-link the peptidoglycans and leaving the bacteria unable to replicate their cell walls. The β-lactams also acylate a group of membrane-bound 60 to 140 kd proteins, designated collectively with the CPases as penicillin-binding proteins (PBPs) (57). The physiological functions of the high molecular weight PBPs are largely unknown, but studies of gene deletion have shown them to be more regularly essential than the CPases for bacterial survival.

Indelicato et al. (58,59) and Yamana et al. (60,61) examined the β-lactam reactivity *in vitro* of a variety of penicillins and cephalosporins in a model designed to quantify their potency as acylators of the bacterial PBPs. pHs of 8 to 10 were used to provide high concentrations of hydroxide, a nucleophile capable of inducing an opening of the β-lactam ring. The nucleophiles of the bacterial proteins are free amino groups positioned to attack and bind to the β-lactam fitted into their carboxy-terminal D-ala-D-ala or similar receptors.

The rank order of reactivity of several penicillins and cephalosporins measured in these studies (58–62) (ceftazidime>cefaclor>cephaloglycin>cephalothin>cephaloridine≥cefazolin>>several penicillins >>cephalexin and other 3-methyl-cephalosporins) does not by itself fit with the antimicrobial potencies of the antibiotics. Factors such as bacterial cell wall penetration and β-lactamase production also affect antimicrobial effectiveness (57).

Similarly, it is possible only in a limited sense to compare data on β-lactam reactivity with the rank order of nephrotoxicity of the cephalosporins (2,7,20,21, 31, 41,63,64): cephaloglycin>cephaloridine>>cefaclor>cefazolin>cephalothin>>> the penicillins, cephalexin, and ceftazidime (no toxicity). The relative stability of the penicillins and the 3-methyl-cephalosporins (like cephalexin) fits well with their uniform lack of toxicity, but the more reactive cephalosporins are not all nephrotoxic. However, when reactivity and intracellular sequestration (Table 4) are considered together, there emerges a more convincing fit with nephrotoxicity. For example, ceftazidime, although very highly reactive, undergoes essentially no concentrative uptake by the tubular cell (9). Cefaclor, which is also highly reactive, is rapidly secreted and has a low renal cortical AUC (7% and 37% of the AUCs of cephaloridine and cephaloglycin, respectively). Cephalothin, although fairly reactive, also has low and transient tubular cell concentrations.

Assuming that these corrections for the AUC are appropriate, there remains one questionable correlation. The combined high *in vitro* reactivity and high tubular cell AUC of cephaloridine do not fit well with its lower toxicity than that of cephaloglycin. An explanation for this discrepancy may be found in cephaloridine's pyridinium ring. The presence of an R_2 cationic nitrogen so near to the anionic carboxyl may restrict cephaloridine's access to its molecular targets, thereby requiring the high and prolonged cellular concentrations needed to produce nephrotoxicity. In support of this speculation, studies of brief *in vivo* exposure have shown cephaloridine to be relatively less reactive than cephaloglycin in the intact kidney (31).

The covalent binding of β-lactam antibiotics to animal proteins has long been of interest in the study of their allergenic properties (65). The penicillins bind to skin and serum proteins, forming the antigenic ligands responsible for allergic sensitization. The cephalosporins are involved in basically the same process. Binding of β-lactams to subcellular constituents has only recently been examined with an emphasis on cytotoxic mechanisms. Browning and Tune (26) compared to binding to rabbit kidney proteins of three β-lactams available in isotopic form: cephaloglycin (highly toxic), cephalothin (minimally nephrotoxic), and benzylpenicillin (no nephrotoxicity).

One-half to 12 hr after intravenous administration of cephaloglycin, renal cortical concentrations were 15 to 30 times of those in liver. Cortical concentrations declined rapidly over the first 3 hr ($t^{1/2} = 0.7$ hr), then much more slowly over the next 9 hr ($t^{1/2} \cong 9$ hr). Total and covalently protein-bound cephaloglycin, cephalothin, and benzylpenicillin were measured in different subcellular fractions of kidney cortex 3 hr after administration of 100 mg/kg BW of each to separate groups of rabbits. This measurement of binding in the *in situ* kidney reflects the net effects of differing AUCs, receptor affinities, and reactivities. Firmly bound cephaloglycin, was comparable in nuclear, mitochondrial, microsomal, and cytosolic proteins, and was 3.5 times that of cephalothin and 7 times that of penicillin.

Studies of binding to cortical microsomes *in vitro*, after 0 to 60 min of incubation, revealed similar binding (cephaloglycin >>cephalothin>penicillin [Fig. 3]). The rate of binding was greatest in the first 20 min but uptake continued throughout the hour. Cephaloglycin binding was reduced 30% to 45% by NADPH, but was unaffected by 1 mM piperonyl butoxide. Unfortunately, other isotopic β-lactams have not been available for similar study.

It was concluded that all three β-lactams bind covalently to a number of tubular cell proteins, without the requirement for metabolic energy of the MFO-activation process. The rank order of binding of these three antibiotics is consistent with the hypothesis that cephalosporin nephrotoxicity is initiated by a process of tubular cell uptake, followed by spontaneous acylation of one or more target proteins. The binding of cephaloglycin (7% of peak cortical concentrations) is so diffuse among subcellular fractions that a specific molecular target was not identified. As in the antimicrobial process, the cephalosporins may impair the functions of multiple cellular proteins. It should not be assumed, however, that the function of every acylated protein is necessarily impaired.

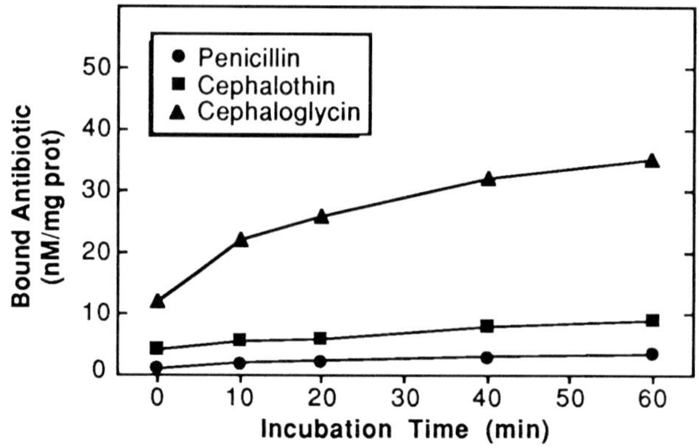

FIG. 3. *In vitro* binding of cephaloglycin (highly nephrotoxic), cephalothin (mildly toxic), and benzylpenicillin (nontoxic) to microsomes from rabbit renal cortex. Microsomes were incubated for 0 to 60 min at 20°C in a medium containing 750 nmol/ml of antibiotic, then trapped on Millipore filters and washed 5 × each with 5 ml of 5% trichloroacetic acid and 5 ml of 55°C methanol. (Data from ref. 26.)

Molecular Targets

Glucose Metabolism; Gluconeogenesis

Goldstein and associates (27) showed a reduction of gluconeogenesis in rat renal cortical slices exposed to cephaloridine for as little as 0.25 hr. Cephaloridine reduced gluconeogenesis from substrates not requiring mitochondrial enzyme activity, suggesting that this effect was not an indirect result of impaired mitochondrial metabolism. Instead, the authors presented evidence of direct inhibition of glucose-6-phosphatase. Although it was concluded that inhibition of gluconeogenesis alone should not produce cellular necrosis, it is tempting to speculate that glucose-6-phosphatase is one of the proteins inactivated through acylation by cephaloridine.

Cytochrome P-450/Microsomal Proteins

Cojocel and associates (28) have measured a decrease of cytochrome P-450 activity in rat renal cotex within 3 hr of injection of a nephrotoxic dose (1,200 mg/kg) of cephaloridine. Accompanying this is a reduction of 50 to 53 kd proteins and the appearance of a 44 kd protein in renal cortical microsomes after three daily injections (66). The mechanism and functional significance of these observations remains to be determined.

Mitochondrial Respiration

Early studies showed a depression of renal mitochondrial respiration from both cephaloridine and cephaloglycin toxicity after *in vivo* exposure in the intact kidney and after *in vitro* exposure of isolated renal tubules (29,30). There are several lines of evidence that this process may be pathogenic in cephalosporin nephrotoxicity: (a) Cephaloridine and cephaloglycin (nephrotoxic) produce respiratory toxicity, whereas cephalexin (nontoxic) does not (31). (b) Respiratory toxicity evolves over 0.5 to 1 hr after cephaloglycin administration, as intracellular antibiotic concentrations decline substantially (20,31). (c) Exposure of cortical slices to cephaloridine decreases their adenosine triphosphate (ATP) content by approximately 1.5 hr (27). (d) Ultrastructural damage to mitochondria and other membranous structures begins between 1 and 5 hr after administration, in a pattern that resembles ischemic and cyanide-induced injury (19,67,68). (e) The respiratory toxicity of cephaloglycin, measured 1 hr after administration, is augmented by an aminoglycoside regimen that has no respiratory toxicity by itself (7). (f) Renal mitochondrial calcification is seen 24 hr after cephaloglycin intoxication (69).

The nephrotoxic cephalosporins produce similar patterns of respiratory toxicity in isolated mitochondria exposed either *in vitro* or *in vivo* (30): (a) With the naturally occurring substrates, respiration with glutamate plus malate is inhibited less than respiration with succinate. (b) Respiration with the artificial electron donors tetramethylphenylenediamine plus ascorbate is depressed little, if at all. (c) State 3 (ATP-generating) respiration is reduced more than the slower, adenosine diphosphate (ADP)-independent respiration.

However, toxicity after exposure *in vitro* differs from that found after exposure *in vivo* in certain important respects (70): (a) Toxicity to isolated normal mitochondria exposed *in vitro* may be seen with any penicillin or cephalosporin, and is immediate in onset; respiratory toxicity from exposure in the intact cell occurs only with the toxic cephalosporins and develops over 0.5 to 1 hr. (b) *In vitro* toxicity is reversed by washing or by increasing concentrations of metabolic substrate, whereas *in vivo* toxicity is not.

The following model was proposed to fit these events (9). Early access of the β-lactams to their mitochondrial targets is nonselective and easily reversed by the metabolic substrates abundant in the intact cell. There follows a slower, irreversible attack by the toxic cephalosporins on these targets. It is proposed that the toxic cephalosporins acylate one or more membrane-bound proteins responsible for transporting metabolic substrates into the mitochondrial inner matrix. Although the β-lactams are exogenous substances, with no obvious basis for recognition by mitochondrial anionic transporters, their transport by basolateral secretory carriers of the tubule cell also lacks a clear evolutionary advantage, and their thousandfold concentration within the tubular cell creates local conditions favoring their acylation of intracellular proteins.

Mitochondrial Substrate Transport

Three observations suggested an effect of the nephrotoxic β-lactams on the transporters that carry anionic substrates into the mitochondrial inner matrix: (a) their natural ability to acylate and inactivate membrane-bound proteins (56) and to acylate tubular cell proteins (26); (b) their consistently greater toxicity to respiration with succinate, which donates electrons to the midregion of the cytochrome chain, than to respiration with glutamate and malate, which donate electrons proximal to that locus, suggesting an action outside the electron transport chain (30,31); (c) the reversal of early *in vitro* respiratory toxicity (Table 6) by increasing concentrations of substrate, reflected as an increased k_m for succinate with an unaffected V_{max} (70). This early competitive inhibition suggested that all β-lactams may fit the mitochondrial carriers for anionic substrate transport, but *in vivo* nephrotoxicity develops only with the comparatively sequestered and reactive ones, which acylate these carriers and cause irreversible injury to substrate uptake.

In Vivo Exposure

As a test of this hypothesis, respiration with and the uptake of succinate were measured in mitochondria exposed *in situ* to nephrotoxic doses (300 mg/kg 1 to 2 hr before sacrifice) of cephaloridine (54), cephaloglycin (32), or imipenem (22). Each of the β-lactams reduced respiration significantly and decreased succinate uptake by up to 70% (Fig. 4). Succinate efflux was unaffected in each case, indicating that reduced net uptake was the result of decreased substrate entry.

Specificity of Mitochondrial Injury

Further studies (71) tested this hypothesis by examining the specificity of the association of reduced substrate transport and reduced respiration. (I) *Specificity of insult*. Compared to the three nephrotoxic β-lactams, other potential or real mitochondrial insults produced different patterns of damage: (a) Cephalexin (54) had no inhibitory effect on respiration or uptake (Fig. 4). (b) Respiratory chain poisons reduced respiration but not uptake. (c) Although ischemia reduced both uptake and

TABLE 6. *Patterns of cephaloglycin toxicity to renal cortical mitochondria*[a]

Exposure	V_{max}[b]	K_m[b]
Control	262 ± 18	4.0 ± 0.3
In vitro	229 ± 13	13.3 ± 3.1
	NS	$p < .005$
In vivo	108 ± 9	2.0 ± 0.2
	$p < .001$	$p < .001$

[a]Data from ref. 70.

[b]Calculated from double reciprocal plots of state 3 respiratory rates against succinate concentrations (2.5–20 mM) in a respiration medium containing 0 vs. 2.5 mM cephaloglycin (*in vitro* exposure), or in mitochondria from rabbits that received 0 vs. 200 mg/kg cephaloglycin 1 hr earlier (*in vivo* exposure).

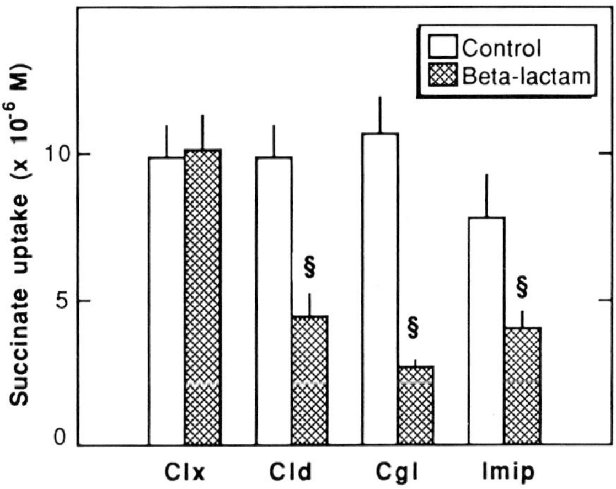

FIG. 4. *In vivo* toxicity of β-lactam antibiotics to succinate uptake by renal cortical mitochondria. Rabbits were injected intravenously with 300 mg/kg of cephaloridine (Cld), cephaloglycin (Cgl), imipenem (Imip), all of which are nephrotoxic, or with 1,000 mg/kg of cephalexin (Clx), which is not toxic, 1 hr before sacrifice. Mitochondria were then isolated and incubated for 5 min in a 20°C bath containing 1.2×10^{-6} M succinate. Data are presented as means ± SE (n = 8–12 each). Significance level by analysis of variance comparing experimental to control mitochondria >99.9% (§).

respiration, it also caused a large increase of substrate efflux. (II) *Specificity of target organ.* Measurements in liver mitochondria showed no effect of cephaloridine or cephaloglycin on either respiration or uptake. (III) *Specificity of molecular target.* Studies of the effects of cephaloridine and cephaloglycin intoxication on other mitochondrial targets in renal cortex showed normalcy of three important functions (Fig. 5): (a) Respiration with pyruvate, which enters the mitochondrion by simple diffusion (72) or by a proton-pyruvate symporter (73), was not reduced. The transport of (b) phosphate and (c) ADP, which are carried into the mitochondrion by their own transporters, and which have critical roles in mitochondrial respiration, was also spared.

In Vitro Exposure

It should follow that *in vitro* β-lactam injury to mitochondrial substrate uptake and respiration becomes irreversible as acylation of the transporters evolves. Earlier efforts at prolonged *in vitro* incubation were confounded by deterioration of function in control mitochondira. Studies were therefore done at 4°C with 0 to 6 hr of *in vitro* exposure to 0 to 3,000 μg/ml of cephaloglycin or imipenem (74). The lower temperature preserved function in controls incubated for the 6 hr. As was found with *in vivo* β-lactam exposure, cephaloglycin and imipenem caused a time- and concentration-dependent irreversible injury to both respiration with and the uptake of succinate by the mitochondrion, while producing little or no injury to ADP uptake.

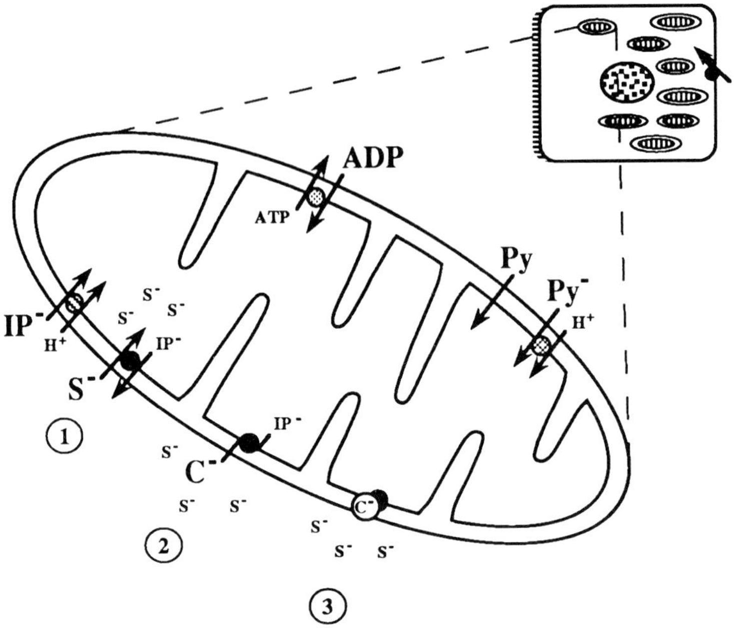

FIG. 5. Effects of nephrotoxic β-lactams on renal tubular mitochondrial function. *1*: Normally, inorganic phosphate (IP^-) is symported into the inner matrix with a proton (H^+) and then antiported in exchange for a metabolic substrate such as succinate (S^-). *2*: The nephrotoxic β-lactams (shown here as C^- for cephalosporin) fit the anionic substrate carrier, initially causing reversible inhibition of transport. *3*: They then acylate the transporter, causing irreversible injury to uptake and secondarily to respiration. The transport of inorganic phosphate, ADP, and pyruvate (Py^-), which enter the mitrochondrion by separate mechanisms, is unaffected.

Isolation of the Oxoglutarate Transporter

We have begun to explore the effects of toxic β-lactam exposure on the 2-oxoglutarate transporter purified by the method of Bisaccia and associates (75). The active carrier protein from mitochondria exposed to 300 mg/kg of cephaloglycin *in vivo* for 1 to 2 hr before isolation has an approximately 35 kd molecular size and appears unaltered compared to normal on one-dimensional polyacrylamide gels. Figure 6 shows two-dimensional gels further characterizing the control and cephaloglycin-exposed proteins. The normal oxoglutarate transporter is seen as the major spot below the line of markers in Fig. 6A. A second protein is seen on the left of the same spot from the β-lactam exposed transporter (Fig. 6B), shifted in the acid direction from a pI of approximately 6.7 to one of around 6.5. Although there are other possible explanations for this new protein, its movement by a distance of approximately two marker points is consistent with a loss of one amino group by acylation plus the addition of one β-lactam carboxyl per carrier molecule. Studies are underway to characterize the functional consequences of this modification of the carrier protein.

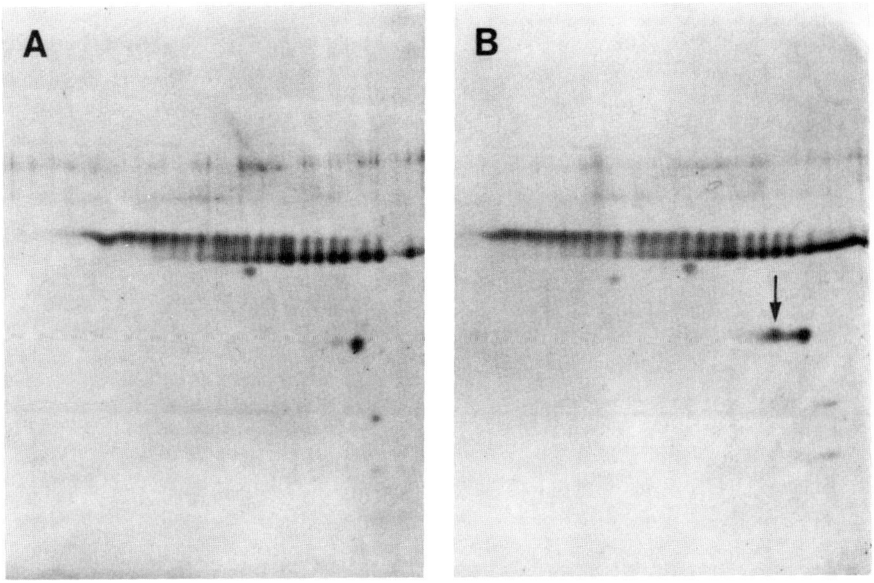

FIG. 6. Two-dimensional (2-D) polyacrylamide gels separating by molecular weight and isoelectric points (pI) normal (*A*) and cephaloglycin-intoxicated (*B*) mitochondrial oxoglutarate carrier proteins. On the *left* are shown molecular weight standards (*top* to *bottom*) of 97.4, 66.2, 45.0, 31.0, and 21.5 kd. A row of 40 kd carbamylated creatine phosphokinase standards (pI = 4.9–7.1, *left* to *right*) is seen above the ~35 kd carrier protein spots in both 2-D gels. The two-spot pI shift of the modified protein, indicated by the *arrow* in panel *B*, is consistent with the acylation of each molecule of the altered carrier protein by a single molecule of cephaloglycin.

Mechanism of Cell Death

It remains to be determined precisely how toxicity to mitochondrial substrate transport can be lethal to the tubule cell. Respiration is reduced with several mitochondrial substrates, presumably by the same process that affects the succinate transporter. A fully toxic dose of cephaloglycin reduces respiration with glutamate and malate by one-half (31), citrate by one-half (this laboratory, unpublished), and succinate by two-thirds in mitochondrial suspensions from whole renal cortex (31). Toxicity to mitochondria of the most affected segments of the proximal tubule should be more complete, and early depletion of cortical ATP (27) indicates a functionally important overall effect on respiration.

Although preservation of the mitochondrial uptake and dehydrogenation of pyruvate (71) allows access of this end product of glycolysis to the tricarboxylic acid (TCA) cycle, respiration cannot be fueled by pyruvate alone if the cycle is disrupted (76). The TCA enzymes are responsible for the catabolism of carbohydrates, fatty acids, and several amino acids (76), all of which enter the cycle by the conjugation of acetylcoenzyme A (acetyl CoA) and oxaloacetate to form citrate (76). Oxaloacetate can enter the mitochondrion directly by the succinate (dicarboxylate) carrier (72), or indirectly through the metabolism of several substrates. Glutamate is a precursor of α-ketoglutarate (oxoglutarate) and therefore of succinate (76). Succinate is a key intermediate in the TCA cycle,[1] as indicated by its rapid mitochondrial transport and metabolism (72,78,79), and is a precursor of oxaloacetate through a series of reactions involving malate as an intermediate (72,76).

Depletion of mitochondrial oxaloacetate through a generalized reduction of substrate uptake will lead to accumulation of the acetyl CoA and its various precursors. High concentrations of acetyl CoA inhibit pyruvate dehydrogenase, thereby blocking ATP production through pyruvate. A resulting accumulation of nonesterified fatty acids could add a further problem. Whereas carbohydrates provide only 10% (fasting) to 30% (fed) of caloric needs, fatty acids are a major source of metabolic energy in renal cortex (80). A cytotoxic role of high intracellular nonesterified fatty acid concentrations has been suggested in several disease states (carnitine deficiency, inborn errors of acylcarnitine metabolism, ischemia, and hypoxia [81–87]).

Mitochondrial transport also plays a direct role in fatty acid catabolism. The long-chain fatty acids cannot cross the inner mitochondrial membrane to be oxidized in the inner matrix unless conjugated to carnitine (81,82). Carnitine, cephaloridine, and cephaloglycin are all zwitterionic at physiological pH (46,82,88), with a carboxyl separated by three or four carbons or nitrogens from a cationic nitrogen (46,81). These structural relationships could facilitate a fit of cephaloridine or cephaloglycin with the regions of the inner membrane that allow fatty acylcarnitine entry.

One could therefore propose two mechanisms by which the impaired mitochondrial substrate transport caused by the toxic β-lactams could inhibit fatty acid catabolism: (a) disruption of the TCA cycle, resulting from injury to the uptake of oxaloacetate and its precursors into the inner matrix (72); and (b) acylation of an acylcarnitine shuttle protein.

Two groups of preliminary studies have been done to test these possibilities: (a) the effects of fasting and carbohydrate loading on the tubular necrosis produced by cephaloglycin; and (b) the effects of *in vivo* cephaloglycin intoxication on mitochondrial palmitoyl carnitine accumulation. Table 7 shows the effects of fasting on the nephrotoxicity of cephaloglycin. Nephrotoxicity was increased by fasting, which increases dependence upon fatty acid catabolism (80), and the augmentation was prevented by glucose, which reverses this increase. An isosmotic isovolemic saline load did not reverse the effects of fasting.

Cephaloglycin, 300 mg/kg IV given 1 hr before sacrifice, produced a small but statistically significant increase of the uptake of trace quantities of ^{14}C-palmitoyl carnitine by isolated mitochondria incubated for 5 min (control 1.02 ± 0.05 vs. cephaloglycin-intoxicated $1.27 \pm 0.06 \times 10^{-5}$ M in mitochondrial water [$n = 12$ each, $p < .001$], from a medium concentration of 0.91×10^{-7} M). The ^{14}C in this isotope is the 1-carbon of the palmitoyl moiety. Thus, the accumulated isotope could reflect one or more of the following, listed in the order of their production:

---

[1]Although succinate is a precursor of heme, and therefore of the cytochromes (77), the cytochrome chain is intact in β-lactam–intoxicated mitochondria at 2 hr (31,70), when cytotoxicity has already begun to develop (19).

TABLE 7. *Effects of fasting and carbohydrate loading on cephaloglycin-induced tubular necrosis*

	Tubular necrosis score[b,c]			
Protocol[a]	0	1	2	3
Control	5	3	0	0
Fasted	2	2	4	0
Fasted + glucose	3	5	0	0
Fasted + saline	1	2	5	0

[a]Rabbits were given a normal diet (control) or denied solid food for 24 hr (fasted). Glucose: 20 ml/kg of a 5% solution infused over a 4-hr period before, and a 10 ml/kg bolus given immediately after, 100 mg/kg of IV cephaloglycin. Saline: the same volume and osmolar load of NaCl before and after the cephaloglycin. Sacrifice 48 hr later for histologic sections of kidney.

[b]Numbers of animals with each proximal tubular necrosis score, from randomly assorted, coded slides (% of tubules necrotic: *0*, 0%, *1*, >0–10%, *2*, >10–25%, *3*, >25%).

[c]Significance levels by exact test, comparing numbers of animals with 0–1 scores (control range) to higher toxicity scores: control vs. fasted, $p = .038$; fasted + glucose vs. fasted + saline, $p = .013$.

palmitoyl carnitine, palmitoyl-CoA, acetyl CoA, a TCA cycle intermediate, or a product of acetate accumulation such as acetoacetate or β-hydroxybutyrate (76).

Augmentation of toxicity by fasting, with a protective effect of glucose but not saline, is consistent with a contributory role of fatty acids in the production of tubular necrosis. The increased mitochondrial ^{14}C from palmitoyl carnitine in cephaloglycin intoxication suggests an accumulation of one or more products of fatty acid catabolism. If the studies of palmitoyl carnitine uptake are supported by further testing, ruling against an injury to the acylcarnitine shuttle, an intramitochondrial decrease of fatty acid catbolism, possibly as a result of depletion of TCA cycle substrates, could provide a plausible explanation for an involvement of fatty acids in β-lactam nephrotoxicity.

CARBAPENEMS: SPECIAL PROPERTIES

Although the pattern of mitochondrial toxicity of imipenem indicates important similarities to the toxic cephalosporins, experience with the carbapenems is too limited to permit the conclusion that they are nephrotoxic by mechanisms identical to those of the cephalosporins. Imipenem differs from the cephalosporins in several respects: (a) although it is secreted by the proximal tubule, imipenem is rapidly hydrolyzed by cytoplasmic and brush border dehydropeptidase I (DHP) to inactive metabolites (8,89); (b) imipenem is very highly reactive, which may allow acylation of mitochondrial anion transporters at comparatively low AUCs (46,90,91); (c) it is marketed in combination with cilastatin, an inhibitor of DHP that also inhibits both its tubular secretion and its nephrotoxicity (8); (d) in an *in vitro* system that bypasses its effect on secretory transport, cilastatin, which has some structural homology with all of the β-lactams (Fig. 1 and 7), partially blocks the mitochondrial toxicity of imipenem, but not of cephaloglycin (74).

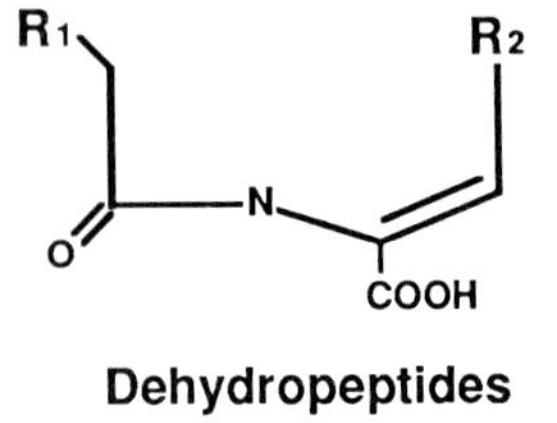

FIG. 7. Core structure of the dehydropeptides, including cilastatin.

Newer carbapenems have been developed that are hydrolyzed significantly less by renal DHP and are less nephrotoxic than imipenem (92,93). The reasons for the lower toxicity of these new carbapenems are not known, but DHP activity does not increase the mitochondrial toxicity of imipenem *in vitro*, ruling against the formation of a toxic by-product of hydrolysis (74).

SUMMARY

The importance of cellular uptake as a contributing factor to β-lactam antibiotic nephrotoxicity has been confirmed by several approaches with each of the toxic β-lactams tested. The suggested role of cytochrome P-450–mediated activation has been largely refuted, except perhaps in the contribution of a cytochrome P-450 reductase to the peroxidative action of cephaloridine. Lipid peroxidation is not a prominent component of the toxicity of cephaloglycin or imipenem, and should not be a primary event in the toxicity of the known toxic cephalosporins other than cephaloridine (25). However, peroxidation does have a role in cephaloridine toxicity.

Toxicity to mitochondrial substrate transport and respiration has been the only consistently observed early effect of the different nephrotoxic β-lactams. Acylation of proteins of the proximal tubular cell, where β-lactam concentrations are 10^2 to 10^4 times antibacterial levels, fits with the rank orders of the nephrotoxic potentials of cephaloglycin, cephalothin, and benzylpenicillin. When viewed in conjunction, the comparative cortical AUCs and reactivities of the cephalosporins also fit with their relative nephrotoxicities. The toxicity of the β-lactams to succinate uptake and respiration in renal cortical mitochondria has features of early reversibility, later irreversibility, and specificity of injury to mitochondrial functions to support the hypothesized acylation of mitochondrial transporters of anionic metabolites. Finally, the oxoglutarate carrier protein from β-lactam intoxicated mitochondria is altered, with a shift in isoelectric point consistent with the addition of a single β-lactam per molecule of protein.

CONCLUSIONS

Nothing that has been demonstrated rules out the possibility of multiple mechanisms of cytotoxic injury by the β-lactams. The lipid peroxidative effects of ceph-

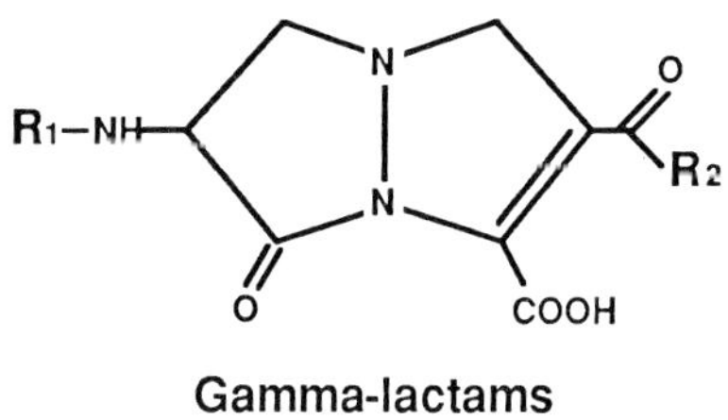

FIG. 8. Basic structure of the γ-lactam antibiotics.

aloridine are impressive, and could be expected from any pyridinium-containing β-lactam that undergoes comparable intracellular sequestration. The mitochondrial toxicity of the β-lactams appears unrelated to peroxidative injury, and we have not yet begun to explore the consequences of acylation of other tubular cell proteins (26). Considering these examples of toxicity by different mechanisms, it is reasonable to expect that newly developed β-lactams may be toxic to the tubular cell by one or more mechanisms if they have high enough intracellular AUCs and their molecular structures convey the potential to do harm.

The newly discovered γ-lactam antibiotics (Fig. 8) may be of interest for the same reasons. The γ-lactams have the basic structure of secreted organic anions (94,95) and a mechanism of antibacterial action much like that of the β-lactams (62,94). The most potent γ-lactams tested so far are more reactive than the most reactive cephalosporins (62). We may, therefore, have in this new class of antibiotics the opportunity to test further the proposed roles of uptake and reactivity in producing nephrotoxicity. Conventional toxicologic studies will require large quantities of each potentially useful γ-lactam, which will be costly to produce. However, if the proposed mechanisms of cytotoxicity are confirmed, methods may be developed to use trace quantities to identify the toxic potential of each γ-lactam.

ACKNOWLEDGMENTS

The work was sponsored by grants from the National Institutes of Health (# DK 33814) and the American Heart Association (# 890665).

REFERENCES

1. Lee CC, Herr EB, Anderson RC. Pharmacological and toxicological studies on cephalothin. *Clin Med* 1963;70:1123–1138.
2. Perkins RL, Apicella MA, Lee IS, Cuppage FE, Saslaw S. Cephaloridine and cephalothin: comparative studies of potential nephrotoxicity. *J Lab Clin Med* 1968;71:75–84.
3. Foord RD. Cephaloridine, cephalothin and the kidney. *J Antimicrob Chemother* 1975;1:119–133.
4. Atkinson RM, Currie JP, Davis B, Pratt DAH, Sharpe HM, Tomich EG. Acute toxicity of cephaloridine, an antibiotic derived from cephalosporin C. *Toxicol Appl Pharmacol* 1966;8:398–406.
5. Welles JS, Bison WR, Harris PN, Small RM, Anderson RC. Toxicity, distribution, and excretion of cephaloridine in laboratory animals. *Antimicrob Agents Chemother* 1966;1965:863–869.
6. Welles JS. Pharmacology and toxicology of cephalosporins. In: Flynn EH, ed. *Cephalosporins and penicillins, chemistry and biology*. New York: Academic Press, 1972;581–608.

7. Bendirdjian J-P, Prime DJ, Browning MC, Hsu C-Y, Tune BM. Additive nephrotoxicity of cephalosporins and aminoglycosides in the rabbit. *J Pharmacol Exp Ther* 1981;218:631–685.
8. Birnbaum J, Kahan FM, Kropp H, MacDonald JS. Carbapenems. A new class of beta-lactam antibiotics. Discovery and improvement of Imipenem/Cilastatin. *Am J Med* 1985;78(suppl 6A):3–21.
9. Tune BM. The nephrotoxicity of cephalosporin antibiotics. Structure-activity relationships. *Comm Toxicol* 1986;1:145–170.
10. Browning MC, Wang PL, Hsu C-Y, Tune BM. Interaction of ischemic and antibiotic-induced injury in the rabbit kidney. *J Infect Dis* 1983;147:341–351.
11. Tune BM, Hsu C-Y. Augmentation of antibiotic nephrotoxicity by endotoxemia in the rabbit. *J Pharmacol Exp Ther* 1985;234:425–430.
12. Tune BM, Hsu C-Y, Fravert D. Mechanisms of the endotoxin-cephalosporin toxic synergy and the protective action of saline in the rabbit kidney. *J Pharmacol Exp Ther* 1988;224:520–525.
13. Klastersky J, Hensgens C, Debusscher L. Empiric therapy for cancer patients: comparative study of ticarcillin-tobramycin, ticarcillin-cephalothin, and cephalothin-tobramycin. *Antimicrob Agents Chemother* 1975;7:640–645.
14. Wade JC, Petty BG, Conrad G, Smith CR, Lipsky JJ, Ellner J, Lietman PS. Cephalothin plus an aminoglycoside is more nephrotoxic than methicillin plus an aminoglycoside. *Lancet* 1978;2:604–606.
15. EORTC International Antimicrobial Therapy Project Group. Three antibiotic regimens in the treatment of infection in febrile granulocytopenic patients with cancer. *J Infect Dis* 1978;137:14–29.
16. Bloch R, Luft FC, Rankin LI, Sloan RS, Yum MN, Maxwell DR. Protection from gentamicin nephrotoxicity by cephalothin and carbenicillin. *Antimicrob Agents Chemother* 1979;15:46–49.
17. Tune BM, Browning MC, Hsu C-Y, Fravert D. Prevention of cephalosporin nephrotoxicity by other cephalosporins and by penicillins without significant inhibition of renal cortical uptake. *J Infect Dis* 1982;145:174–180.
18. English J, Gilbert DN, Kohlhepp S, Kohnen PW, Mayor G, Houghton DC, Bennett WM. Attenuation of experimental tobramycin nephrotoxicity by ticarcillin. *Antimicrob Agents Chemother* 1985; 27:897–902.
19. Silverblatt F, Turck M, Bulger R. Nephrotoxicity due to cephaloridine: a light- and electron-microscopic study in rabbits. *J Infect Dis* 1970;122:33–44.
20. Tune BM, Fravert D. Mechanisms of cephalosporin nephrotoxicity. A comparison of cephaloridine and cephaloglycin. *Kidney Int* 1980;18:591–600.
21. Wang PL, Prime DJ, Hsu C-Y, Tune BM. Effects of ureteral obstruction on the toxicity of cephalosporins in the rabbit kidney. *J Infect Dis* 1982;145:574–581.
22. Tune BM, Fravert D, Hsu C-Y. Thienamycin nephrotoxicity: mitochondrial injury and oxidative effects of imipenem in the rabbit kidney. *Biochem Pharmacol* 1989;38:3779–3783.
23. Tune BM. Effect of organic acid transport inhibitors on renal cortical uptake and proximal tubular toxicity of cephaloridine. *J Pharmacol Exp Ther* 1972;181:250–256.
24. McMurtry RJ, Mitchell JR. Renal and hepatic necrosis after metabolic activation of 2-substituted furans and thiophenes, including furosemide and cephaloridine. *Toxicol Appl Pharmacol* 1977;42: 285–300.
25. Kuo C-H, Maita K, Slieght SD, Hook JB. Lipid peroxidation: a possible mechanism of cephaloridine-induced nephrotoxicity. *Toxicol Appl Pharmacol* 1983:67:78–88.
26. Browning MC, Tune BM. The reactivity and binding of beta-lactam antibiotics in rabbit renal cortex. *J Pharmacol Exp Ther* 1983;226:640–644.
27. Goldstein RS, Contardi LR, Pasino DA, Hook JB. Mechanisms mediating cephaloridine inhibition of gluconeogenesis. *Toxicol Appl Pharmacol* 1987;87:297–305.
28. Cojocel C, Kramer W, Mayer D. Depletion of cytochrome P-450 and alterations of activities of drug metabolizing enzymes induced by cephaloridine in the rat kidney cortex. *Biochem Pharmacol* 1988; 37:3781–3785.
29. Tune BM, Wu KY. Longerbeam D, Holtzman D. Renal transport and toxicity of cephalosporins, including effects on tubular and mitochondrial respiration. In: Lemieux G, ed. *Proceedings of the Seventh International Congress of Nephrology*. Basel: S. Karger, 1978;279–287.
30. Tune BM, Wu KY, Fravert D, Holtzman D. Effect of cephaloridine on respiration by renal cortical mitochondira. *J Pharmacol Exp Ther* 1979;210:98–100.
31. Tune BM, Fravert D. Cephalosporin nephrotoxicity. Transport, cytotoxicity and mitochondrial toxicity of cephaloglycin. *J Pharmacol Exp Ther* 1980;215:186–190.
32. Tune BM, Sibley RK, Hsu C-Y. The mitochondrial respiratory toxicity of cephalosporin antibiotics. An inhibitory effect on substrate uptake. *J Pharmacol Exp Ther* 1988;245:1054–1059.

33. Tune BM, Burg MB, Patlak CS. Characteristics of *p*-aminohippurate transport in proximal renal tubules. *Am J Physiol* 1969;217:1057–1063.
34. Tune BM, Fernholt M. Relationship between cephaloridine and *p*-aminohippurate transport in the kidney. *Am J Physiol* 1973;225:1114–1117.
35. Brogard JM, Comte F, Pinget M. Pharmacokinetics of cephalosporin antibiotics. *Antibiot Chemother* 1978;25:123–162.
36. Tune BM, Wu KY, Longerbeam DF, Kempson RL. Transport and toxicity of cephaloridine in the kidney. Effect of flurosemide, *p*-aminohippurate and saline diuresis. *J Pharmacol Exp Ther* 1977; 202:472–478.
37. Tune BM. Cephalosporin nephrotoxicity. Mechanisms and modifying factors. In: Porter G, ed. *Nephrotoxic mechanisms of drugs and environmental toxins*. New York: Plenum, 1982;151–164.
38. Tune BM, Fernholt M, Schwartz A. Mechanism of cephaloridine transport in the kidney. *J Pharmacol Exp Ther* 1974;191:311–317.
39. Wold JS, Turnipseed SA, Miller BL. The effect of renal cation transport on cephaloridine nephrotoxicity. *Toxicol Appl Pharmacol* 1979;45:115–122.
40. Williams PD, Hitchcock MJM, Hottendorf GH. Effect of cephalosporins on organic ion transport in renal membrane vesicles from rat and rabbit kidney cortex. *Res Commun Chem Pathol Pharmacol* 1985;47:357–369.
41. Tune BM. Relationship between the transport and toxicity of cephalosporins in the kidney. *J Infect Dis* 1975;132:189–194.
42. Pasino DA, Miura K, Goldstein RS, Hook JB. Cephaloridine nephrotoxicity: strain and sex differences in mice. *Fundam Appl Toxicol* 1985;5:1153–1160.
43. Wold JS, Joost RR, Owen NV. Nephrotoxicity of cephaloridine in newborn rabbits: role of the renal anionic transport system. *J Pharmacol Exp Ther* 1977;201:778–785.
44. Tune BM, Wu KY, Kempson RL. Inhibition of transport and prevention of toxicity of cephaloridine in the kidney. Dose-responsiveness of the rabbit and the guinea pig to probenecid. *J Pharmacol Exp Ther* 1977;202:466–471.
45. Wold JS, Turnipseed SA. The effect of renal cation transport inhibitors on the *in vivo* and *in vitro* accumulation and efflux of cephaloridine. *Life Sci* 1980;27:2559–2564.
46. Hoover JRE. Beta-lactam antibiotics: structure-activity relationships. In: Demain AL, Solomon NA, eds. *Handbook of experimental pharmacology, vol 67/II. Beta-lactam antibiotics*. Berlin: Springer-Verlag, 1983;119–245.
47. Tune BM, Kuo D-H, Hook JB, Hsu C-Y, Fravert D. Effects of piperonyl butoxide on cephalosporin nephrotoxicity in the rabbit. An effect on cephaloridine transport. *J Pharmacol Exp Ther* 1983; 224:520–524.
48. Kuo C-H, Tune BM, Hook JB. Effect of piperonyl butoxide on organic anion and cation transport in rabbit kidneys. *Proc Soc Exp Biol Med* 1983;174:165–171.
49. Kuo C-H, Hook JB. Depletion of renal cortical glutathione and nephrotoxicity by cephaloridine, cephalothin and gentamicin in male Sprague-Dawley rats. *Life Sci* 1982;31:255–260.
50. Kuo C-H, Hook JB. Depletion of renal glutathione content and nephrotoxicity of cephaloridine in rabbits, rats, and mice. *Toxicol Appl Pharmacol* 1982;63:292–302.
51. Cojocel C, Hannemann J, Baumann K. Cephaloridine-induced lipid peroxidation by reactive oxygen species as a possible mechanism of cephaloridine nephrotoxicity. *Biochem Biophys Acta* 1985;834: 402–410.
52. Cojocel C, Laeschke KH, Inselmann G, Baumann K. Inhibition of cephaloridine-induced lipid peroxidation. *Toxicology* 1985;35:295–305.
53. Goldstein RS, Pasino DA, Hewitt WR, Hook JB. Biochemical mechanisms of cephaloridine nephrotoxicity: time and concentration dependence of peroxidative injury. *Toxicol Appl Pharmacol* 1986; 87:297–305.
54. Tune BM, Fravert D, Hsu C-Y. The oxidative and mitochondrial toxic effects of cephalosporin antibiotics in the kidney. A comparative study of cephaloridine and cephaloglycin. *Biochem Pharmacol* 1989;38:795–802.
55. Cojocel C, Hannemann J, Inselmann G, Laeschke KH, Baumann K. Lipid peroxidation, a possible mechanism of cephalosporin induced nephrotoxicity. *Pflugers Arch* 1984;400(suppl):R19.
56. Tipper DJ, Strominger JL. Mechanism of action of penicillins: a proposal based on their structural similarity to acyl-D-analyl-D-alanine. *Proc Natl Acad Sci USA* 1965;541:1133–1141.
57. Waxman DJ, Strominger JL. Penicillin binding proteins and the mechanism of action of beta-lactam antibiotics. *Annu Rev Biochem* 1983;52:825–869.
58. Indelicato JM, Norvillas TT, Pfeiffer RR, Wheeler WJ, Wilham WL. Substituent effects upon the

base hydrolysis of penicillins and cephalosporins. Comparative intramolecular nucleophilic amino attack in cephalosporins. *J Med Chem* 1974;17:523–527.
59. Indelicato JM, Dinner A, Peters LR, Wilham WL. Hydrolysis of 3-chloro-3-cephems. Intramolecular nucleophillic attack in cefaclor. *J Med Chem* 1977;20:961–963.
60. Yamana T, Tsuji A, Kanayama K, Nakano O. Comparative stabilities of cephalosporins in aqueous solution. *J Antibiot* 1974;27:1000–1002.
61. Yamana T, Tsuji A. Comparative stability of cephalosporins in aqueous solution: kinetics and mechanisms of degradation. *J Pharm Sci* 1976;65:1563–1574.
62. Indelicato JM, Pasini CE. The acylating potential of gamma-lactam antibacterials: base hydrolysis of bicyclic pyrazolidinones. *J Med Chem* 1988;31:1227–1230.
63. Capel-Edwards K, Pratt DAH. Renal tolerance of ceftazidime in animals. *J Antimicrob Chemother* 1981;8(suppl B):241–245.
64. EORTC International Antimicrobial Therapy Cooperative Group. Ceftazidime combined with a short or long course of amikacin for empirical therapy of gram-negative bacteremia in cancer patients with granulocytopenia. *N Engl J Med* 1987;317:1692–1698.
65. Browning MC, Tune BM. Toxicology of the beta-lactam antibiotics. In: Demain AL, Solomon NA, eds. *Handbook of experimental pharmacology, Vol 67/II. Beta-lactam antibiotics*. Berlin: Springer-Verlag, 1983;371–397.
66. Kramer W, Cojocel C, Mayer D. Specific alterations of rat renal microsomal proteins induced by cephaloridine. *Biochem Pharmacol* 1988;37:4135–4140.
67. Trump BF, Bulger RE. Studies of cellular injury in isolated flounder tubules. IV. Electron microscopic observations of changes during the phase of altered homeostasis in tubules treated with cyanide. *Lab Invest* 1968;18:731–739.
68. Venkatachalam MA, Bernard DB, Donohoe JF, Levinsky NG. Ischemic damage and repair in the rat proximal tubule: differences among the S_1, S_2, and S_3 segments. *Kidney Int* 1978;14:31–49.
69. Silverblatt F. Pathogenesis of nephrotoxicity of cephalosporins and aminoglycosides: a review of current concepts. *Rev Infect Dis* 1982;4:S360–S365.
70. Bendirdjian J-P, Prime DJ, Browning MD,Tune BM. The mitochondrial respiratory toxicity of cephalosporins. Molecular properties and pathogenic significance. In: Fillastre JP, ed. *Nephrotoxicity, ototoxicity of drugs*. Rouen: Editions INSERM, 1982;303–319.
71. Tune BM, Hsu C-Y. The renal mitochondrial toxicity of cephalosporins: specificity of the effect on anionic substrate uptake. *J Pharmacol Exp Ther* 1990;252:65–69.
72. Tzagoloff A. Mitochondrial transport systems. In: Tzagoloff A, ed. *Mitochondria*. New York: Plenum, 1982;199–233.
73. Alberts B, Bray D, Lewis J, Raff M, Roberts K, Watson JD. Energy conversion: mitochondria and chloroplasts. In: Alberts B, Bray D, Lewis J, Raff M, Roberts K, Watson JD. *Molecular biology of the cell*, 2nd ed. New York: Garland, 1989;342–404.
74. Tune BM, Hsu C-Y. The renal mitochondrial toxicity of beta-lactam antibiotics: in vitro effects of cephaloglycin and imipenem. *J Am Soc Nephrol* 1990;1:815–821.
75. Bisaccia F, Indiveri C, Palmieri F. Purification and reconstitution of two anion carriers from rat liver mitochondria: the dicarboxylate and the 2-oxoglutarate carrier. *Biochim Biophys Acta* 1988;933: 229–240.
76. Stryer L. Citric acid cycle. In: Stryer L, ed. *Biochemistry*, 3rd ed. New York: WH Freeman, 1988; 373–397.
77. Orten JM, Neuhaus OW. Blood. In: Orten JM, Neuhaus OW, eds. *Human biochemistry*. St Louis: CV Mosby, 1982;434–475.
78. Klingenberg M. Overview on mitochondrial metabolite transport systems. *Methods Enzymol* 1979; 56:245–252.
79. Estabrook RW. Mitochondrial respiratory control and the polarographic measurement of ADP: O ratios. *Methods Enzymol* 1967;10:41–47.
80. Wiedemann MJ, Krebs HA. The fuel of respiration in rat renal cortex. *Biochem J* 1969;112: 149–166.
81. Stryer L. Fatty acid metabolism. In: Stryer L, ed. *Biochemistry*, 3rd ed. New York: WH Freeman, 1988;469–494.
82. Borum PR. Carnitine. *Annu Rev Nutr* 1983;3:233–259.
83. Neely JR, Feuvray D. Metabolic products and myocardial ischemia. *Am J Pathol* 1981;102: 282–291.
84. Boime I, Smith EE, Hunter EJ Jr. The role of fatty acids in mitochondrial changes during liver ischemia. *Arch Biochem Biophys* 1970;139:425–443.

85. Idell-Wenger JA, Grotyohann LW, Neely JR. Coenzyme A and carnitine distribution in normal and ischemic hearts. *J Biol Chem* 1978;253:4310–4318.
86. Smith MW, Collan Y, Kahng MW, Trump BJ. Changes in mitochondrial lipids of rat kidney during ischemia. *Biochim Biophys Acta* 1980;618:192–201.
87. Whitmer JT, Idell-Wenger JA, Rovetto MJ, Neely JA. Control of fatty acid metabolism in ischemic and hypoxic hearts. *J Biol Chem* 1978;253:4305–4309.
88. Inui K-I, Takano M, Okano T, Hori R. H^+ gradient-dependent transport of aminocephalosporins in rat renal brush border membranes. H^+/organic cation transport system. *J Pharmacol Exp Ther* 1985;233:181–185.
89. Kropp H, Sundelof JG, Hajdu R, Kahan FM. Metabolism of thienamycin and related carbapenem antibiotics by the renal dipeptidase, dehydropeptidase-I. *Antimicrob Agents Chemother* 1982;22: 62–70.
90. Kahan JS, Kahan FM, Goegelman R, Currie SA, Jackson M, Stapley EO, Miller TW, Miller AK, Hendlin D, Mochales S, Hernandez S, Woodruff HB, Birnbaum J. Thienamycin, a dew beta-lactam antibiotic. I. Discovery, taxonomy, isolation and physical properties. *J Antibiot* 1978;32:1–12.
91. Kropp H, Sundelof JG, Kahan JS, Kahan FM, Birnbaum J. MK0787 (*N*-formimidoyl thienamycin): evaluation of *in vitro* and *in vivo* activities. *Antimicrob Agents Chemother* 1980;17:993–1000.
92. Brughera M, Scampini G, Ferrari ML, Nava A, Mazué G. Toxicologic profile of FCE 22101 and its orally available ester FCE 22891. *J Antimicrob Chemother* 1989;23(suppl C):129–135.
93. Topham JC, Murgatroyd LB, Jones DV, Goonetilleke UR, Wright J. Safety evaluation of meropenem in animals: studies on the kidney. *J Antimicrob Chemother* 1989;24(suppl A):287–306.
94. Allen NE, Hobbs JN Jr, Preston DA, Turner JR, Wu CYE. Antibacterial properties of the bicyclic pyrazolidinones. *J Antibiot* 1990;43:92–99.
95. Møller JV, Sheikh MI. Renal organic anion transport system: pharmacological, physiological, and biochemical aspects. *Pharm Rev* 1983;34:315–358.

Toxicology of the Kidney, Second Edition,
edited by Jerry B. Hook and Robin S. Goldstein.
Raven Press, Ltd., New York © 1993.

10

The Nephrotoxicity of Antineoplastic Drugs

Richard F. Borch

Department of Pharmacology, University of Rochester Medical Center, School of Medicine and Dentistry, Rochester, New York 14642

Most of the drugs currently in use as anticancer agents are characterized by their potent cytotoxicity and their low therapeutic index. Nephrotoxicity, however, is a relatively infrequent side effect despite the high renal blood flow and tubular concentrating ability of the kidney, facilitating delivery of high dose intensities. In addition, the kidney is a vulnerable target for the free radical and highly electrophilic intermediates generated by the metabolism of many of these drugs. The nephrotoxicity of agents commonly used in chemotherapy has been extensively reviewed (1–7). The emphasis of this chapter will be primarily on the recent investigations of the mechanisms of kidney damage resulting from the agents presented in Table 1.

ASSESSMENT OF KIDNEY DAMAGE

During chemotherapy, the systematic evaluation of renal function is crucial for both drugs primarily excreted through the kidney and drugs that are known to induce nephrotoxicity. The most common and the most widely used parameter for measuring renal function is creatinine clearance. However, due to the problems inherent in collecting reliable 24-hr urine measurements, the creatinine clearance factor is frequently calculated based upon serum creatinine, age, and weight. In patients undergoing chemotherapy, a poor correlation was found between the measured and calculated clearances ($r = 0.40$). Thus, for this population, the calculated clearance is not a useful parameter in assessment of renal function (8). In addition, creatinine clearance is relatively insensitive to low levels of renal damage.

Several more sensitive methods have been developed to evaluate early tubule injury by chemotherapeutic agents. Increased urinary excretion of *N*-acetyl-β-D-glucosaminidase (NAG) and alanine aminopeptidase (AAP), enzymes preferentially localized on proximal tubule cells, and β_2-microglobulin, a small protein that is freely filtered and almost completely reabsorbed in the proximal tubule, has been used to determine proximal tubule damage following chemotherapy (9,10). Immu-

TABLE 1. *Anticancer drugs exhibiting clinical nephrotoxicity*

Adriamycin
Celiptinium
Methotrexate
Mitomycin C
Streptozotocin
Semustine
Cisplatin

nochemical and enzyme-linked immunosorbent assay (ELISA) detection assays with high specificity for proximal tubule cellular antigens excreted in urine have also been developed (11,12). For example, urine adenosine deaminase–binding protein (ADB) was measured using an ADB-specific monoclonal antibody. Using this assay, urinary ADB increased over fivefold following administration of cisplatin. Similar results were obtained following exposure to ifosfamide and methotrexate. For all three agents, the increase in ADB preceded an increase in serum creatinine (13). Immunochemical analysis using distal tubule–specific antigens in urine has been used to determine injury to distal tubules (14).

ADRIAMYCIN

Adriamycin (doxorubicin) is an anthracycline antibiotic that is used for treatment of solid as well as of disseminated tumors. The dose-limiting toxicity of Adriamycin is manifested as a cumulative and irreversible dose-dependent cardiomyopathy that leads to congestive heart failure (CHF). At present, there is no evidence for primary Adriamycin-induced nephrotoxicity at the clinical doses currently in use. Any renal effects observed in patients are similar to those seen in CHF of other etiologies.

In rats, Adriamycin induces a nephrotic syndrome exemplified by acute glomerular injury and sustained proteinuria. The characteristic features include epithelial cell detachment, cytoplasmic vacuolization, glomerular epithelial cell alterations, glomerular anionic charge loss, and foot process fusion (15). Nonselective glomerular lesions in the juxtamedullary nephrons result in proteinuria (16). Proteinuria does not seem to occur in the cortical glomeruli. Stimulation of glomerular metabolism by Adriamycin also appears to be selective for juxtaglomerular glomeruli (17). The early glomerular effects of Adriamycin, increased water permeability and reduced adenosine triphosphatase (ATPase) activity, are oxygen dependent and are inhibited by *N*-acetylcysteine. The increase in sieving coefficient for albumin is not dependent upon oxygen (18).

Recent investigations suggest that platelet activating factor (PAF) may be a mediator of Adriamycin-induced nephrotoxicity. PAF, synthesized by mesangial cells, induces the loss of glomerular anionic charge. In rats treated with Adriamycin, PAF antagonists have been shown to prevent ultrastructural glomerular alterations and proteinuria (15). The interactions of Adriamycin with other drugs may be important in understanding the underlying mechanisms of Adriamycin-induced nephropathy. In a study using the combination of Adriamycin and nitrosourea CCNU, results suggest that the CCNU-induced cholestasis modifies the Adriamycin-induced biliary excretion. The compensatory increase in renal Adriamycin excretion results in earlier and more severe glomerular alterations (19).

CELIPTINIUM

Celiptinium (9-hydroxy-2-methylellipticinium acetate) is a novel DNA interacting agent used in treatment of metastatic breast cancer. Lack of significant observed hematologic toxicity is an attractive feature of this chemotherapeutic agent. However, in approximately 5% of patients, renal insufficiency has been detected. Acute renal failure appears to correlate with dose intensity, whereas chronic renal failure seems to be related to cumulative dose (20). Autopsy reports indicate that renal lesions are tubular and consist primarily of epithelial necrosis. No interstitial or glomerular abnormalities have been observed.

In rats treated with deliptinium, acute toxicity studies indicate increases in urinary enzymes characteristic of proximal tubule injury. These include irreversible diffuse renal lesions with tubular necrosis, luminal dilation, and interstitial infiltrates (21). In addition, celiptinium exposure induced lipid overload in cortical tubule cells and significant changes in lipid peroxidation in the renal cortex (22). Peroxidative damage was found mainly in brush border membranes and to some extent in the mitochondrial and microsomal membranes (23), suggesting that celiptinium-induced lipid peroxidation in the proximal tubule cell contributes to the pathogenesis of celiptinium nephrotoxicity.

METHOTREXATE AND RELATED AGENTS

Methotrexate, a well-established chemotherapeutic agent, has significant effects on a wide variety of solid tumors, including head and neck cancers, breast cancer, and osteogenic sarcoma (24). Its main dose-limiting side effects are myelosuppression and gastrointestinal toxicity. Both methotrexate and its 7-hydroxy metabolite are excreted through the kidney by tubular secretion and glomerular filtration. This results in high luminal concentrations of both compounds. Drug doses in excess of 1 g/m^2 can result in luminal concentrations that exceed the solubility limit. The subsequent crystallization leads to tubular obstruction accompanied by a 50% reduction in glomerular filtration rate (25). In addition, acute deterioration of kidney function was accompanied by tubular damage, as indicated by significant increases in urinary β_2-microglobulin and NAG excretion. Diltiazem, a calcium channel blocker, had no visible effect on urinary enzyme excretion or on serum creatinine levels (26). Both methotrexate and its metabolite are weak organic acids that are significantly more soluble at neutral pH than in the weakly acidic environment of the tubular lumen. Thus, the obstructive nephropathy observed in patients undergoing methotrexate treatment can be dramatically reduced with intensive hydration and alkalinization of the urine (27).

Maintaining adequate renal function is crucial in patients undergoing methotrexate treatment. When clearance is diminished, plasma methotrexate concentrations increase, thereby leading to increased renal and nonrenal toxicity. Nephrotoxicity can be significantly greater in response to methotrexate in conjunction with other compounds. Special attention must be given to these indications when the drug is administered in combination with other nephrotoxic agents such as cisplatin (28). Treatment with leucovorin (tetrahydrofolate) appears to counter the cytotoxic effects of methotrexate in proliferating tissues (29). However, renal function does not seem to be restored by this drug.

Other antifolate agents related to methotrexate have been developed with the intent of enhancing anticancer activity while reducing toxicity. In several preclinical models, trimetrexate, a second-generation folate antagonist, has shown superior antitumor activity to that of methotrexate. The compound is eliminated primarily through metabolism but 10% to 20% is excreted in the urine (30). Thus far, in early clinical trials, trimetrexate has shown minimal nephrotoxicity both when administered alone and in combination with cisplatin (31). Urine flow and the renal clearance of trimetrexate were significantly increased in combination chemotherapy with cisplatin, whereas nonrenal clearance was unaffected. Although tremetrexate clearance seems to correlate with urine flow, the mechanism that alters clearance is not known.

Dichloromethotrexate has been under investigation for many years in the hope that its predominantly nonrenal elimination would be advantageous over methotrexate, especially in combination with other chemotherapeutic agents, such as cisplatin. However, for dichloromethotrexate, hepatotoxicity was the dose-limiting factor and its clearance from plasma was inversely related to the extent of liver damage (32). Therefore, further development of this drug seems unlikely. In preclinical trials, *N*10-propargyl-5,8-dideazafolic acid (CB 3717), a potent inhibitor of thymidylate synthetase, exhibits impressive antitumor activity. However, significant dose-dependent nephrotoxicity accompanied by dose-independent hepatotoxicity was observed in phase I trials (33,34).

MITOMYCIN C

Mitomycin C, another antibiotic, undergoes reductive conversion to reactive intermediates that then alkylate and cross-link DNA (35,36). The half-life of mitomycin C in plasma is less than 15 min and its clearance is due primarily to rapid metabolism in the liver and other tissues. Renal excretion accounts for less than 10% (37). The most significant toxicity observed in patients is myelosuppression and is related to the cumulative dose. Clinically, nephrotoxicity occurs both in fulminant and in indolent forms (38). Most commonly, the disease is characterized by the delayed onset of a hemolytic-uremic syndrome accompanied by renal microangiopathic hemolytic anemia (39). The induction mechanism of this syndrome by mitomycin C is not known. Although rats treated with mitomycin C exhibit proximal tubule damage and leakage of adenosine triphosphate (ATP) (40), when the drug is perfused directly into the rat kidney, the resulting endothelial cell damage and microangiopathic lesions are indistinguishable from the hemolytic-uremic syndrome described in patients (41). Clinically, mitomycin C–induced nephrotoxicity has an incidence of 2% to 10%. For example, in one study, 14 out of 143 patients showed signs of renal damage and 6 of these died as a result of renal failure (38). Unfortunately, patient sensitivity to mitomycin C is highly variable; at this time, predictive laboratory tests are unavailable, and the progression of renal damage is irreversible.

Studies indicate that mitomycin C–induced renal toxicity is dependent upon the cumulative dose, with very low incidence at doses less than 50 mg/m^2, and approximately 25% frequency at doses greater than 70 mg/m^2 (42). In one recent case report, for example, mitomycin C–induced nephrotoxicity and resulting renal failure necessitated the establishment of chronic hemodialysis for the patient (43).

NITROSOUREAS

Streptozotocin

Streptozotocin, an alkylating agent, is used for the treatment of carcinoid and islet cell tumors (44). The agent is cleared quite rapidly through renal excretion. Nephrotoxicity is generally the dose-limiting factor and is usually mild and reversible. It is characterized by a decrease in creatinine clearance, seen in 20% to 30% of patients, and by the onset of proteinuria 2 to 3 weeks following treatment in 50% to 70% of patients. Although proteinuria is the first clinical sign of nephrotoxicity, the primary lesion is at the level of the proximal tubules (45,46). Although streptozotocin-induced renal toxicity is not strictly dose-dependent, incidence increases dramatically with cumulative doses in excess of 4 g/m^2. Normal kidney function is restored within weeks of termination of treatment, especially if this occurs immediately at the first indication of onset of proteinuria.

Other Nitrosoureas

Carmustine (BCNU), lomustine (CCNU), and semustine (methyl-CCNU), all lipophilic nitrosoureas, are antitumor agents used in treatment of brain and gastrointestinal cancers. These agents are metabolized rapidly and the intermediary compounds are eliminated primarily through the urine (47). The incidence of nephrotoxicity at a clinically significant level appears to be much lower for carmustine and lomustine than it is for semustine (48,49). Semustine-induced renal toxicity is related to cumulative dose of the drug, is mainly at the proximal tubule, and can be delayed for 1 or 2 years following therapy (48). There is a gradual decrease in creatinine clearance followed by progressive and irreversible kidney failure. Clinical manifestations include interstitial fibrosis, glomerulosclerosis, and tubular degeneration. Restricting the total administered dose to no more than 1,200 mg/m^2 can minimize the risk of renal failure. Although the mechanisms of semustine-induced toxicity have not yet been determined, preclinical results suggest that the nephrotoxic agent is the alkylating rather than the carbamoylating metabolite. Rats pretreated with buthionine sulfoximine (BSO) showed increased renal damage compared with animals treated with semustine alone (50). At similar concentrations, chlorozotocin is known to be more toxic than semustine despite its lower efficacy as a carbamoylating agent (51).

CISPLATIN

Cisplatin ranks as one of the most commonly used drugs in the treatment of solid tumors (52). Its mechanism of action is similar to those of alkylating agents. Cisplatin interacts with the nucleophilic sites on DNA that can result in both inter- and intrastrand cross-linking. Myelosuppression, gastrointestinal toxicity, neurotoxicity, and nephrotoxicity are the most frequently observed adverse reactions. Although cisplatin-induced nephrotoxicity has been recently reviewed in several sources (5,6,53), the present emphasis will be on the studies of mechanisms and modulation of renal toxicity.

The kidney is the critical organ in the metabolism of cisplatin. It is responsible for most of the platinum excretion and is a major site for accumulation as well as for retention. In currently used protocols, the kidney is the major determinant of dose-limiting toxicity. During the first 4 hr following treatment by bolus injection, approximately half of the total dose is eliminated renally and pharmacokinetic analysis of both total and free platinum in patients reveals a biphasic pattern. For total platinum, the half-life of the alpha component is 48 min and of the beta component, 20 to 80 hr. For both components, the half-life of free platinum is less than 50 min. These observations suggest that the slow terminal phase is associated with protein-bound platinum. Within 3 hr of bolus injection, approximately 90% of the platinum becomes bound to protein. Fractional clearance of cisplatin by the kidney is greater than 1 (54), whereas clearance of ultrafilterable platinum is nonlinear (55). These observations suggest a renal handling mechanism involving net tubular secretion, saturable absorption, and glomerular filtration. Data using perfused rat kidney indicate that although filtration is not an essential requirement for induction of renal toxicity, cisplatin transport from a basolateral site is important (56).

Acute proximal tubule dysfunction indicates the onset of renal toxicity by cisplatin. Although blood flow in the kidney and glomerular filtration rate (GFR) are not altered following drug administration, proximal absorption rates of water and sodium are diminished and fluid delivery out of the proximal tubule is increased dramatically (53,57,58). The observed reduction in the rate of sodium reabsorption may be a result of inhibition of sodium entry at the apical membrane (59). Increased renal excretion in patients of NAG and β_2-microglobulin, both of which are proximal tubule markers, is indicative of initial proximal tubule damage. Although reabsorption of water and sodium increases in the more distal segments, this does not compensate for the decrease in proximal tubule reabsorption and results in net diuresis. Seventy-two hours following administration, GFR and renal blood flow are dramatically decreased, possibly the result of increased vascular resistance and decreased filtration pressure (60). Impaired sodium transport in the thick ascending limb of Henle and further deterioration of distal and proximal reabsorption results in increased polyuria (61). Although diminished kidney function as measured by creatinine clearance seems to be cumulative, decreased GFR is dependent upon single dose. Cisplatin-induced acute renal failure cannot be inhibited by verpamil or by captopril (62,63). These observations suggest that the renin-angiotensin system does not play an important role in the reduction of GFR by cisplatin (64). However, atrial natriuretic factor can modulate, but not completely reverse, the cisplatin-induced decrease in GFR (65). Renal magnesium depletion is observed in all patients undergoing cisplatin treatment (66) and magnesium supplementation is a standard and necessary component of the accompanying hydration therapy. Although the mechanisms of cisplatin-induced decrease in magnesium reabsorption are not clear, some data indicate involvement of the loop of Henle (67).

Mechanisms of Renal Toxicity

Despite extensive studies and numerous hypotheses, the specific mechanisms that result in selective damage to the proximal tubule remain unclear. Selective toxicity may be in part due to transport-dependent drug localization. Platinum preferentially accumulates in the pars recta of the proximal tubule, also the site of maximal necrosis. Correlations have also been observed between kidney damage in patients and platinum concentrations in the cortex (68). Studies of cisplatin interactions with both the anion and cation transport systems in Sperber chicken preparations (69), rat tubule membrane preparations (70), and rat kidney cortical slices (71) suggest that both transporters may contribute to cisplatin concentration. In patients administered cisplatin by continuous infusion, net tubular secretion of platinum can be inhibited by probenecid (72). Renal tubule transport of cisplatin, however, does not account for the observed selective nephrotoxicity. Platinum analogues, carboplatin and iproplatin, have comparable fractional renal clearances to cisplatin but do not cause nephrotoxicity (73).

Renal toxicity attributed to cisplatin may be due to the presence of one or more metabolites. These may be generated within the tubule cells or may be produced in other tissues and transported to the kidney. Studies of toxicity and pharmacokinetics of cisplatin metabolites have been performed using rat models (74–76). Mixed metabolites, when administered to tumor-bearing rats and also to mice, were more nephrotoxic than cisplatin on a molar basis but showed minimal antineoplastic activity. Specific metabolites responsible for the renal effects were not identified.

In the rat, methionine pretreatment increased cisplatin-dependent toxicity (77). However, the 1:1 methionine/cisplatin adduct was not nephrotoxic (75). *In vitro* studies with porcine proximal tubule cells (LLC-PK_1) suggest that extracellular metabolites are not necessary for cisplatin-induced tubule damage (78). One-hour incubation with cisplatin under conditions that permit the existence of stable extracellular cisplatin produced a similar level of cytotoxicity to that observed *in vivo*. When cisplatin is preincubated with methionine, cysteine, or glutathione, treatment of LLC-PK_1 cells with the mixtures diminished toxicity (79).

The binding of cisplatin to specific proteins affects biological activity in varying ways. Although binding to immunoglobulins does not appear to affect activity (80), cisplatin binding causes cross-linking and inactivation of α_2-macroglobulin (81). Cisplatin can bind both irreversibly through a cysteine sulfhydryl moiety (82) and via a nonspecific reversible interaction (73) to inhibit essential enzyme activities within the proximal tubule. Cisplatin-induced inhibition of several enzymes has been investigated *in vitro* (83). These include, most notably, ATPase (84–86) and γ-glutamyl transpeptidase (87). Carboplatin and iproplatin, nontoxic analogues of cisplatin, do not inhibit ATPase (88), whereas diethyldithiocarbamate, a renal protector, restores the activity of γ-glutamyl transpeptidase (87) and of macroglobulin (81). Significant inhibition of specific enzyme activities by cisplatin has not been reported *in vivo* (88,89). Na-K–ATPase activity was diminished in the inner stripe of the outer medulla and in the renal cortex of rats treated with cisplatin. However, since this inhibition becomes apparent 5 to 7 days following treatment, it may be a result of the toxicity rather than a mechanism by which toxicity is induced (61). Enzyme inhibition by cisplatin has not been established as a mechanism for induction of nephrotoxicity.

Recent data suggest that inhibition of synthesis of renal macromolecules may be important in cisplatin-induced toxicity. When rabbit renal proximal tubule cells are exposed to cisplatin *in vitro*, after 24 hr, a dose-dependent decrease in cell viability is observed. Although ATPase, alkaline phosphatase, and succinic dehydrogenase activities remained essentially unchanged 6 hr after exposure, DNA, RNA, and protein synthesis were significantly diminished (86). Similarly, incubation of LLC-PK_1 cells with cisplatin for 1 hr resulted in decreased nucleic acid and protein synthesis (78). The effect on DNA synthesis occurred at both nontoxic and toxic doses and was independent of cisplatin concentration. Inhibition of RNA and protein synthesis, however, increased with cisplatin dose and inversely correlated with cell viability. The renal protector, diethyldithiocarbamate, administered for 1 hr immediately following cisplatin treatment, improved cell viability, and restored protein synthesis, but did not affect cisplatin-inhibited RNA synthesis. Thus, the effects of cisplatin on protein synthesis may be an important mechanism in the induction of toxicity in proximal tubule cells.

Cisplatin has been shown to result in oxidative damage in several studies with an indirect correlation with renal toxicity. The agent increased malondialdehyde production and decreased gluconeogenesis, *p*-aminohippurate and tetraethylammonium uptake in a dose- and time-dependent manner in rabbit and rat kidney slices. Antioxidants diminished these effects on cation and anion uptake as well as on malondialdehyde production. No significant change was observed in cisplatin-inhibited gluconeogenesis (90,91). Cisplatin induces lipid peroxidation and depletes glutathione (GSH) in rat kidney cortical slices. Antioxidants counteract the effects on peroxidation but not on GSH depletion. These observations suggest that lipid peroxidation results from a mechanism distinct from effects on GSH levels (92). Cisplatin treatment of rat kidney cells *in vitro* produced an increase in lipid peroxides followed by leakage of enzymes into the medium (93). Mannitol is used in standard protocols as a modulator of cisplatin toxicity because of its osmotic diuretic effect. In addition, mannitol counteracts the cisplatin-induced increase in lipid peroxidation in rat cortex slices (94). These studies also indicate that the potentiation of cisplatin renal toxicity by methionine may be in part due to its ability to increase peroxidation sensitivity. It has also been suggested that metallothionein modulation of cisplatin nephrotoxicity is a result of its antioxidant properties (95).

Mitochondria are thought to be a possible target of cisplatin toxicity in renal tubule cells (96). Morphological changes appeared in mouse mitochondria 72 hr after cisplatin exposure, and biochemical effects were observed shortly thereafter (97). Diminished concentration of *p*-aminohippurate has been correlated with ultrastructural changes in mitochondria from rat cortical slices (98). Recent data from rabbit tubule cells show that mitochondrial injury is an early event observed even when oxygen consumption and potassium transport are still within normal limits (99). Cisplatin inhibits calcium uptake, and GSH depletion enhances this effect by unknown mechanisms (100). In rat kidney cell calcium homeostasis is affected by cisplatin through stimulation of endoplasmic reticulum calcium pump activity. However, nonnephrotoxic platinum analogues show no effect on the calcium pump. The increase occurs within 4 hr following cisplatin exposure and precedes morphological and biochemical changes, indicating that disruption of calcium homeostasis may be an important early event (101).

Modulation of Cisplatin Nephrotoxicity

The high incidence of clinically important cisplatin-induced renal toxicity has stimulated the development of pharmacological strategies to modulate the toxicity of this drug. These have been discussed in several recent reviews (102,103). Extensive hydration in combination with mannitol diuresis is now a standard part of cisplatin chemotherapy. This protocol, in most cases, provides adequate kidney protection for doses up to 100 mg/m^2. Increase of the cisplatin dose to 200 mg/m^2 per course has been achieved by administration in hypertonic (3%) saline and given in divided doses of 40 mg/m^2/day on days 1 to 5 (104,105) or 100 mg/m^2/day on days 1 and 8 (106,107). Although these regimens markedly reduce the cisplatin-induced nephrotoxicity, neurotoxicity and myelosuppression are severe. The cellular mechanisms by which isotonic hydration and/or hypertonic saline treatment reduce nephrotoxicity remain unclear.

Several nucleophilic sulfur-containing compounds have been tested for their ability to modulate cisplatin-induced nephrotoxicity. Based on the well-known affinity of sulfur ligands for platinum (II) complexes, these agents presumably react with and thus inactivate toxic platinum metabolites. Sodium thiosulfate (TS) forms highly stable platinum (II) adducts, and its safety in humans is well established, making it a leading candidate for cisplatin chemoprotection. Preliminary animal studies indicate that TS effectively inhibits nephrotoxicity when administered between 1 hr before and 30 min following cisplatin treatment (108). However, significant inhibition of antitumor activity (108–110) as well as cytotoxicity (111) was also reported. The mechanism of renal protection appears to be based on TS concentration in proximal tubule cells and subsequent reaction with cytotoxic platinum metabolites (112,113). At pharmacologic concentrations, the reaction rate of TS with cisplatin is very slow (88). However, cisplatin inactivation by TS has been observed in blood (114,115). Thiosulfate modulates cisplatin-induced cytotoxicity in LLC-PK_1 porcine proximal tubule cells when incubated just prior to cisplatin exposure but is ineffective when used immediately following treatment. Since experimental conditions preclude formation of extracellular platinum metabolites, these results suggest that cisplatin is the major toxic species to enter the tubule cell, and that TS is required intracellularly before cisplatin exposure to provide significant protection (78). The primary clinical role of TS as a chemoprotector has focused on the simultaneous administration of high-dose intraperitoneal cisplatin and intravenous TS in the treatment of intraperitoneal disease (116–118). Although concomitant intravenous TS and intravenous cisplatin did not increase the therapeutic index of the antineoplastic agent in animal models (119,120), clinical modulation of renal nephrotoxicity has been observed with this regimen (121–123).

WR-2721 (S-2-(3-aminopropylamino)ethylphosphorothioic acid) is a phosphatase thioester prodrug of the diaminothiol WR1065. It was initially developed as a radiation protector and has been studied extensively in radiation therapy (124). The selectivity of WR-2721 is thought to be due to alkaline phosphate hydrolysis of WR-2721 and selective accumulation of WR-1065 in normal tissues (125,126). In the rodent models WR-2721 modulates nephrotoxicity without diminishing antitumor activity (127,128). However, pretreatment of V79 cells with the metabolite WR-1065 markedly reduced cisplatin toxicity *in vitro* (129). Clinically, WR-2721 is administered by rapid infusion (15 min) at doses of 740 to 910 mg/m^2. Reversible hypotension and emesis are dose-limiting. WR-2721 shows modest efficacy in modulating the clinical renaltoxicity of cisplatin as well as reducing myelosuppression, neurotoxicity, and ototoxicity (129,130). In addition, reports indicate that WR-2721 may potentiate cisplatin's antitumor activity against metastatic melanoma (131).

Sodium diethyldithiocarbamate (DDTC), a bidentate chelating agent, anionic at physiological pH, is unique among the cisplatin modulating agents in its effectiveness when administered after the chemotherapeutic agent both *in vivo* (132–134) and *in vitro* (78). The selectivity of this drug is thought to be based upon its ability to reverse platinum complexes with the cysteine and methionine residues of cell proteins but not platinum-DNA cross-links (81,87,88,135). This theory assumes that DNA is not the cytotoxic target in the kidney. *In vitro* studies with porcine proximal tubule cells show that DDTC modulation of cisplatin-induced toxicity does not correlate with inhibition of DNA synthesis but does correlate with inhibition of protein synthesis (78). Several *in vivo* and *in vitro* studies have demonstrated that DDTC does not inhibit cisplatin antitumor activity (111,133,134).

Clinical studies with DDTC as a cisplatin modulator have reported conflicting results. In phase I trials (136), high-dose DDTC administered following cisplatin infusion afforded complete renal protection against cisplatin doses up to 120 mg/m^2. In a phase I cisplatin dose-escalation study, high-dose DDTC completely inhibited renal toxicity at cisplatin doses up to 160 mg/m^2. Here ototoxicity became the dose-limiting factor (137). High-dose DDTC administration in combination with a cisplatin dose of 200 mg/m^2 divided on days 1 and 8 also provided protection against nephrotoxicity (138). In contrast, no effect was observed in toxicity when low-dose DDTC was used with 120 mg/m^2 cisplatin in a randomized trial (139). DDTC showed no effect on the pharmacokinetics of filterable platinum in patients (139,140). Rapid intravenous administration of high-dose DDTC (4 g/m^2 over 1 hr) produced a variety of symptoms, including diaphoresis, facial burning, flushing, and anxiety, which were modulated, but not completely blocked, by premedication with sedatives. These reactions moderated with time and disappeared after the termination of the infusion. Reduction of infusion rate and the DDTC dose ($\leq$400 $mg/m^2/hr$ for 4 hr) eliminated the side effects. At this dose DDTC is presently under evaluation in two phase II multicenter trials.

The renal handling of cisplatin and its metabolites has been investigated with the intent that agents modulating cisplatin uptake may provide protection for the organ. The focus has been on the role of tubular secretion and reabsorption in intracellular concentration of platinum. The effects of probenecid anion transport inhibition are controversial. In the rat this agent increases the clearance ratio of ultrafilterable platinum (73,141,142) and inhibited platinum uptake in kidney slices (71). However, probenecid has been shown to both increase (76) and decrease (143) cisplatin-induced renaltoxicity in the rat. In human studies, probenecid administration initiated 1 day prior to a 24-hr cisplatin infusion resulted in a greater than 40% reduction of the fractional clearance of cisplatin (54,72). In a phase I cisplatin dose-escalation study, when probenecid was administered as a chemoprotector, no renal impairment was observed at doses from 100 to 160 mg/m^2 (144).

Several other modulators of cisplatin-induced toxicity have been developed and studied. Mercaptoethanesulfonate (mesna) has been both effective (145,146) and ineffective (147) as a renal chemoprotector. *In vitro* data indicate that mesna pretreatment provides partial protection, but that concomitant or subsequent treatment is ineffective (78). Recent kinetic studies confirm mesna's low reactivity toward platinum complexes (113).

Glutathione (GSH) is the most abundant intracellular nonprotein thiol. Although at intracellular concentrations its reaction rate with cisplatin is very slow, the reaction with aquated metabolites is instantaneous (88). GSH administration in mice decreased cisplatin-induced nephrotoxicity and lethality (148,149). Glutathione isopropyl ester was more effective than the free acid form based upon its facile intracellular hydrolysis to GSH and its improved transport properties (150). GSH modulation of nephrotoxicity has also been observed in clinical studies (151). Buthionine sulfoximine (BSO), a selective inhibitor of γ-glutamylcysteine synthase, decreases intracellular GSH levels. BSO pretreatment increased cisplatin-induced nephrotoxicity in mice, suggesting that intracellular GSH may be an important regulator (150,152). In rats, however, BSO has been shown to decrease the renaltoxicity of cisplatin. The degree of nephrotoxicity did not correlate with GSH levels, suggesting that the mechanism of this effect is unlikely to be related to GSH depletion (153).

The role of renal metallothionein (MT) in modulating cisplatin nephrotoxicity is somewhat controversial. The effects expected from MT induction are based upon the accessibility of 20 cysteine residues within this low molecular weight (6 to 7 kd) protein. In the native state, all of the residues are coordinated to divalent metal ions. Although platinum complexes will react with MT, over time the rates are not rapid enough to account for the modulation of toxicity through chelation mechanism (154–156). The majority of the evidence for MT as a renal chemoprotector is indirect. Pretreatment of animals with MT-inducing metals decreased cisplatin-induced nephrotoxicity and lethal toxicity in several studies (95,157,158), although the MT levels did not correlate well with the degree of protection (159). In other studies, however, the renal protection afforded by MT induction was negligible (149). In proximal tubule cells MT induction had no apparent effect on cisplatin cytotoxicity *in vitro* (79), and increased platinum binding to MT following MT induction has not been reported (95,149,155,160). As an explanation for the protective effects of MT, its antioxidant properties have been proposed as a mechanistic alternative to platinum chelation (95).

Coadministration of sodium selenite with cisplatin appears to diminish nephrotoxicity in several model systems (161–164). Similar results have been reported using ebselen, an organic selenium derivative that releases nucleophilic selenols in thiol-rich tissues (165). Mice given selenium-deficient diets showed increased sensitivity to the toxic and lethal effects of cisplatin, indicating that selenium levels in the kidney may be important in regulating cisplatin toxicity (166). The mechanism of renal protection is not clear but may be related either to nucleophilic reactions with toxic platinum metabolites or to the antioxidant properties of selenium.

CONCLUSIONS

Cancer chemotherapy represents a critical intervention designed to modify the course of potentially terminal diseases. The treatments are aggressive and the level of tolerated drug-induced toxicity would be unacceptable in most other clinical situations. A successful outcome of chemotherapy requires the administration of agents known to be highly cytotoxic to cells derived from normal host tissues. Surprisingly, these drugs, for the most part, do not cause irreversible clinically detectable nephrotoxicity. However, their widespread clinical use has led to the development of strategies designed to limit and control toxicity.

Cisplatin, a highly effective antineoplastic agent for treatment of solid tumors, showed severe renal toxicity induction in early trials. Its usefulness as an anticancer drug was nearly eliminated. However, as novel approaches to counteract and modulate cisplatin-induced nephrotoxicity were developed, the maximum tolerated dose continues to increase. Unfortunately, our understanding of the cellular and biochemical mechanisms that modulate drug-induced toxicity has lagged behind clinical protocols. Further studies of these mechanisms are essential for the development of new, selective chemotherapeutic agents as well as for the more effective use of existing compounds in the treatment of cancer.

REFERENCES

1. Weiss RB, Poster DS. The renal toxicity of cancer chemotherapeutic agents. *Cancer Treat Rev* 1982;9:37–56.
2. Garnick MB, Mayer RJ, Abelson HT. Acute renal failure associated with cancer treatment. In: Brenner BM, Lazarus JM, eds. *Acute renal failure*. Philadelphia: Saunders, 1983;527–554.
3. Ries F, Klastersky J. Nephrotoxicity induced by cancer chemotherapy with special emphasis on cisplatin toxicity. *Am J Kidney Dis* 1986;8:368–379.
4. Fillastre JP, Viotte G, Morin JP, Moulin B. Nephrotoxicity of antitumoral agents. *Adv Nephrol* 1988;17:175–218.
5. Fillastre JP, Raguenez-Viotte G. Cisplatin nephrotoxicity. *Toxicol Lett* 1989;46:163–175.
6. Daugaard G, Abildgaard U. Cisplatin nephrotoxicity. *Cancer Chemother Pharmacol* 1989;25:1–9.
7. Narins RG, Carley M, Bloom EJ, Harrison DS. The nephrotoxicity of chemotherapeutic agents. *Semin Nephrol* 1990;10:556–564.
8. McDermott DF, Galindo A, Sherman RL, Jaffe EA, Coleman M, Pasmantier MW. Inadequacy of predicted creatinine clearance as a guide to chemotherapy. *Cancer Treat Rep* 1987;71:1067–1069.
9. Bumah PK, Howell A, Whitby H, Harpur ES, Gescher A. Assessment of renal function during high-dose cisplatin therapy in patients with ovarian carcinoma. *Cancer Chemother Pharmacol* 1982;8:281–284.
10. Goren MP, Wright RK, Osborne S. Two automated procedures for *N*-acetyl-β-D-glucosaminidase determination evaluated for detection of drug-induced tubular nephrotoxicity. *Clin Chem* 1986;32: 2052–2055.
11. Falkenberg FW, Mai U, Puppe C, et al. Kidney-derived urinary antigens assayed with monoclonal antibodies for the detection of renal damage. *Clin Chim Acta* 1986;160:171–182.
12. Mutti A, Lucertini S, Valcavi P, Neri TM, Fornari M, Alinovi R, Franchini I. Urinary excretion of brush-border antigen revealed by monoclonal antibody: early indicator of toxic nephropathy. *Lancet* 1985;2:914–917.
13. Goren MP, Wright RK, Horowitz ME, Pratt CB. Cancer chemotherapy-induced tubular nephrotoxicity evaluated by imunochemical determination of urinary adenosine deaminase binding protein. *Am J Clin Pathol* 1986;86:780–783.
14. Falkenberg FW, Mondorf U, Pierard D, et al. Identification of fragments of proximal and distal tubular cells in the urine of patients under cytostatic treatment by immunoelectron microscopy with monoclonal antibodies. *Am J Kidney Dis* 1987;9:129–137.
15. Egido J, Robles A, Ortiz A, Ramirez F, Gonzalez E, Mampaso F, Sanchez Crespo M, Braquet P, Hernando L. Role of platelet-activating factor in adriamycin-induced nephropathy in rats. *Eur J Pharmacol* 1987;138:119–123.
16. Soose M, Haberstroh U, Rovira-Halach G, Brunkhorst R, Stolte H. Heterogeneity of glomerular

barrier function in early Adriamycin nephrosis of MWF rats. *Clin Physiol Biochem* 1988;6:310–315.
17. Kastner S, Wilks MF, Gwinner W, Soose M, Bach PH, Stolte H. Metabolic heterogeneity of isolated cortical and juxtamedullary glomeruli in Adriamycin nephrotoxicity. *Clin Physiol Biochem* 1991;14:48–54.
18. Barbey MM, Fels LM, Soose M, Poelstra K, Gwinner W, Bakker W, Stolte H. Adriamycin affects glomerular renal function: evidence for the involvement of oxygen radicals. *Free Radic Res Commun* 1989;7:195–203.
19. Raguenez-Viotte G, Lahoue M, Ducastelle T, Morin JP, Fillastre JP. CCNU-Adriamycin association induces earlier and more severe nephropathy in rats. *Arch Toxicol* 1988;61:282–291.
20. Ryckelynck JP, Heron JF, Juret P. Toxicite renale du 9-hydroxy-2-methylellipticinium. *Nephrologie* 1984;5:59–63.
21. Raguenez-Viotte G, Dadoun C, Buchet P, Ducastelle T, Fillastre JP. Renal toxicity of the antitumor drug *N*2-methyl-9-hydroxyellipticinium acetate in the Wistar rat. *Arch Toxicol* 1988;61:292–297.
22. Dadoun C, Raguenez-Viotte G. Celiptium-induced nephrotoxicity and lipid peroxidation in rat renal cortex. *Cancer Chemother Pharmacol* 1990;27:178–186.
23. Raguenez-Viotte G, Thomas N, Fillastre JP. Subcellular localization of celiptium-induced peroxidative damage in rat renal cortex. *Arch Toxicol* 1991;65:244–251.
24. Bleyer WA. The clinical pharmacology of methotrexate: new applications of an old drug. *Cancer* 1978;41:36–51.
25. Jaffe N, Traggis D. Toxicity of high-dose methotrexate (NSC-740) and citrovorum factor (NSC-3590) in osteogenic carcinoma. *Cancer Chemother Rep* 1975;part 36:31–36.
26. Deray G, Khayat D, Cacoub P, et al. The effects of diltiazem on methotrexate-induced nephrotoxicity. *Eur J Clin Pharmacol* 1989;37:337–340.
27. Pitman SW, Frei E. Weekly methotrexate-calcium leucovorin rescue: effect of alkalinization on nephrotoxicity; pharmacokinetics in the CNS; and use in CNS non-Hodgkin's lymphoma. *Cancer Treat Rep* 1977;61:695–701.
28. Goren MP, Wright RK, Horowitz ME, Meyer WH. Enhancement of methotrexate nephrotoxicity after cisplatin therapy. *Cancer* 1986;58:2617–2621.
29. Abelson HT, Fosburg MT, Beardsley GP, Goorin AM, Gorka C, Link M, Link D. Methotrexate-induced renal impairment: clinical studies and rescue from systemic toxicity with high-dose leucovorin and thymidine. *J Clin Oncol* 1983;1:208–216.
30. Lin JT, Bertino JR. Trimetrexate: a second-generation folate antagonist in clinical trial. *J Clin Oncol* 1987;5:2032–2040.
31. Hudes GR, LaCreta F, Walczak J, Tinsley P, Litwin S, Comis RL, O'Dwyer PJ. Pharmacokinetic study of trimetrexate in combination with cisplatin. *Cancer Res* 1991;51:3080–3087.
32. Hantel A, Rowinsky EK, Noe DA, et al. Clinical and pharmacologic reappraisal of dichloromethotrexate. *J Natl Cancer Inst* 1988;80:1547–1553.
33. Calvert AH, Alison DL, Harland SJ, et al. A phase I evaluation of the quinazoline antifolate thymidylate synthase inhibitor, *N*10-propargyl-5, 8-dideazafolic acid, CB 3717. *J Clin Oncol* 1986;4:1245–1252.
34. Sessa C, Zucchetti M, Ginier M, Willems Y, Dincalci M, Cavalli F. Phase I study of the antifolate *N*10-propargyl-5, 8-dideazafolic acid, CB 3717. *Eur J Cancer Clin Oncol* 1988;24:769–775.
35. Szybalski WA, Iyer VN. Crosslinking of DNA by enzymatically or chemically activated mitomycins and porfiromycin, bifunctionally "alkylating" antibiotics. *Fed Proc* 1964;23:946–957.
36. Tomasz M, Chawla AK, Lipman R. Mechanism of monofunctional and bifunctional alkylation of DNA by mitomycin C. *Biochemistry* 1988;27:3182–3187.
37. Crooke ST, Bradner WT. Mitomycin C: a review. *Cancer Treat Rev* 1976;3:121–139.
38. Hanna WT, Krauss S, Regester RF, Murphy WM. Renal disease after mitomycin C therapy. *Cancer* 1981;48:2583–2588.
39. Giroux I, Bettez P, Giroux L. Mitomycin C nephrotoxicity: a clinical-pathologic study of 17 cases. *Am J Kidney Dis* 1985;6:28–39.
40. Verweij J, Kerpel-Fronius S, Stuurman M, van Triet AJ, van Hattum L, de Vries J, Pinedo HM. Mitomycin C–induced organ toxicity in Wistar rats: a study with special focus on the kidney. *J Cancer Res Clin Oncol* 1988;114:137–141.
41. Cattell V. Mitomycin-induced hemolytic uremic kidney. *Am J Pathol* 1985;121:88–95.
42. Verweij J, de Vries J, Pinedo HM. Mitomycin C–induced renal toxicity, a dose dependent side effect? *Eur J Cancer Clin* 1987;23:195–199.

43. Poch E, Gonzalez-Clemente JM, Torras A, Darnell A, Botney A, Revert L. Silent renal microangiopathy after mitomycin C therapy. *Am J Nephrol* 1990;10:514– 517.
44. Weiss RB. Streptozotocin: a review of its pharmacology, efficacy and toxicity. *Cancer Treat Rep* 1982;66:427–438.
45. Sadoff I. Nephrotoxicity of streptozotocin (NSC-85998). *Cancer Chemother Rep* 1970;54:457 459.
46. Schein PS, O'Connell MJ, Blom J, et al. Clinical antitumor activity and toxicity of streptozotocin (NSC 85998). *Cancer* 1974;34:993–1000.
47. Olivero VT. Toxicology and pharmacology of the nitrosoureas. *Cancer Chemother Rep* 1973;4: 13–20.
48. Wasserman TH, Slavik M, Carter SK. Clinical comparison of the nitrosoureas. *Cancer* 1975;36: 1258–1264.
49. Weiss RB, Posada JG Jr, Kramer RA, Boyd MR. Nephrotoxicity of semustine. *Cancer Treat Rep* 1983;67:1105–1112.
50. Kramer RA, Schuller HM, Smith AC, Boyd MR. Effects of buthionine sulfoximine on the nephrotoxicity of 1-(2-chloroethyl)-3-(trans-4-methylcyclohexyl)-1-nitrosourea (MeCCNU). *J Pharmacol Exp Ther* 1985;234:498–506.
51. Kramer RA, Boyd MR, Dees JH. Comparative nephrotoxicity of 1-(2-chloroethyl)-3-(trans-4-methylcyclohexyl)-1-nitrosourea (MeCCNU) and chlorozotocin: functional-structural correlations in the Fischer 344 rat. *Toxicol Appl Pharmacol* 1986;82:540–550.
52. Borch RF. The platinum antitumor drugs. In: Powis G, Prough RA, eds. *Metabolism and action of anticancer drugs*. London: Taylor and Francis, 1987;163–193.
53. Daugaard G. Cisplatin nephrotoxicity: experimental and clinical studies. *Danish Med Bull* 1990; 37:1–12.
54. Jacobs C. The handling of platinum by the human kidney. In: McBrien DCH, ed. *Biomedical mechanisms of platinum antitumor drugs*. Oxford: IRL Press, 1986;147–170.
55. Reece PA, Stafford I, Russell J, Hill PG. Nonlinear renal clearance of ultrafilterable platinum in patients treated with cis-diamminedichloroplatinum (II). *Cancer Chemother Pharmacol* 1985;15: 295–299.
56. Miura K, Goldstein RS, Pasino DA, Hook JB. Cisplatin nephrotoxicity: role of filtration and tubular transport of cisplatin in isolated perfused kidneys. *Toxicology* 1987;44:147–158.
57. Daugaard G, Abildgaard U, Holstein-Rathlou N-H, Amtorp O, Olsen HP, Dikhoff TG. Acute effect of cisplatin on renal hemodynamics and tubular function in dog kidneys. *Renal Physiol* 1986; 9:308–316.
58. Daugaard G, Holstein-Rathlou N-H, Leyssac PP. Effect of cisplatin on proximal convoluted and straight segments of the rat kidney. *J Pharmacol Exp Ther* 1988;224:1081–1085.
59. Field MJ, Bostrom TE, Seow F, Gyory AZ, Cockayne DJ. Acute cisplatin nephrotoxicity in the rat. Evidence for impaired entry of sodium into proximal tubule cells. *Eur J Physiol* 1989;414:647–650.
60. Winston JA, Safirstein R. Reduced renal blood flow in early cisplatin-induced acute renal failure in the rat. *Am J Physiol* 1985;249:F490–F496.
61. Seguro AC, Shimizu MH, Kudo LH, dos Santos Rocha A. Renal concentration effect induced by cisplatin. The role of thick ascending limb and papillary collecting duct. *Am J Nephrol* 1989;9:59–65.
62. Offerman JJG, Meijer S, Sleijfer DTH, Mulder NH, Donker AJM, Schraffordt-Koops H, Van der Hem GK. The influence of verapamil on renal function in patients treated with cisplatin. *Clin Nephrol* 1985;24:249–255.
63. Offerman JJG, Mulder NH, Sleijfer DTh, Meijer S, Van der Hem GK. Influence of captopril on cis-dichlorodiammineplatinum-induced renal toxicity. *Am J Nephrol* 1985;14:262–268.
64. Sarfirstein R, Winston J, Moel D, Dikman S, Guttenplan J. Cisplatin nephrotoxicity: insights into mechanism. *Int J Androl* 1987;10:325–346.
65. Capasso G, Anastasio P, Giordano D, Albarano L, De Santo NG. Beneficial effects of atrial natriuretic factor on cisplatin-induced acute renal failure in the rat. *Am J Nephrol* 1987;7:228–234.
66. Schilsky RL, Anderson T. Hypomagnesemia and renal magnesium wasting in patients given cisplatin. *Ann Intern Med* 1979;90:929–931.
67. Mavichak V, Wong NLM, Quamme GA, Magil AB, Sutton RAL, Dirks JH. Studies on the pathogenesis of cisplatin-induced hypomagnesemia in rats. *Kidney Int* 1985;28:914–921.
68. Stewart DH, Mikhael NZ, Nanji AA, et al. Renal and hepatic concentrations of platinum: relationship to cisplatin time, dose, and nephrotoxicity. *J Clin Oncol* 1985;3:1251–1256.

69. Bird JE, Walser MM, Quebbeman AJ. Protective effect of organic cation transport inhibitors on cis-diamminedichloroplatinum-induced nephrotoxicity. *J Pharmacol Exp Ther* 1984;231:752–758.
70. Williams PD, Hottendorf GH. Effect of cisplatin on organic ion transport in membrane vesicles from rat kidney cortex. *Cancer Treat Rep* 1985;69:875–880.
71. Sarfirstein R, Miller P, Guttenplan JB. Uptake and metabolism of cisplatin by rat kidney. *Kidney Int* 1984;25:753–758.
72. Jacobs C, Coleman CN, Rich L, Hirst K, Weiner MW. Inhibition of cis-dichlorodiammineplatinum secretion by the human kidney with probenecid. *Cancer Res* 1984;44:3632–3635.
73. Daley-Yates PT, McBrien DCH. The renal fractional clearance of platinum antitumor compounds in relation to nephrotoxicity. *Biochem Pharmacol* 1985;34:1423–1428.
74. Daley-Yates PT, McBrien DCH. Cisplatin metabolites: a method for their separation and for measurement of their renal clearances in vivo. *Biochem Pharmacol* 1983;32:181–184.
75. Daley-Yates PT, McBrien DCH. Cisplatin metabolites in plasma, a study of their pharmacokinetics and importance in the nephrotoxic and antitumor activity of cisplatin. *Biochem Pharmacol* 1984;33: 3063–3070.
76. Daley-Yates PT, McBrien DCH. Enhancement of cisplatin toxicity by probenecid. *Cancer Treat Rep* 1984;68:445–446.
77. Alden WW, Repta AJ. Exacerbation of cisplatin-induced nephrotoxicity by methionine. *Chem Biol Interact* 1984;48:121–124.
78. Montine TJ, Borch RF. Quiescent LLC-PK1 cells as a model for cis-dichlorodiammineplatinum (II) nephrotoxicity and modulation by thiol rescue agents. *Cancer Res* 1988;48:6017–6024.
79. Montine TJ, Borch RF. Role of endogenous thiols in an in vitro model of cis-dichlorodiammine-platinum (II) induced nephrotoxicity. *Biochem Pharmacol* 1990;39:1751–1757.
80. Robins AB. The binding of platinum ethylenediamine dichloride to proteins, in vitro and in vivo. *Chem-Biol Interact* 1982;38:349–356.
81. Gonias SL, Oakley AC, Walther PJ, Pizzo SV. Effects of diethyldithiocarbamate and nine other nucleophiles on the intersubunit protein cross-linking and inactivation of purified human α_2-macroglobulin by cis-dichlorodiammineplatinum (II). *Cancer Res* 1984;44:5764–5769.
82. Gonias SL, Pizzo SV. Complexes of serum albumin and cis-dichlorodiammineplatinum (II). *J Biol Chem* 1983;258:5764–5769.
83. Aull JL, Allen RL, Bapat AR, Daron HH, Friedman ME, Wilson JF. The effects of platinum complexes on seven enzymes. *Biochim Biophys Acta* 1979;571:352–358.
84. Daley-Yates PT, McBrien DCH. The inhibition of renal ATPase by cisplatin and some biotransformation products. *Chem Biol Interact* 1982;40:325–334.
85. Nechay BR, Neldon SL. Characteristics of inhibition of human renal adenosine triphosphatases by cisplatin and chloroplatinic acid. *Cancer Treat Rep* 1984;68:1135–1141.
86. Tay LK, Bregman CL, Masters BA, Williams PD. Effects of cis-diamminedichloroplatinum (II) on rabbit kidney in vivo and on rabbit renal proximal tubule cells in culture. *Cancer Res* 1988;48: 2538–2543.
87. Bodenner DL, Dedon PC, Keng PC, Borch RF. Effect of diethyldithiocarbamate on cis-platinum-induced cytotoxicity, DNA cross-linking, and g-glutamyl transpeptidase inhibition. *Cancer Res* 1986;46:2745–2750.
88. Dedon PC, Borch RF. Characterization of the reactions of platinum antitumor agents with biologic and nonbiologic sulfur-containing nucleophiles. *Biochem Pharmacol* 1987;36:1955–1964.
89. Litterst CL. Cisplatinum: a review, with special reference to cellular and molecular interactions. *Agents Actions* 1984;15:520–524.
90. Hannemann J, Baumann K. Cisplatin-induced lipid peroxidation and decrease of gluconeogenesis in rat kidney cortex: different effects of antioxidants and radical scavengers. *Toxicology* 1988;51: 119–132.
91. Hannemann J, Baumann K. Nephrotoxicity of cisplatin, carboplatin and transplatin. A comparative in vitro study. *Arch Toxicol* 1990;64:393–400.
92. Nakano S, Gemba M. Potentiation of cisplatin-induced lipid peroxidation in kidney cortical slices by glutathione depletion. *Jpn J Pharmacol* 1989;50:87–92.
93. Fukuishi N, Gemba M. Use of cultured renal epithelial cells for the study of cisplatin toxicity. *Jpn J Pharmacol* 1989;50:247–249.
94. Sugihara K, Nakano S, Gemba M. Effect of cisplatin on in vitro production of lipid peroxides in rat kidney cortex. *Jpn J Pharmacol* 1987;44:71–76.
95. Boogaard PJ, Slikkerveer A, Nagelkerke JF, Mulder GJ. The role of metallothionein in the reduction of cisplatin-induced nephrotoxicity by Bi^{+3}-pretreatment in the rat in vivo and in vitro. Are

antioxidant properties of metallothionein more relevant than platinum binding? *Biochem Pharmacol* 1991;41:369–375.
96. Gordon JA, Gattone VH. Mitochondrial alterations in cisplatin induced acute renal failure. *Am J Physiol* 1986;250:F991–998.
97. Singh G. A possible cellular mechanism of cisplatin-induced nephrotoxicity. *Toxicology* 1989;58: 71–80.
98. Appenroth D, Gambaryan S, Gerhardt S, Kersten L, Braunlich H. Age dependent differences in the functional and morphological impairment of kidney following cisplatin administration. *Exp Pathol* 1990;38:231–239.
99. Brady HR, Kone BC, Stromski ME, Zeidel ML, Giebisch G, Gullans SR. Mitochondrial injury: an early event in cisplatin toxicity to renal proximal tubules. *Am J Physiol* 1990;258:F1181–1187.
100. Kameyama Y, Gemba M. Cisplatin-induced injury to calcium uptake by mitochondria in glutathione-depleted slices of rat kidney cortex. *Jpn J Pharmacol* 1991;55:174–176.
101. DeWitt LM, Jones TW, Moore L. Stimulation of the renal endoplasmic reticulum calcium pump: a possible biomarker for platinate toxicity. *Toxicol Appl Pharmacol* 1988;92:157–169.
102. Borch RF, Markman M. Biochemical modulation of cisplatin toxicity. *Pharmacol Ther* 1987;41: 371–380.
103. Gandara DR, Perez EA, Wiebe V, DeGregorio MW. Cisplatin chemoprotection and rescue: pharmacologic modulation of toxicity. *Semin Oncol* 1991;18(1, suppl 3):49–55.
104. Ozols RF, Corden BJ, Jacob J, Wesley MN, Ostchega Y, Young RC. High-dose cisplatin in hypertonic saline. *Ann Intern Med* 1984;100:19–24.
105. Ozols RF, Ostchega Y, Myers CE, Young RC. High-dose cisplatin in hypertonic saline in refractory ovarian cancer. *J Clin Oncol* 1985;3:1246–1250.
106. Gandara DR, DeGregorio MW, Wold HG, et al. High-dose cisplatin in hypertonic saline; reduced toxicity of a modified dose schedule and correlation with plasma pharmacokinetics. A Northern California Oncology Group (NCOG) pilot study in non-small cell lung cancer. *J Clin Oncol* 1986; 4:1787–1793.
107. Gandara DR, Perez EA, Phillips WA, Lawrence HJ, DeGregorio M. Evaluation of cisplatin dose intensity: current status and future prospects. *Anticancer Res* 1989;9:1121–1128.
108. Howell SB, Taetle R. Effect of sodium thiosulfate on cis-dichloridiammineplatinum (II) toxicity and antitumor activity in L1210 leukemia. *Cancer Treat Rep* 1980;64:611–616.
109. Uozumi J, Ishizawa M, Iwanmoto Y, Baba T. Sodium thiosulfate inhibits cis-diamminedichloroplatinum (II) activity. *Cancer Chemother Pharmacol* 1984;15:93–96.
110. Catino JJ, Francher DM, Schurig JE. Evaluation of cis-diamminedichloroplatinum (II) combined with metoclopramide or sodium thiosulfate on L1210 leukemia in vitro and in vivo. *Cancer Chemother Pharmacol* 1986;18:1–4.
111. Felder TB, Wasserman K, Shah R, Paredes J, Hong WK, Newman RA. Effect of diethyldithiocarbamate (DDTC) and sodium thiosulfate on the cytotoxicity and pharmacology of cisplatin. *Proc Am Assoc Cancer Res* 1987;28:31.
112. Shea M, Koziol JA, Howell SB. Kinetics of thiosulphate, a cisplatin neutralizer. *Clin Pharmacol Ther* 1989;35:419–425.
113. Leeuwenkamp OR, van der Vijgh WJF, Neijt JP, Pinedo HM. Reaction kinetics of cisplatin and its monoaquated species with the (potential) renal protecting agents (di)mensa and thiosulphate. Estimation of the effect of protecting agents on the plasma and peritoneal AUCs of cisplatin. *Biochem Pharmacol* 1990;27:111–114.
114. Abe R, Akiyoshi T, Baba T. Inactivation of cisdiamminedichloroplatinum (II) in blood by sodium thiosulphate. *Oncology* 1990;47:65–69.
115. Iwamoto Y, Kawano T, Ishizawa M, Aoki K, Kuroiwa T, Baba T. Inactivation of cis-dichlorodiammineplatinum (II) in blood and protection of its toxicity by sodium thiosulfate in rabbits. *Cancer Chemother Pharmacol* 1985;15:228–232.
116. Abe R, Akiyoshi T, Baba T. Two-route chemotherapy using cisplatin and its neutralizing agent, sodium thiosulphate, for intraperitoneal cancer. *Oncology* 1990;47:422–426.
117. Markman M, Cleary S, Howell SB. Nephrotoxicity of high-dose intracavitary cisplatin with intravenous thiosulfate protection. *Eur J Cancer Clin Oncol* 1985;21:1015–1018.
118. Markman M, Howell SB, Cleary S, Lucas WE. Intraperitoneal chemotherapy with high dose cisplatin and cytarabine for refractory ovarian carcinoma and other malignancies principally involving the peritoneal cavity. *J Clin Oncol* 1985;3:925–931.
119. Amadal S, Fodstad O, Pihl A. Sodium thiosulphate fails to increase the therapeutic index of

intravenously administered cisdiamminedichloroplatinum (II) in mice bearing murine and human tumors. *Cancer Chemother Pharmacol* 1988;21:129–133.
120. Inoue M, Shimizu C, Shimizu H, Tanizawa O. Neutralizing effect of sodium thiosulfate on antitumor efficacy of cisplatin for human carcinoma xenografts in nude mice. *Gynecol Oncol* 1991; 40:34–37.
121. Pfeifle CE, Howell SB, Felthouse RD, Woliver TBS, Andrews PA, Markman M, Murphy MP. High-dose cisplatin with sodium thiosulfate protection. *J Clin Oncol* 1985;3:237–244.
122. Hirosawa A, Niitani H, Hayashibara K, Tsuboi E. Effects of sodium thiosulfate in combination therapy of cis-dichlorodiammineplatinum and vindesine. *Cancer Chemother Pharmacol* 1989;23: 255–258.
123. Markman M, D'Acquistino R, Iannotti N, et al. Phase-1 trial of high-dose intravenous cisplatin with simultaneous intravenous sodium thiosulfate. *J Cancer Res Clin Oncol* 1991;117:151–155.
124. Brown DQ, Graham WJ, McKenzie LJ, Pittock JW, Shaw LM. Can WR2721 be improved upon? *Pharmacol Ther* 1988;39:157–168.
125. Calabro-Jones PM, Aguilera JA, Ward JF, Smoluk GD, Fahey RC. Uptake of WR2721 derivatives by cells in culture: identification of the transported form of the drug. *Cancer Res* 1988;48:3634–3640.
126. Shaw LM, Glover D, Turrisi A, et al. WR2721 pharmacokinetics. *Pharmacol Ther* 1988;39:195–201.
127. Yuhas JM, Culo F. Selective inhibition of nephrotoxicity of cis-dichlorodiammineplatinum (II) by WR-2721 without altering its antitumor properties. *Cancer Treat Rep* 1988;64:57–64.
128. Jordan SW, Yuhas JM, Glick J. Modulation of cis-platinum renal toxicity by the radioprotective agent WR 2721. *Exp Mol Pathol* 1982;36:297–305.
129. Glover D, Glick JH, Weiler C, Fox K, Turrisi A, Kligerman MM. Phase I/II trial of WR-2721 and cis-platinum. *Int J Radiat Oncol Biol Phys* 1986;12:1509–1512.
130. Glover D, Grabelsky S, Fox K, Weiler C, Cannon L, Glick J. Clinical trials of WR-2721 and cis-platinum. *Int J Radiat Oncol Biol Phys* 1989;16:1201–1204.
131. Glover D, Glick JH, Weiler C, Fox K, Guerry D. WR-2721 and high-dose cisplatin: an active combination in the treatment of metastatic melanoma. *J Clin Oncol* 1987;5:574–578.
132. Borch RF, Pleasants ME. Inhibition of cis-platinum nephrotoxicity by diethyldithiocarbamate in a rat model. *Proc Natl Acad Sci USA* 1979;76:6611–6614.
133. Borch RF, Katz JC, Lieder PH, Pleasants ME. Effect of diethyldithiocarbamate on tumor response to cis-platinum in a rat model. *Proc Natl Acad Sci USA* 1980;77:5541–5444.
134. Bodenner DL, Dedon PC, Keng PC, Katz JC, Borch RF. Selective protection against cis-dichlorodiammineplatinum (II)-induced toxicity in kidney, gut, and bone marrow by diethyldithiocarbamate. *Cancer Res* 1986;46:2751–2755.
135. Pizzo SV, Roche PA, Feldman SR, Gonias SL. Further characterization of the platinum-reactive component of the α_2-macroglobulin-receptors recognition site. *Biochem J* 1986;238:217–225.
136. Qazi R, Change AYC, Borch RF, Montine T, Dedon P, Loughner J, Bennett JM. Phase I clinical and pharmacokinetic study of diethyldithiocarbamate as a chemoprotector of cisplatin toxicity. *J Natl Cancer Inst* 1988;80:1486–1488.
137. Berry JM, Jacobs C, Sikic B, Halsey J, Borch RF. Modification of cisplatin toxicity with diethyldithiocarbamate. *J Clin Oncol* 1990;8:1585–1590.
138. Gandara DR, DeGregorio MW, Perez E, Holleran W, Denham A, Lawrence HJ, Borch R. Diethyldithiocarbamate (DDTC) rescue following very high dose cisplatin (200 mg/m^2/cycle): preliminary results of a phase 1 trial and pharmacokinetic observations. *Proc Am Soc Clin Oncol* 1988; 7:107(abstract).
139. Paredes J, Hong WK, Felder TB, et al. Prospective randomized trial of high-dose cisplatin and fluorouracil infusion with or without sodium diethyldithiocarbamate in recurrent and/or metastatic squamous cell carcinoma of the head and neck. *J Clin Oncol* 1988;6:955–962.
140. Degregorio MW, Gandara DR, Holleran WM, et al. High-dose cisplatin with diethyldithiocarbamate (DDTC) rescue therapy: preliminary pharmacologic observations. *Cancer Chemother Pharmacol* 1989;23:276–278.
141. Daley-Yates PT, McBrien DCH. The mechanism of renal clearance of cisplatin (cis-dichlorodiammineplatinum [II]) and its modification by furosemide and probenecid. *Biochem Pharmacol* 1982; 31:2243–2246.
142. Osman NM, Litterst CL. Effect of probenecid and *N'*-methylnicotinamide on renal handling of cis-dichlorodiammineplatinum-II in rats. *Cancer Lett* 1983;19:107–111.

143. Ross DA, Gale GR. Reduction of the renal toxicity of cis-dichlorodiammine platinum(II) by probenecid. *Cancer Treat Rep* 1979;63:781–787.
144. Jacobs C, Kaubisch S, Halsey J, Lum BL, Gosland M, Coleman CN, Sikic BI. The use of probenecid as a chemoprotector against cisplatin nephrotoxicity. *Cancer* 1991;67:1518–1524.
145. Kempf SR, Ivankovic S, Wiessler M, Schmal D. Effective prevention of the nephrotoxicity of cisplatin (CDDP) by administration of sodium 2-mercaptoethanesulfonate (MESNA) in rats. *Br J Cancer* 1985;52:937–939.
146. Kempf SR, Ivankovic S. Nephrotoxicity and carcinogenic risk of cisplatin (CDDP) prevented by sodium 2-mercaptoethanesulfonate (MESNA): experimental results. *Cancer Treat Rev* 1987;14: 365–372.
147. Millar BC, Siddik ZH, Millar JL, Jinks S. Mesna does not reduce cisplatin nephrotoxicity in the rat. *Cancer Chemother Pharmacol* 1985;15:307–309.
148. Zunino F, Pratezi G, Micheloni A, Cavalletti E, Sala F, Tofanetti O. Protective effect of reduced glutathione against cisplatin-induced renal and systemic toxicity and its influence on the therapeutic activity of the antitumor drug. *Chem Biol Interact* 1989;70:89–101.
149. Suzuki CIM, Cherian MG. The interactions of cisdiamminedichloroplatinum (II) and metallothionein and glutathione in rat liver and kidney. *Toxicology* 1990;64:113–127.
150. Anderson ME, Naganuma A, Meister A. Protection against cisplatin toxicity by administration of glutathione ester. *FASEB J* 1990;4:3251–3255.
151. Di Re F, Bohm S, Oriana S, Spatti GB, Zunino F. Efficacy and safety of high-dose cisplatin and cyclophosphamide with glutathione protection in the treatment of bulky advanced epithelial ovarian cancer. *Cancer Chemother Pharmacol* 1990;25:355–360.
152. Ishikawa M, Takayanagi Y, Sasaki K. Enhancement of cisplatin toxicity by buthionine sulfoximine, a glutathione-depleting agent, in mice. *Res Commun Chem Pathol Pharmacol* 1990;67: 131–141.
153. Mayer RD, Lee KE, Cockett AT. Improved use of buthionine sulfoximine to prevent cisplatin nephrotoxicity in rats. *J Cancer Res Clin Oncol* 1989;115:428–432.
154. Zelazowski AJ, Garvey JS, Hoeschele JD. In vivo and in vitro binding of platinum to metallothionein. *Arch Biochem Biophys* 1984;229:246–252.
155. Mason R, Edwards IR, McLaren SJ. Interaction of platinum with metallothionein-like ligands in the rat kidney after administration of cis-dichlorodiammineplatinum II. *Chem Biol Interact* 1984; 49:165–176.
156. Bongers J, Bell JU, Richardson DE. Platinum (II) binding to metallothionein. *J Inorg Biochem* 1988;34:55–62.
157. Naganuma A, Satoh M, Imura N. Prevention of lethal and renal toxicity of cis-dichlorodiammineplatinum (II) by induction of metallothionein synthesis without compromising its antitumor activity in mice. *Cancer Res* 1987;47:983–987.
158. Hamada T, Nishiwaki Y, Kodama T, et al. Prevention of renal toxicity of cisplatin by administration of bismuth subnitrate. *Jpn J Cancer Chemother* 1989;16:3587–3593.
159. Naganuma A, Satoh M, Koyama Y, Imura N. Protective effect of metallothionein inducing metals on lethal toxicity of cis-dichlorodiammineplatinum (II) in mice. *Toxicol Lett* 1985;24:203–207.
160. Sommer S, Thorling EB, Jakobsen A, Steiness A, Ostergaard K. Can bismuth decrease the kidney toxic effect of cisplatinum? *Eur J Clin Oncol* 1989;25:1903–1904.
161. Naganuma A, Satoh M, Imura N. Effect of selenite on renal toxicity and antitumor activity of cis-dichlorodiammineplatinum (II) in mice inoculated with Ehrlich ascites tumor cells. *J Pharmacobiodyn* 1984;7:217–220.
162. Ohkawa K, Tsukada Y, Dohzono H, Koike K, Terashima Y. The effects of coadministration of selenium on cisplatin-induced toxicity and antitumor activity. *Br J Cancer* 1988;58:38–41.
163. Baldew GS, van den Hamer CJA, Los G, Vermeulen NPM, de Goeij JJM, McVie JG. Selenium-induced protection against cis-diamminedichloroplatinum (II) nephrotoxicity in mice and rats. *Cancer Res* 1989;49:3020–3023.
164. Satoh M, Naganuma A, Imura N. Optimum schedule of selenium administration to reduce lethal and renal toxicities of cis-diamminedichloroplatinum in mice. *J Pharmacobiodyn* 1989;12:246–253.
165. Baldew GS, McVie JG, van der Valk MA, Los G, de Goeij JJ, Vermeulen NP. Selective reduction of cis-diamminedichloroplatinum (II) nephrotoxicity by ebselen. *Cancer Res* 1990;50:7031–7036.
166. Satoh M, Naganuma A, Imura N. Deficiency of selenium intake enhances manifestation of renal toxicity of cis-diamminedichloroplatinum in mice. *Toxicol Lett* 1987;38:155–160.

Toxicology of the Kidney, Second Edition,
edited by Jerry B. Hook and Robin S. Goldstein.
Raven Press, Ltd., New York © 1993.

11

Analgesic Nephrotoxicity

Geoffrey G. Duggin

Toxicology Unit, Royal Prince Alfred Hospital, Camperdown NSW 2050, Australia

Acetaminophen (paracetamol) is one of the most widely consumed antipyretic analgesics in the world. In most Western countries the per capita consumption now significantly exceeds that of aspirin. It has increased in popularity over the past three decades principally because it is an effective analgesic and antipyretic but also because of its minimal side effects at therapeutic dosages. Significant problems arise however in the context of acute drug overdose with doses greater than 300 mg/kg body weight, where hepatotoxicity and nephrotoxicity are the principal manifestations. Chronic abuse, in combination with other antipyretic analgesics, particularly aspirin, can produce analgesic nephropathy. There have been occasional reports of chronic kidney damage from acetaminophen alone, but most of these cases have been poorly substantiated. In the vast majority of cases the disease is caused by the chronic excessive ingestion of the analgesic combination. The mechanism of acute and chronic toxicity have quite separate mechanisms and will be considered separately.

CLINICAL FEATURES OF ACUTE ACETAMINOPHEN TOXICITY

The incidence of acute renal failure associated with acetaminophen overdose ranges from 0.6% to 1.6% (1,2). Acetaminophen-induced acute renal failure is most frequently seen in the context of acetaminophen overdose, accompanied by severe hepatic dysfunction. However, the development of acetaminophen-induced acute renal failure in the absence of liver failure (defined as deep jaundice, encephalopathy, or severe bleeding diathesis) is now a well-recognized clinical entity (1–8). Prescott and colleagues (2) reported a total of 33 cases of acute renal failure in 2,060 cases of paracetamol overdose in the period from 1969 to 1980 inclusive. Eighteen of these cases developed acute renal failure in the absence of hepatic failure or encephalopathy (2).

An early study of 160 patients with fulminant hepatic failure failed to demonstrate a higher incidence of renal failure in patients who had taken an overdose of acetaminophen, compared to other causes of hepatic failure (9). In this study the onset and duration of renal failure was related to the hepatic damage rather than acetaminophen-induced nephrotoxicity (9); that is, the renal failure followed 2 to 3 days after the onset of hepatic failure, indicating the development of the hepatorenal failure rather than the nephrotoxicity.

In the absence of liver failure, the reported cases of acetaminophen-induced acute renal failure appear to have characteristic features in their presentation. The onset of acute renal failure was delayed, occurring up to 7 days following ingestion, as opposed to the acute hepatic damage, which was maximal by 2 to 4 days (10). Although hepatic damage was evident histologically in those cases subjected to a liver biopsy, liver function had usually recovered rapidly, and hepatic dysfunction rarely caused any problems in management (1,2). The acute renal failure was characterized by a rising creatinine greater than 300 μmol/l and was predominantly oliguric in presentation (1,2,4,6). The duration of oliguria was variable, ranging from 3 to 12 days. The urinary biochemistry typically demonstrated a low urinary osmolality and a normal elevated fractional excretion of sodium, consistent with acute tubular necrosis rather than with hepatorenal etiology for the acute renal failure (1,2,4,6).

Renal biopsies showed a histological picture of patchy acute tubular necrosis (1–4,6–8). Bjorck and colleagues (7) have also reported the presence of endothelial cell necrosis along with focal tubular epithelial cell necrosis in three patients with acetaminophen-associated acute renal failure. The significance of the endothelial cell damage is not clear, because in the cases reported acetaminophen was taken in combination with other analgesics, alcohol, or penicillin (7). It is possible that other factors may have contributed to the endothelial cell damage.

In addition to the acute renal failure associated with excessive amounts of the drug, therapeutic doses of acetaminophen have been reported to cause nephrotoxicity (3,11,12). This most commonly occurs when acetaminophen is taken in combination with alcohol (11,12). Chronic ethanol ingestion results in hepatic enzyme induction and is often associated with a reduced amount of glutathione secondary to the poor nutritional status of many alcoholics. The net effect is the alteration of hepatic metabolism of acetaminophen in the setting of a more vulnerable kidney predisposed to the development of nephrotoxicity. What role ethanol-induced enzyme induction plays in renal microsomal enzyme systems and subsequent metabolism of acetaminophen and its metabolites has not been studied.

BIOCHEMICAL MECHANISMS OF ACUTE ANALGESIC NEPHROTOXICITY

It has been postulated that acetaminophen induces acute tubular necrosis through depletion of glutathione and other sulfhydryl groups necessary to prevent the covalent binding of the reactive intermediate *N*-acetyl-*p*-benzoquinoneimine to cellular proteins, the same mechanisms involved in hepatic toxicity (1–4). Administration of *N*-acetylcysteine has been reported to prevent the nephrotoxicity as well as the hepatotoxicity associated with acetaminophen overdose (1,2). However, Davenport and Finn (8) have documented two cases where acute renal failure secondary to acetaminophen occurred in the absence of liver failure, despite full courses of *N*-acetylcysteine. This would suggest that arylation of cellular proteins by the reactive metabolite *N*-acetyl-*p*-benzoquinoneimine is not the only mechanism by which acetaminophen may produce acute renal failure.

Activation of Acetaminophen

Acute toxicity of acetaminophen is dependent on metabolic activation of acetaminophen to toxic metabolites, which then produce hepatic necrosis and/or renal cortical necrosis (13–15). Acetaminophen can be metabolized by different metabolic pathways: cytochrome P-450 mixed-function oxidases (MFO), deacetylases, and peroxidases, including prostaglandin H synthase. Each of these different enzyme systems can contribute to the development of acute acetaminophen-induced renal failure. The hepatic MFOs appear to play a significant role in the normal metabolism of acetaminophen (13). The MFOs are also present in the renal cortex, but this enzyme activity has lower activity when compared to the activity of hepatic MFO (16,17). Deacetylase, which converts acetaminophen into *p*-aminophenol, a potent nephrotoxicant, is significantly more active in the renal cortex than in the liver (18). Prostaglandin H synthase, and possibly other peroxidases, can convert acetaminophen and *p*-aminophenol into reactive intermediates through peroxidative reactions (17,19–21), which in turn can potentiate renal nephrotoxicity. In the renal cortex, cytochrome P-450 plays an important role in the peroxidative activation of acetaminophen and *p*-aminophenol (19,20,22). Reactive metabolites that bind covalently to cellular constituents and cause severe depletion of cellular glutathione (GSH) and lipid peroxidation are able to initiate cell damage leading eventually to cell death.

Deacetylase Participation

Deacetylases play an important role in the development of acetaminophen-induced toxicity in the renal cortex (18,23). Deacetylase converts acetaminophen into the more nephrotoxic *p*-aminophenol in the renal cortex (18). Further activation of *p*-aminophenol, either spontaneously or enzymatically, would lead to the generation of reactive metabolite(s) such as *p*-benzoquinoneimine, which are more nephrotoxic than acetaminophen or *p*-aminophenol (23). Deacetylase activity is greater in the renal cortex than in the liver, and it therefore probably plays a greater role than cytochrome P-450 in the formation of the reactive metabolites of acetaminophen in the kidney. The susceptibility of certain strains of rats and the resistance of certain other strains of rats to the nephrotoxicity of acetaminophen has been demonstrated to correlate well with the higher levels of activity of renal cortical deacetylases in the susceptible strains of rats than in the resistant strains (22).

Cytochrome P-450 Mixed-Function Oxidases Involvement

Cytochrome P-450 is an essential component of the MFOs that participate in the activation of acetaminophen and *p*-aminophenol (24). There are multiple isozymes of cytochrome P-450, and certain specific isozymes are involved in the conversion of acetaminophen into the reactive intermediate, *N*-acetyl-*p*-benzoquinoneimine (25,26). In the kidney, the total cytochrome P-450 concentration is approximately one-third that of the liver and has a heterogeneous distribution. Cytochrome P-450 is present in the renal cortex and in trace amounts in the renal outer medulla; it is not detectable in the renal inner medulla (16,17). The distribution of various isozymes of cytochrome P-450 within the kidney would influence the extent of activation of acetaminophen and *p*-aminophenol in the cortex and in the outer medulla. Ethanol has been demonstrated to induce a specific isozyme of cytochrome P-450 in the rabbit liver (25). It is not certain whether ethanol-inducible cytochrome P-450 is responsible for the activation of acetaminophen in the cortex of the human kidney. Clinical observations (27) and animal experiments (15) on the acute toxicity of acetaminophen have demonstrated that whereas the renal cortex is affected, the renal inner medulla remains undamaged.

Peroxidases—Including Prostaglandin H Synthase Reactions

MFOs require nicotinamide-adenine dinucleotide phosphate, reduced (NADPH) and molecular oxygen for catalyzing the activation of acetaminophen and *p*-aminophenol. However, cytochrome P-450 can oxidize acetaminophen through a one-electron pathway to the semiquinoneimine *N*-acetyl-*p*-benzoquinoneimine (NAPQI) and through a two-electron pathway into the quinoneimine (30). *p*-Aminophenol can undergo oxidative activation by autooxidation requiring oxygen or by catalytic conversion mediated by MFOs or peroxidative activation by cytochrome P-450. The reactive metabolite of *p*-aminophenol is likely to be *p*-benzoquinoneimine (PQI). Peroxidase reactions of cytochrome P-450 (19,20), prostaglandin H synthase (19,20), and horseradish peroxidase (20,21) have been demonstrated to mediate the activation of acetaminophen and *p*-aminophenol into respective reactive metabolites. In the rabbit kidney cortex, cytochrome P-450 was found to be more active than prostaglandin H synthase in the peroxidative conversion of acetaminophen into metabolites that bind to cellular proteins (19). Cytochrome P-450–mediated peroxidative activation of both acetaminophen and *p*-aminophenol can continue to occur once NADPH and GSH are depleted from the cell. In acute toxicity this is likely to occur after the initial conversion of a substantial amount of either acetaminophen or *p*-aminophenol into their respective quinoneimines.

Metabolic Deactivation

There are three endogenous compounds that protect the cell from the reactive metabolites of compounds such as acetaminophen and *p*-aminophenol. They are

GSH, NADPH, and ascorbic acid. The toxicity of acetaminophen is manifested only when cellular GSH concentration falls below a critical level (31,32). Protection by GSH against the toxicity of the acetaminophen metabolite NAPQI has several mechanisms. GSH can react with NAPQI forming a glutathione conjugate that will then be excreted, usually as the mercapturic acid derivative (33–35). GSH can react with NAPQI to reform acetaminophen itself (33–35). In the presence of GSH, certain isozymes of glutathione *S*-transferase can convert NAPQI into a glutathione conjugate more readily than when NAPQI reacts directly with GSH (36). It has also been suggested that GSH protects against lipid peroxidation resulting from further reactions of NAPQI (37). The levels of activities of other GSH-related enzymes also are likely to contribute to the susceptibility of the renal cortex to the acute toxicity of acetaminophen and *p*-aminophenol. Selenium-dependent glutathione peroxidase plays a major role in converting the peroxides hydrogen peroxide and hydroperoxy fatty acids, formed after lipid peroxidation, into water and hydroxy fatty acids, respectively. Certain glutathione *S*-transferase isozymes also have glutathione peroxidase activity (selenium-independent), whereby they can convert hydroperoxy fatty acids into hydroxy fatty acids. GSH is required for the activity of glutathione peroxidase. Depletion of GSH by NAPQI and PQI would prevent glutathione peroxidase from removing hydrogen peroxide and hydroperoxy fatty acids, and these would then be able to participate in the cytochrome P-450–mediated peroxidase-type activation of both acetaminophen and *p*-aminophenol.

Detoxication of NAPQI by NADPH can occur through direct reaction with NAPQI to form acetaminophen (38). NADPH has been shown to prevent the covalent binding of *p*-aminophenol to kidney proteins (39). NADPH is an essential component for NADPH cytochrome P-450 reductase, which is also involved in acetaminophen metabolism, as will be discussed in a subsequent section. Therefore, depletion of renal cortical NADPH will potentiate renal toxicity. Vitamin C (ascorbic acid) has been shown to prevent toxicity produced by the reactive metabolites of acetaminophen (40) and *p*-aminophenol (39). The mechanism has not been elucidated but is probably related to the antioxidant properties of ascorbic acid.

Metabolite Reactions

The *p*-aminophenol metabolite PQI is likely to be more reactive than NAPQI, which is generated directly from acetaminophen (22). The toxicity of these metabolites could be due to covalent binding to cellular macromolecules as well as to further conversion of these quinoneimines generating more reactive intermediates (41,42). The reactive metabolites of acetaminophen and *p*-aminophenol, NAPQI and PQI, respectively, have characteristics similar to quinone metabolites and therefore could undergo most of the reactions of quinones (41), including lipid peroxidation, the generation of excess oxidized glutathione, and changes in cytosolic Ca^{2+} flux. The net effect is increased cell damage and cell death.

NADPH-Cytochrome P-450 Reductase Involvement

It has been demonstrated that NAPQI can undergo reductive activation through a one-electron reduction mediated by NADPH–cytochrome P-450 reductase (NCPR) into a semiquinoneimine (30). It is possible that PQI could also form a semiquinoneimine derivative via the same reaction, but at present there is no supportive experimental evidence to show that PQI can undergo such a conversion, possibly because of the highly reactive nature and very short half-life of NCPR. The NCPR-mediated reduction requires NADPH. Hence, NADPH can participate in the metabolism of acetaminophen during its activation to NAPQI, during the conversion of NAPQI into acetaminophen, and in the reductive activation of NAPQI into *N*-acetyl-semiquinoneimine (NASQI) mediated by NCPR. NCPR has been found to occur at low concentrations in different regions of the kidney (16). Semiquinoneimine radicals, like the semiquinone radicals, could react with molecular oxygen, releasing the parent quinoneimines and forming superoxide anions (41). Recent work suggests that NASQI does not react with oxygen, and it was suggested that this could be due to the electron-withdrawing effect of the *N*-acetyl group (41,42). NASQI may react directly with cellular macromolecules, resulting in covalent binding, and initiate radical-induced lipid peroxidation. In the case of the semiquinoneimine (SQI) generated from *p*-aminophenol, it appears that direct reaction between SQI and molecular oxygen is still possible and that this would produce reactive oxygen species as well as initiate lipid peroxidation. These reactions could be responsible for the high nephrotoxicity of *p*-aminophenol in the renal cortex and could contribute to the acute toxicity of acetaminophen due to high-level participation of deacetylases producing *p*-aminophenol (18).

DT-Diaphorase Involvement

DT-diaphorase (DTD), a quinone reductase, is regarded as a possible control device for the detoxication of quinones (43). So far this has not been demonstrated to occur in the case of quinoneimines, and further investigation in this area is required to establish whether this can occur. Within the kidney there is a heterogeneous distribution of DTD, with very low activity in the renal cortex, moderate activity in the renal outer medulla, and the highest levels of activity in the renal inner medulla (44). Low levels of activity of DTD in the renal cortex could mean that insufficient DTD is available to prevent or modify the generation of toxicity by the quinoneimines. Since DTD requires NADPH for its activity, the depletion of NADPH would further reduce DTD's ability to counteract the toxicity by the quinoneimines. In order to establish the possible role of DTD in reducing NAPQI into acetaminophen and PQI into *p*-aminophenol, it has to be demonstrated that NADPH and DTD are more efficient together than NADPH is alone for the same conversion.

Calcium Influence on Toxicity

The depletion of GSH and NADPH through the reaction with the reactive metabolites of acetaminophen and *p*-aminophenol would generate elevated levels of oxidized glutathione (GSSG) and NADP leading to increases in cytosolic Ca^{2+} concentration (45). Elevations in intracellular Ca^{2+} would potentiate the development of cellular toxicity and eventually lead to cell death (45). The mechanism(s) associated with acetaminophen and *p*-aminophenol–induced changes in intracellular Ca^{2+} flux are probably analogous to that documented in experimental quinone toxicity (44,45).

Methods of Preventing Nephrotoxicity

There have been numerous studies on the compounds that prevent hepatotoxicity following ingestion of toxic quantities of acetaminophen (46). These studies have not addressed the question of prevention of nephrotoxicity. However, if the generation of a radical intermediate is involved in both organs, it is probable that *N*-acetylcysteine and other sulfhydryls are effective in preventing renal damage.

CHRONIC NEPHROTOXICITY

Analgesic nephropathy is a unique drug-induced kidney disease. It is characterized by renal papillary necrosis and interstitial nephritis resulting from prolonged excessive consumption of combination antipyretic analgesics.

Antipyretic analgesics have found widespread use as everyday remedies in almost every country in the world. It was not until 1953, however, that Spuehler and Zollinger (47) described the renal disease associated with the chronic consumption of combination analgesics containing phenacetin.

There is now overwhelming evidence that consumption of combination analgesics is causally associated with renal disease. Clinical and epidemiologic studies indicate an increased incidence of renal disease in people who abuse analgesics. Nordenfelt and Ringertz (48) found that 29% of people who had consumed an estimated kilogram or greater of phenacetin in a combination analgesic had evidence of renal damage. Others have reported the incidence of renal impairment to vary between 3% and 90%, being greater in each instance than in the normal population with which they were compared. The apparent discrepancies result from the different methods used to determine renal function, the amount of drugs consumed, and the different combinations of analgesics. The incidence of analgesic abuse in patients with renal disease further supports a causal relationship. Murray and Goldberg (49) reported that 20% of patients with chronic interstitial nephritis abused analgesics.

Data from the Australia and New Zealand Dialysis and Transplant Registry (50) in the late 1970s, when combination analgesics were widely available, also showed that patients who abused combination analgesics developed renal disease, and approximately 20% of patients on the Australian program for dialysis and transplant were there as a result of analgesic-induced kidney disease. The correlation between the severity of renal disease and the extent of analgesic abuse had been demonstrated by Gault et al. (51), who found a linearly increased relationship between the amount of analgesic consumed and the severity of renal disease, as assessed by creatinine clearance and renal biopsy. The incidence of patients with analgesic nephropathy per country remarkably parallels the per capita consumption of phenacetin in that country (49).

Until 1964, it was widely accepted that phenacetin was the agent primarily responsible for the disease. This was largely based on clinical data from Western Europe, particularly Switzerland and Sweden. Gilman (52), in an editorial, questioned the validity of the theory that phenacetin caused the disease. This resulted in considerable controversy as to which drug was responsible for the disease.

Most investigators have concentrated on a single drug being responsible for the disease. As there is a striking association between the abuse of combination analgesics and the disease, this raises the possibility of synergistic toxicity with the combination of these drugs (53). Clinical evidence to support this contention is provided by Ferguson et al. (54), who studied patients attending a clinic for rheumatism. Patients who had consumed in excess of 1 kg of aspirin alone had a 0.3% incidence of papillary necrosis, whereas patients who had consumed in excess of 1 kg of combination analgesics containing aspirin and phenacetin or paracetamol had a 10.6% incidence of the disease. A prospective study by Dubach et al. (55) in Switzerland provided evidence that combination analgesics containing phenacetin produced evidence of renal disease. The study involved 623 people employed in watch factories in Switzerland. These subjects were found to have phenacetin metabolites (measured as paracetamol) present in their urine, and were compared to an age-, sex-, and occupation-matched control group that had no drug present. Over the 4-year period of study, 3.8% of the phenacetin group developed an abnormal urine concentrating capacity, against 0.8% of the control group. The incidence of raised serum creatinine was 2.9% in the phenacetin group and 0.4% of the low-consumption group. The data were even more significant when the phenacetin group was subdivided into those showing high and low consumption; 5.4% of the high-consumption group and 0.4% of the low-consumption group had raised serum creatinine levels.

The pathology of the disease has been reviewed extensively (56,57). Lindeneg et al. (58) suggested that the disease commenced in the renal papillae and resulted in necrosis of this anatomically discrete tissue. This then may lead to secondary nephron damage.

Hypotheses for a Pathophysiological Mechanism

For a drug to induce selective damage to the renal papillae, the drug or its derivative must satisfy one or both of the following criteria (59): the tissue must have unique metabolic or functional features that render it sensitive to the drug (47), and the drug must be concentrated selectively within that tissue.

Intrarenal Distribution of Analgesics

A limited number of drugs have been studied with respect to their distribution in the kidney. Most reports have been confined to the concentration within the total tissue, and most authors have not determined any compartmental distribution within the kidney. This is particularly important in the kidney, as this organ has an intratubular compartment in addition to the usual intracellular and interstitial compartments. Hence, it is possible for two compounds to have total tissue concentrations, one compound being distributed evenly throughout all compartments and the second being concentrated only within a single compartment. This is particularly important when considering drug toxicity, because it is probable that the mechanism of toxicity involves an intracellular site of action.

Phenacetin

Barraclough and Nilam (60) reported that the tubular transport of phenacetin was influenced by vasopressin and that under conditions of antidiuresis there was an increased concentration of phenacetin in the medulla, relative to the cortex. Their method of determining phenacetin, however, has been shown to be unsuitable for urinary and kidney tissue samples, as the method simultaneously determines both phenacetin and a metabolite (61). In a study (62) using a specific high-performance liquid chromatography method for determining phenacetin (63), it was demonstrated that under conditions of both diuresis and antidiuresis, no corticopapillary concentration gradient developed. Further analysis of these data has indicated that phenacetin is distributed uniformly in the intratubular, intracellular, and interstitial compartments of both the cortex and medulla.

Paracetamol (Acetaminophen)

There are only two studies on the renal distribution of paracetamol. Bluemle and Goldberg (64), in a study of dogs, examined the renal cortical, corticomedullary junction and medullary concentrations of paracetamol, following the administration of phenacetin. Their data indicated that during antidiuresis there was a significant corticopapillary concentration gradient, and that during diuresis, no gradient developed. The gradient was similar to that developed for the polar conjugates of paracetamol. They concluded that paracetamol and its conjugates were transported in a manner similar to urea and underwent countercurrent multiplication. The possibility was not considered, however, that the compounds might exist at different concentrations in different compartments within the medulla. In the distal nephron within the renal medulla, one would expect the highly polar conjugates of paracetamol to be confined to the tubular lumen. The concentration would be high within this compartment because of the proximal tubular secretion of these conjugates and the reabsorption of water along the length of the tubule. The moderately polar parent drug, paracetamol, might be expected to diffuse into the cells and interstitial fluid. Duggin and Mudge (65) tested this hypothesis in a study in dogs, using inulin as a marker because it is an inert nonreabsorbable compound. Concentrations in the urine were used for reference in the calculation of the volume of distribution within the medulla. The volume of distribution for the conjugates of paracetamol in the medulla was similar to that of inulin, but the volume of distribution of paracetamol in the medulla was on the average 2.3 times larger than that of inulin during both antidiuresis and diuresis. Thus, because inulin is confined to the intratubular and interstitial compartments, paracetamol must be distributed within the cells of the medulla. The medullary concentration reached as high as seven times the cortical concentration during antidiuresis, but this gradient was absent in diuresis.

Salicylate

Despite the large number of studies on the renal excretion and renal tubular transport of salicylate, there have been but few studies on its renal concentration and intrarenal distribution. Quintanilla and Kessler (66) studied the renal clearance in dogs and also performed a limited number of investigations on the renal cortical and medullary concentrations. They found a concentration in the cortex of 0.5 times the plasma, and the medullary concentration to be the same as the plasma concentration, making a corticopapillary concentration gradient of 1:2. Bluemle and Goldberg (64) studied the renal cortical, corticomedullary junction, and medullary concentration of salicylate during diuresis and antidiuresis. Their data may be questioned, however, because of the analytic method used (67). This is suitable for determining the salicylated concentration in plasma, but unsuitable for determining urine or tissue concentrations, because of the presence of interfering metabolites. Caterson and Duggin (68) studied rabbits following the IV administration of salicylate or aspirin. Using a specific high-performance liquid chromatography method for determining salicylate (69), they showed that during diuresis the mean salicylate concentration in the cortex was 1.8 times that of the plasma; in the renal medulla, the concentration was 3.4 times the plasma. The resultant corticomedullary gradient was 1.0:1.9. During antidiuresis, the mean concentration in the cortex was 6 times that in the plasma, and in the medulla it was 13.2 times, giving a corticomedullary concentration ratio of 1.0:2.2. They also compared the intrarenal distribution of salicylate with that of inulin. Salicylate was distributed within the tubules and the cells of the medulla. The volume of distribution increased with an acid urine and was decreased with an alkaline urine. As with aspirin, the pH dependence might be expected to be particularly important in man, in whom the urine is normally acid, particularly during antidiuresis. Beyer and Gelanden (70) studied the concentration of salicylate in the dog and found a corticopapillary concentration ratio of 1.5 to 2.0 during diuresis and 2.0 to 3.0 during antidiuresis. Although they did not study the intrarenal distribution further, their data would support that of Caterson and Duggin (68).

Biochemical Mechanisms

With chronic administration, acetaminophen achieves a higher concentration in the cells of the renal inner medulla compared to the renal cortex and plasma (62). This relatively higher concentration is important in the subsequent development of chronic nephrotoxicity. The prostaglandin (PG) H synthase enzyme complex, which appears to be the main mediator of chronic nephrotoxicity, is predominantly located in the inner medulla (16,17,71,72,73). The hydroperoxidase component reduces the hydroperoxy group of PGG_2 to the alcohol producing the endoperoxide PGH_2, with the oxidation of a suitable electron donor (48). Acetaminophen has been shown to act as a suitable substrate in this enzyme reaction (19,33). Mohandas and Duggin (74) have demonstrated *in vitro* that the prostaglandin synthesis is enhanced by acetaminophen at low concentrations, comparable to those that would be achieved during chronic ingestion (up to 0.5 mM), and inhibited at higher concentrations (as would be seen in acute overdose situations). The prostaglandin hydroperoxidase component of the enzyme complex converts acetaminophen to its reactive metabolite probably by one electron oxidation reaction and hydrogen abstraction to form the phenoxy radical of acetaminophen, which then undergoes further oxidation to the more reactive intermediate NAPQI (33). This metabolite reacts rapidly with GSH with the regeneration of acetaminophen or the formation of a stable conjugate.

The sharing of the conversion of PGG_2 to PGH_2, by both glutathione peroxidase and prostaglandin hydroperoxidase would influence the extent of co-oxidative activation of acetaminophen, since depletion of GSH by binding to NAPQI would decrease glutathione peroxidase participation in this reaction as opposed to prostaglandin hydroperoxidase, which does not require GSH as a substrate. The increased prostaglandin hydroperoxidase activity would increase the co-oxidation of acetaminophen and formation of active metabolites (75).

The cellular concentration of GSH is critical in preventing damage initiated by the reactive acetaminophen metabolites. The metabolite NAPQI may form a conjugate or is reduced back to acetaminophen with the production of oxidized glutathione (GSSG) (33). GSSG is reduced by glutathione reductase requiring $NADPH^+$. Thus, depletion of cellular GSH may occur due to decreased availability of $NADPH^+$, low activity of glutathione reductase in the renal medulla, or the movement of excess GSSG out of the cell, in addition to conjugation with metabolites (75). In addition, extracellular GSSG is not readily available to the renal inner medulla cells due to very low levels of γ-glutamyl transpeptidases on the cell membranes as opposed to high enzyme concentration in renal cells in the cortex (75).

Compound analgesics containing aspirin and phenacetin have a synergistic effect in the development of chronic nephrotoxicity. Aspirin inhibits the action of cyclooxygenase but not prostaglandin hydroperoxidase in the prostaglandin synthase complex (76). The therapeutic concentrations of acetaminophen will stimulate prostaglandin hydroperoxidase with increased activation of acetaminophen to more reactive metabolites. Aspirin is deacetylated to salicylate, which has a potent effect in depleting renal glutathione levels but not affecting the glutathione content of other organs. The specificity of salicylate in depleting renal glutathione is in part related to the extremely high tissue concentration in the kidney relative to other organs. The net effect is increased covalent binding to renal macromolecules and initiation of cellular injury (77).

Analgesic nephropathy is the end result of chronic ingestion of compound analgesics containing phenacetin (or acetaminophen), aspirin, and caffeine. It is difficult to clearly apportion the nephrotoxic role of each constituent in this syndrome. However, the experimental evidence discussed above support the predominant role of acetaminophen and/or its metabolites in the generation of analgesic nephropathy, with the injury induced by chronic acetaminophen exposure being potentiated by one or more of the agents in the compound analgesic.

What role excessive acetaminophen ingestion may play in the progression of other renal diseases is unknown. In a study by Sandlier et al. (78), an association between chronic renal failure (of any cause) and excess acetaminophen usage was reported. Due to the nature of the study, cause and effect were not established and the conclusions must be interpreted with caution. Further experimental work is required to establish what contribution acetaminophen may play in the progression of chronic renal disease, apart from that seen with chronic acetaminophen nephrotoxicity and/or analgesic nephropathy.

ACKNOWLEDGMENTS

The collaboration with Drs. Janardanan Mohandas and Robert Walker in many of the studies is gratefully acknowledged, as is the clerical assistance of Mrs. Louise Stratton.

REFERENCES

1. Cobden I, Record CO, Ward MK, Kerr DNS. Paracetamol-induced acute renal failure in the absence of fulminant liver damage. *Br Med J* 1982;284:21–22.
2. Prescott LF, Proudfoot AT, Gregeen RJ. Paracetamol-induced acute renal failure in the absence of fulminant liver damage. *Br Med J* 1982;284:421–422.
3. Gabriel R. Paracetamol-induced acute renal failure in the absence of fulminant liver damage. *Br Med J* 1982;284:505–506.
4. Gabriel R, Caldwell J, Hartley RB. Acute tubular necrosis, caused by therapeutic doses of paracetamol? *Clin Nephrol* 1983;18:269–271.
5. Kher K, Makker S. Acute renal failure due to acetaminophen ingestion without concurrent hepatotoxicity. *Am J Med* 1987;82:1280–1281.

6. Curry RW, Robinson JD, Sughue MJ. Acute renal failure after acetaminophen ingestion. *JAMA* 1982;247:1012–1014.
7. Bjorck S, Svalander CT, Aurell M. Acute renal failure after analgesic drugs including paracetamol (acetaminophen). *Nephron* 1988;50:55–56.
8. Davenport A, Finn R. Paracetamol (acetaminophen) poisoning resulting in acute renal failure without hepatic coma. *Nephron* 1988;50:55–56.
9. Wilkinson SP, Moodie H, Arroyo VA, Williams R. Frequency of renal impairment in paracetamol overdosage compared to other causes of acute liver failure. *J Clin Pathol* 1977;30:141–143.
10. Meredith TJ, Vale JA. *Paracetamol-poisoning. Poisoning: diagnosis and treatment.* London: Update Books, 1981;104–112.
11. Kaysen GA, Pond SM, Roper MH, Menke DJ, Marrama MA. Combined hepatic and renal injury in alcoholics during therapeutic use of acetaminophen. *Arch Intern Med* 1985;145:2019–2023.
12. Denisen H, Kaczynski J, Wallerstedt S. Paracetamol medication and alcohol abuse: a dangerous combination for the liver and kidney. *Scand J Gastroenterol* 1987;22:701–704.
13. Potter WZ, Davis DD, Mitchell JR, Jollow DJ, Gillette JR, Brodie BB. Acetaminophen-induced hepatic necrosis. III. Cytochrome P-450-mediated covalent binding in vitro. *J Pharmacol Exp Ther* 1973;187:203–210.
14. Boyer TD, Rouff SL. Acetaminophen-induced hepatic necrosis and renal failure. *JAMA* 1971; 218:440–441.
15. McMurtry RJ, Snodgrass WR, Mitchell JR. Renal necrosis, glutathione depletion, and covalent binding after acetaminophen. *Toxicol Appl Pharmacol* 1978;46:87–100.
16. Zenzer TV, Mattammal MB, David BB. Differential distribution of the mixed-function oxidase activities in rabbit kidney. *J Pharmacol Exp Ther* 1978;207:719–725.
17. Mohandas J, Duggin GG, Horvath JS, Tiller DJ. Metabolic oxidation of acetaminophen (paracetamol) mediated by cytochrome P-450 mixed-function oxidase and prostaglandin endoperoxidase synthetase in rabbit kidney. *Toxicol Appl Pharmacol* 1981;61:252–259.
18. Carpenter HM, Mudge GH. Acetaminophen nephrotoxicity: Studies on renal acetylation and deacetylation. *J Pharmacol Exp Ther* 1981;218:161–167.
19. Mohandas J, Duggin GG, Horvath JS, Tiller DJ. Regional differences in peroxidatic activation of paracetamol (acetaminophen) mediated by cytochrome p450 and prostaglandin endoperoxide synthetase in rabbit kidney. *Res Commun Chem Pathol Pharmacol* 1981;34:69–80.
20. Potter DW, Hinson JA. Mechanisms of acetaminophen oxidation to *N*-acetyl-*p*-benzo-quinoneimine by horseradish peroxidase and cytochrome P-450. *J Biol Chem* 1987;262:966–973.
21. Josephy PD, Eling TE, Mason RP. Oxidation of *p*-aminophenol catalyzed by horseradish peroxidase and prostaglandin synthase. *Mol Pharmacol* 1983;23:461–466.
22. Newton JF, Pasino DA, Hook JB. Acetaminophen nephrotoxicity in the rat: quantitation of renal metabolic activation in vivo. *Toxicol Appl Pharmacol* 1985;78:39–46.
23. Newton JF, Kuo CH, DeShone GM, Hoefle D, Bernstein J, Hook JB. The role of *p*-aminophenol in acetaminophen-induced nephrotoxicity: effect of *bio*(*p*-nitro-phenyl) phosphate on acetaminophen and p-aminophenol nephrotoxicity and metabolism in Fischer 344 rats. *Toxicol Appl Pharmacol* 1985;81:416–430.
24. De Vries J. Hepatotoxic metabolic activation of paracetamol and its derivatives phencetin and benorilate: oxygenation or electron transfer? *Biochem Pharmacol* 1981;30:399–402.
25. Morgan ET, Koop DR, Coon MJ. Comparison of six rabbit liver cytochrome P-450 isozymes in formation of a reactive metabolite of acetaminophen. *Biochem Biophys Res Commun* 1983;112:8–13.
26. Steele CM, Masson HA, Battershill JM, Gibson GG, Ioannides C. Metabolic activation of paracetamol by highly purified forms of cytochrome P-450. *Res Commun Chem Pathol Pharmacol* 1983;40:109–119.
27. Brown RAG. Hepatic and renal damage with paracetamol overdosage. *J Clin Pathol* 1968;21:793.
28. Pezzano M, Richard C, Lampl E, Pelletier G, Fabre M, Rimailho A, Auzepy P. Hepatic and renal toxicity of paracetamol in chronic alcoholic patients. *Presse Med* 1988;17:21–24.
29. Rahimtula AD, O'Brien PJ. Hydroperoxide catalyzed liver microsomal aromatic hydroxylation reactions involving cytochrome P-450. *Biochem Biophys Res Commun* 1974;60:440–447.
30. Van De Stratt R, Vromans RM, Bosman P, De Vries J, Vermeulen NPE. Cytochrome P-450-mediated oxidation of substrates by electron-transfer; role of oxygen radicals and of 1- and 2-electron oxidation of paracetamol. *Chem Biol Interact* 1988;64:267–280.
31. Mitchell JR, Jollow DJ, Potter WZ, Gillette JR, Brodie BB. Acetaminophen-induced hepatic necrosis. IV. Protective role of glutathione. *J Pharmacol Exp Ther* 1973;187:211–217.

32. Mudge GH, Gemborys MW, Duggin GG. Covalent binding of metabolites of acetaminophen to kidney protein and depletion of renal glutathione. *J Pharmacol Exp Ther* 1978;206:218–226.
33. Moldeus P, Andersson B, Rahimtula A, Berggren M. Prostaglandin synthetase catalyzed activation of paracetamol. *Biochem Pharmacol* 1982;31:1363–1368.
34. Potter DW, Hinson JA. Reactions of *N*-acetyl-*p*-benzo-quinoneimine with reduced glutathione, acetaminophen, and NADPH. *Mol Pharmacol* 1986;30:33–41.
35. Orrenius S, Moldeus P. The multiple roles of glutathione in drug metabolism. *Trends Pharmacol Sci* 1984;432–435.
36. Ketterer B, Coles B, Meyer DJ. The role of glutathione in detoxication. *Environ Health Perspect* 1983;49:59–69.
37. Wendel A, Feuerstein S, Konz KH. Acute paracetamol intoxication of starved mice leads to lipid peroxidation in vivo. *Biochem Pharmacol* 1979;28:2051–2055.
38. Dahlin DC, Miwa GT, Lu AYH, Nelson SD. *N*-acetyl-*p*-benzo-quinoneimine: a cytochrome P-450-mediated oxidation product of acetaminophen. *Proc Natl Acad Sci USA* 1984;81:1327–1331.
39. Calder IC, Yong AC, Woods RA, Crowe CA, Ham KN, Tange JD. The nephrotoxicity of *p*-aminophenol. II. The effect of metabolic inhibitors and inducers. *Chem Biol Interact* 1979;21:245–254.
40. Lake BG, Harris RA, Phillips JC, Gangoli SD. Studies on the effects of *L*-ascorbic acid on acetaminophen-induced hepatoxicity. I. Inhibition of the covalent binding of acetaminophen metabolites to hepatic microsomes in vitro. *Toxicol Appl Pharmacol* 1981;60:229–240.
41. Powis G, Hodnett EM, Santone KS, See KL, Melder DC. Role of metabolism and oxidation-reduction cycling in cytotoxicity of antitumor quinoneimines and quinonedimines. *Cancer Res* 1987; 47:2363–2370.
42. Mason RP, Fischer V. Free radicals of acetaminophen: Their subsequent reactions and toxicological significance. *Fed Proc* 1986;45:2493–2499.
43. Lind C, Hochstein P, Ernster L. DT-disphorase as a quinone reductase: a cellular control device against semiquinone and superoxide radical formation. *Arch Biochem Biophys* 1982;216:178–185.
44. Mohandas J, Chennell AF, Duggin GG, Horvath JS, Tiller DJ. DT-diaphorase: differential distribution in rabbit kidney and possible protection against quinone toxicity in the inner medulla. *Res Commun Chem Pathol Pharmacol* 1984;43:463–475.
45. Thor H, Smith MT, Hartzell P, Bellomo G, Jewell SA, Orrenius S. The metabolism of menadione (2-methyl-1,4-naphthoquinone) by isolated hepatocytes—a study of the implications of oxidative stress in intact cells. *J Biol Chem* 1982;257:12419–12425.
46. Prescott LF. Paracetamol overdosage. Pharmacological considerations and chemical management. *Drugs* 1983;25290–25314.
47. Spuehler O, Zollinger HU. Die chronische interstitielle nephritis. *Z Klin Med* 1953;151:1–50.
48. Nordenfelt O, Ringertz N. Phenacetin takers dead with renal failure. *Acta Med Scand* 1961;170: 385–402.
49. Murray T, Goldberg M. Analgesic abuse and renal disease. *Annu Rev Med* 1976;26:537–550.
50. Second Report of the Australia and New Zealand Transplant Registry. Australian Kidney Foundation, 1979;8.
51. Gault MH, Blennerhassett J, Muehrcke RC. Analgesic nephropathy: a clinicopathologic study using electron microscopy. *Am J Med* 1971;51:740–756.
52. Gilman A. Analgesic nephrotoxicity: a pharmacological analysis (editorial). *Am J Med* 1964;36: 167–173.
53. Duggin GG. Analgesic induced kidney disease. *Aust J Pharmacol Sci* 1977;6,2:44–49.
54. Ferguson I, Johnson F, Reay B, Wigley R. Aspirin, phenacetin and the kidney: A rheumatism clinic study. *Med J Aust* 1977;1:950–954.
55. Dubach UC, Levy PS, Rosner B, Baumeler H, Muller A, Peier A, Ehrenspencer T. Relation between regular intake of phenacetin-containing analgesics and laboratory evidence for urorenal disorders in a working female population of Switzerland. *Lancet* 1975;1:539–543.
56. Gloor FJ. Changing concepts in pathogenesis and morphology of analgesic nephropathy as seen in Europe. *Kidney Int* 1978;13:27–33.
57. Burry A. Pathology of analgesic nephropathy: Australian experience. *Kidney Int* 1978;13:34–40.
58. Lindeneg O, Fischer S, Pederson J, Nissen NI. Necrosis of the renal papillae and prolonged abuse of phenacetic. *Acta Med Scand* 1959;165:321–332.
59. Goodman LS, Gilman A. *The pharmacological basis of therapeutics*, 5th ed. New York: Macmillan, 1975;325.

60. Barraclough MA, Nilam F. Effect of vasopressin on the renal tubular reabsorption and corticopapillary concentration gradient of phenacetin and its metabolites. *Experientia* 1972;28:1065–1066.
61. Brodie BB, Axelrod J. The fate of acetophenetidin (phenacetin) in man and methods for the estimation of acetophenetidin and its metabolites in biological material. *J Pharmacol Exp Ther* 1949; 97:58–67.
62. Duggin GG, Mudge GH. Phenacetin: renal tubular transport and intrarenal distribution in the dog. *J Pharmacol Exp Ther* 1976;199:1–9.
63. Duggin GG. Phenacetin estimation from biological samples by high performance liquid chromatography. *J Chromatogr* 1976;6:214–217.
64. Bluemle W, Goldberg M. Renal accumulation of salicylate and phenacetin: possible mechanisms in the nephropathy of analgesic abuse. *J Clin Invest* 1968;47:2507–2514.
65. Duggin GG, Mudge GH. Analgesic nephropathy: renal distribution of acetaminophen and its conjugates. *J Pharmacol Exp Ther* 1976;199:1–9.
66. Quintanilla A, Kessler RH. Direct effects of salicylate on renal function in the dog. *J Clin Invest* 1973;52:3143–3153.
67. Trinder P. Rapid determination of salicylate in biological fluids. *Biochem J* 1954;57:301–305.
68. Caterson RJ, Duggin GG. Intrarenal distribution of salicylate. *Proc Aust Soc Med Res* 1978;11: 1–57.
69. Caterson RJ, Duggin GG, Horvath JS, Tiller DJ. Simultaneous determination of aspirin and salicylate by high performance liquid chromatography. *Aust J Pharmacol Sci* 1978;7,4:111–112.
70. Beyer KH Jr, Gelanden RT. Renal concentration gradients of salicylic acid and its metabolic congeners in the dog. *Arch Intern Pharmacol Ther* 1978;2312:180–195.
71. Zenser TV, Mattammal MB, Brown WW, Davies BD. Enzyme nephropathy. *Kidney Int* 1980; 18:553–561.
72. Boyd J, Eling TE. Prostaglandin endoperoxide synthetase-transport and intrarenal distribution in the dog. *J Pharmacol Exp Ther* 1976;199:10–16.
73. Mohandas J, Duggin GG, Horvath JS, Tiller DJ. Metabolic oxidation of acetaminophen (paracetamol) mediated by cytochrome p-450 mixed function oxidase and prostaglandin endoperoxide synthetase in rabbit kidney. *Toxicol Appl Pharmacol* 1981;61:252–259.
74. Duggin GG, Mohandas J. Biochemical mechanisms of acetaminophen (paracetamol) induced hepatic and renal toxicity. In: Yoshida H, Hagihara Y, Ebashi S, eds. *Advances in pharmacology and therapeutics II, vol 5. Toxicology and experimental models.* Oxford: Pergamon Press, 1982;77–86.
75. Mohandas J, Marshall JJ, Duggin GG, Horvath JS, Tiller DJ. Differential distribution of glutathione and glutathione-related enzymes in the rabbit kidney. *Biochem Pharmacol* 1984;33:1801–1807.
76. Zenser TV, Mattammal MB, Brown WW, Davies BD. Effect of aspirin on metabolism of acetaminophen and benzidine by renal inner medullary prostaglandin hydroperoxidase *J Clin Lab Med* 1983;101:58–65.
77. Duggin GG. Mechanisms in the development of analgesic nephropathy. *Kidney Int* 1980;18:553–561.
78. Sandler DP, Smith JC, Weinberg CR, Buckalew VM. Dennis systems involved in the formation of reactive metabolites in the renal medulla: Cooxidation via prostaglandin H synthase. *Fundam Appl Toxicol* 1984;4:922–929.

Toxicology of the Kidney, Second Edition,
edited by Jerry B. Hook and Robin S. Goldstein.
Raven Press, Ltd., New York © 1993.

12

Nephrotoxicity of Cyclosporine and Other Immunosuppressive and Immunotherapeutic Agents

Lorraine C. Racusen and *Kim Solez

*Department of Pathology, The Johns Hopkins University School of Medicine, Baltimore, Maryland 21205; and *Department of Pathology, The University of Alberta, Edmonton, Alberta, Canada T6G 2R7*

Solid organ and bone marrow transplantation have been revolutionized by the availability of new immunosuppressive agents developed over the past 10 to 15 years. The first and most widely used is cyclosporin A (CsA) a fungal metabolite with immunosuppressive properties, first described by Borel in 1972. The drug acts on the immune system to selectively inhibit T-cell activation and interleukin-2–mediated events. In the cell, this hydrophobic molecule binds to a cytoplasmic receptor, cyclophilin, one of a family of intracellular proteins, the immunophilins (1); cyclophilin appears to be identical to peptidyl-prolyl isomerase, which catalyzes the interconversion of the cis- and trans-rotamases of peptidyl-prolyl bonds of peptides and proteins (2,3). FK506, a recently discovered macrolide fungal product, also inhibits T-cell activation, interacting with a cytoplasmic binding protein, FKBP, which also has rotamase activity but is distinct from cyclophilin (4,5). The monoclonal antibody OKT_3 has been used in immunosuppressive protocols to destroy effector T cells and prevent or treat acute rejection (6,7).

A major side effect of cyclosporine, and potentially of FK506 and other agents as well, is renal toxicity. At least, with cyclosporine, immunosuppressive and nephrotoxic actions of the drug are tightly linked (8). Immunosuppressive protocols have reduced this toxic side effect to some extent, but it still remains a significant problem. CsA has proven so useful and effective, however, that it will likely continue to be used for some time to come, making study of renal pathology and pathophysiology produced by the drug of continued clinical as well as theoretical importance. In this chapter, the effects of CsA on renal structure and function in humans and in experimental models are reviewed. In addition, clinical and experimental toxicity of other newer immunosuppressive agents are considered.

Interleukin-2 (IL-2) represents another class of immunotherapeutic agents, developed to stimulate the immune system. IL-2 is a cytokine that activates polymorphonuclear leukocytes as an early effect, and stimulates generation of lymphokine-activated killer cells. This latter property has led to the use of IL-2 in cancer chemotherapy (9,10). However, treatment with IL-2 is associated with severe and potentially life-threatening complications, including acute renal failure. Nephrotoxicity of IL-2 in both clinical use and in experimental models is also discussed in this chapter, as well as nephrotoxicity due to therapy with interferon and/or recombinant human tumor necrosis factor.

CLINICAL NEPHROTOXICITY OF IMMUNOSUPPRESSIVE AGENTS

Cyclosporine

It is not clear that the nephrotoxic and immunosuppressive effects of cyclosporine can be completely separated; therefore, there may not be a real "therapeutic window" in the sense of a completely nontoxic but effective dose range for the drug. If sensitive and accurate serial measurements of glomerular filtration rate were employed in all cyclosporine-treated patients, it is likely that the rate of detected renal dysfunction would approach 100%. Most transplant patients have demonstrated an improvement in renal function when they are converted from cyclosporine to azathioprine immunosuppression, as long as rejection does not occur (11,12). This finding supports the idea that cyclosporine therapy reduces renal function in most patients. In many cases, however, the renal dysfunction produced by cyclosporine is mild and probably clinically unimportant, at least over the short term.

Four discrete syndromes of clinically significant renal dysfunction caused by cyclosporine in the native or grafted kidney have been identified (13–15):(a) acute reversible renal functional impairment, usually occurring early in the course of treatment, (b) delayed renal allograft function, (c) acute vasculopathy (thrombotic microangiopathy), and (d) chronic nephropathy with interstitial fibrosis. Various combinations of these syndromes may occur, and they can also be combined with transplant rejection or other types of renal disease not directly related to cyclosporine therapy.

Acute Reversible Renal Functional Impairment

This syndrome is probably most similar to acute nephrotoxicity models in animals. It was first reported in patients receiving cyclosporine following bone marrow transplantation (16). Cyclosporine was administered parenterally in high doses (up to 20 mg/kg/day), and acute impairment often occurred in patients who were also receiving other known nephrotoxic drugs. Acute renal failure (ARF) was sometimes dramatic in onset and protracted. Patients treated with a lower dose of cyclosporine have a less dramatic onset of renal failure and a lower incidence of oliguria.

In heart allograft recipients treated with cyclosporine, acute oliguric renal failure frequently occurs within the first 4 days posttransplant. Reporting on the University of Pittsburgh experience, Greenberg et al. (14) observed significant azotemia in 25 of 43 patients, with full-blown ARF in 5 of these. Urine sodium is characteristically less than 10 mEq/l and the oliguria is normally self-limiting with normal urine output returning by day 5 or 6 (13,14,17). Although peak serum creatinine levels tend to coincide with the highest trough serum cyclosporine levels during the first week posttransplant, the absolute magnitude of the renal functional impairment correlates more closely with the degree of impaired renal function observed prior to cardiac transplantation than with serum cyclosporine levels, suggesting that patients with inadequate renal reserve are more susceptible to acute reversible renal functional impairment brought about by cyclosporine (13). Similar episodes of ARF have been reported following liver transplantation, particularly when intravenous cyclosporine was used (18).

Although vasopressors were often in use during this period of acute reversible renal functional impairment in cyclosporine-treated heart allograft recipients, the patients did not appear to be volume-depleted or in a severe low-output state by clinical examination or cardiac-output measurements (14). In fact, most patients had a significant persistent weight gain during the early posttransplant period. Nonetheless, the renal dysfunction observed did have features suggestive of a volume depletion "prerenal azotemia." Serum urea nitrogen rose proportionately more than serum creatinine, and the kidney retained its ability to reabsorb sodium and to produce a concentrated urine. In these respects, the renal dysfunction was like that reported in nonhypotensive sepsis in which azotemia occurs despite good hydration (19). In the study of Greenberg et al. (14), slight azotemia also occurred in the azathioprine-treated cardiac allograft group (mean BUN of 32 mg/dl on day 4), suggesting that a small but significant portion of the azotemia observed in the cyclosporine-treated group relates to the post–cardiac transplant status of the patients rather than to cyclosporine toxicity.

Characteristic of this syndrome of acute reversible renal functional impairment brought about by cyclosporine is the very rapid return of renal function when cyclosporine levels are reduced (20). As discussed by Myers (21), the return of renal function tends to coincide with the normalization of serum cyclosporine levels, with the slope of declining levels and declining serum creatinine concentrations being approximately equal. The relationship between acute cyclosporine nephrotoxicity and circulating levels of the drug is controversial. However, nephrotoxicity is generally observed in association with rising or elevated serum levels exceeding 200 ng/ml and is common in patients with levels exceeding 400 ng/ml. Toxicity due to cyclosporine alone is rarely observed with serum cyclosporine levels of less than 200 ng/ml (22,23).

The distinction between acute cyclosporine nephrotoxicity and acute renal transplant rejection is frequently difficult. Klintmalm et al. (24) and Flechner et al. (25) have compared the clinical characteristics of these two situations. Acute rejection is rare after 4 months posttransplant. In renal allograft recipients, the increase in serum creatinine accompanying cyclosporine toxicity is generally slower, rising to 25% above baseline by approximately 1 week. Oliguria is less common than in acute rejection, and fever is highly unusual. In contrast, acute rejection is usually characterized by at least one of the following findings: oliguria, an increase in weight of more than 0.5 kg, fever exceeding 37.5°C, and a rapidly increasing serum creatinine level. Serum cyclosporine levels are generally higher during acute nephrotoxicity (>200 ng/ml), and often have fallen preceding the onset of rejection. In Keown et al.'s (23) series, a mean trough serum level during acute rejection within the first 3 months posttransplant was 165 ng/ml compared with 210 ng/ml during periods of stable allograft function.

Percutaneous needle biopsies of the grafted kidney as well as fine-needle aspirates have been used to distinguish between cyclosporine nephrotoxicity and acute rejection. Some typical appearances obtained through these two techniques are illustrated in color plates in Burdick et al. (26). The presence of an intimal arteritis (27,28) (Fig. 1) or of Leu7$^+$ intratubular lymphocytes (29) are reliable indicators of the presence of acute rejection. Arteriolar hyalinosis (Fig. 2) is frequently observed in cyclosporine nephrotoxicity but is not seen in all cases (30–32). In a recent biopsy study, this was the only lesion clearly differentiating cases of cyclosporine nephrotoxicity from control cases with normal function (33). "Isometric" vacuolization of proximal tubular cells (Fig. 3) appears to be more prominent in fine-needle

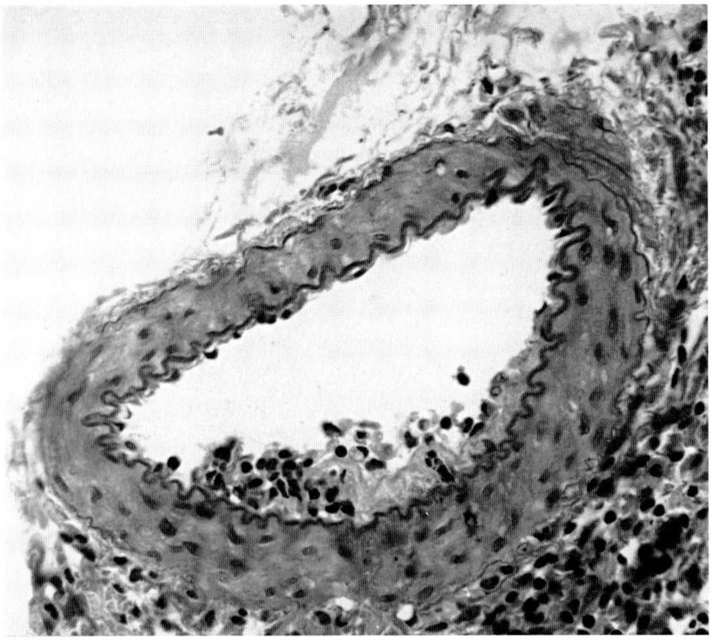

FIG. 1. A vessel in a renal transplant biopsy showing infiltration of the intima by mononuclear inflammatory cells, so-called intimal arteritis or endothelialitis. (Reprinted from Burdick et al. Characteristics of early routine renal allograft biopsies. *Transplantation* 1984;38:679–684.)

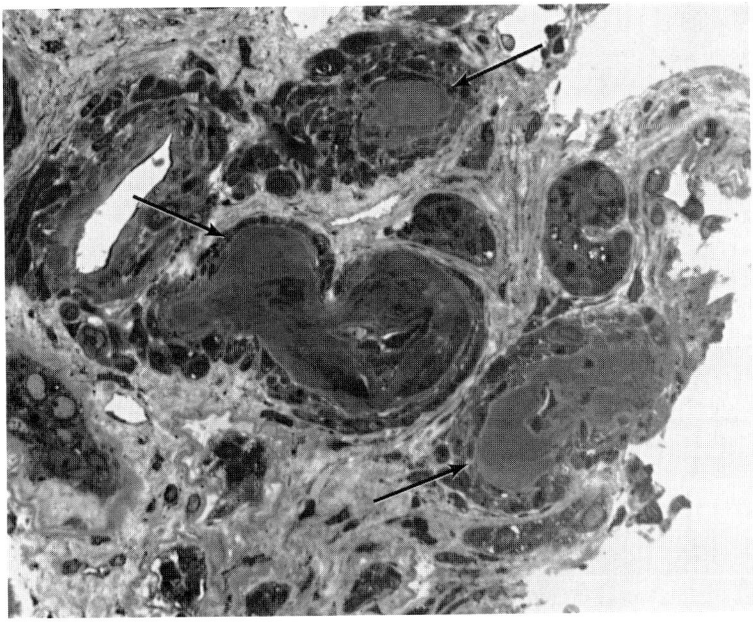

FIG. 2. Arterioles in a renal biopsy from a cardiac allograft recipient on cyclosporine for 440 days. Vessels show loss of myocytes and mural hyalinosis, with a number of discrete nodular deposits (*arrows*). (Reprinted from Keown et al., ref. 13, with permission.)

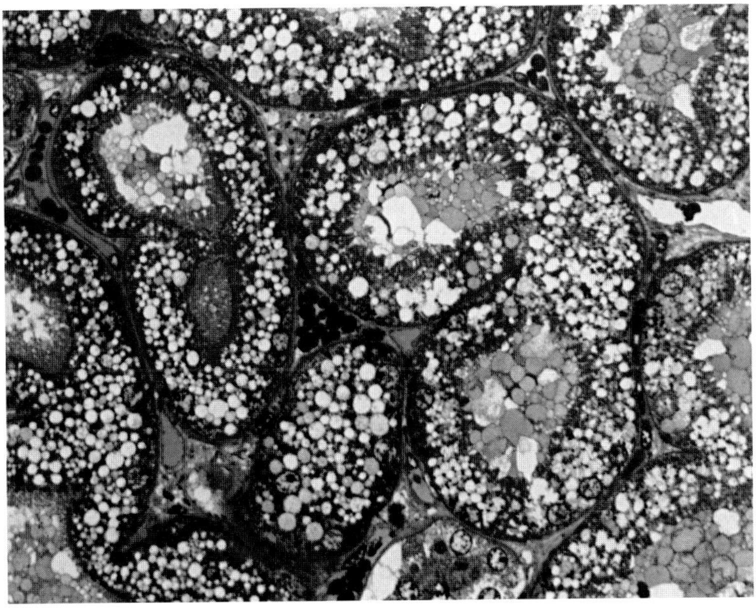

FIG. 3. Renal proximal tubules showing extensive "isometric" vacuolization typical of that seen in renal biopsies from cyclosporine-treated patients. (Reprinted from Keown et al., ref. 13, with permission.)

aspirates than in biopsies. This change has been reported to be present in 11 out of 12 cases of CsA toxicity studies by fine-needle aspiration (34). Although tubular vacuolization and the presence of cytoplasmic inclusions are characteristic of cyclosporine therapy, they are not specific for cyclosporine nephrotoxicity. A substantial interstitial infiltrate of inflammatory cells can occur in the absence of rejection, and it is frequently present even in stable, well-functioning renal allografts (28). On a histological basis, cyclosporine nephrotoxicity is often a diagnosis of exclusion made when definite signs of acute rejection are not present. Salaman and Griffin (35) have described the use of fine-needle intrarenal manometry to distinguish rejection from cyclosporine nephrotoxicity. Acute rejection is associated with intense inflammation and interstitial edema, and therefore the renal interstitial pressure is elevated. Cyclosporine nephrotoxicity is associated with renal vasoconstriction without interstitial edema, and therefore interstitial pressure is low (35). It is certainly possible for rejection and cyclosporine nephrotoxicity to coexist, and the distinction between these two entities often depends on the response to therapy. If a reduction in the dose of cyclosporine results in a fall of serum creatinine, this suggests cyclosporine nephrotoxicity. If, on the other hand, there is resolution of renal function following the administration of steroids or antilymphocyte globulin, this suggests the presence of acute rejection.

Myers et al. (36) has recently put forward the view that the acute reversible renal functional impairment is caused by afferent arteriolar vasoconstriction that with time leads to the hyaline arteriolopathy mentioned above. Eventually, this arteriolar lesion leads to a "striped" interstitial fibrosis and more chronic renal functional impairment (see below). There is some evidence that the renin-angiotensin system may be involved in the arteriolar vasoconstriction (37). In the early phases, the vasoconstriction can be reversed by dopamine and nifedipine (38,39).

Delayed Renal Allograft Function

It is now well established that cyclosporine prolongs the duration of ischemic posttransplant ARF in renal allografts. Belitsky et al. (40) found that delayed function in patients receiving cyclosporine is related to the duration of cold storage of the graft. Countries such as Australia that do not use beating-heart donors have a significantly higher incidence of initial nonfunction. Shiel et al. (41) showed that the incidence of initial nonfunction rose from 60% to 83% with cyclosporine therapy, and the mean duration of posttransplant failure, which had been 13 days on steroid-azathioprine immunosuppression, nearly doubled to 23 days.

In the Canadian multicenter trial, initial nonfunction did not appear to be an entirely benign condition even though most grafts eventually did regain function. Patients with initial nonfunction had a significantly longer hospital stay and increased number of treated "rejection episodes," a higher cumulative steroid dose, a higher serum creatinine 6 months posttransplant, and a lower graft survival (42). However, it is likely that factors such as early rejection and surgical complications were responsible for some of the nonfunction observed; thus, it cannot be concluded that uncomplicated ischemic injury was associated with an adverse outcome.

Acute Vasculopathy (Thrombotic Microangiopathy)

There has been some confusion between the changes of cyclosoprine-induced arteriolopathy and the vascular changes of acute rejection. Differences between these two are clearly depicted in Figs. 1 and 2 (also see color Figs. 2A and B in Burdick et al., 26). The intimal arteritis of acute rejection (Fig. 1) involves arcuate and interlobular arteries, in which there is a cellular intimal thickening with lymphocytes incorporated into the intimal mass. Cyclosporine arteriolopathy (Fig. 2), on the other hand, affects arterioles and glomerular capillaries and has no intrinsic inflammatory cell component. Arterioles show various combination of hyaline and fibrinoid change, often with identifiable fibrinogen deposition by immunofluorescence. Glomerular capillaries show thrombosis with endothelial cell desquamation or nuclear pyknosis. Certainly, vascular lesions can occur that represent a combination of rejection and cyclosporine toxicity, and this may be the situation with the lesions described by Sommer et al. (43). We have observed glomerular capillary thrombosis in biopsy specimens taken 1 hr after anastomoses from renal transplant patients pretreated with parenteral cyclosporine. For the first 80 Johns Hopkins Hospital renal transplant patients pretreated with cyclosporine, 7 have shown glomerular capillary thrombosis and/or endothelial injury in the 1-hr posttransplant biopsy (Fig. 4). In these cases, we excluded not only hyperacute rejection and perfusion injury as possible causes of the changes seen, but also such phenomena as the presence of cold-reactive IgM antibodies (44) or red cell cold agglutinins (45). By the process of exclusion, therefore, since unexplained capillary thrombosis had not occurred in our experience in the precyclosporine era, we concluded that cyclosporine was the likely cause of these changes. It is of interest that all 7 cases of glomerular capillary thrombosis in 1-hr posttransplant biopsies occurred in the winter months, and we have not observed this phenomenon before November or after mid-March. The seasonal predilection is like that seen in scleroderma renal failure (46), which is also characterized by intrarenal thrombosis.

Of the 7 patients in whom glomerular capillary thrombosis and/or endothelial injury were observed in the 1-hr posttransplant biopsy, one had primary nonfunction without signs of rejection and ultimately had the transplant removed, another had prolonged transplant dysfunction and never obtained a serum creatinine below 2.7 mg/dl, and the remainder had delayed function but ultimately lowered their serum creatinines below 2.7 mg/dl at times ranging from 14 to 150 days posttransplant (mean 74 days).

Parmar et al. (47) have recently described four cases of severe glomerular endothelial cell injury and microvascular thrombosis detected in routine 1-hr posttransplant biopsies, associated clinically with initial allograft nonfunction followed by irreversible renal failure. The four allografts were cadaveric kidneys from two do-

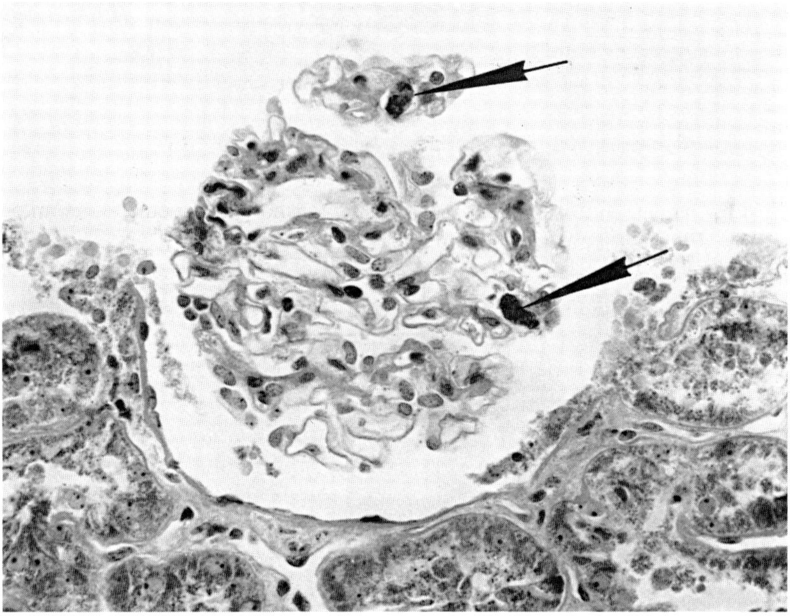

FIG. 4. A glomerulus with capillary loops containing fibrin thrombi (*arrows*). (Reprinted from Racusen and Solez, ref. 138, with permission.)

nors with severe brain injury. The clinical course was not unlike cases of allograft nonfunction ascribed to "acute tubular necrosis," except that recovery was incomplete in all cases. Follow-up biopsies at variable intervals of 2 to 15 weeks showed resolving lesions. Other potential causes, including hyperacute rejection, perfusion injury, large vessel thromboses, and the presence of cold agglutinins were ruled out; none of the patients were treated with cyclosporine before onset of the syndrome and performance of the initial allograft biopsy (47). The authors postulate that the severe injury to the brain released humoral mediators that damaged the microvascular endothelium in the donors prior to harvesting. This study serves as a reminder that the clinical transplant setting is complex, and that there are a variety of factors, some including cyclosporine, defined, and others as yet undefined, that may contribute to endothelial injury in these patients.

Although intrarenal thrombosis has not been described by others as early as 1 hr posttransplant, there are numerous reports of thromboembolic complications occurring later in the posttransplant period in cyclosporine-treated renal allograft recipients (48–50). The first report of cyclosporine-induced vasculopathy was that of Shulman et al. (50) in bone marrow allograft recipients. These vascular changes may relate to the endothelial damaging and thrombogenic effects of cyclosporine observed in animal models.

Grace et al. (51) have demonstrated increased platelet aggregation and thromboxane release in patients and normal volunteers treated with CsA. The calcium channel blocker nifedipine appeared to eliminate these effects.

Chronic Nephropathy with Interstitial Fibrosis

It is a common, widely accepted observation that renal allograft recipients on chronic cyclosporine therapy generally show some evidence of long-term nephrotoxicity with serum creatinine levels of 2.0 mg/dl or higher (52). Renal biopsy specimens from patients treated with cyclosporine for a year or more, in which renal function impairment of this type is often observed, show a striped form of interstitial fibrosis (Fig. 5). However, as emphasized by Keown et al. (13), in renal allografts it is often difficult to differentiate the changes of chronic cyclosporine toxicity from those of so-called chronic rejection. Chronic nephrotoxicity is somewhat easier to study in the cardiac allograft recipients who are transplanted at a time when they have healthy native kidneys (14,53). As is shown in Fig. 6, taken from Myers (21), the prevailing level of serum creatinine among cyclosporine-treated 1-year survivors of heart transplantation at Stanford University is significantly higher than that in the historical control group treated with steroids and azathioprine. Serum creatinine concentration was below 1.4 mg/dl in most of the azathioprine-treated recipients, but exceeded 1.4 mg/dl in almost all of the cyclosporine patients. The mean serum creatinine concentration in the cyclosporine group of 2.1 mg/dl was significantly greater than the corresponding value of 1.2 in the azathioprine group ($p<.001$). About one-third of the patients in each group were selected at random for inulin clearance studies. As can be seen in the lower portion of Fig. 6, inulin clearance was in a normal range (>80 ml/min/1.73 m^2) in most of the azathioprine-treated group, but was significantly reduced in all but one of the cyclosporine-treated patients. As with the serum creatinine levels, there was little overlap between the two groups. The mean glomerular filtration rate (GFR) in the cyclosporine-treated group was decreased by almost 50% (53 ± 4 vs. 91 ± 4 ml/min/1.73 m^2, $p<.001$) (21,53). Other features of chronic nephropathy in cyclosporine-treated heart transplant recipients included severe hypertension, mild proteinuria, and tubular dysfunction. A similar chronic cyclosporine toxicity has also been detected in liver transplant recipients (54). The markedly impaired GFR in stable long-surviving renal transplant patients receiving cyclosporine is probably a manifestation of the same type of chronic nephrotoxicity (55). The renal failure brought about by chronic cyclosporine nephrotoxicity may not reverse when cyclosporine is discontinued (56).

There is evidence that the structural basis of chronic cyclosporine nephrotoxicity is unique. In cardiac allograft recipients who developed end-stage renal disease on this basis, kidney size and weight were increased, not decreased, as in most types of chronic renal failure (B. Myers, personal communication). Mesangial matrix was also increased (34). Jackson et al. (57) have found evidence for proliferation of interstitial fibroblasts in rats treated with high-dose cyclosporine (100 mg/kg/day), and a similar phenomenon may occur in humans.

In studies of cardiac allograft recipients, Greenberg et al. (14) have emphasized that although both acute reversible and chronic cyclosporine nephrotoxicity occur with high prevalence, the acute form does not appear to be a specific risk factor for the chronic form. In their study, two-thirds of cyclosporine-treated patients had

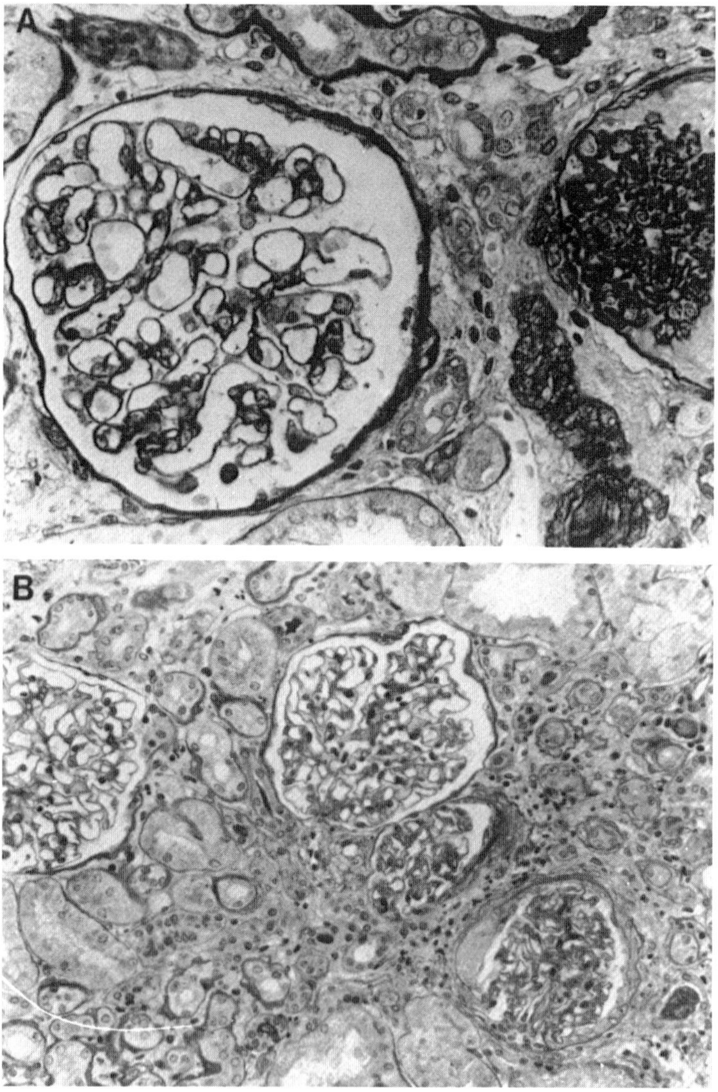

FIG. 5. Interstitial fibrosis and sclerosing glomerular changes in a renal biopsy from a patient with a cardiac transplant. **A:** Periodic acid-Schiff (PAS)-Alcian blue stain showing a collapsed sclerotic glomerulus. **B:** Small collapsed glomeruli and enlarged hypertrophic glomeruli, with zone of interstitial fibrosis and tubular atrophy. (Reprinted from Myers et al., ref. 36, with permission.)

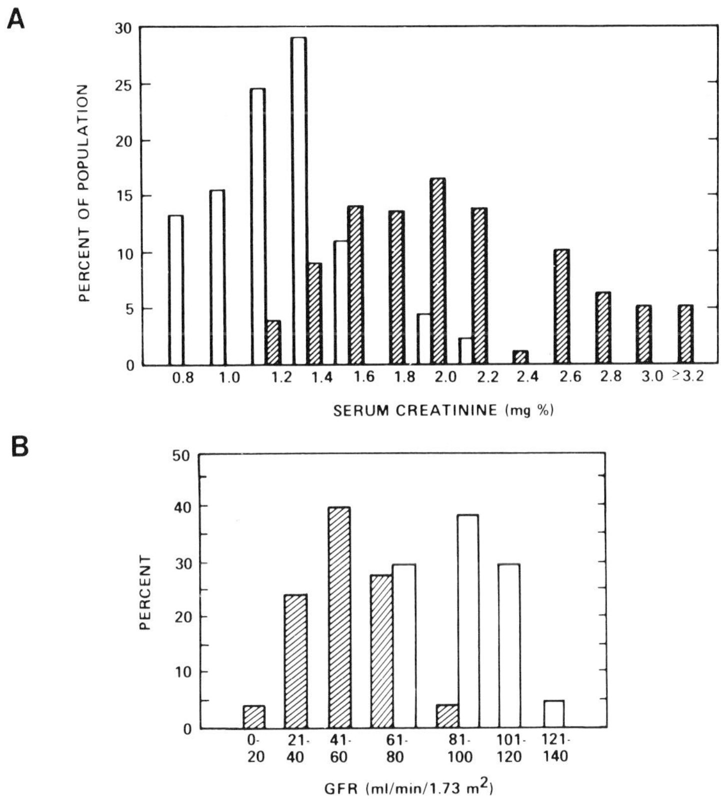

FIG. 6. Bar graphs showing serum creatinine **(A)** and glomerular filtration rate as measured by inulin clearance **(B)** in patients immunosuppressed with azathioprine (*open bars*) or cyclosporine (*hatched bars*), expressed as percent of the patient population at each value. (Reprinted from Myers, ref. 21, with permission.)

renal dysfunction at 1 year in both the group that had experienced posttransplant ARF and the group that had maintained normal renal function in the perioperative period. In renal allograft recipients there is a relationship between cumulative cyclosporine dose and chronic nephrotoxicity, whereas acute nephrotoxicity is related to trough cyclosporine blood levels (13,27,58). Thus, one would not necessarily expect the same patients to be affected by both types of toxicity. In many patients the sustained mild-to-moderate decrease in GFR brought about by cyclosporine therapy does not appear to progress over time (59).

Myers et al. (60) and Bertani et al. (61) have recently drawn attention to the significant effects of cyclosporine on glomerular structure and function. Apparently, as a result of the obliterative hyaline arteriolopathy caused by cyclosporine, there is a progressive downstream collapse and sclerosis of glomeruli in biopsies from cardiac allograft recipients (Fig. 5). Analysis of dextran transport with an isoporous membrane model suggested that cyclosporine significantly reduced glomerular capillary pressure (60). Both groups (60,61) noted that a bimodal distribution of glomerular size developed, with an increased number of both abnormally small and abnormally large glomeruli; the latter probably represent compensatory hypertrophy. As end-stage renal failure sets in, there is a shift in the glomerular population, with a greater and greater number becoming abnormally small. Hyperplasia of the juxtaglomerular apparatus was also observed (61). This is less consistently observed in renal allografts treated with cyclosporine (36), suggesting that the finding in cardiac allograft recipients cannot necessarily be generalized to other situations.

Summary of Studies of Clinical Cyclosporine Nephrotoxicity

The four types of nephrotoxicity seen with cyclosporine are probably related, but it is not clear that episodes of acute reversible dysfunction increase the likelihood of chronic toxicity. The acute vasculopathy may manifest itself within 1 hr after transplantation and appears frequently to be a self-limited process. Further experimental studies are clearly needed to improve our understanding of clinical nephrotoxicity, and to devise ways of avoiding or lessening it. Morphologically, cyclosporine nephrotoxicity appears fundamentally different from the nephrotoxicity of other drugs. However, there remains a significant problem differentiating cyclosporine nephrotoxicity from acute rejection.

FK506

The best characterized of the new immunosuppressive agents, FK506, appears to have a mechanism of action similar to that of cyclosporine (62–65). The two agents are reported to have synergistic immunosuppressive and nephrotoxic properties. The high incidence of renal functional impairment observed when both agents are used together has led some authors to suggest that combination therapy should be avoided (66).

In human liver and kidney transplant patients, proximal tubular vacuolization has been reported as well as changes of acute tubular necrosis. Glomerular capillary and arteriolar thrombi have been reported in four renal allograft recipients (67). Although these four patients had other factors that may have contributed to the observed thrombosis (prior cyclosporine therapy in three cases, fungal sepsis in the fourth), they represented half the kidney allograft patients in the reported series (67). It remains possible that FK506 has endothelial-cell toxicity similar to that of cyclosporine (see Experimental Toxicity, below) despite the absence of direct *in vitro* evidence (68,69).

Interleukin-2

The relative effectiveness of IL-2 in treating metastatic renal-cell carcinoma (72,73) might suggest the possibility of direct renal tubular toxicity. However, it appears that most of the compound's nephrotoxic effects are actually indirect (72–82). The renal functional impairment frequently encountered after IL-2 therapy has usually been attributed to a systemic capillary leak with hypotension and prerenal azotemia (72–77). Rhabdomyolysis secondary to convulsions also has been cited as a cause (78). IL-2 really has no direct effect on endothelium, but stimulates release of other cytokines, including IL-1, tumor necrosis factor (TNF), lymphocytotoxin, and interferon-γ that cause endothelial-cell activation and vascular leakiness to macromolecules (79,80). Samlowski et al. (81) reported heavy shedding of renal tubular cells into the urine of patients 2 to 4 days after initiation of IL-2 therapy. Onset of these cytologic features of tubular injury preceded significant hypotension or elevation in serum creatinine, suggesting a direct tubular toxic effect.

Mercatello et al. (82) have recently reported on the characteristics of the renal functional impairment encountered in patients treated with a combination of IL-2 and interferon-α. In 16 patients treated with this combined regimen for renal cell carcinoma, renal plasma flow remained constant despite a 25% decrease in GFR, 20% decrease in systemic blood pressure, and a 50% decrease in urine output. Despite the preservation of renal blood flow, the renal failure was associated with a decrease in fractional excretion of sodium (from 1.37% to 0.56%) and a 30% increase in heart rate, features suggestive of "prerenal azotemia." Microalbuminuria was also observed. The authors postulate that the renal functional impairment is due either to a decrease in the efferent to afferent resistance ratio, leading to a decrease in glomerular capillary pressure, or to a decrease in K_f, or both. They point out that nonsteroidal anti-inflammatory agents, frequently used to minimize side effects of the immunotherapy, could considerably worsen the renal functional impairment observed in these protocols (82).

OKT_3 and TNF

The immunosuppressive agent OKT_3, a monoclonal anti–T-cell antibody, causes cytokine release similar to that of IL-2 and may manifest a similar type of nephrotoxicity in poorly hydrated patients (83–85). The higher peak creatinine during renal allograft rejection episodes treated with OKT_3 has been attributed to these effects (83). Cytologic studies have suggested the possibility of a direct tubular toxic effect (86). TNF_a may be the key mediator of OKT_3 toxicity (87).

The systemic administration of recombinant human tumor necrosis factor is characterized by side effects very similar to those for IL-2, largely attributed to a capillary leak syndrome and prerenal azotemia (88,89). In reported series, 13% to 21% of patients developed some element of renal insufficiency. The presence of enzymuria in over half the patients provided some evidence of at least subclinical direct tubular toxicity (88).

Interferon

The acute renal failure occasionally encountered in patients treated with interferon-α or -γ appears to be different from that seen with other types of immunotherapy. Proteinuria is frequently a prominent part of the presentation (90,91), and the renal failure is often severe (92), leading to death in one reported case (93). An acute interstitial nephritis was observed in one patient treated with interferon-α for mycosis fungoides (90). In another report, a patient treated with interferon-γ for acute lymphoblastic leukemia developed proteinuria and renal failure with a combination of focal glomerular sclerosis and acute tubular necrosis on biopsy, with cast formation and extensive regenerative changes in tubular epithelium (94). Both proteinuria and renal failure resolved after interferon therapy was terminated.

FROM THE CLINIC TO THE LABORATORY

Clearly, important observations have been made on the renal effects of immunotherapeutic agents in patients receiving these regimens, and the pathogenesis of renal pathology and pathophysiology has been addressed to some extent in clinical studies. However, experimental model systems are necessary to completely elucidate mechanisms of nephrotoxicty, enabling careful control of experimental variables not possible to achieve clinically. Invasive techniques enable direct study of hemodynamics and glomerular and tubular function *in vivo* in experimental animals, or in the isolated perfused kidney. Cell culture systems can be used to directly assess effects of the immunotherapeutic agent on specific cell populations in a carefully controlled milieu. Numerous *in vivo* and *in vitro* model systems have been used to study mechanisms of nephrotoxicity of cyclosporine, and to a lesser extent other immunotherapeutic agents. Results of these studies are summarized in the following discussion.

Using experimental models, considerable advances have been made in our understanding of the pathophysiology and important pathology of cyclosporine nephrotoxicity, and at least some of the general mechanisms defined for cyclosporine toxicity may apply to other immunotherapeutic agents as well. There are differences between clinical and experimental cyclosporine nephrotoxicity, some of which are related to the higher doses administered in some animal models, and factors such as plasma volume depletion and reduced oral intake, which become important variables in some animal models. However, it is likely that many of the basic experimental observations discussed below are relevant to the clinical state. Of the four types of cyclosporine nephrotoxicity seen in patients, acute reversible renal insufficiency has proven to be the most easily reproducible in experimental animals. The other types of clinical nephrotoxicity have proven more difficult to model. Delayed renal allograft function as a manifestation of cyclosporine toxicity has not been modeled. The overt acute vasculopathy described in some patients is seen only in the spontaneously hypertensive rat, and in a new model, discussed below, in which cyclosporine is administered with *Escherichia coli* lipopolysaccharide—a common thread may be preexisting endothelial injury. Substantial progress has been made in developing models of chronic nephropathy with interstitial fibrosis, models that should yield critical information on the pathogenesis of this generally irreversible form of renal injury.

Other immunotherapeutic agents that cause clinical renal dysfunction and/or injury are relatively new, and fewer models have been developed and studies performed with these agents. Although progress has been made in defining acute effects of these agents, as discussed below, no studies of their long-term impact on renal function have been performed, nor have long-term clinical assessments been made. Effects of these agents on the kidney will remain an area of active experimental interest for some time to come.

EXPERIMENTAL TOXICITY OF IMMUNOTHERAPEUTIC AGENTS

Despite preclinical testing in rodents, dogs, and the rhesus monkey, the full nephrotoxic potential of cyclosporine was not recognized until it was used as an immunosuppressive agent in humans, and it appears that the human is one of the species most sensitive to nephrotoxic side effects of this widely used immunosuppressive agent. Moreover, no one animal model reflects the spectrum of nephrotoxic effects of the drug seen in patients. Nevertheless, animal models, as well as *in vitro* studies, have proven useful in elucidating the mechanisms of cyclosporine nephrotoxicity. In contrast, although significant toxic effects of FK506 have been reported in experimental models (see below), initial human clinical transplantation trials have revealed relatively less nephrotoxicity with this agent in humans. In this section, we will review experimental studies of effects of cyclosporine and other newer immunotherapeutic agents on the kidney.

Cyclosporine Nephrotoxicity

In experimental studies, cyclosporine has been shown to have effects on structure and function of the renal tubule, renal vasculature and hemodynamics, and on the renal interstitium. Which of these effects is/are most relevant clinically has been debated, and doubtless varies with the type of clinical cyclosporine-induced renal dysfunction being considered, and with an array of clinical variables including acute and cumulative dose, patient age, the presence of preexisting or concomitant ischemic injury, and other factors.

The Renal Tubule

Early studies in rat models suggested that CsA is a primary tubular toxin, and that tubular effects of the drug explained its effects on renal function. Blair et al. (95) described isometric vacuolization of tubular cells, accumulation of eosinophilic bodies often representing giant mitochondria, and microcalcification in proximal tubules after up to 21 days of CsA (100 mg/kg/day po) (95), findings confirmed by other investigators (96–98). However, tubular cell vacuolization was also described following treatment with the parenteral CsA vehicle (99–101), and could be dissociated from a reduction in glomerular filtration rate (97,102–105), especially in acute toxic injury. Effects on the proximal tubule tend to be most prominent in the S_3 segment (106), becoming more widespread at very high doses. However, functional defects in the proximal tubule are relatively slight, and some experimental studies have shown increased reabsorption of Na, and reduction of fractional excretion, probably as a result of compensatory mechanisms (101,105). In micropuncture studies of rats treated with a low dose of CsA (15 mg/kg/day po $\times$ 5–7 days), electrolyte transport also remained normal in the loop of Henle as well as in the whole kidney (107). In the distal tubule, a hyperkalemic renal tubular acidosis is seen. Hypomagnesemia occurs due to renal magnesium wasting, but the tubular site of the failure of magnesium reabsorption has not been identified (108).

With chronic administration of cyclosporine in experimental animals, tubular changes are seen in both cortex and medulla. Rosen et al. (109) in studies of rats treated for 3 to 10 weeks with CsA (12.5 mg/kg/day) have recently described striking morphological alterations predominantly in the medullary rays of the cortex. Changes included vacuolization in proximal tubular and thick ascending limb cells; vacuoles appeared to originate in part from the basolateral membranes, with concomitant loss of mitochondria. These changes progressed with time, with decrease in medullary ray cellular mass. In the medulla, there was atrophy of medullary thick ascending limb (mTAL) cells and cast formation, most prominent in the inner stripe of the outer medulla. At 10 weeks, large numbers of calcified casts were seen in occasional animals especially in the deep outer stripe. On electron microscopy (EM), atrophic cells showed ultrastructural simplification with associated obliteration of tubular lumina. Histiocytes were observed infiltrating the walls of mTALs. Salt depletion exacerbated the injury, although uninephrectomized animals appeared to be protected from this combined effect. The investigators emphasized that these changes were localized and best seen on perfusion-fixed material on 1-μm plastic sections of the kidney; similar injury may have been underappreciated in other studies of chronic CsA-induced renal injury (109). Micropuncture studies in rats have demonstrated significantly higher electrolyte concentrations in thick ascending limb fluid in rats treated with acute infusion of CsA (5 mg/kg) or short-term CsA (15 mg/kg/day $\times$ 5–7 days), suggesting a possible mTAL transport defect (110). Increased calcium accumulation in renal cells in CsA-treated rodents is most marked in the renal medulla (111). Whether the morphological and functional alterations in the medulla and mTAL are primary, contributing to reduction of GFR perhaps in part via tubuloglomerular feedback, or whether they are secondary to cortical alterations and/or hemodynamic changes with hypoperfusion, is unknown.

In the intact animal or isolated perfused organ, it is difficult to separate direct tubular toxic effects from tubular effects due to hemodynamic changes. *In vitro* studies of tubular cells and/or segments provide an opportunity to study direct effects of the drug on tubular epithelium. The relevance of these observations to *in vivo* nephrotoxicity must be extrapolated with caution, however, with special attention to the concentrations of drug utilized *in vitro*; blood levels of the drug are generally kept below 200 ng/ml in patients, though they may rise to 1,000 ng/ml and above in some settings, and may be severalfold higher in tissues.

An early *in vitro* study of effects of CsA on cultured human renal tubular cells demonstrated vacuolization in response to the drug (112). Wilson and Hreniuk (113) screened effects of CsA on cells from proximal convoluted tubule, proximal straight tubule, cortical thick ascending limb, and cortical collecting tubules. Time-dependent toxicity, measured by LDH release and nigrosin uptake, was seen at doses of 100 ng/ml CsA and above; proximal tubular cells seemed most sensitive to the drug. Toxic effects appeared calcium-dependent and mediated by nonlysosomal cysteine proteases (113). Scoble et al. (114) have used LLC-PK_1 cells as a model of the proximal tubule. They documented cell uptake of CsA and found increasing cell vacuolization at 2 and 12 μg/ml CsA. At 12 μg/ml they also noted inhibition of cell growth and of activity of the sodium glucose cotransporter (114).

Jackson et al. (115) have examined interactions of cyclosporine with renal proximal tubule cells and cellular membranes. They found that CsA bound to isolated rat renal brush border membranes in a saturable manner, with analysis suggesting a partitioning effect rather than specific binding. Uptake into rabbit renal tubular segments was rapid and saturable at 100 μM. However, incubation with 10 μM (12 μg/ml) for 16 hr, or for 2 hr with and without hypoxia, produced no effect on basal and uncoupled tubule respiratory rates, tubule K^+ or Ca^{2+} concentrations, or adenine nucleotide levels, indicating no acute tubular toxic effects despite cellular uptake at these high concentrations.

In these studies, CsA also inhibited rat renal cortical mitochondrial respiration in a dose-dependent manner, with a threshold of 8 μM CsA. These results are comparable to those reported by Jung and Pergande (116) in isolated rat kidney mitochondria, as well as in human kidney mitochondria (1–25 μg CsA/ml) (117). These studies suggest that CsA can cause impaired mitochondrial function, though only at very high concentrations. Strzelecki et al. (118) have reported that oxidation of succinate by rat kidney cortical mitochondria is markedly inhibited by toxic levels of CsA (25–50 nmol/mg protein). Mitochondria isolated from rats treated with CsA *in vivo* showed impaired adenosine diphosphate (ADP)-stimulated respiration at a toxic (75 mg/kg/day po) but not an immunosuppressive (25 mg/kg/day po) dose. An important result of this study was that CsA appears to have similar effects on mitochondria *in vitro* and *in vivo*.

Although there may be effects of CsA on mitochondrial respiration, Elzinga et al. (119), using a rat model of nephrotoxicity induced by 25 mg/kg body weight ip ×

14 days, found only minor effects of CsA on respiration (and only pyruvate-malate supported respiration) of mitochondria isolated from these animals, and a slight depression of Ca^{2+} accumulation. These minor alterations were found despite severe depression in GFR and typical renal morphological changes, arguing against an important primary toxic effect of CsA on renal tubule cells.

CsA is known to be a potent inhibitor of the inner membrane permeability transition in liver mitochondria induced by a variety of agents, with complete inhibition at 150 pmol CsA/mg protein; in liver, CsA did not inhibit Ca^{2+} uptake or mitochondrial phospholipase A, and results were consistent with CsA interaction with a membrane pore or pore regulator (120). In model membrane bilayers, CsA has been shown to reduce both temperature and maximum heat capacity of the dipalmitoyl phosphatidyl-choline gel-to-liquid crystalline phase transition, and markedly reduce the amplitude of the pretransition to less than 20% compared to values in the pure lipid (121,122). However, in an erythrocyte preparation, CsA did not cause erythrocyte hemolysis or inhibit hypotonic hemolysis, suggesting that the compound does not necessarily cause functional changes in cell membranes (121). The changes in mitochondrial function noted above at very high doses of the drug are probably due to alterations in mitochondrial membrane structure (115).

Although cyclosporine does not inhibit Na-glucose cotransport in the renal tubule, it has been shown to bind to a polypeptide component of the renal cotransporter, competing at the Na-dependent high-affinity phlorizin binding site (123). Additional data suggested a cyclosporine-induced alteration of transporter turnover. The authors hypothesized that CsA binds to a newly synthesized component of the transporter, inhibiting its assembly so that components, which accumulate in subapical vessels and lysosomes, build up in the cell. Moreover, in proximal straight tubules, the authors also observed vacuolization of endoplasmic reticulum (ER), and in these cells, monoclonal antibody to the cotransporter reacted with membranes of this dilated ER as well as Golgi vesicles. The authors suggest that these results might explain the concentration of CsA in renal tissue, as it binds to this polypeptide.

Recent studies have suggested that cyclosporine may indeed interfere with normal protein synthesis and/or processing in renal cells. Buss et al. (124) have reported inhibition of renal microsomal protein chain elongation following *in vivo* cyclosporine treatment. Cytoplasm of renal cells from cyclosporine-treated rats inhibited microsomal protein synthesis in control microsomes. However, since these effects reach their nadir after renal dysfunction is established and recover well before renal functional recovery, alterations in renal microsomal protein synthesis are unlikely to be the direct cause of acute nephrotoxicity, although they may slow cellular recovery from injury and contribute to chronic tubular changes (125). The discovery that the ubiquitous intracellular cyclosporine-binding protein cyclophilin is identical to peptidyl-prolyl-cis-trans-isomerase has led to speculation that protein folding during synthesis, which is facilitated by this isomerase, may be perturbed by cyclosporine (2,3). These effects on protein conformation and function could be responsible for its immunosuppressive, and potentially its nephrotoxic, properties.

However, Schreiber (1) has pointed out that since only a small fraction of the isomerase would be inhibited at effective immunosuppressive doses, inhibition of the enzyme is an insufficient explanation for immunosuppressive action of the drug on T-lymphocytes (1). The possible role of changes in protein conformation, perhaps related to effects on this isomerase, in renal toxicity of the drug remains to be studied. Finally, Walker et al. (126,127) have shown that CsA significantly inhibits protein kinase C activity in renal cells *in vivo* and *in vitro*. Since this enzyme is involved in phosphorylation of cellular proteins and enzymes, these effects on the function of this enzyme, perhaps combined with a demonstrated inhibition of mixed-function oxidase complex in renal cells produced by the drug (126), could interfere with regulation of intracellular functions and cell response to injury (127).

Cyclosporine effects on DNA and protein synthesis in renal epithelial cells may interfere with recovery from injury and/or development of compensatory hypertrophy and hyperplasia. Effects of CsA in uninephrectomized animals have been employed as a model system particularly relevant to renal transplantation, where the donor kidney is removed from an individual with, generally, two functioning kidneys, and placed in the recipient where it must take over all renal function, in the process undergoing compensatory changes in response to what amounts to a reduction in functioning renal mass. Animal models of reduced renal mass are particularly useful to study effects of CsA on compensatory renal adaptation since renal changes in these models are not complicated by ischemia or rejection, which may supervene in the transplant setting.

Following *in vivo* unilateral nephrectomy, a number of investigators have shown suppression of compensatory changes in CsA-treated animals (128–130). Indeed, by comparing three groups of CsA-treated animals—no surgery, laparotomy only, and uninephrectomy—treated with 25 mg/kg/day for 4 weeks, Whiting et al. (131) demonstrated worsening of renal function and increased tubular morphological changes in uninephrectomized animals, despite similar tissue CsA levels, suggesting that the kidney undergoing adaptive hemodynamic and growth changes may be more susceptible to CsA nephrotoxicity. Inhibition of compensatory renal growth by CsA has been recently investigated *in vivo* with careful pair-feeding to control for effects of reduced oral intake. In these studies, Batlle et al. (130) found that kidneys of uninephrectomized animals treated for the 3 weeks following surgery with CsA, 12 mg/kg/day ip, increased in weight to the level of those in pair-fed controls, but renal cortical RNA and protein content were markedly reduced. The increase in weight in these studies was felt to be due to tissue edema. In long-term studies, Brunner et al. (132) have reported that low-dose CsA (5–20 mg/kg/day) begun several weeks after ablation was actually beneficial in preventing glomerular sclerosis and vasculopathy, perhaps due to a decreased blood pressure.

In summary, only mild tubular injury can be demonstrated in the majority of renal tubules even when relatively sophisticated methods of study such as analysis of mitochondrial function are employed, in most experimental models of CsA nephrotoxicity, unless very high doses/concentrations of drug are used. These minimal tubular changes are found even when GFR is substantially reduced, suggesting that tubular injury is not the major pathogenic factor. The studies of Rosen et al. (109), however, demonstrate that particularly with relatively prolonged administration of CsA, localized tubular changes occur that may be difficult to demonstrate but could have considerable functional significance; changes limited to one or a few nephron segments may not be detectable if whole-kidney or whole-cortex preparations of, e.g., mitochondria, are assessed. Moreover, subtoxic alterations in renal cells may become significant in the setting of other factors modifying renal function such as hemodynamic changes and/or ischemia.

Overt tubular cell injury, including frank necrosis, with CsA treatment is more commonly seen in the ischemically injured kidney. The combination of mild ischemia and CsA treatment has been used by a number of investigators as a strategy to develop experimental models of CsA-induced renal injury (99,133–136). These models have particular relevance to renal transplantation, where some level of ischemic injury is probably present in all transplanted organs, especially from cadaveric donors; however, it may also be relevant to other organ transplant settings where there is circulatory insufficiency. The tendency of CsA to exacerbate ischemic injury contributes to the prolonged primary nonfunction as well as the more severe and prolonged "acute tubular necrosis" seen in transplanted kidneys (see below). Even a low dose of parenteral CsA (5 mg/kg) can exacerbate renal ischemic injury when given after, although not before, the ischemic insult (136).

It is not clear to what extent this interaction of CsA and ischemia is due to direct effects on renal tubular cells with enhanced mitochondrial dysfunction, substrate depletion, and/or interference with cell repair mechanisms, or to hemodynamic effects. Walker et al. (126) have shown that cyclosporin A reduces renal content of glutathione and produces a significant increase in lipid peroxidation in renal cortical membrane fractions *in vitro*. In this setting, hypoxia and/or no-flow/reflow could lead to increased oxidant injury. As noted above, cell repair in response to injury could be impaired by cyclosporine inhibition of intracellular protein and enzyme synthesis and function (124–127). Alternatively, or perhaps in addition, it has been suggested that the vasoconstriction induced by cyclosporine could contribute to renal ischemia, increasing the chance of developing acute tubular cell injury. We will move now to a consideration of the hemodynamic effects of cyclosporine, thought by many investigators to be the primary mechanism of CsA nephrotoxicity.

Renal Vasculature and Hemodynamics

Effects of CsA on the renal vasculature are well established. Hemodynamic effects are probably responsible for, or contribute to, all of the various clinical syndromes recognized as CsA nephrotoxicity, including chronic nephropathy. Experimental models have proven very useful in defining vascular effects of cyclosporine, and in defining the mechanisms producing these effects.

Decreased blood flow can be demonstrated in many organs with cyclosporine administration, including heart, lung, liver, spleen, and kidney (137). Many investigators have documented acute and/or chronic reductions in renal blood flow and increase in renal vascular resistance in experimentl animals *in vivo* in response to cyclosporine (reviewed in 138–140). Marked renal vasoconstriction is also seen in the isolated perfused kidney when CsA is added to the perfusate (141). Of interest, the polyoxyethylated castor oil that served as the initial parenteral vehicle for cyclosporine, which has poor aqueous solubility, also acutely reduced renal blood flow and increased renal vascular resistance *in vivo* (142,143) and in the isolated perfused kidney (141); unlike effects of CsA, the hemodynamic effects of this parenteral vehicle appeared to be transient (142). Gillum et al. (144) have recently shown that partial ablation of renal mass and high-protein feeding partially protected against the fall in GFR and renal plasma flow (RPF), and the morphological changes induced by CsA, 25 mg/kg/day × 28 days, presumably by inducing relative renal vasodilation (144).

Micropuncture studies of glomerular hemodynamics following acute infusion of CsA (50 mg/kg) by Barros et al. (145) have revealed increases in both afferent and efferent arteriolar resistance, and proportionate reductions in glomerular plasma flow and whole kidney and single-nephron GFR. Since there was a greater increment in efferent arteriolar resistance, filtration fraction and mean glomerular capillary hydraulic pressure increased in these studies. Despite a 33% increase in ΔP however, single-nephron GFR (SNGFR) fell, in part because glomerular K_f was decreased by approximately 70% (145). Glomerular hemodynamics have also been studied after "short-term chronic" treatment with CsA (30 mg/kg SQ × 8 days). Thomson et al. (146) found reduction in SNGFR due to decreased in single-nephron plasma flow (SNPF) and ΔP, but with no decrease in glomerular membrane hydraulic permeablity. There was no significant difference in overall nephron vascular resistance between CsA-treated rats and pair-fed vehicle controls, but afferent arteriolar resistance increased disproportionately to efferent resistance in CsA-treated animals, contributing to the lower glomerular capillary hydrostatic pressures (146). Discrepancies between this study and that of Barros et al. described above are almost surely due to different dose and duration of treatment. Schor et al. (147) have recently reported findings similar to those of Thomson et al. (146) with 25 mg/kg CsA ip × 9 days, confirming that glomerular hemodynamic patterns after acute and chronic CsA are different. Using vascular casting, English et al. (148) have provided an elegant morphological demonstration of progressive afferent arteriolar vasoconstriction in perfused kidneys removed from rats treated with CsA, 50 mg/kg/day. Winston et al. (149) have studied glomerular hemodynamics during compensatory renal growth in a uninephrectomy model in rats. They found that reductions in whole kidney and SNGFR in CsA-treated animals were due solely to reduction in K_f, with no evidence of renal vasoconstriction. Using isolated glomeruli and acute exposure to high concentrations of CsA (10^{-4} M), Wiegmann et al. (150) have documented a dose-dependent decrease in glomerular volume consistent with mesangial contraction, and highly significant decreases in K_f and glomerular hydraulic conductivity.

Zimmerhackl et al. (151) have been able to assess effects of cyclosporine on the entire renal vasculature by using a hydronephrotic rat kidney model. The kidneys of these rats lack tubular structures, enabling visualization of vascular structures and removing tubular injury as an experimental variable. Using television microscopy, they observed that acute infusion of CsA (30–50 mg/kg) caused severe constriction of arcuate arteries in CsA-treated rats. Application of 10^{-7} to 10^{-5} M CsA directly to the kidney surface did not produce vasoconstriction, suggesting that this was not a direct effect of CsA but was mediated via other mechanisms.

What are the mechanisms of these altered hemodynamics? Depletion of effective circulating volume may contribute to the hemodynamic effects of cyclosporine, at least in experimental models. Gerkens et al. (152) documented an effect of salt intake on cyclosporine-induced renal functional impairment in rats, suggesting a possible prerenal component, and other investigators have suggested that decreased circulatory volume may play a role in reduction of renal function in CsA-treated animals (153,154). Devarajan et al. (155) recently reported results of studies assessing the role of blood volume and sodium balance in producing CsA-induced alterations in renal hemodynamics, using a low-dose model in young male rats (10 mg/kg/day im × 7 days). They found that acute volume expansion (10% body weight as saline) at the end of the CsA treatment period completely normalized renal blood flow (RBF) and GFR, and largely restored renal autoregulatory ability. Chronic volume expansion (10% BW/day saline ip) beginning 3 days before and extending through CsA treatment partially prevented the fall in GFR and RBF and the increase in renal vascular resistance produced by CsA, as well as improving autoregulation. Plasma and red cell volumes were reduced with CsA treatment; acute repletion of the deficit with an iso-oncotic solution restored GFR and RBF to control values. Extracellular fluid volume (inulin space) was not different in CsA and control rats. Control and experimental groups were in positive Na^+ balance, though dietary intake was somewhat lower and stool Na losses were higher in CsA-treated animals (155). These results are certainly consistent with a significant role of prerenal mechanisms related to hypovolemia in "initiating, sustaining, or aggravating" CsA-induced vasoconstriction. Finally, Thomson et al. (146), in hemodynamic studies in rats treated with CsA (30 mg/kg/day SQ × 8 days), found that plasma volume expansion caused SNGFR, ΔP, and SNPF to rise in both CsA and pair-fed vehicle-treated controls, but without eliminating differences in these parameters between animal groups. Thus, despite a potential role for prerenal mechanisms in CsA-induced alterations in renal blood flow and function, there are clearly also more direct renal effects of CsA on determinants of renal hemodynamics and GFR.

Adrenergic renal nerves have been implicated in the renal functional effects of CsA. Murray et al. (156) found that prior renal denervation largely prevented the decrease in renal blood flow and in inulin clearance in response to an acute infusion of 20 mg/kg CsA; the α-adrenergic antagonist phenoxybenzamine also prevented the decrease in RBF (156). In a more chronic model (20 mg/kg/day ip × 7 days), the α-adrenergic antagonist prazosin also prevented CsA-induced fall in RBF and GFR (157). Moss et al. (158) have demonstrated generalized activation of sympathetic nerves in CsA-treated rats (10 mg/kg over 30 min), with significant increases in renal afferent and efferent nerve activity. In rats with unilateral denervation, CsA reduced urine flow rate, sodium excretion, and GFR in the innervated kidney, basal GFR and RPF were increased in the denervated kidney and were not altered by CsA. In their short-term chronic model (30 mg/kg SQ × 8 days), Thompson et al. (146) have found that prior renal denervation resulted in increased GFR, SNGFR, SNPF, and transglomerular pressure, although it did not alter reduction in glomerular capillary pressure with CsA or eliminate hemodynamic differences between CsA-treated and pair-fed control animals. Renal denervation also ameliorated CsA-induced reduction of GFR in uninephrectomized rats receiving 12.5 mg/kg/day ip × 21 days, causing an increase in RBF and a reduction in renal vascular resistance (130). Interestingly, in these studies, innervated CsA-treated rats had reduced GFR with *normal* RBF, demonstrating that denervation may ameliorate CsA-induced effects by mechanisms other than mere reversal of CsA-induced pathophysiological events. Xue et al. (159) have reported that the contraction of isolated rat aorta induced *in vitro* by CsA (5×10^{-6} M) was significantly inhibited by phenoxybenzamine, suggesting mediation of this effect by adrenergic nerves.

Although CsA effects on renal nerves may have relevance to the pathophysiology of CsA nephrotoxicity in the native kidney, the relevance of this mechanism to toxicity in the renal allograft has been questioned, since the transplanted organ is denervated. As Moss et al. (158) have pointed out, however, there would be hypersensitivity to circulating catecholamines in the denervated organ. It also appears that within a few months of transplant, renal allografts are significantly reinnervated (160). It is possible, then, that neural mechanisms may play a role in nephrotoxicity even in the renal allograft.

The renin-angiotensin system has also been implicated in the changes in renal hemodynamics and function in CsA-treated animals. Indeed, it is likely that the hemodynamic effects of renal nerve stimulation are mediated at least in part by angiotensin II (161–163). In experimental animals, plasma renin rises in response to acute CsA infusion (156,164), and may also rise with chronic administration (156,165–167); the latter effect, however, may be due to volume depletion in the CsA-treated animals. In humans, peripheral renin is reported to be unchanged or depressed (168,169), though if total renin rather than active renin is measured, total renin is increased due to increased circulating prorenin, the activation of which appears to be depressed (170). Renin release has been shown to be increased on *in vitro* incubation with CsA in renal cortical slices (171), and in primary cultures of isolated juxtaglomerular cells (172). Renin synthesis and release in JGA cells both appeared to be elevated, with later increase in prorenin levels, suggesting inhibition of conversion and/or release. A number of investigators have noted hyperplasia of the JGA in experimental animals during CsA therapy (173–175). However, this is an inconstant finding in humans.

Using captopril, the angiotensin-converting enzyme inhibitor, Barros et al. (145) were able to abolish the renal vasoconstriction produced by acute infusion of CsA (50 mg/kg iv). On the other hand, Murray et al. (156) reported no effect of captopril pretreatment on the fall in RBF with short-term chronic CsA (20 mg/kg × 7 days) in conscious rats. Likewise, Kaskel et al. (153) and Gerkens and Smith (176) found no effect of captopril pretreatment of renal dysfunction induced by short-term treatment with CsA.

Failure to prevent CsA effects by angiotension converting enzyme (ACE) inhibition, especially with chronic administration, would suggest that if tubuloglomerular feedback is involved in producing experimental CsA toxicity, angiotensin II may not be the principal mediator. To examine the possibility that adenosine may function as the mediator, Gerkens and Smith (176) pretreated rats with theophylline, and found no effect on the elevations in SUN and creatinine in their experimental model. As discussed above, and in a recent brief review by Mason et al. (37), proximal tubular reabsorption is essentially normal or even increased in most models of CsA nephrotoxicity, removing the abnormalities in distal salt delivery that would activate tubuloglomerular feedback.

The loss of renal autoregulatory ability in CsA-treated animals appears to be due to a direct effect on preglomerular myogenic mechanisms rather than to impairment of tubuloglomerular feedback (177). Although systemic arterial pressure is unchanged or reduced in experimental animals following cyclosporine administration, particularly after high doses, hypertension is frequently seen clinically in patients receiving the drug. The only animal model in which CsA produces hypertension is in the spontaneously hypertensive rat; in these animals, CsA accelerates the development of hypertension, with evidence of direct arteriolar injury (96). This model may be relevant to the arteriolopathy seen in some patients treated with CsA, but is probably not completely relevant to the hypertension developing in patients without this lesion. Recent experimental studies by Golub and coworkers (178), however, have shown an altered vascular response of systemic vessels in cyclosporine-treated spontaneously hypertensive rats. Following CsA 5 or 20 mg/kg/day × 4 days, systemic blood pressure and *in vitro* tail artery contactile response to nerve stimulation and, in the high-dose group, to norepinephrine, increased. Xue et al. (159) have reported a slow contraction of rings of isolated rat aorta on exposure to CsA (5×10^{-6} M), an effect significantly inhibited by verapamil as well as phenoxybenzamine. In recent studies by Muller-Schweinitzer (179,180), CsA appeared to activate renin or a renin-like substance in peripheral and renal veins and arteries, increasing local angiotensin formation, which may contribute to CsA-induced hypertension.

Antidiuretic hormone has also been implicated in the acute glomerular functional impairment produced by CsA. Barros et al. (145), in studies using acute infusion of CsA (50 mg/kg) found that GFR and glomerular plasma flow (GPF) decreased significantly less in Brattleboro rats (lacking endogenous antidiuretic hormone [ADH]) than in Munich-Wistar rats, although there was still a significant effect of CsA. Antidiuretic hormone is known to produce renal vasoconstriction and to reduce K_f presumably by mesangial cell contraction (181), both effects seen in CsA-treated rats. Kremer et al. (182) used rat glomerular mesangial cells in primary culture to assess CsA effects on an ADH-induced rise in intracellular Ca and stimulation of prostaglandin production. They found that CsA 1 to 10 μg/ml for up to 90 min enhanced the rise in intracellular Ca^{2+} and inhibited both basal and ADH-stimulated production of the vasodilatory prostaglandin PGE_2 (182). In cultured rat mesangial cells *in vitro*, preincubation with 10 μg/ml CsA significantly increased the AVP-induced rise in intracellular Ca^{2+} and the percentage of contracting mesangial cells as assessed by digital imaging analysis. Pretreatment with CsA appeared to increase Ca^{2+} uptake into ADH-sensitive stores, such as the endoplasmic reticulum; verapamil, a calcium channel blocker, had no effect on this CsA-induced uptake (183).

Cultured rat mesangial cells and isolated glomeruli have also been used to examine the role of platelet activating factor (PAF) in producing mesangial cell contraction. Rodriguez-Puyol et al. (184) found that PAF antagonists completely inhibited CsA-induced decrease in planar surface area and inhibited decrease in whole glomerular cross-sectional area. In contrast, verapamil was only partially effective in inhibiting effects of CsA (1 μm). In addition, CsA increased glomerular PAF production over twofold, an effect not inhibited by verapamil. Dos Santos et al. (185) have studied effects of a PAF antagonist *in vivo* using micropuncture techniques, and found that pretreatment of rats with the antagonist prevented renal vasoconstriction and the fall in SNGFR and glomerular K_f following acute infusion of CsA; total GFR was unaffected, suggesting significant effects of the PAF antagonist only in superficial nephrons (185). Another PAF antagonist has been reported to lessen the interstitial fibrosis developing in rats receiving chronic cyclosporine (186).

The role of the vasoregulatory prostaglandins in CsA nephrotoxicity has been the subject of intense investigation, with results suggesting an important role for an imbalance of vasodilatory and vasoconstrictor prostaglandins in the pathogenesis of CsA-induced renal dysfunction. Since PGE_2 is a stimulator of renin secretion, Baxter et al. (187) *in vivo* and Kurtz et al. (172) *in vitro* in isolated JGA cells assessed PG release in studies demonstrating CsA-induced stimulation of renin secretion; PGE_2 release was not enhanced in these models. As noted above, Kremer et al. (182) found that an ADH-stimulated increase in PGE_2 production was inhibited by CsA in mesangial cell cultures. Stahl and Kudelka (188) reported reduction of (basal) PGE_2 formation in isolated glomeruli and papillae of rat kidneys with chronic treatment with oral CsA. Stahl et al. (189) have also found inhibition of angiotensin II– or calcium ionophore–induced PGE_2 formation in cultured rat mesangial cells, at CsA concentrations as low as 800 ng/ml; this effect appeared to be due to inhibition of release of arachidonic acid substrate from cell membranes rather than to inhibition of cyclooxygenase. Decreased synthesis of PGE_2 and $PGF_{1\alpha}$ have also been reported in isolated glomeruli from CsA-treated rats (190). Exogenous PGE_2 (or variant) has been shown to reduce or prevent CsA nephrotoxicity in rat models (191,192).

Other investigators, however, have found *increases* in vasodilatory prostaglandins, presumably as a compensatory mechanism, with CsA treatment. Murray et al. (156) reported that CsA, given acutely or on a more chronic regimen *in vivo*, increased urinary excretion of 6-keto-PGF_1, and that cyclooxygenase inhibitors exacerbated the CsA-induced decrease in RBF and increase in RVR (156). A similar increase in 6-keto-$PGF_{1\alpha}$ was reported with acute CsA administration to conscious rabbits (164). In a chronic postischemic, denervated rat model of CsA nephrotoxicity (50 mg/kg/day × 12–14 days), Coffman et al. (193) found increased urinary excretion of 6-keto-$PGF_{1\alpha}$ and increased tissue production of PGE_2 as well as 6-keto-$PGF_{1\alpha}$ in kidneys removed from CsA-toxic animals and perfused *in vitro*.

Discrepancies in the results of analysis of vasodilatory prostaglandins in these various models are due in part to differences in dose and duration of CsA treatment. Since there are a number of potential sites of prostaglandin synthesis, including endothelial and smooth muscle cells, glomerular cells, tissue macrophages and lymphocytes, monocytes, and platelets, results with isolated glomeruli or in cultured cells may be different than with renal slices or the intact animal. Moreover, urinary excretion of prostaglandins may not necessarily reflect localized tissue levels (193).

Coffman et al. (193), in addition to finding increased production of vasodilatory prostaglandin with CsA treatment, also reported increased production and excretion of thromboxane (TX), a vasoconstrictor prostaglandin in their model. Elzinga et al. (194) looked at renal cortical TXB_2 content in studies on the modification of CsA toxicity by the use of fish oil rather than olive oil as the vehicle for the drug. They found significant preservation of GFR and reduction in tubular cell morphological changes in animals given CsA in fish oil. These results were associated with significantly reduced levels of cortical TXB_2, presumably due to the 3-omega fatty acids in fish oil that are known to inhibit cyclooxygenase. These investigators have also reported selective enhancement of thromboxane in kidneys and in peritoneal macrophages in CsA-treated rats (12.5 mg/kg/day ip × 2 weeks); modest reductions in PGE_2 and prostacyclin were also seen. These effects were suppressed by a diet rich in fish oil, and the decreased GFR and tubular vacuolization seen in these animals were also decreased on this regimen (195). In clinical studies, van der Heide et al. (196) have recently reported that 3 months of dietary fish oil supplementation improved GFR and reduced renal vascular resistance in patients with stable renal function on a stable dose of CsA for at least 3 months.

Perico et al. (197) have specifically assessed the functional significance of the increased synthesis of thromboxane A_2 induced by CsA. Using a selective thromboxane synthetase inhibitor, they found a marked reduction in urinary TXB_2, and a significant increase in GFR in CsA-treated rats (40 mg/kg qod × 6 weeks). No effects on renal plasma flow were seen, leading to the conclusion that TXA_2 may be reducing GFR by altering K_f, presumably via mesangial cell contraction. These investigators have also recently reported that a TXA_2 receptor antagonist partially prevented the decline in GFR and RPF induced by acute CsA administration (50 mg/kg iv). In the same model, an antagonist to the receptor for LTC_4/D_4, sulfidopeptide leukotrienes shown to decrease GFR and increase RVR *in vivo* and *in vitro*, also partially prevented CsA-induced hemodynamic effects. A combination of the TXA_2 and LTC_4/D_4 receptor antagonists completely abolished acute CsA-induced effects in rats (198).

Recent studies suggest that effects of vasoconstrictor compounds such as thromboxane on renal hemodynamics may be mediated via substances released from endothelial cells. In particular, the most potent vasoconstrictor substance yet identified, endothelin, has recently been discovered and characterized (199). It is a peptide released from endothelial cells, has powerful systemic and renal vasoconstrictor effects (199–201), and has been implicated in postischemic renal vasoconstriction (202). Badr et al. (203) have characterized renal effects of endothelin; these effects include increases in afferent and efferent arteriolar resistances, decrease in SNGFR and a decrease in K_f, changes similar to those produced by CsA. In recent studies, Kon et al. (204) have examined the role of endothelin in cyclosporine-induced glomerular dysfunction. Utilizing continuous infusion of rabbit antiporcine endothelin into a first-order branch of the main renal artery of Munich-Wistar rats, they then performed micropuncture on glomeruli infused versus not infused with antiendothelin in the same kidney. CsA reduced SNGFR and glomerular plasma flow rate associated with increased afferent arteriolar resistance and decreased glomerular capillary pressure; these changes were markedly attenuated by the antiendothelin antibody. In additional animals, they demonstrated marked elevations of endothelin with CsA treatment (204). Perico et al. (205) have also found that endothelin appears to mediate CsA-induced renal vasoconstriction in the rat. Awazu et al. (206), using isolated glomerular membranes, have recently shown that CsA promotes glomerular endothelin binding *in vivo*. CsA also diminishes ACH-mediated vasodilatation in microvessels of rat kidneys, perhaps by decreasing nitric oxide synthesis (207).

Altered release of vasoactive substances from endothelial cells is probably due to endothelial injury. There is evidence that CsA may induce endothelial and vascular injury in experimental models, analogous to the CsA-induced clinical arteriolopathy reported in occasional renal transplant patients and the HUS-like syndrome in rare patients (see above). Neild and coworkers described a Schwartzman-like reaction in CsA-treated rabbits with serum sickness; these investigators later demonstrated depression of prostacyclin synthesis *in vitro* by vasculature of CsA-treated rabbits, apparently due to decreased levels of PGI_2 stimulating factor (208). CsA has also been shown to exacerbate development of arteriolopathy in the spontaneously hypertensive rat (96). Faraco et al. (209) have recently proposed a new model for the microangiopathic lesion produced by CsA. They infused lipopolysaccharide (LPS) from *E. coli* into rabbits pretreated for 10 days with parenteral CsA (25 mg/kg im) or its vehicle. LPS animals developed typical signs of endotoxemia and a significant rise in serum creatinine. Kidneys were harvested after the 5-hr infusion, and histologic examination revealed that 84.75% of glomeruli in CsA + LPS animals contained fibrin deposits compared to 5.4% of glomeruli in vehicle + LPS rats, and none in vehicle or CsA rats not given LPS. By light and electron microscopy, lesions in glomeruli in CsA + LPS animals resembled the HUS-like lesions described clinically. Since both LPS and CsA stimulate procoagulant activity in endothelial cells, the authors suggest that these agents, and potentially other inflammatory mediators induced by LPS may interact in vessels and glomeruli in the clinical setting as well as in this experimental model.

Using cultured endothelial cells from bovine aorta, Zoja et al. (210) demonstrated that exposure to CsA produced time- and dose-dependent cell injury with early detachment followed by cell lysis; they also demonstrated time- and dose-dependent increase in prostacyclin and thromboxane A_2. Lau et al. (211) have also described CsA-induced changes in endothelial cells of the microvasculature of the rat. Cell replication in culture was depressed significantly at 250 and 1,000 ng/ml CsA, but with no evidence of increased cell death. There were morphological changes in the cells including nucleolar changes and formation of cytoplasmic vesicles, and prostacyclin release was increased as well.

As discussed, obvious arteriolopathic lesions are seen in only one experimental model, the spontaneously hypertensive rat (96), although perhaps also in the LPS-treated rabbit (209). However, when careful ultrastructural studies were performed on perfusion-fixed kidneys harvested from Wistar rats treated with high doses of CsA (100 mg/kg/day po × 10 days), individual necroses of myocytes in the media of afferent arterioles were seen. Similar changes were found sporadically in interlobular arteries near the origin of afferent arterioles. Twenty-five percent of the CsA-treated rats (and all of the control rats) had no such alterations. Affected myocytes showed karyolysis, large vacuoles, loss of cell organelles, and swollen mitochondria. All other vessels were unaltered (212). Rats were normotensive, so the changes were not due to hypertension. However, it is not clear that significant sustained vasoconstriction rather than a direct effect of the drug caused these alterations.

CsA may have additional vascular effects in vessels with significant endothelial injury, with implications for the development of chronic vascular insufficiency. Ferns et al. (213) have shown that in rabbits with de-endothelialized carotid arteries, treatment with CsA was associated with an increase in total intimal thickening in these vessels due to numerous foam cells, incorporation of H^3-thymidine by neointimal monocytes/macrophages, and intimal smooth muscle vacuolization. The authors suggested that CsA may contribute to graft-related atherosclerosis. The renal allograft, especially from a cadaveric donor, is very likely to sustain endothelial injury due to a variety of factors including altered hemodynamics and/or vascular rejection. CsA could certainly contribute to vascular pathology in such a setting.

Endothelin and a number of other vasoconstrictor hormones act at least in part via elevated levels of intracellular Ca^{2+}, and there is some experimental evidence that Ca^{2+} may mediate renal effects of cyclosporine. Dieperink et al. (214) found that concomitant treatment of CsA-treated rats (25 mg/kg/day po × 13 days) with nifedipine improved inulin clearance, renal blood flow, and renal arterial pressure, and improved proximal and distal tubular reabsorption; acute infusion of the calcium channel blocker after the 13-day protocol did not reverse CsA-induced changes. Barros et al. (145), in studies of glomerular hemodynamics with acute CsA infusion, found that verapamil significantly decreased the effects of CsA on GFR and renal plasma flow. In studies in the hydronephrotic rat kidney, the vasoconstrictor effect of CsA on the arcuate arteries was partially reversed by the calcium channel blocker nitrendipine (151). As noted above, recent experimental studies have shown increased Ca^{2+} mobilization in vasopressin-treated glomerular mesangial cells exposed to CsA (182), an effect not blocked by verapamil. In contrast, Scoble et al. (114) have reported that verapamil *potentiated* the increased CsA toxicity produced by increasing Ca^{2+} concentrations in the medium bathing LLC-PK_1 cells, a cell line derived from proximal tubule. Cyclosporine uptake (at 2 μg/ml in the medium) could be blocked by verapamil but only at very high toxic doses of the calcium channel blocker. Therefore, it is likely that the functionally significant alterations in cellular calcium induced by CsA and modulation of toxicity by calcium channel blockers takes place at the level of renal vessels/glomeruli rather than at the renal tubule, although Wilson and Hreniuk (113) found that toxic effects of CsA on cultured tubular cells were Ca^{2+}-dependent.

In summary, the acute or subacute effects of CsA on renal hemodynamics may be mediated by a number of factors, with current experimental evidence most strongly implicating an imbalance in vasoconstrictor and vasodilator prostaglandins. Vasoconstrictor effects may well be mediated by endothelin and/or PAF release and at the cellular level by increased intracellular Ca^{2+}; there is some experimental evidence that thromboxanes may modulate endothelin gene expression and synthesis (140). As recently suggested, CsA toxicity may ultimately be regarded as a disorder of transmembrane signal transduction (215). Prerenal factors, renal nerves, and/or interactions among these various factors may also play a role.

The relevance of these mechanisms to chronic CsA-induced nephrotoxicity as seen in humans and some experimental models remains to be established. The interstitial fibrosis seen in chronic nephrotoxicity, which may at least in part be due to vascular insufficiency, is discussed below.

Chronic Cyclosporine Nephrotoxicity and the Renal Interstitium

An understanding of the pathogenesis of chronic cyclosporine nephrotoxicity, described initially in cardiac allograft recipients, has been hampered by the lack of an experimental model of chronic injury. In the past few years, however, a number of investigators have developed models of long-term cyclosporine administration, usually given over several months, with progressive deterioration in renal function and the histologic pattern of striped interstitial fibrosis described in patients with evidence of chronic toxicity (109,216–218).

At high doses of CsA, focal areas of tubular atrophy and interstitial fibrosis may be seen with less than 2 weeks of treatment. Jackson et al. (57) noted these changes as well as an increase in interstitial cells and reduction of renal blood flow and GFR within 4 to 10 days on CsA doses of 100 mg/kg/day SQ in low-sodium diet rats. There was increased incorporation of H^3-thymidine into DNA in inner and outer cortex and inner and outer medulla. Using histoautoradiography and morphometric analysis, they demonstrated that interstitial cell proliferation accounted for most of the increased labeling.

Rosen et al. (109) using a rat model and lower doses of CsA (12.5 mg/kg × 3–10 weeks) have emphasized thick ascending limb cell atrophy with fibroblast proliferation and collagen formation in the inner stripe of the outer medulla and the medullary rays, with S_2 to S_3 segment degenerative changes as well. Morphological changes predicted renal failure, though a causal effect was not established. The authors emphasized that injury occurred in areas of limited oxygen availability and was aggravated by salt depletion, suggesting a role for chronic hypoperfusion.

The interstitial fibrosis seen with chronic treatment may be related to a direct stimulatory effect of CsA. Wolf et al. (219) have recently shown that CsA stimulates transcription and procollagen secretion in cultured tubulointerstitial fibroblasts and proximal tubular cells. Similarly, Nast et al. (220) in studies of rats treated with CsA 25 mg/kg/day SQ for 1 or 4 weeks, found elevated cortical procollagen-α_1 (I) mRNA levels at 1 week, before morphological evidence of the focal cortical tubular atrophy and interstitial fibrosis which had developed by 4 weeks in these animals. Procollagen-α_1 (III) and α_1 (IV) and B-actin mRNA levels were not increased (220). Of possible relevance to the fibrosis seen in the kidney, CsA increases connective tissue in nonrenal tissue, notably gingival tissue (221–223). Kopp and Klotman (224) have recently reviewed what is known of mechanisms of matrix protein accumulation in cyclosporine nephrotoxicity.

In recent long-term studies in Sprague-Dawley rats, Backman et al. (225) monitored rats ingesting about 5 mg/kg/day of cyclosporine for up to 66 weeks, examining renal histology at 21, 32, and 66 weeks, using quantitative morphometry. At 21 weeks, mild focal segmental glomerular sclerosis and nephron atrophy were reported in CsA-treated rats but not in vehicle-treated controls. By 66 weeks, 33% of the glomeruli of CsA-treated rats contained segmental sclerotic lesions, versus 7.5% of control; nephron atrophy and interstitial fibrosis were also significantly greater than in controls. No significant vascular lesions were seen in any group, even by EM. Vacuolization of the proximal tubule was an infrequent feature. The striking glomerular lesions reported in this study are not a prominent feature of the chronic nephropathy described in models with shorter-term CsA administration. However, segmentally or globally sclerotic glomeruli have been described in clinical chronic cyclosporine nephropathy, ascribed to structural arteriolar damage and/or sustained vasoconstriction (60,61). The absence of structural vascular lesions in the long-term experimental study of Backman et al. would suggest that vasoconstriction is the primary mechanism in their model.

Cyclosporin G

Cyclosporin G is a fungal metabolite similar in structure to cyclosporin A (226). Paller and Ferris (227) found that acute infusion with CsG reduced GFR and RBF by approximately 50%; CsG given for 4 to 7 days (20 mg/kg/day ip) significantly reduced creatinine clearance. No direct comparison with CsA was made in these studies (227). Some studies have suggested that this compound is less nephrotoxic per given dose than CsA (228–231). However, in studies comparing 50 mg/kg/day, CsA or CsG po for 14 days, Duncan et al. (232) found comparable decreases in clearances of urea nitrogen and creatinine, and increases in enzymuria, indicative of tubular injury. In a recent study, Tejani et al. (229) studied nephrotoxicity of cyclosporin A and G in Sprague-Dawley rats given 25 mg/kg/day SQ for 21 days. By day 22, RPF and GFR (measured by inulin clearance) were significantly decreased in CsA-treated rats, but unchanged from controls in CsG rats; serum creatinines were not different among groups. On histology, vacuolization of proximal tubular cells and microcalcification at the corticomedullary junction were seen with significantly greater frequency with CsA. They noted the discrepancy in their results and the studies of Duncan et al. (232) and ascribed differences in findings to differing dose regimens, and the different clearance methods employed in the two studies.

Although dose-for-dose CsG may be less nephrotoxic than CsA, it is also a less effective immunosuppressant (230). Moreover, CsG has apparent hepatotoxicity, which has limited enthusiasm for its widespread clinical use.

FK506

This fungal product has been used successfully for liver, pancreas, and kidney transplantation in humans. Clinical side effects of the drug include nephrotoxicity, as discussed above. Results of animal studies confirm the nephrotoxic potential of the drug, though some studies suggest that FK506 is less nephrotoxic than CsA. Todo et al. (233) reported serious side effects in allografted dogs treated with FK506. These included fibrinoid necrosis of the media of medium-sized arteries, especially in the heart and GI tract; however, these changes were also found with equal frequency and severity in control animals. In dogs with liver transplants, isometric vacuolization of proximal tubules was seen in the kidney, but no renal functional studies were done. (As discussed above, in cyclosporine nephrotoxicity such vacuolization may not correlate with renal dysfunction.) In the study of Todo et al., analysis of extrarenal tissues in primates with renal transplants revealed less evidence of systemic toxicity in monkeys and baboons than in dogs, but the kidneys were not examined for toxic effects (138). In studies in a Lewis rat renal ischemia model, Nalesnik et al. (234) reported less nephrotoxicity with FK506 than with cyclosporine.

Kumano et al. (235) assessed functional and morphological changes induced by FK506 in the kidneys of heminephrectomized rats. FK506 was given at 1, 2.5, or 5 mg/kg by gavage for 21 days. Creatinine clearances were reduced in a dose-dependent manner (10% to 25% decrease). There was no change in FeNa, but FeK decreased. Inulin and *p*-aminohippuric acid (PAH) clearances at 21 days revealed decreased GFR and RPF, with an increase in renal vascular resistance. Histology revealed vacuolization in proximal tubules and arteriolar smooth muscle, as well as eosinophilic "inclusions" in the media of vessels and in tubules. Tubular atrophy and focal interstitial fibrosis were also seen. Daily doses of the calcium channel blocker diltiazem improved renal functional parameters, whereas captopril and prazosine did not. Diltiazem also lessened vascular lesions, assessed semiquantitatively. In glomeruli isolated from normal rats, these authors also found an increase in the ratio of vasoconstrictor to vasodilator prostaglandins released on exposure to FK506. These studies suggest a role for alterations in renal hemodynamics, perhaps via altered intracellular calcium and glomerular prostaglandin synthesis, in the renal response to FK506 (235,236).

Ochiai et al. (237) studied a renal allograft model in dogs and suggested that combination treatment with FK506 and cyclosporine prolonged recipient survival time and resulted in less frequent and severe histologic vascular changes. However, in humans it appears that FK506 potentiates the nephrotoxicity of CsA and such a combination should be used with caution, as noted above.

Interleukin-2

Acute renal failure is an important complication of IL-2 therapy. Clinically, ARF has generally been ascribed to hypotension and prerenal azotemia developing in the setting of a generalized capillary leak syndrome (see above). Anderson and Hayes (238) have reported toxic effects of human recombinant interleukin-2 in rats. Mortality in treated animals was due to severe anemia and/or hepatic damage. Mild elevations in SUN were detected; no other tests of renal function were performed. Renal histopathologic lesions occurred at high doses (60 and 150 r IL-2 $\times 10^6$ units/kg/day iv) and consisted of cytoplasmic inclusions in proximal tubules, felt to be hemoglobin. Doses of 3.75 r IL-2 $\times 10^6$ units/kg/injection (ip or iv) bid produced cytoplasmic inclusions and a lymphocytic infiltrate; the same total daily dose given as a single bolus produced only mild lymphoid infiltrate. Because of the paucity of histopathologic findings in the kidney, the rise in SUN was attributed to prerenal azotemia.

Welbourn et al. (239), in studies of multiorgan edema produced by IL-2, have documented significant edema of the kidney in rats when IL-2 (10^5–10^6 units) was given as a 1-hr infusion. Plasma thromboxane increased significantly as well, and polymorphonuclear leukocyte (PMNL) sequestration was demonstrated in the lung. These effects were not seen with rapid bolus injection. Renal function and renal or urinary prostanoids were not measured. These investigators have since shown that phalloidin, which stabilizes actin filaments, and antamanide, an analogue of phalloidin, reduce edema formation, perhaps by stabilizing the microvascular permeability barrier. Antamanide reduced kidney edema, although phalloidin, which reduced lung edema, did not. Both agents also lowered plasma thromboxane B_2, but did not prevent neutrophil sequestration in the lung. No renal functional studies were performed (240). In studies of a model of IL-2 toxicity in rats, Rubinger et al. (241) reported increase in urinary thromboxane associated with decreased GFR and increased fractional excretion of Na, an effect exacerbated by high-dose indomethacin.

Interleukin-2 alone does not increase endothelial permeability *in vitro* (242,243). Vascular effects seen with IL-2 therapy, which may lead directly or indirectly to renal dysfunction, appear at this time to be most likely mediated by neutrophils and thromboxane, and perhaps other cytokines (79,80).

Other Agents

In experimental studies, Morel-Maroger et al. (244) have described the development of a progressive glomerulonephritis in newborn Swiss mice receiving daily injections of murine interferon. This finding may relate to the proteinuria observed in man (see above). Maessen et al. (245) looked at direct cytotoxic effects of interferon and/or recombinant interleukin-1 on cultured human kidney epithelial cells. They found that both agents caused cell injury as measured by lactate dehydrogenase release and inhibition of protein synthesis, suggesting a direct tubulotoxic effect.

REFERENCES

1. Schreiber SL. Chemistry and biology of the immunophilins and their immunosuppressive ligands. *Science* 1991;251:283–287.
2. Fischer G, Wittmann-Liebold B, Lang K, Kiefhaber T, Schmid FX. Cyclophilin and peptidyl-prolyl cis-trans isomerase are probably identical proteins. *Nature* 1989;337:476–478.
3. Takahashi N, Hayano T, Suzuki M. Peptidyl-prolyl cis-trans isomerase is the cyclosporin A-binding protein cyclophilin. *Nature* 1989;337:473–475.
4. Harding MW, Galat A, Uehling DE, Schreiber SL. A receptor for the immunosuppressant FK506 is a cis-trans peptidyl-prolyl isomerase. *Nature* 1989;341:758–760.
5. Siekierka JJ, Hung SHY, Poe M, Lin CS, Sigal NH. A cytosolic binding protein for the immunosuppressant FK506 has peptidyl-prolyl isomerase activity but is distinct from cyclophilin. *Nature* 1989;341:755–757.
6. Thistlethwaite JR, Heffron TG, Stuart JK, Buckingham M, Stuart FP. Selective OKT_3 induction therapy in adult cadaveric donor renal transplants. *Am J Kidney Dis* 1989;14:28–34.
7. Ortho Multicenter Transplant Study Group. A randomized clinical trial of OKT_3 monoclonal antibody for acute rejection of cadaveric renal transplants. *N Engl J Med* 1985;313:337–342.
8. Kahan BD. (Review) Cyclosporine. *N Engl J Med* 1989;321:1725–1738.
9. Rosenberg SA, Lotze MT, Muul LM, et al. A progress report on the treatment of 175 patients with advanced cancer using lymphokine-activated killer cells and interleukin-2 or high-dose interleukin-2 alone. *N Engl J Med* 1987;316:889–897.
10. Lotze MT, Matory YL, Rayner AA, et al. Clinical effects and toxicity of interleukin-2 in patients with cancer. *Cancer* 1986;58:2764–2772.
11. Morris PJ, Allen RD, Thompson JF, Chapman JR, Ting A, Dunnill MS, Wood RFM. Cyclosporine conversion versus conventional immunosuppression: long-term follow-up and histological evaluation. *Lancet* 1987;1:586–591.
12. Hoitsma AJ, van Lier HJJ, Wetzels JFM, Berden JHM, Koene RAP. Cyclosporine treatment with conversion after three months versus conventional immunosuppression in renal allograft recipients. *Lancet* 1987;1:584–586.
13. Keown PA, Stiller CR, Wallace AC. Nephrotoxicity of cyclosporin A. In: Williams GM, Burdick JF, Solez K, eds. *Kidney transplant rejection: diagnosis and treatment.* New York: Marcel Dekker, 1986;423–457.
14. Greenberg A, Egel JW, Thompson ME, et al. Early and late forms of cyclosporine nephrotoxicity: studies in cardiac transplant recipients. *Am J Kidney Dis* 1987;9:12–22.
15. Bennett WM. Clinical aspects of cyclosporine nephrotoxicity. In: Hitano M, ed. *Nephrology: Proceedings of the XIth International Congress of Nephrology*, Tokyo: Springer-Verlag, 1991; 564–575.
16. Powles RL, Barrett AJ, Clink H, Kay HEM, Sloane J, McElwain TJ. Cyclosporin A for the treatment of graft-versus-host disease in man. *Lancet* 1978;2:1327–1331.
17. Devineni R, McKenzie N, Wall W, Campbell C, Stiller C, Keown P, Kostuk W. Renal function in patients receiving cyclosporine for orthotopic cardiac transplantation. *Transplant Proc* 1985;17: 1256–1257.
18. Powell-Jackson PR, Young B, Calne RY, Williams R. Nephrotoxicity of parenterally administered cyclosporine after orthotopic liver transplantation. *Transplantation* 1983;36:505–508.

19. Walker JF, Cumming AD, Lindsay RM, Solez K, Linton AL. The renal response produced by nonhypotensive sepsis in a large animal model. *Am J Kidney Dis* 1986;8:88–97.
20. Henny FC, Klehbloesem CH, Moolenaar AJ, Paul LC, Breimer DD, van Es LA. Pharmacokinetics and nephrotoxicity of cyclosporine in renal transplant recipients. *Transplantation* 1985;40:261–265.
21. Myers BD. Cyclosporine nephrotoxicity (review). *Kidney Int* 1986;30:964–974.
22. Kahan B, Reid M, Newberger J. Pharmacokinetics of cyclosporin A in human transplantation. *Transplant Proc* 1983;15:446–453.
23. Keown PA, Stiller CR, Sinclair NR, et al. The clinical relevance of cyclosporine blood levels as measured by radioimmunoassay. In: Kahan BD, ed. *Cyclosporine: biological activity and clinical applications*. Orlando, FL: Grune & Stratton, 1984;222.
24. Klintmalm G, Ringden O, Groth CG. Clinical and laboratory signs in nephrotoxicity and rejection in cyclosporine-treated renal allograft recipients. In: Kahan BD, ed. *Cyclosporine: biological activity and clinical applications*. Orlando, FL: Grune & Stratton, 1984;599.
25. Flechner SM, Van Buren C, Kerman RH, Kahan BD. The nephrotoxicity of cyclosporine in renal transplant recipients. In: Kahan BD, ed. *Cyclosporine: biological activity and clinical applications*. Orlando, FL: Grune & Stratton, 1984;473.
26. Burdick JF, Williams GM, Solez K, Racusen LC. *Kidney transplant rejection: diagnosis and treatment*, 2nd ed. New York: Marcel Dekker, 1991.
27. Burdick JF, Beschorner WB, Smith WJ, McGraw D, Bender WL, Williams GM, Solez K. Characteristics of early routine renal allograft biopsies. *Transplantation* 1984;38:679–684.
28. Solez K, McGraw DJ, Beschorner WE, Kone BC, Racusen LC, Whelton A, Burdick JF. Reflections on use of the renal biopsy as the "gold standard" in distinguishing transplant rejection from cyclosporine nephrotoxicity. *Transplant Proc* 1985;17:123–133.
29. Beschorner WE, Burdick JF, Williams GM, Solez K. The presence of Leu 7 reactive lymphocytes in renal allografts undergoing acute rejection. *Transplant Proc* 1985;17:618–622.
30. Neild GH, Taube DH, Hartley RB, et al. Morphological differentiation between rejection and cyclosporin nephrotoxicity in renal allografts. *J Clin Pathol* 1986;39:152–159.
31. Myers BD, Sibley RN, Tomlanovich L, et al. The long-term course of cyclosporine-associated chronic nephropathy. *Kidney Int* 1988;33:590–600.
32. Mihatsch MJ, Ryffel B. Evolution of cyclosporin nephrotoxicity. In: Hitano M, ed. *Nephrology: Proceedings of the XIth International Congress of Nephrology*. Tokyo: Springer-Verlag, 1991; 576–589.
33. Solez K, Racusen L, Marcussen N, Slatnik I, Keown P, Burdick JF, Olsen S. Pathology of "acute tubular necrosis", normal function and cyclosporine nephrotoxicity in renal allograft recipients treated with cyclosporine. (Submitted).
34. Nast CC, Blifeld C, Danovitch GM, Fine RN, Ettenger RB. Evaluation of cyclosporine nephrotoxicity by renal transplant fine needle aspiration. *Mod Pathol* 1989;2:577–582.
35. Salaman JR, Griffin PJ. Fine-needle intrarenal manometry: a new test for rejection in cyclosporin-treated recipients of kidney transplants. *Lancet* 1983;2:709–711.
36. Myers BD, Sibley R, Newton L, et al. The long-term course of cyclosporine-associated chronic nephropathy. *Kidney Int* 1988;33:590–600.
37. Mason J, Muller-Schweinitzer E, Dupont M, Casellas D, Mihatsch M, Moore L, Kaskel F. Cyclosporine and the renin-angiotensin system. *Kidney Int* 1991;39:S28–S32.
38. Conte G, Dal Canton A, Sabbatini M, et al. Acute cyclosporine renal dysfunction reversed by dopamine infusion in healthy subjects. *Kidney Int* 1989;36:1086–1092.
39. Propper DJ, Whiting PH, Power DA, Edward N, Catto GRD. The effect of nifedipine on graft function in renal allograft recipients treated with cyclosporin A. *Clin Nephrol* 1989;32:62–67.
40. Belitsky P, for the Canadian Transplant Study Group. Initial nonfunction of cyclosporine-treated cadaver renal allografts preserved by simple cold storage. *Transplant Proc* 1985;17:1485–1488.
41. Shiel AGR, Hall BM, Tiller DJ, et al. Australian trial of cyclosporine (CsA) in cadaveric donor renal transplantation. In: Kahan BD, ed. *Cyclosporine: biological activity and clinical applications*. Orlando, FL: Grune & Stratton, 1984;307.
42. Stiller G, for the Canadian Transplant Study Group. The Canadian Trial of cyclosporine: cyclosporine therapy compared to standard immunosuppression in renal transplants. An exploration of nephrotoxicity. In: Kahan BD, ed. *Cyclosporine: biological activity and clinical applications*. Orlando, FL: Grune & Stratton, 1984;263.
43. Sommer BG, Innes JT, Whitehurst RM, Sharma HM, Ferguson RM. Cyclosporine-associated renal arteriopathy resulting in loss of allograft function. *Am J Surg* 1985;149:756–764.

44. Lobo PI, Sturgill BC, Bolton WK. Cold-reactive alloantibodies and allograft malfunction occurring immediately posttransplant. *Transplantation* 1984;37:76–81.
45. Schweizer RT, Bartus SA, Perkins HA, Belzer FO. Renal allograft failure and cold red blood cell autoagglutinins. *Transplantation* 1982,33:77–79.
46. Cannon PJ, Hassar M, Case DB, Casarella WJ, Sommers SC, Leroy EC. The relationship of hypertension and renal failure in scleroderma to structural and functional abnormalities of the renal cortical circulation. *Medicine* 1974;53:1–46.
47. Parmar MS, Kjellstrand CM, Solez K, Halloran PF. Glomerular endothelial stripping in paired cadaver kidneys: Evidence for diffuse endothelial injury in some cadaver donors. (Submitted).
48. Vanrenterghem Y, Lerut T, Roels L, et al. Thromboembolic complications and haemostatic changes in cyclosporin-treated cadaveric kidney allograft recipients. *Lancet* 1985;1:999–1002.
49. Neild G, Reuben R, Hartley B, Cameron JS. Glomerular thrombi in renal allografts associated with cyclosporin therapy. *Kidney Int* 1985;27:345.
50. Shulman H, Striker G, Deeg HJ, Kennedy M, Storb R, Thomas ED. Nephrotoxicity of cyclosporin A after allogeneic marrow transplantation. Glomerular thromboses and tubular injury. *N Engl J Med* 1981;305:1392–1395.
51. Grace AA, Barradas MA, Mikhailidis DP, Jeremy JY, Moorhead JF, Sweny P, Dandora P. Cyclosporine A enhances platelet aggregation. *Kidney Int* 1987;32:889–895.
52. Calne RY, Wood AJ. Cyclosporin in cadaveric renal transplantation: 3-year follow-up of a European multicentre trial (letter). *Lancet* 1985;2:549.
53. Myers BD, Ross J, Newton L, Luetscher J, Perlroth M. Cyclosporine-associated chronic nephropathy. *N Engl J Med* 1984;311:699–705.
54. McCauley J, Van Thiel DH, Starzl TE, Puschett JB. Acute and chronic renal failure in liver transplantation. *Nephron* 1990;55:121–128.
55. Ross EA, Wilkinson A, Hawkins RA et al. The plasma creatinine concentration is not an accurate reflection of the glomerular filtration rate in stable renal transplant patients receiving cyclosporine. *Am J Kidney Dis* 1987;10:113–117.
56. Rao KV, Crasson JT, Kjellstrand CM. Chronic irreversible nephrotoxicity from cyclosporin A. *Nephron* 1985;41:75–77.
57. Jackson NM, Hsu C-H, Visscher GE, Venkatachalam MA, Humes HD. Alterations in renal structure and function in a rat model of cyclosporine nephrotoxicity. *J Pharmacol Exp Ther* 1987;242: 749–756.
58. Kahan BD. Cyclosporine nephrotoxicity: pathogenesis, prophylaxis, therapy, and prognosis. *Am J Kidney Dis* 1986;8:323–331.
59. Bantle JP, Paller MS, Boudreau RJ, Olivari MT, Ferris TF. Long-term effects of cyclosporine on renal function in organ transplant recipients. *J Lab Clin Med* 1990;115:233–240.
60. Myers BD, Newton L, Boshkos C, et al. Chronic injury of human renal microvessels with low-dose cyclosporine therapy. *Transplantation* 1988;46:694–703.
61. Bertani T, Ferrazzi P, Schieppati A, et al. Nature and extent of glomerular injury induced by cyclosporine in heart transplant patients. *Kidney Int* 1991;40:243–250.
62. Harding MW, Galat A, Uehling DE, Schreiber SL. A receptor for the immunosuppressant FK506 is a cis-trans peptidyl-prolyl isomerase. *Nature* 1989;341:758–760.
63. Kay J, Moore AL, Doe SEA, Benzie CR, Schonbrunner R, Schmid FX, Halestrap AP. The mechanism of action of FK506. *Transplant Proc* 1990;22:96–99.
64. Suzuki N, Sakane T, Tsunematsu T. Effects of a novel immunosuppressive agent, FK506, on human B-cell activation. *Clin Exp Immunol* 1990;79:240–245.
65. Tocci MJ, Matkovich DA, Collier KA, et al. The immunosuppressive FK506 selectively inhibits expression of early T-cell activation genes. *J Immunol* 1984;143:718–726.
66. Fung JJ, Todo S, Jain A, McCauley J, Alessiani M, Scott C, Starzl TE. Conversion from cyclosporine to FK506 in liver allograft recipients with cylosporine-related complications. *Transplant Proc* 1990;22:6–12.
67. Demetris AJ, Fung JT, Todo S, Banner B, Zerbe T, Syn G, Starzl TE. Pathologic observations in human allograft recipients treated with FK506. *Transplant Proc* 1990;22:25–34.
68. Brown Z, Neild GH. FK506 and haemolytic uremic syndrome. *Lancet* 1990;1:412.
69. McCauley J, Bronsther O, Fung J, Todo S, Starzl TE. Treatment of cyclosporine-induced haemolytic uraemic syndrome with FK506. *Lancet* 1989;2:1516.
70. Butkowski RM, Goodman P, Crawford ED, Sergi JS, Redman BG, Whitehead RP. Phase II trial of high-dose intermittent interleukin-2 in metastatic renal cell carcinoma: A Southwest Oncology Group Study. *J Natl Cancer Inst* 1990;82:143–146.

71. Fisher RL, Coltman CA Jr, Doroshow JH, et al. Metastatic renal cancer treated with interleukin-2 and lymphokine-activated killer cells: a phase II clinical trial. *Ann Intern Med* 1988;108: 518–523.
72. Belldegrun A, Webb DE, Austin HA III, et al. Effect of interleukin-2 on renal function in patients receiving immunotherapy for advanced cancer. *Ann Intern Med* 1984;106:1006.
73. Chochat P, Floret D, Bouffet E, et al. Renal effects of continuous infusion of recombinant interleukin-2 in children. *Pediatr Nephrol* 1991;5:33–37.
74. Nasr G, McKolanis J, Pais R, et al. A phase I study of interleukin-2 in children with cancer, and evaluation of clinical and immunologic status during therapy. A Pediatric Oncology Group study. *Cancer* 1989;64:783–786.
75. Hamblin TJ. Interleukin-2: Side effects are acceptable. *Br Med J* 1990;30:275–276.
76. Rosenberg SA, Lotze MT, Muul LM, et al. Observation on the systemic administration of autologous lymphokine-activated killer cells and recombinant interleukin-2 to patients with metastatic cancers. *N Engl J Med* 1985;313:1485–1492.
77. Rosenstein M, Ettinghausen SE, Rosenberg SA. Extravasation of intravascular fluid mediated by the systemic administration of recombinant interleukin-2. *J Immunol* 1986;137:1735–1742.
78. Sarna GP, Figlin RA, Pertckeck M, Altrock B, Kradjian SA. Systemic administration of recombinant methionyl human interleukin 2 (Ala 125) to cancer patients. Clinical results. *J Biol Response Mod* 1989;8:16–24.
79. Butler LD, Mohler KM, Layman NK, Cain RL, Riedl PE, Puckett LD, Bendele AM. Interleukin-2 induced systemic toxicity: induction of mediators and immunopharmacologic intervention. *Immunopharmacol Immunotoxicol* 1989;11:445.
80. Cotran RS, Pober JS, Gimbrone MA, et al. Endothelial activation during interleukin-2 immunotherapy: a possible mechanism for the vascular leak syndrome. *J Immunol* 1988;140:1883–1888.
81. Samlowski W, Schumann JL, Birchfield GR, Ward JH, Schumann GB. Cytologic evidence of nephrotoxicity in patients receiving high-dose interleukin-2. In: *Abstracts of the XIth International Congress of Nephrotoxicity*. Tokyo: 1990:436A.
82. Mercatello A, Aoumeur H-A, Negrier S, et al. Acute renal failure with preserved renal plasma flow induced by cancer immunotherapy. *Kidney Int* 1991;40:309–314.
83. Goldman M, van Laethem J-L, Abramowicz D, DePauw L, Kinnaert P, Vereersrraeten P. Evolution of renal function during treatment of kidney graft rejection with OKT3 monoclonal antibody. *Transplantation* 1990;50:158–159.
84. Maessen JG, Bourman WA, Ko G. Direct cytotoxic effect of cytokines in kidney parenchyma. A possible mechanism of allograft destruction. *Transplant Proc* 1989;21:309–310.
85. Simpson MA, Madras PN, Cornaby AJ, Etienne T, Dempsey RA, Clowes GHA, Monaco AP. Sequential determinations of urinary cytology and plasma and urinary lymphokines in the management of renal allograft recipients. *Transplantation* 1989;47:218–223.
86. Danowitch GM, Nast C, Rosenthal T, Ettenger R, Wilkinson AH. Features of aspiration biopsy cytology during treatment of acute rejection with OKT3. *Abstracts: XIIIth International Congress of the Transplantation Society*. San Francisco, August 1990;141.
87. Gaston RS, Deierhoi MH, Patterson T, et al. OKT3 first-dose reaction: association with T cell subsets and cytokine release. *Kidney Int* 1991;39:141–148.
88. Moritz T, Niederle N, Baumann J, et al. Phase I study of recombinant human tumor necrosis factor a in advanced malignant disease. *Cancer Immunol Immunother* 1989;19:144–150.
89. Steinmetz T, Schaadt M, Gahl R, Schenk V, Diehl V, Pfreundschuh M. Phase I study of 24-hour continuous infusion of recombinant human tumor necrosis factor. *J Biol Response Mod* 1988;7: 417–423.
90. Ault BH, Stapleton F-B, Gaber L, Martin A, Roy S III, Murphy SB. Acute renal failure during therapy with recombinant human gamma interferon. *N Engl J Med* 1988;319:1397–1400.
91. Cooper MR, Fefer A, Thompson J, et al. Interferon alpha 2h/melphalan/prednisone in previously untreated patients with multiple myeloma. A phase I-II trial. *Invest New Drugs* 1987;5:41–46.
92. Fiedler W, Zellor W, Peimann CJ, Weh HJ, Hossfeld DK. A phase II combination trial with recombinant human tumor necrosis factor and gamma interferon in patients with colorectal cancer. *Klin Wochenschr* 1991;59:261–268.
93. Mahaley MS, Bertsch L, Cash S, Gillespie GY. Systemic gamma-interferon therapy for recurrent glioma. *J Neurosurg* 1988;69:826–829.
94. Averbuch SD, Austin HA III, Sherwin SA, Antonovych T, Bunn PA Jr, Longo DL. Acute interstitial nephritis with the nephrotic syndrome following recombinant leukocyte alpha-interferon therapy for mycosis fungoides. *N Engl J Med* 1984;310:32–35.

95. Blair JT, Thompson AW, Whiting PH, Davidson RJL, Simpson JG. Toxicity of the immune suppressant cyclosporin A in the rat. *J Pathol* 1982;138:163–177.
96. Ryffel B, Donatsch P, Madorin M, et al. Toxicological evaluation of cyclosporin A. *Arch Toxicol* 1983;53:107–141.
97. Siegl H, Ryffel B, Petric R, Shoemaker P, Muller A, Donatsch P, Mihatsch M. Cyclosporine, the renin-angiotensin-aldosterone system, and renal adverse reactions. *Transplant Proc* 1983;15: 2719–2725.
98. Thomson AW, Whiting PH, Simpson JG. Cyclosporine: immunology, toxicity and pharmacology in experimental animals. *Agents Actions* 1984;15:306–327.
99. Kone BC, Racusen LC, Whelton A, Solez K. Acute renal failure produced by combining cyclosporine and brief renal ischemia in the Munich Wistar rat. *Clin Nephrol* 1986;25:S171–S174.
100. Chow SS, Thorner P, Baumal R, Wilson DR. Cyclosporine and experimental renal ischemic injury. *Transplantation* 1986:41:152–156.
101. Dieperink H, Starklint H, Leyssac PP. Nephrotoxicity of cyclosporine—an animal model: study of the nephrotoxic effect of cyclosporine on overall renal and tubular function in conscious rats. *Transplant Proc* 1983;15:2736.
102. Cunningham C, Gavin MP, Whiting PH, Burke MD, MacIntyre F, Thomson AW, Simpson JG. Serum cyclosporine levels, hepatic drug metabolism and renal tubulotoxicity. *Biochem Pharmacol* 1985;33:2857–2861.
103. Thomson AW, Whiting PH, Blair JT, Davidson RJL, Simpson JG. Pathological changes developing in the rat during a 3-week course of high dosage cyclosporin A and their reversal following drug withdrawal. *Transplantation* 1981;32:271–277.
104. Yagisawa T, Takahashi K, Teraoka S, Yamaguchi Y, Toma H, Agishi T, Ota K. Cyclosporine tissue levels and morphological and functional changes in organs of cyclosporine-treated rats. *Transplant Proc* 1986;18:1272–1277.
105. Schwass DE, Sasaki AW, Houghton DC, Benner KE, Bennett WM. Effect of phenobarbital and cimetidine on experimental cyclosporine nephrotoxicity: preliminary observations. *Clin Nephrol* 1986;25:S117–S120.
106. Duncan JI, Thomson AW, Aldridge RD, Simpson JG, Whiting PH. Cyclosporine-induced renal structural damage: influence of dosage, strain, age and sex with reference to the rat and guinea pig. *Clin Nephrol* 1986;25:S14–S17.
107. Muller-Suur R, Davis SD. Effect of cyclosporine A on renal electrolyte transport: whole kidney and Henle loop study. Effect of cyclosporine on the diluting capacity of the rat kidney. *Clin Nephrol* 1986;25:S57–S61.
108. Rahman MA, Ing TS. Cyclosporine and magnesium metabolism. *J Lab Clin Med* 1989;114:211–214.
109. Rosen S, Greenfeld Z, Brezis M. Chronic cyclosporine-induced nephropathy in the rat. *Transplantation* 1990;49:445–452.
110. Gnutzmann KH, Hering K, Gutsche H-U. Effect of cyclosporine on the diluting capacity of the rat kidney. *Clin Nephrol* 1986;25:S31–S36.
111. Borowitz JL. Cyclosporine increases calcium in kidney medulla. *Life Sci* 1988;42:1215–1222.
112. Trifillis AL, Kahng MW. Effects of cyclosporine A on cultured human kidney cells: lipid peroxidation and cytosolic calcium. *Transplant Proc* 1988;20:717–721.
113. Wilson PD, Hreniuk D. Nephrotoxicity of cyclosporine in renal tubule cultures and attenuation by calcium restriction. *Transplant Proc* 1988;20:709–711.
114. Scoble JE, Senior JCM, Chan P, Varghese Z, Sweny P, Moorhead JF. In vitro cyclosporine toxicity. The effect of verapamil. *Transplantation* 1989;47:647–650.
115. Jackson NM, O'Connor RP, Humes HD. Interactions of cyclosporine with renal proximal tubule cells and cellular membranes. *Transplantation* 1988;46:109–114.
116. Jung K, Pergande M. Influence of cyclosporin A on the respiration of isolated rat kidney mitochondria. *FEBS Lett* 1985;183:167–169.
117. Jung K, Reinholdt C, Scholz D. Inhibitory effects of cyclosporine on the respiratory efficiency of isolated human kidney mitochondria. *Transplantation* 1987;43:162–163.
118. Strzelecki T, Kuman S, Khauli R, Menon M. Impairment by cyclosporine of membrane-mediated functions in kidney mitochondria. *Kidney Int* 1988;34:234–240.
119. Elzinga LW, Mela-Riker LM, Widener LL, Bennett WM. Renal cortical mitochondrial integrity in experimental cyclosporine nephrotoxicity. *Transplantation* 1989;48:102–106.
120. Broekemeier KM, Dempsey ME, Pfeiffer DR. Cyclosporin A is a potent inhibitor of the inner membrane permeability transition in liver mitochondria. *J Biol Chem* 1989;264:7826–7830.

121. O'Leary TJ, Ross PD, Lieber MR, Levin IW. Effects of cyclosporine A on biomembranes: vibrational spectroscopic, calorimetric and hemolysis studies. *Biophys J* 1986;49:795–801.
122. Wiedmann TS, Trouard T, Shekar SC, Polikandritou M, Rahman Y-E. Interaction of cyclosporin A with dipalmitoylphosphatidylcholine. *Biochim Biophys Acta* 1990;1023:12–18.
123. Ziegler K, Frimmer M, Fritzsch G, Koepsell H. Cyclosporin binding to a protein component of the renal Na^+-D-glucose cotransporter. *J Biol Chem* 1990;265:3270–3277.
124. Buss WC, Steparek J, Bennett WM. A new proposal for the mechanism of cyclosporine nephrotoxicity: inhibition of renal microsomal protein chain elongation following in vivo cyclosporin A. *Biochem Pharmacol* 1989;38:4085–4093.
125. Bennett WM, Houghton DC, Buss WC. Cyclosporine-induced renal dysfunction: correlations between cellular events and whole kidney function. *JASN* 1991;1:1212–1219.
126. Walker RJ, Lazzaro VA, Duggin GG, Horvath JS, Tiller DJ. Cyclosporin-induced alterations in renal metabolism: the role of lipid peroxidation and enzyme inhibition in cyclosporine nephrotoxicity. *Transplantation* 1990;50:487–492.
127. Walker RJ, Lazzaro VA, Duggin GG, Horvath JS, Tiller DJ. Cyclosporin A inhibits protein kinase C activity: a contributing mechanism in the development of nephrotoxicity? *Biochem Biophys Res Commun* 1989;160:409–415.
128. Schurek HJ, Neumann KH, Jesinghaus WP, Aeikens B, Wonigeit K. Influence of cyclosporine A on adaptive hypertrophy after unilateral nephrectomy in the rat. *Clin Nephrol* 1986;25:S144–S147.
129. Feingold R, Winston J, Safirstein R. Cyclosporine inhibits compensatory renal growth. *Clin Res* 1986;34:595A.
130. Batlle DC, Gutterman C, Keilani T, Peces R, LaPointe M. Effect of cyclosporin A on renal function and kidney growth in the uninephrectomized rat. *Kidney Int* 1990;37:21–28.
131. Whiting PH, Duncan JI, Gavin MP, Heys SD, Simpson JG, Asfar SK, Thomson AW. Renal function in rats treated with cyclosporin following unilateral nephrectomy. *Br J Exp Pathol* 1985; 66:535–542.
132. Brunner FP, Hermle M, Mihatsch MJ, Thiel G. Effect of cyclosporine in rats with reduced renal mass. *Clin Nephrol* 1986;25:S148–S154.
133. Iaina A, Herzog D, Cohen D, et al. Cyclosporine and short ischaemia: a new model of experimental acute renal failure in rats. *Proc EDTA-ERA* 1984;21:849–852.
134. Kanzai G, Stowe N, Steinmuller D, Ho-Hsieh H, Novick A. Effect of cyclosporine upon the function of ischemically damaged kidneys in the rat. *Transplantation* 1986;41:782.
135. Jablonski P, Harrison C, Howden BH, Rae D, Tavalis G, Marshall VC, Tange JD. Cyclosporine and the ischemic rat kidney. *Transplantation* 1986;41:147–151.
136. Bia MJ, Tyler KA. Effect of cyclosporine on renal ischemic injury. *Transplantation* 1987;43:800–804.
137. McKenzie N, Devineni R, Vezina W, Keown P, Stiller C. The effect of cyclosporine on organ blood flow. *Transplant Proc* 1986;17:1973–1975.
138. Racusen LC, Solez K. Cyclosporine nephrotoxicity. *Int Rev Exp Pathol* 1988;30:107–157.
139. Mason J. The pathophysiology of Sandimmune (cyclosporine) in man and animals. Part 1. *Pediatr Nephrol* 1990;4:554–574.
140. Perico N, Remuzzi G. Mechanisms and mediators of cyclosporine-induced renal vascular changes. In: Hitano M, ed. *Nephrology: Proceedings of the XIth International Congress of Nephrology.* Tokyo: Springer-Verlag, 1991;543–554.
141. Besarab A, Jarrell BE, Hirsch S, Carabasi RA, Cressman MD, Green P. Use of the isolated perfused kidney model to assess the acute pharmacologic effects of cyclosporine and its vehicle, cremophor el. *Transplantation* 1987;44:195–201.
142. Racusen LC, Kone BC, Solez K. Early renal pathophysiology in an acute model of cyclosporine nephrotoxicity in rats. *Ren Fail* 1987;10:29–37.
143. Thiel G, Hermle M, Brunner FP. Acutely impaired renal function during intravenous administration of cyclosporine A: a cremophore side-effect. *Clin Nephrol* 1986;25:S40–S42.
144. Gillum DM, Truong L, Suki WN. Effects of uninephrectomy and high protein feeding in cyclosporine nephropathy. *Kidney Int* 1989;36:194–200.
145. Barros EJG, Boim MA, Ajzen H, Raimas OL, Schor N. Glomerular hemodynamics and hormonal participation in cyclosporine nephrotoxicity. *Kidney Int* 1987;32:19–25.
146. Thomson SC, Tucker BJ, Gabbai F, Blantz RC. Functional effects on glomerular hemodynamics of short-term chronic cyclosporine in male rats. *J Clin Invest* 1989;83:960–969.
147. Schor N, Roim MA, Barros EJG, Santos OFP. Glomerular hemodynamic effects of cyclosporine.

In: Hitano M, ed. *Nephrology: Proceedings of the XIth International Congress of Nephrology*. Tokyo: Springer-Verlag, 1991;534–542.
148. English J, Evan A, Houghton DC, Bennett WM. Cyclosporine-induced acute renal dysfunction in the rat. *Transplantation* 1987;44:135–141.
149. Winston J, Feingold R, Safirstein R. Glomerular hemodynamics in cyclosporine nephrotoxicity following nephrectomy. *Kidney Int* 1989;35:1175–1182.
150. Wiegmann TB, Sharma R, Diederich DA, Savin V. In vitro effects of cyclosporine on glomerular function. *Am J Med Sci* 1990;299:149–152.
151. Zimmerhackl LB, Fretschner M, Steinhausen M. Cyclosporin reduces renal blood flow through vasoconstriction of arcuate arteries in the hydronephrotic rat model. *Klin Wochenschr* 1990;68: 166–174.
152. Gerkens JF, Bhagwandken SH, Dosen PJ, Smith AJ. The effect of salt intake on cyclosporine-induced impairment of renal function in rats. *Transplantation* 1984;38:412–417.
153. Kaskel FJ, Devarajan P, Arbeit LA, Partin JS, Moore LC. Cyclosporine nephrotoxicity: sodium excretion, autoregulation, and angiotensin II. *Am J Physiol* 1987;252:F733–F742.
154. Ryffel B, Mihatsch MJ. Cyclosporine nephrotoxicity. *Toxicol Pathol* 1986;14:73–92.
155. Devarajan P, Kaskel FJ, Arbeit LA, Moore LC. Cyclosporine nephrotoxicity: blood volume, sodium conservation, and renal hemodynamics. *Am J Physiol* 1989;256:F71–F78.
156. Murray BM, Paller MS, Ferris TF. Effect of cyclosporine administration on renal hemodynamics in conscious rats. *Kidney Int* 1985;28:767–774.
157. Murray BM, Paller MS. Beneficial effects of renal denervation and prazosin on GFR and renal blood flow after cyclosporine in rats. *Clin Nephrol* 1986;25:S37–S39.
158. Moss NG, Powell SL, Falk RJ. Intravenous cyclosporine activates afferent and efferent renal nerves and causes sodium retention in innervated kidneys in rats. *Proc Natl Acad Sci USA* 1985;82: 8222–8226.
159. Xue H, Bukoski D, McCarron DA, Bennett WM. Induction of contraction in isolated rat aorta by cyclosporine. *Transplantation* 1987;43:715–718.
160. Gazdar AF, Dammin GJ. Neural degeneration and regeneration in human renal transplants. *N Engl J Med* 1970;283:222–224.
161. Blantz RC, Konnen KS, Tucker BJ. Angiotension II effects upon the glomerular microcirculation and ultrafiltration coefficient of the rat. *J Clin Invest* 1976;57:419–434.
162. Tucker BJ, Mundy CA, Blantz RC. Adrenergic and angiotensin II influences on renal vascular tone in chronic sodium depletion. *Am J Physiol* 1987;21:F811–F817.
163. Kopp U, Aurell M, Sjolander M, Ablad B. The role of prostaglandins in the alpha- and beta-adrenoreceptor mediated renin release response to graded renal nerve stimulation. *Pfugers Arch* 1981;391:1–8.
164. Caterson RJ, Duggin GG, Critchley L, Baxter C, Horvath JS, Hall BM, Tiller DJ. Renal tubular transport of cyclosporine A (CsA) and associated changes in renal function. *Clin Nephrol* 1986;25: S30–S33.
165. Perico N, Benigni A, Bosco E, et al. Acute cyclosporine A nephrotoxicity in rats: which role for renin-angiotensin system and glomerular prostaglandins? *Clin Nephrol* 1986;25:S83–S88.
166. Perico N, Zoja C, Benigni A, Ghilardi F, Gualandris L, Remuzzi G. Effect of short-term cyclosporine administration in rats on renin-angiotensin and thromboxane A_2: possible relevance to the reduction in glomerular filtration rate. *J Pharmacol Exp Ther* 1986;239:229–235.
167. Siegl H, Ryffel B, Petric R, Shoemaker P, Muller A, Donatsch P, Mihatsch M. Cyclosporine, the renin-angiotensin-aldosterone system, and renal adverse reactions. *Transplant Proc* 1983;15: 2719–2725.
168. Myers BD, Ross J, Newton L, Leutscher J, Perlroth M. Cyclosporine-associated chronic nephropathy. *N Engl J Med* 1984;311:699–705.
169. Bantle JP, Nath KA, Sutherlant DE, Najarian JS, Ferris TF. Effects of cyclosporine on the renin-angiotensin-aldosterone system and potassium excretion in renal transplant recipients. *Arch Intern Med* 1985;145:505–508.
170. Myers BD, Sibley R, Newton L, et al. The long-term course of cyclosporine-associated chronic nephropathy. *Kidney Int* 1988;33:590–600.
171. Duggin GG, Baxter C, Hall BM, Horvath JS, Tiller DJ. Influence of cyclosporine A on intrarenal control of GFR. *Clin Nephrol* 1986;25:S43–S45.
172. Kurtz A, Bruna RD, Kuhn K. Cyclosporine A enhances renin secretion and production in isolated juxtaglomerular cells. *Kidney Int* 1988;33:947–953.

173. Gillum DM, Truong L, Tasby J, Migliore P, Suki WN. Chronic cyclosporine nephrotoxicity. A rodent model. *Transplantation* 1988;46:285–292.
174. Verpooten GA, Wybo I, Pattyn VM, et al. Cyclosporine nephrotoxicity: comparative cytochemical study of rat kidney and human allograft biopsies. *Clin Nephrol* 1986;25:S18–S22.
175. Nitta K, Friedman AL, Nicastri AD, Paik S, Friedman EA. Granular juxtaglomerular cell hyperplasia caused by cyclosporine. *Transplantation* 1987;44:417–421.
176. Gerkens JF, Smith AJ. Effect of captopril and theophylline treatment on cyclosporine-induced nephrotoxicity in rats. *Transplantation* 1985;40:213–214.
177. Kaskel FJ, Devarajan P, Birzgalis A, Moore LC. Inhibition of myogenic autoregulation in cyclosporine nephrotoxicity in the rat. *Renal Physiol Biochem* 1989;12:250–259.
178. Golub MS, Lustig S, Berger ME, Lee DBN. Altered vascular responses in cyclosporine-treated rats. *Transplantation* 1989;48:116–118.
179. Muller-Schweinitzer E. Changes in the venous compliance in bradykinin and angiotensin II and its significance for the vascular effects of cyclosporine A. *Naunyn Schmiedebergs Arch Pharmacol* 1988;338:699–703.
180. Muller-Schweinitzer E. Interaction of cyclosporine A with the renin-angiotensin system in canine veins. *Naunyn Schmiedebergs Arch Pharmacol* 1989;340:252–257.
181. Schor N, Ichikawa J, Brenner BM. Mechanisms of action of various hormones and ultrafiltration in the rat. *Kidney Int* 1981;20:442–451.
182. Kremer S, Margolis B, Harper P, Skorecki K. Cyclosporine induced alterations in vasopressin signalling in the glomerular mesangial cell. *Clin Invest Med* 1989;12:201–206.
183. Meyer-Lehnert H, Schrier RW. Cyclosporine A enhances vasopressin-induced Ca^{2+} mobilization and contraction in mesangial cells. *Kidney Int* 1988;34:89–97.
184. Rodriguez-Puyol D, Lamas S, Olivera A, et al. Actions of cyclosporin A on cultured rat mesangial cells. *Kidney Int* 1989;35:632–637.
185. dos Santos OFP, Boim MA, Bregman R, et al. Effect of platelet-activating factor antagonist on cyclosporine nephrotoxicity. *Transplantation* 1989;47:592–595.
186. Pirotzsky E, Colliez P, Guilmard C, Schaeverbeke J, Broquet P. Cyclosporin-induced nephrotoxicity: preventive effect of a PAF-acether antagonist BN52063. *Transplant Proc* 1988;665–669.
187. Baxter CR, Duggin GG, Hall BM, Horvath JS, Tiller DJ. Stimulation of renin release from rat renal cortical slices by cyclosporin A. *Res Commun Chem Pathol Pharmacol* 1984;43:417–423.
188. Stahl RAK, Kudelka S. Chronic cyclosporine A treatment reduces prostaglandin E_2 formation in isolated glomeruli and papilla of rat kidneys. *Clin Nephrol* 1986;25:S78–S82.
189. Stahl RAK, Adler S, Baker PJ, et al. Cyclosporin A inhibits prostaglandin E_2 formation by rat mesangial cells in culture. *Kidney Int* 1989;35:1161–1167.
190. Bunke M, Wilder L, McLeish K. Effect of cyclosporine on glomerular prostaglandin production. *Transplant Proc* 1988;20:646–649.
191. Makowka L, Lopatin W, Gilas L, Falk J, Phillips MJ, Falk R. Prevention of cyclosporine (CyA) nephrotoxicity by synthetic prostaglandins. *Clin Nephrol* 1986;25:S89–S94.
192. Ryffel B, Donatsch P, Hiestand P, Mihatsch MJ. Prostaglandin E_2 reduces nephrotoxicity and immunosuppression of cyclosporine in rats. *Clin Nephrol* 1986;25:S95–S99.
193. Coffman TM, Carr DR, Farger WE, Klotman P. Evidence that renal prostaglandin production and thromboxane production is stimulated in chronic cyclosporine nephrotoxicity. *Transplantation* 1987;43:282–285.
194. Elzinga L, Kelley VE, Houghton DC, Bennett WM. Modification of experimental nephrotoxicity with fish oil as the vehicle for cyclosporine. *Transplantation* 1987;43:271–274.
195. Rogers TS, Elzinga L, Bennett WM, Kelley VE. Selective enhancement of thromboxane in macrophages and kidneys in cyclosporine-induced nephrotoxicity. *Transplantation* 1988;45:153–156.
196. van der Heide JJH, Bilo HJG, Tegzess AM, Donker AJM. The effects of dietary supplementation with fish oil on renal function in cyclosporine-treated renal transplant recipients. *Transplantation* 1990;49:523–527.
197. Perico N, Benigni A, Zoja C, Delaini F, Remuzzi G. Functional significance of exaggerated renal thromboxane A_2 synthesis induced by cyclosporin A. *Am J Physiol* 1986;251:F581–F587.
198. Perico N, Pasini M, Gaspari F, Abbate M, Remuzzi G. Co-participation of thromboxane A_2 and leukotriene C_4 and D_4 in mediating cyclosporine-induced acute renal failure. *Transplantation* 1991;52:873–878.
199. Schlondorff D. The glomerular mesangial cell: an expanding role for a specialized pericyte. *FASEB J* 1987;1:272–281.
200. Fukuda Y, Hirata Y, Yoshimi H, Kojima T, Kobayashi Y, Yanigasawa M, Masaki T. Endothelin

is a potent secretagogue for atrial natriuretic peptide in cultured rat atrial myocytes. *Biochem Biophys Res Commun* 1988;155:167–172.
201. Hirata Y, Yoshimi H, Takata S, Watanabe X, Kumagi S, Nakajima K, Sakakibara S. Cellular mechanism of action by a novel vasoconstrictor endothelin in cultured vascular smooth muscle cells. *Biochem Biophys Res Commun* 1988;154:868–875.
202. Harris AK, Wild P, Stopak D. Silicone rubber substrata: a new wrinkle in the study of cell locomotion. *Science* 1980;208:177–179.
203. Badr KF, Murray JJ, Breyer MD, et al. Mesangial cell, glomerular and renal vascular responses to endothelin in the rat kidney. Elucidation of signal transduction pathways. *J Clin Invest* 1989;83: 336–342.
204. Kon V, Sugiura M, Inagami T, Harvie BR, Ichikawa I, Hoover RL. Role of endothelin in cyclosporine-induced glomerular dysfunction. *Kidney Int* 1990;37:1487–1491.
205. Perico N, Dadan J, Remuzzi G. Endothelin mediates the renal vasoconstriction induced by cyclosporine in the rat. *JASN* 1990;1:76–83.
206. Awazu M, Sugiura M, Inagami T, Ichikawa I, Kon V. Cyclosporine promotes glomerular endothelin binding in vivo. *JASN* 1991;1:1253–1258.
207. Takenaka T, Hashimoto Y, Epstein M. Diminished ACH-induced vasodilatation in renal microvessels of CsA-treated rats. *JASN* 1992;3:42–50.
208. Neild GH, Rocchi G, Imberti L, Fumagalli F, Brown Z, Remuzzi G, Williams DG. Effect of cyclosporine on prostacyclin synthesis by vascular tissue in rabbits. *Transplant Proc* 1983;15: 2398–2400.
209. Faraco PR, Hewitson TD, Kincaid-Smith P. An animal model for the study of the microangiopathic form of cyclosporine nephrotoxicity. *Transplantation* 1991;51:1129–1131.
210. Zoja C, Furci L, Ghilardi F, Zilio P, Benigni A, Remuzzi G. Cyclosporin-induced endothelial cell injury. *Lab Invest* 1986;55:455–462.
211. Lau DCW, Wong K-L, Hwang WS. Cyclosporine toxicity on cultured rat microvascular endothelial cells. *Kidney Int* 1989;35:604–613.
212. Fasel J, Kaissling B, Ludwig KS. Light and electron microscopic changes in the kidney of Wistar rats following treatment with cyclosporine A. *Ultrastruct Pathol* 1987;11:435–448.
213. Ferns G, Reidy M, Ross R. Vascular effects of cyclosporine A in vivo and in vitro. *Am J Pathol* 1990;137:403–413.
214. Dieperink H, Leyssac PO, Starklint H, Jorgensen KA, Kemp E. Antagonist capacities of nifedipine, captopril, phenoxybenzamine, prostacyclin and indomethacin on cyclosporin A induced impairment of rat renal function. *Eur J Clin Invest* 1986;16:540–548.
215. Skorecki KL, Rutledge WP, Schrier RW. (Review) Acute cyclosporine nephrotoxicity—prototype for a membrane signalling disorder. *Kidney Int* 1992;42:1–10.
216. Bertani T, Perico N, Abbate M, Battaglia C, Remuzzi G. Renal injury induced by long-term administration of cyclosporin A to rats. *Am J Pathol* 1987;127:569–579.
217. Simpson JG, Saunders NJ, Thompson KJ, Whiting PH. Chronic renal damage caused by cyclosporine. *Transplant Proc* 1988;20:792–799.
218. Gillum DM, Truong L, Tasby J, Migliore P, Suki WN. Chronic cyclosporine toxicity. *Transplantation* 1988;461:285–292.
219. Wolf G, Killen PD, Neilson EG. Cyclosporin A stimulates transcription and procollagen secretion in tubulointerstitial fibroblasts and proximal tubular cells. *JASN* 1990;1:918–922.
220. Nast C, Adler SG, Artishevsky A, Kresser CT, Ahmed K, Anderson PS. Cyclosporine induces elevated procollagen alpha 1 (I) mRNA levels in the rat renal cortex. *Kidney Int* 1991;39: 631–638.
221. Pisanty S, Shoshan S, Chajek T, Maftsir G, Sacks B, BenEzra D. The effect of cyclosporin A treatment on gingival tissue of patients with Behcet's disease. *J Periodontol* 1988;59:599–603.
222. Pisanty S, Rahamim E, Ben-Ezra D, Shoshan S. Prolonged systemic administration of cyclosporin A affects gingival epithelium. *J Periodontol* 1990;61:138–141.
223. Thompson HL, Burbelo PD, Gabriel G, Yamada Y, Metcalfe DD. Murine mast cells synthesize basement membrane components: a potential role in early fibrosis. *J Clin Invest* 1991;87:619–623.
224. Kopp JB, Klotman PE. Cellular and molecular mechanisms of cyclosporin nephrotoxicity. *JASN* 1990;1:162–179.
225. Backman L, Sundelin B, Bohman S-O. Chronic renal lesions in rats after long-term treatment with cyclosporine A. *Transplant Proc* 1990;22:133–134.
226. Traber L, Loosli HR, Hofmann H, Kuhn M, Wartburg A. Isolierung and strukturemittlung der neuen cyclosporine E, F, G, H, und I. *Helv Chir Acta* 1982;65:1655–1677.

227. Paller MS, Ferris TF. Effects of Nva2-cyclosporine on glomerular filtration rate and renal blood flow in the rat. *Transplantation* 1987;43:893–895.
228. Hiestand PC, Gunn HC, Gale JM, Ryffel B, Borel JF. Comparison of the pharmacological profiles of cyclosporine, (Nva2)-cyclosporine and (Val2) dihydro-cyclosporine. *Immunology* 1985;55:249–255.
229. Tejani A, Lancman I, Pomrants A, Khawar M, Chen C. Nephrotoxicity of cyclosporine A and cyclosporine G in a rat model. *Transplantation* 1988;45:184–187.
230. Hoyt EG, Hagberg RC, Billingham ME, Baldwin JC, Jamieson SW. Analysis of the immunosuppressive and nephrotoxic effects of cyclosporin G. *J Heart Transplant* 1988;7:111–118.
231. Kawashima H, Mochizuki M, Okumura A, et al. Cyclosporine G and D in experimental autoimmune uveoretinitis in the rat. *Jpn J Ophthalmol* 1989;33:425–440.
232. Duncan JI, Whiting PH, Simpson JH, Thomson AW. Nephrotoxicity of cyclosporin G in rats (letter). *Lancet* 1985;2:1004–1005.
233. Todo S, Ueda Y, Demetris JA, et al. Immunosuppression of canine, monkey, and baboon allografts by FK506: with special reference to synergism with other drugs and to tolerance induction. *Surgery* 1988;104:239–249.
234. Nalesnik M, Lai HS, Murase N, Todo S, Starzl TE. The effect of FK506 and cyclosporine A on the Lewis rat renal ischemia model. *Transplant Proc* 1990;22:87–89.
235. Kumano K, Wang G, Sakai T. Functional and morphological changes in rat kidney induced by FK506 (FK). *JASN* 1990;1:613.
236. Kumano K, Wang G, Endo T, Kuwao S. FK506-induced nephrotoxicity in rats. *Transplant Proc* 1991;23:512–515.
237. Ochiai T, Sakamoto K, Gunji Y, et al. Effects of combination treatment with FK506 and cyclosporine on survival time and vascular changes in renal-allograft-recipient dogs. *Transplantation* 1989;48:193–197.
238. Anderson TD, Hayes TJ. Toxicity of human recombinant interleukin-2 in rats. *Lab Invest* 1989;60: 331–346.
239. Welbourn R, Goldman G, Kobzik L, Valeri CR, Shepro D, Hechtman HB. Involvement of thromboxane and neutrophils in multiple-system organ edema with interleukin-2. *Ann Surg* 1990;212: 728–733.
240. Welbourn R, Goldman G, Kobzik L, Valeri CR, Hechtman HB, Shepro D. Attenuation of IL-2-induced multisystem organ edema with phalloidin and antamanide. *J Appl Physiol* 1991;70:1364–1368.
241. Rubinger D, Cohen E, Shiloni E, Rathaus M, Bernheim J, Popovtzer MM. Increased thromboxane (TXB_2) mediates the adverse renal effects of interleukin-2 (IL-2) in rats. *JASN* 1990;1:448.
242. Damle N, Doyle L. IL-2-activated human killer lymphocytes but not their secreted products mediate increase in albumin flux across cultured endothelial monolayers. *J Immunol* 1989;142:2660–2669.
243. Klausner J, Morel N, Paterson I, et al. The rapid induction by interleukin-2 of pulmonary microvascular permeability. *Ann Surg* 1989;209:119–128.
244. Morel-Maroger L, Slopes JC, Vinter J, Woodrow D, Gresser I. An ultrastructural study of the development of nephritis in mice treated with interferon in the neonatal period. *Lab Invest* 1978;39: 513–522.
245. Maessen JG, Buurman WA, Knotstra G. Direct cytotoxic effect of cytokines in kidney parenchyma: a possible mechanism of allograft destruction. *Transplant Proc* 1989;21:300–310.

Toxicology of the Kidney, Second Edition,
edited by Jerry B. Hook and Robin S. Goldstein.
Raven Press, Ltd., New York © 1993.

13

Pathogenesis and Therapeutic Aspects of Radiocontrast-Induced Renal Dysfunction

George L. Bakris

Renal Division, University of Texas, Health Science Center, San Antonio, Texas 78284-7882

Various types of radiocontrast media have been used over the past 70 years for diagnostic visualization of various organs. A consequence of these agents, however, is radiocontrast-mediated nephropathy. Radiocontrast medium–induced nephropathy (renal failure) will be defined in this chapter as a significant increase in serum creatinine ($\geq$ 50% above baseline) within 48 hr after radiocontrast medium administration. If hemodialysis was ultimately required to manage certain patients, it is stated; otherwise, it must be assumed that this mode of therapy was not required.

Two separate studies document the fact that at least 10% of all cases of acute renal failure in the hospital setting are caused by radiographic studies involving the use of various radiocontrast media (1,2). Furthermore, the third most common cause of hospital acquired renal failure results from radiocontrast medium administration for various diagnostic studies (2). Thus, with the wide clinical use of these agents, insight into the mechanisms of renal dysfunction and possibly prophylactic measures to prevent renal failure in high-risk patients requiring radiocontrast studies is of paramount importance.

Numerous studies have been performed over the past few decades to examine the mechanisms that mediate radiocontrast medium–induced renal failure as well as possible prophylactic measures to ameliorate or prevent this problem. This chapter presents an overview of the history, risk factors, and mechanisms involved in renal dysfunction following administration of radiocontrast agents. It further focuses on both clinical and laboratory studies that compare the renal effects of ionic and nonionic radiocontrast agents. In addition, studies evaluating the possible prophylactic role of pharmacologic agents that have been shown to attenuate radiocontrast medium–induced declines in renal dysfunction will be discussed.

HISTORY

Radiocontrast agents were first used for *in vivo* angiographic studies in the early 1920s (3). The agents used during this period included strontium bromide, thorium dioxide, and sodium bromide. Although excellent radiocontrast agents, unfortunately both the strontium and thorium derivatives were associated with malignant diseases and prolonged radioactivity many years after their use (4,5). Organic diiodinated preparations were initially used during the early 1920s when Swick demonstrated that these compounds were reliable agents for intravenous urographic studies (5). These diiodinated agents were widely used until the mid-1950s when triiodinated compounds such as sodium diatrizoate were introduced. These triiodinated agents were found to be less toxic and more viscous than the diiodinated compounds.

The major chemical difference between the triiodinated radiocontrast agents and those previously used was the presence of three atoms of iodine per molecule as opposed to one or two. As a result of increasing the number of iodine atoms per compound, these triiodinated radiocontrast agents did not represent the ideal contrast agent, i.e., they were not water soluble, nor did they possess a low osmolarity. These highly osmotic agents, however, have been widely used over the past three decades, and consequently, implicated as a cause of renal failure (6–11).

Investigations toward less osmotic and less toxic radiocontrast agents have culminated with the development of the low osmolar (nonionic) radiocontrast agents. These agents are termed "nonionic" because an organic side chain has replaced the carboxyl group, and hence, these agents do not ionize in solution. They also differ from the ionic radiocontrast agents in the number of osmotic particles per iodine atom (roughly 50% less than ionic agents), which accounts for low osmolarity (5,12). The historic evolution of radiocontrast agents over the past 70 years is summarized in Table 1.

PHARMACOLOGY AND PHYSIOLOGY

The radiocontrast agents currently used in medical practice are the two, four, six triiodinated benzoic acid derivatives. This is true for both ionic and nonionic radio-

TABLE 1. *The evolution of clinically used radiocontrast media*

Agent	Year first used
Sodium iodide	1918[a], 1923
Strontium bromide	1923
Thorium dioxide	1923
Monoiodinated compounds	1929
Lopax and others	
Diiodinated compounds	Early 1930s
Diodrast, Skiodan, Diodon, and others	
Triiodinated compounds	Mid-1950s
Sodium diatrizoate, diatrizoate meglumine, etc.	
Low-osmolar (nonionic) compounds	Late 1970s, early 1980s
Metrizamide, iohexol, iopamidol and others	

[a]Initially suggested for use as radiocontrast agent.

contrast media. The major difference among these compounds lies in their divergent osmolarities and not in their iodine content or viscosity. A comparison among the various radiocontrast media is summarized in Table 2.

The most popular ionic compounds are the diatrizoate derivatives (13). These compounds are water soluble and have a low pK_a due to their carboxyl group. They exist as anions in biological systems, and hence, are only in the extracellular space (14). They are not significantly protein bound and are almost entirely (99%) renally excreted; the remaining 1% of their excretion is accounted for by gastrointestinal and biliary losses, which become more pronounced in renal failure (15,16).

Injection of radiocontrast agents results in a rapid equilibration across capillary membranes except for an intact blood-brain barrier. Radiocontrast medium can enter the cerebrospinal fluid, however, through the fenestrae in the choroid plexus (17). During the first phase of distribution following radiocontrast medium administration, there is a marked increase in intravascular osmolality causing a rapid fluid shift across capillary membranes toward the hypertonic (intravascular) compartment (13,18). Furthermore, the kinetics of radiocontrast medium distribution depend upon multiple factors including organ blood flow, capillary density and permeability, interstitial diffusion distances, and other factors (19,20). Thus, the distribution of infused ionic radiocontrast medium varies depending upon these factors (Fig. 1).

The acute change in serum osmolality induced by these agents, results in a number of vascular and peripheral, neurologically mediated phenomena. These include vasodilation, the sensation of heat and pain, and involuntary movements occasionally seen in patients that receive these agents. These effects may be mediated by adenosine or other local mediators that radiocontrast media are known to effect.

Triiodinated compounds are freely filtered by the glomerulus and neither secreted nor absorbed by the tubules (18). In other words, these agents are similar to inulin.

TABLE 2. *Physical properties of some radiocontrast agents*

	Osmolarity (mOsm/l)	Iodine (%)	Viscosity 37° ($M_pA.S$)
Ionic			
Iothalamate meglumine (Conray 60)	1,217	28	4.0
Sodium diatrizoate (Hypaque)[a]	1,470	30	2.5
Meglumine-sodium diatrizoate (Renografin 76)	1,690	37	9.1
Iothalamate-sodium (Conray 400)	1,965	40	4.5
Nonionic			
Iotrol[a]	300	30	9.1
Metrizamide	450	28	5.0
Iopamidol[a]	570	28	3.8
Iohexol	620	28	4.8

This is an abbreviated list adapted from refs. 5, 12, and 13. Name in parentheses is the tradename. Range of molecular weights for radiocontrast media mentioned above is 636 (diatrizoate) to 1626 (Iotrol).

[a]Most commonly used radiocontrast agents.

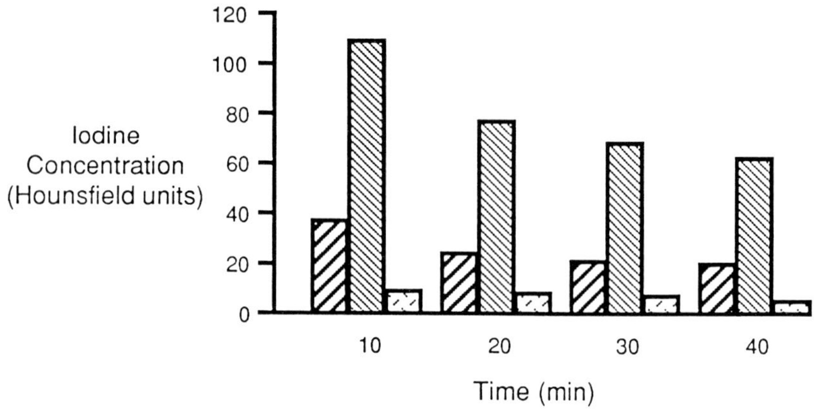

FIG. 1. The distribution to various tissues over time of an ionic radiocontrast medium (diatrizoate sodium). Note: 25 Hounsfield units equal 1 mg/ml. *Dark hatched bars*, liver; *light hatched bars*, kidney; *dotted bars*, muscle. (Adapted from Burgener and Hamlin, ref. 20.)

Thus, after bolus intravenous injection of various ionic radiocontrast media, an equilibration of these agents occurs in the extracellular space and simultaneous excretion by glomerular filtration ensues in subjects with normal kidneys. Once equilibration is achieved, the amount of contrast media entering the tubule is determined in large part by two factors: plasma concentration and glomerular filtration rate (14,18). In persons with normal renal function, the half-life of radiocontrast media is between 30 and 60 min (14,18). Furthermore, the peak time for excretion of radiocontrast media is about 3 min following intravenous injection. Peak urine iodine concentrations occur approximately 1 hr after radiocontrast medium administration (21–23).

Urine flow rates, as well, are increased with meglumine salts but not with sodium salts. This results in higher urinary concentrations of the sodium-associated radiocontrast media as compared to the meglumine derivatives (24). In fact, the initial concentration of radiocontrast medium in the tubule is the same as the plasma level. In the proximal tubule, as a result of sodium and water reabsorption, the concentration of radiocontrast medium increases five- to tenfold. This increased concentration may help explain, in part, enhanced toxicity to this portion of the renal tubule.

Proximal tubular sodium and water reabsorption is independent, however, of hydration and is influenced by diuretics and osmotic load (16,25). Furthermore, in states of dehydration, the concentration of a radiocontrast medium can be further increased in the collecting system secondary to the increased levels of antidiuretic hormone, which is increased in volume-depleted states. It is conceivable, therefore, that the concentration of a radiocontrast medium leaving the tubule may be up to 50 or 100 times that entering the tubule (16–25).

Radiocontrast agents are not protein bound, and possess relatively low molecular weights; thus, they are readily dialyzable. A number of studies have evaluated the dialyzability of both ionic and nonionic radiocontrast agents (26–30). These studies demonstrate that the mean half-life of radiocontrast agents is roughly doubled in dialysis patients when compared to normal subjects. Furthermore, the clearance of these agents by hemodialysis, at a blood flow between 172 and 250 ml per min varies from 65% to 80% following a 4-hr treatment. It is important to note, however, that between 25% and 36% of any given radiocontrast medium has already been eliminated by extrarenal routes (gastrointestinal and biliary systems) prior to institution of dialysis (28,30).

Unfortunately, no study, to date, has addressed the issue of the actual need for dialysis following a radiographic procedure in a renal failure patient. It is generally accepted clinical practice, however, for dialysis to follow immediately after a radiocontrast procedure to eliminate the hyperosmolar radiocontrast medium. The new lower osmolar agents, however, may not require this therapy and as has been stated, about one-third of any given radiocontrast medium has already been eliminated prior to initiation of dialysis. Until a prospective, randomized study is performed to assess the validity of hemodialysis following a procedure that utilizes a radiocontrast medium in renal failure subjects, the issue will remain unresolved.

The variability of renal vascular effects that follow injection of radiocontrast medium depend upon the dosage and route of administration (14,18). Figure 2 demonstrates the time course and variability in renal vascular responsiveness be-

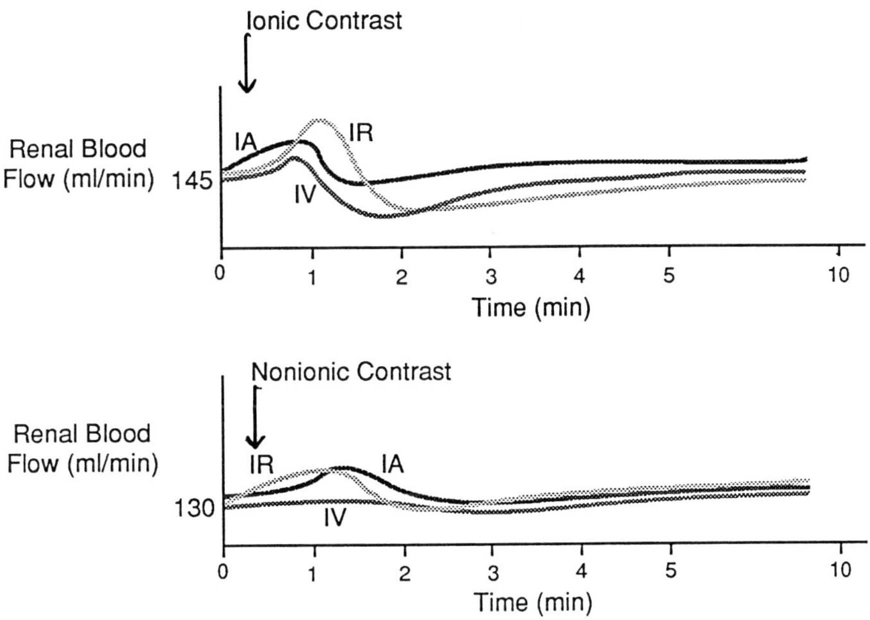

FIG. 2. The renal vascular effects of an ionic (sodium diatrizoate) and nonionic (iopamidol) radiocontrast medium in the normal dog. Note: Results obtained from two separate dogs in the author's laboratory. IA, intraarterial; IR, intrarenal; IV, intravenous.

tween an intrarenal, intraarterial (thoracic aorta), and intravenous bolus injection of an ionic and nonionic radiocontrast medium in the normal dog. These observations on renal vascular effects of radiocontrast media from my laboratory are also supported by other investigators (31–33). As can be noted, administration of radiocontrast medium characteristically gives a biphasic renal blood flow response. There is an initial transient vasodilation followed by a more sustained vasoconstrictor response that persists for up to 10 min. The mechanisms for these renal hemodynamic changes will be discussed later in this chapter.

In addition to the renal vascular changes, changes in peripheral arterial flows are also dependent upon the osmotic concentration of the radiocontrast medium utilized. Figure 3 demonstrates the contrasting effects in the femoral and renal circulations following administration of either a high- or low-osmolar radiocontrast agent. Clearly, less dramatic renal hemodynamic and peripheral arterial effects are seen with nonionic (low osmolar) radiocontrast agents.

MECHANISMS OF NEPHROTOXICITY

Nephrotoxicity secondary to radiocontrast agents can be broadly grouped under two categories: renal hemodynamic alterations and tubular injury. An overall schematic representation of the changes in these parameters and their consequences following high-osmolar radiocontrast medium administration are summarized in Fig. 4. It can be seen from this figure that the principal factor that leads to both these changes is the high osmotic properties of radiocontrast agents (33–35).

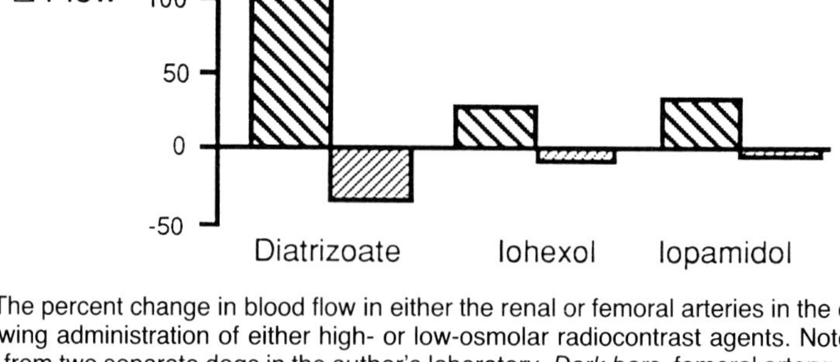

FIG. 3. The percent change in blood flow in either the renal or femoral arteries in the euvolemic dog following administration of either high- or low-osmolar radiocontrast agents. Note: Results obtained from two separate dogs in the author's laboratory. *Dark bars*, femoral artery; *light bars*, renal artery.

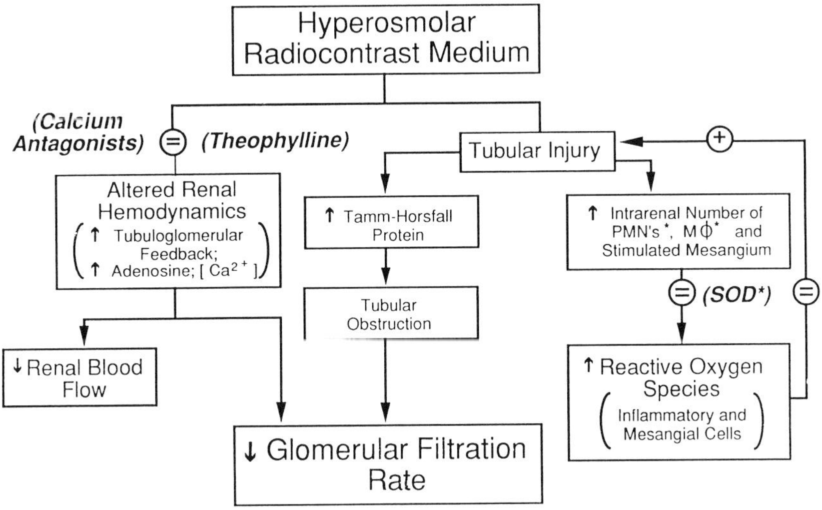

FIG. 4. A proposed model of the mechanisms involved in radiocontrast medium–induced renal dysfunction. SOD, superoxide dismutase; PMN, polymorphonuclear leukocytes; Mϕ, macrophages; ⊜ , inhibits; ⊕ , potentiates; *SOD does not affect renal hemodynamic response to contrast medium but preserves GFR.

A number of studies have evaluated the possible mechanisms for the renal hemodynamic alterations that follow radiocontrast medium administration in both animal models as well as man (14,36–43). These studies demonstrate that renal arterial injection of a high-osmolar radiocontrast agent, or hypertonic saline, results in a biphasic response in renal blood flow characterized by a transient increase followed by a prolonged decrease. This decrease in renal blood flow is approximately 30% to 40% and correlates positively with the osmolality of the solution injected (35,36,44,45). These changes in renal blood flow can be appreciated by a review of Fig. 2.

High-osmolar radiocontrast media also lead to direct tubular and cellular injury. A number of *in vitro* studies have evaluated the relative effects of high-osmotic radiocontrast agents as well as mannitol on proximal tubular cell integrity and metabolism (46,47). These studies clearly demonstrate that administration of high-osmolar radiocontrast agents results in total cellular disintegration within the period of a few minutes. Furthermore, recent observations demonstrate that when the low-osmolar radiocontrast agent iopamidol is administered to human mesangial cells, only relatively minor changes in cellular integrity occur (unpublished observation). This cellular preservation is also true of proximal tubular cells exposed to nonionic radiocontrast medium (48).

The remaining discussion in this section will focus on specific factors implicated in both altered renal hemodynamics and tubular injury that have been associated with radiocontrast medium injury.

Calcium

A number of studies have investigated various aspects of renal hemodynamics with regard to the vasoconstrictor response following radiocontrast medium administration (31–42). These studies attempted to ablate the vasoconstrictor response associated with radiocontrast medium injection by utilizing various methods including inhibition of the renin-angiotensin system, α-adrenergic antagonists, vasodilators, as well as vasodilating prostaglandins, none of which attenuated this vascular effect. The first study to demonstrate almost total elimination of this vasoconstrictor response following radiocontrast medium injection was performed in 1984. Studies infusing various low-dose calcium antagonists and a calcium chelator into the renal artery of a euvolemic dog resulted in obliteration of the vasoconstrictor response to intrarenal injection of an ionic radiocontrast medium (39). These studies were later corroborated by a group of French investigators (40). The clinical importance of this observation has been demonstrated in clinical studies utilizing various calcium antagonists to prevent the renal hemodynamic changes that follow radiocontrast medium injection. These studies will be discussed in the prophylaxis section of the chapter.

In addition to inhibiting calcium entry into cells and blocking vasoconstriction, calcium antagonists also inhibit inherent renal autoregulatory mechanisms, i.e., tubuloglomerular feedback and afferent arteriolar "myogenic" response (49–51). Radiocontrast medium, by delivering a large osmotic load to the macula densa in the area of the distal tubule, results in stimulation of the tubuloglomerular feedback processes, and hence, reduces glomerular filtration rate. Calcium antagonists, in addition to a direct vascular effect, have been generally shown to inhibit this feedback process (49–51). Hence, these agents would attenuate any decreases in glomerular filtration rate seen after radiocontrast injection. No published studies, however, are available that specifically examine this autoregulatory process with regard to radiocontrast agents.

The effects of hypertonic saline and other hypertonic solutions have been examined with regard to this autoregulatory process. These studies provide support for the hypothesis that hyperosmolar radiocontrast agents would stimulate the tubuloglomerular feedback mechanism, and hence, reduce glomerular filtration rate (44). Thus, hyperosmotic radiocontrast agents may be postulated to increase tubuloglomerular feedback and in this way lead to vasoconstriction and decreases in glomerular filtration rate. Calcium antagonists or calcium chelators inhibit this response and thus attenuate drops in renal blood flow and glomerular filtration rate following administration of contrast agents. It should also be noted that all studies mentioned in this section were performed in normal animal models, and hence, cannot necessarily be extrapolated to pathophysiological states.

Adenosine

Adenosine is a well-known vasodilator in the peripheral circulation; however, in the renal cortex it has clearly been shown to be a vasoconstrictor (52–55). Given the hypothesis that the renal hemodynamic response to adenosine infusion is similar to that seen during the vasoconstrictor and recovery phase following radiocontrast medium injection, we undertook studies to evaluate the role of adenosine with regard to its effect on the renal vasoconstrictor response following intrarenal ionic radiocontrast medium injection (38,55). Studies were performed in four groups of normal dogs utilizing the adenosine antagonist, theophylline, and the adenosine potentiator, dipyridamole (38). Doses of these agents were infused so as not to effect renal blood flow or arterial pressures. The results of our studies clearly demonstrate that adenosine has a role in mediating the vasoconstrictor response associated with radiocontrast medium administration. These studies were recently corroborated by a group of French investigators who found similar renal hemodynamic effects in the presence of theophylline following radiocontrast medium administration (40).

Adenosine has also been shown to play a critical role in maintenance of renal autoregulatory responses, specifically tubuloglomerular feedback (52,55). Specifically, inhibition of adenosine has been shown to attenuate the tubuloglomerular feedback mechanism (52,53). Thus, the renal hemodynamic alterations (vasoconstriction) seen following radiocontrast medium injection may be secondary to either an increase in renal adenosine concentration, consequently stimulating tubuloglomerular feedback, or a direct effect of adenosine on the renal vasculature. Thus, adenosine appears to play an important role in altering renal hemodynamics following injection of ionic radiocontrast medium. The need for additional studies to evaluate the effects of both ionic and nonionic radiocontrast agents on the tubuloglomerular feedback mechanism as well as the interaction with adenosine is obvious.

Reactive Oxygen Species

Reactive oxygen species include the superoxide anion, hydrogen peroxide, hydroxyl radical, and singlet oxygen. A number of reviews have been written on the renal effects of these species, which have very short half-lives and yet are implicated in contributing to renal demise under various experimental conditions, e.g., ischemic acute renal failure, acute glomerulonephritis, and toxic renal diseases (56–58).

Reactive oxygen species are released by a variety of different cells including polymorphonuclear leukocytes, macrophages, and the glomerular mesangium (56, 58,59). These reactive oxygen species help in primarily destroying and phagocytosing bacteria and other invasive organisms in biological systems. Their production can be inhibited by glucocorticoids, and specific scavengers such as superoxide dismutase, glutathione, and dimethyl sulfoxide (56–61).

In vitro investigations utilizing electron spin resonance techniques demonstrate that administration of an ionic radiocontrast medium (diatrizoate sodium) to human mesangial cells increases production of reactive oxygen species (Fig. 5; unpublished observation). The reactive oxygen species produced by radiocontrast medium include both superoxide and hydroxyl radical species, which can be suppressed with superoxide dismutase and dimethyl sulfoxide, respectively (56–58).

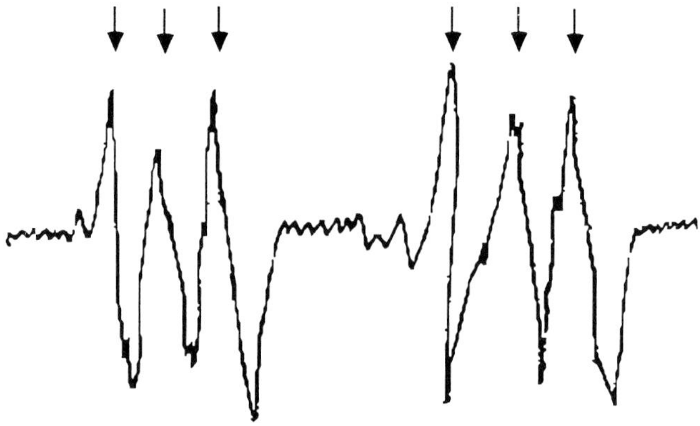

FIG. 5. The electron spin resonance spectra following administration of an ionic radiocontrast medium (sodium diatrizoate) administered to human mesangial cells and the resultant generation of reactive oxygen species measured by electron spin resonance. *Arrows* indicate generation of reactive oxygen species. (Methodology adapted from Baud et al., ref. 59.)

We performed studies in normal, mildly volume-depleted dogs to evaluate the role of reactive oxygen species in contributing to the decline in renal hemodynamics following intrarenal ionic radiocontrast medium administration (41). These studies demonstrated that the oxygen free radical scavenger, superoxide dismutase, inhibited the fall in glomerular filtration rate but had no effect on renal blood flow. In addition, renal biopsies performed within 2 hr of intrarenal radiocontrast medium administration confirm a large influx of polymorphonuclear leukocytes and macrophages in both the glomerular and tubular areas (unpublished observations). Thus, we hypothesized that these cells, in addition to mesangial cells, release oxygen free radicals and actually potentiate the tubular injury initially induced by the hyperosmotic properties of radiocontrast agents (Fig. 4).

Recent studies in the rat provide further evidence to support these findings. Yoshioka et al. (62) found that the cellular content of superoxide dismutase was much lower in volume-depleted rats when compared with euvolemic animals. Furthermore, the volume-depleted group showed the greatest declines in glomerular filtration rate following ionic radiocontrast administration. Thus, reactive oxygen species are to play a role in contributing to tubular toxicity following ionic radiocontrast medium administration. The potential clinical benefit of free radical scavengers, however, has not been shown in any clinical trial.

Tamm-Horsfall Protein

Tamm-Horsfall protein is a large glycoprotein normally found only in the ascending limb of the loop of Henle extending into the very early portion of the distal tubule (63). This protein is released following tubular destruction to this area of the nephron and forms the matrix of urinary casts (63,64). The solubility of the Tamm-Horsfall protein in the urine depends on the pH, salt concentration, and concentration of proteins in the urine as well as other factors (63).

A number of studies have demonstrated increases in urinary levels of Tamm-Horsfall protein following ionic radiocontrast medium administration (63–66). Given the available evidence that reactive oxygen species are generated, intrarenally, following radiocontrast medium injection, and that these reactive oxygen species may be implicated in tubular injury, we undertook a series of experiments to evaluate the role of reactive oxygen species in contributing to increases in urinary Tamm-Horsfall protein following hyperosmolar radiocontrast medium administration (67). Studies conducted in normal, mildly volume-depleted dogs demonstrate that inhibition of oxygen free radicals with superoxide dismutase clearly attenuate the release of Tamm-Horsfall protein and ameliorate declines in glomerular filtration rate following hyperosmolar radiocontrast medium administration (Fig. 6). In addition to this finding, we observed a much lower quantity of urinary casts, following radiocontrast medium injection, in those kidneys that received superoxide dismutase (unpublished observation).

Preliminary studies in euvolemic dogs ($n=3$) that received intrarenal injections of the nonionic, low-osmolar radiocontrast agent iopamidol demonstrate a much smaller increase in urinary Tamm-Horsfall protein excretion as well as reactive oxygen species generation when compared to hyperosmolar radiocontrast agents (unpublished observation). Furthermore, there were relatively smaller declines in renal blood flow and glomerular filtration rate with the low-osmolar agents. Thus,

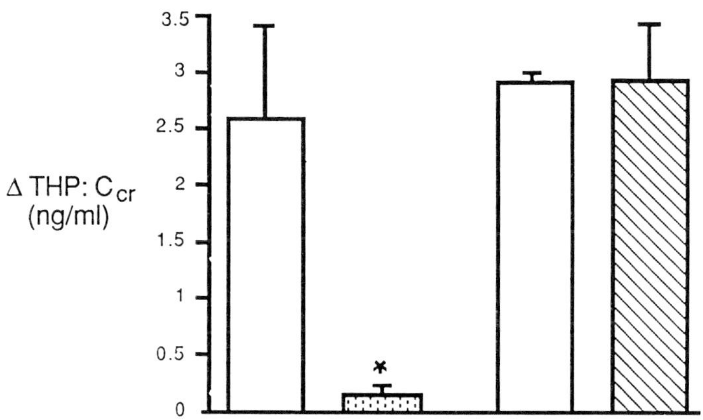

FIG. 6. The effects of an intrarenal injection of the ionic radiocontrast medium (sodium diatrizoate) on urinary Tamm-Horsfall protein (THP). Data expressed as mean ± SEM and represent change in ratio of Tamm-Horsfall protein to creatinine clearance (C_{cr}). *$p<.05$ compared with baseline. *Open bars*, baseline; *dotted bars*, superoxide dismutase; *light crosshatch bars*, heat inactivated superoxide dismutase.

reactive oxygen species appear to play a role in tubular injury and subsequent release of Tamm-Horsfall protein into the urine. The clinical implications of these findings have not yet been explored. The clinical relevance of these findings, however, must be viewed with some skepticism since these studies were performed in dogs with normal renal function and no preexisting renal disease.

Renal Metabolism

Numerous studies have investigated the effects of high- and low-osmolar radiocontrast agents on cellular enzyme activity, prostaglandin production, sodium-potassium–adenosine triphosphatase (Na-K–ATPase) activity and renal oxygen metabolism (68–83). In general, the enzymatic studies indicate that there is no reliable urinary enzymatic indicator of radiocontrast medium injury with the possible exception of the proximal tubular enzymes alanine aminopeptidase and γ-glutamyl transpeptidase (69). These two enzymes were found in significantly higher concentrations in the urine of patients as early as 24 hr following nonionic radiocontrast medium studies. Interestingly, these enzymes were elevated in the absence of any significant increase in serum creatinine. Furthermore, this trend was present with both ionic (diatrizoate) and nonionic (iohexol) contrast agents. Unfortunately, these studies did not provide follow-up data ($>$ 72 hr post–radiocontrast medium administration) to assess the clinical predictability of these enzyme markers on development of renal dysfunction.

Although Na-K–ATPase activity is clearly inhibited by hyperosmolar radiocontrast agents (70–72), the mechanism for this inhibition is unclear. However, data from our laboratory suggests that oxygen free radical generation that follows radiocontrast medium injection may play a role. Two separate investigators document depression of Na-K–ATPase activity in both the heart and ischemic kidney associated with increased oxygen free radical generation (75,76). We performed *in vitro* studies on canine renal slices and measured both Na-K–ATPase activity as well as mitochondrial ATPase activity after exposure to either ionic (diatrizoate sodium) or nonionic (iohexol) radiocontrast medium in the presence and absence of superoxide dismutase. We found a significant reduction in ouabain-sensitive Na-K–ATPase but not mitochondrial ATPase (Fig. 7, unpublished observations). Furthermore, this reduction in Na-K–ATPase activity was attenuated in the presence of superoxide dismutase.

The clinical correlation of these cellular studies demonstrating a decrease in Na-K–ATPase activity was also noted in our dog studies. Natriuresis following radiocontrast medium administration (diatrizoate sodium) in the dogs that received superoxide dismutase was comparatively less than controls (41). Thus, it appears that the mechanism of Na-K–ATPase inhibition associated with radiocontrast medium may be related to the ability of radiocontrast agents to generate reactive oxygen species.

The effects of radiocontrast medium as well as other hypoxic factors on medullary thick ascending limb of Henle's loop have been evaluated (77–80). In a uni-

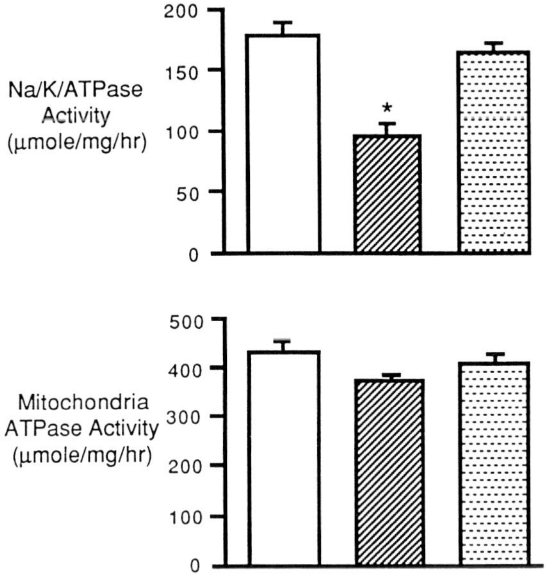

FIG. 7. The effects of ionic radiocontrast medium (diatrizoate sodium) on Na-K–ATPase and mitochondrial ATPase activity in normal dog kidney. *p<.05 compared with baseline. *Open bars*, baseline; *dark crosshatched (middle) bars*, contrast medium alone; *dotted bars*, contrast medium with superoxide dismutase.

laterally nephrectomized rat model that was treated with indomethacin and given an ionic radiocontrast medium (iothalamate), a significant fall was noted in creatinine clearance after 24 hr (79). In addition, histologic studies in this model demonstrate that the loop of Henle had the greatest amount of histologic injury. Thus, these and other investigators have speculated that the loop of Henle, because of its very poor oxygen supply, is the most susceptible area of the nephron to hypoxic injury following ionic radiocontrast medium injection (77,79,80). Interestingly, *in vitro* studies that have evaluated factors that diminished tubular work (inhibition of Na-K–ATPase activity, etc.) demonstrate a relative protective effect against medullary hypoxic injury (70–72,77,78). Thus, paradoxically, ionic radiocontrast medium has both a direct tubular toxic effect as well as an inhibitory effect on Na-K–ATPase activity. In this way, its effect on Na-K–ATPase activity may help partially counterbalance its toxic tubular effects.

Lastly, numerous studies have evaluated the modulatory role of prostaglandins of the E series on renal hemodynamics following radiocontrast medium administration (78,80–83). Prostaglandin E_2 has been shown to prevent hypoxic injury to the medullary area of the kidney by inhibiting oxygen consumption (78). Further studies in normal dogs, however, demonstrate that prostaglandin inhibition does not result in radiocontrast medium–induced renal dysfunction regardless of the osmotic content of the agent used (82,83). Prostaglandin inhibition in rabbits with a decreased renal mass, however, clearly demonstrates a potentiation in the vasoconstrictor response that follows radiocontrast medium injection (81). Thus studies evaluating the effects of various radiocontrast agents on renal physiology need to be performed in pathophysiologically relevant models to attain clinical meaningfulness.

MODELS OF CONTRAST NEPHROPATHY

Evaluation of the renal toxic and hemodynamic effects of radiocontrast agents has been largely performed in normal dogs, rabbits, or rats. Thus, any assertions from these studies to renal hemodynamic alterations in pathophysiological states (i.e., congestive heart failure, diabetic nephropathy, cirrhosis) is, at best, speculative. To date, only one clinically relevant animal model has been developed to investigate the renal hemodynamic effects of radiocontrast agents. This dog model was also used to study possible prophylactic measures that would prevent detrimental renal hemodynamic changes following radiocontrast medium administration.

Margulies and (42) coworkers evaluated the renal hemodynamic effects of the radiocontrast medium Vascoray in dogs with congestive heart failure. Congestive heart failure was induced after 8 days of pacing the dogs at a ventricular rate of 250 beats per min. Radiocontrast medium was given as an intravenous infusion in the presence and absence of an infusion of atrial natriuretic factor. This study demonstrates that an intravenous infusion of radiocontrast medium in the setting of heart failure results in a significant and more persistent decline in creatinine clearance than under normal circumstances. These investigators noted that the decline in renal function occurred only in the group of dogs with congestive heart failure and that this decline was attenuated by atrial natriuretic factor infusion. Please note that this study utilized an infusion rather than a bolus injection of radiocontrast medium. Based on previous studies, the decline in renal function would be predicted to be greater if a bolus injection had been given (18,20). Thus, to date, this is the only published pathophysiological model in the dog that allows for study of altered renal hemodynamics following radiocontrast medium administration. Additional studies in man by the same investigators noted that intraarterial infusion of atrial natriuretic peptide attenuated declines in renal hemodynamics that follow arteriography (84).

Another model of contrast nephropathy is described in the rabbit by Vari and coworkers (81), who attempt to explain the mechanisms involved in renal dysfunction following hyperosmolar radiocontrast medium injections. They utilize a 1–⅚ nephrectomized rabbit model that has received large doses of nonsteroidal anti-inflammatory agents followed by large bolus injections of hyperosmolar radiocontrast medium. This model has potential usefulness in the investigation of renal hemodynamics; however, no therapeutic interventions were performed to assess "protection" from radiocontrast medium-induced renal dysfunction. It does focus directly on the pathophysiology of end-stage renal disease and the possible protective physiological mechanisms involved in maintaining renal hemodynamics following radiocontrast medium injection. Thus, this study is insightful with regard to the mechanisms of radiocontrast medium–induced nephropathy in end-stage renal disease. Unfortunately, it is known that patients with significant preexisting renal dysfunction are at much higher risk for exacerbation of this problem following radiocontrast medium administration. Thus, the use of therapeutic intervention would have been appropriate in this study.

Finally, a number of studies in a variety of rat models have been performed under various conditions including administration of radiocontrast medium following dehydration, nonsteroidal anti-inflammatory agents, and 1–$\frac{5}{6}$ renal ablation (77, 78,80). Unfortunately, the rat is particularly refractory to renal hemodynamic changes following large doses of ionic radiocontrast agents. Furthermore, some of the studies reported using this model are difficult, if not impossible, to reproduce (R. Vari, unpublished observations). Hence, with the exception of the congestive heart failure model in the dog, and possibly the renal failure model in the rabbit, there are no meaningful pathophysiological animal models by which to study the possible ameliorative effects of various therapeutic agents on renal hemodynamics that portend injection of radiocontrast medium.

RISK FACTORS

It is difficult to arrive at an actual incidence of contrast-associated renal dysfunction or failure. This is largely due to varying definitions among the various studies. A number of studies investigating the incidence of renal failure following either venous or angiographic procedures report values anywhere from 0% to 0.5% in a random population to 92% in a high risk population, e.g., patients with diabetes or heart failure with and without renal insufficiency (1,2,6,7,11,84–139). A review of these studies illustrates the importance of uniform definitions and clear identification of patient populations in order to meaningfully compare one study with another.

In a classic study by Byrd and Sherman, a number of clinical risk factors were outlined to define patients who are at risk of developing radiocontrast medium–induced nephrotoxicity (9). From this study, subjects with advanced age, prior renal insufficiency (serum creatinine > 1.6 mg/dl), dehydration, and hyperuricemia all had a greater than 50% risk for developing contrast nephropathy. Multiple-contrast exposure within 24 hr or diabetes mellitus had a 33% or 37% risk, respectively. Over the past decade, a number of well-done retrospective and prospective studies have evaluated some of these risk factors in patients undergoing arteriographic studies (84–114,138,139). In addition, some studies have compared the possible differences between ionic and nonionic radiocontrast medium administration on renal function in patients with these and other risk factors (102–107,109,112, 114,116).

A recent study by Parfrey et al. (99) documents that the population at highest risk for developing radiocontrast medium–induced nephrotoxicity following angiographic study were diabetic patients with renal insufficiency (100). These investigators found that given equal hydration status, neither diabetes nor renal insufficiency alone, although yielding a somewhat higher risk for renal failure than the normal population, resulted in a statistically greater incidence of renal dysfunction following radiocontrast medium injection than did the normal population. This and other studies clearly support the notion that adverse renal effects following radiocontrast medium administration largely depend upon the underlying disease state and preexisting renal function prior to radiocontrast injection rather than other factors. Thus, if previous studies documenting various risk factors were viewed in this light, it becomes clear that the current state of renal function in a given patient along with other concomitant diseases known to affect renal function (heart failure, diabetes, cirrhosis, etc.) would clearly result in a higher risk for renal failure following any radiocontrast medium administration.

A number of both venous and angiographic studies in populations with various risk factors have been performed to evaluate the effects of hyperosmolar and low-osmolar radiocontrast agents (7,100–140). It is clear that diabetics with moderate renal impairment are at the highest risk for radiocontrast medium–induced renal failure (9,97,98,100,102–104,123,124,126,128,130,133). Numerous *in vitro* and *in vivo* studies demonstrate that low-osmolar radiocontrast agents result in less dramatic renal hemodynamic changes and preserve cellular integrity better than high-osmotic agents (Fig. 2) (46,48,82,85,137,138–140). It is noteworthy, however, that recent prospective clinical studies fail to show a difference in the incidence of radiocontrast medium–induced renal failure in these high-risk populations (100–104). Furthermore, a summary of 14 angiographic studies comparing high- versus low-osmolar radiocontrast agents on renal function document no consistent benefit with low-osmolar radiocontrast agents (105–116,119,120). A large, prospective double-blind trial involving 26 medical centers throughout the country has just been completed comparing the effects of a high- versus low-osmolar radiocontrast agents in patients undergoing coronary angiography. The risk factors studied included renal insufficiency and/or diabetes. The data from this study, however, are not available at this time and will be of critical importance in assessing whether low-osmolar contrast media attenuate declines in renal function when compared to high-osmolar agents.

PROPHYLAXIS

A number of both retrospective and prospective studies have evaluated various therapeutic maneuvers in an attempt to attenuate the decline in renal function following administration of various radiocontrast media. These include administration of loop diuretics at various times periods throughout the contrast study; administration of osmotic diuretics, e.g., mannitol, as well as the combination of mannitol and a loop diuretic prior to and during the contrast study; and finally, administration of various calcium antagonists prior to radiocontrast administration (2,125,141–150). Unfortunately, many of these attempts at prophylaxis have been less than satisfying.

Since dehydration has been touted as a risk factor, saline infusions have an appealing rationale in minimizing radiocontrast-associated nephropathy. This notion is largely a result of many retrospective studies that have shown an association between radiocontrast-induced renal dysfunction in volume-depleted subjects (9,127, 151,152). Three subsequent prospective studies, however, fail to support this association (86,87,94). Saline infusion (0.9%) has been shown, however, in a prospective study to prevent renal failure following angiography when administered at a rate of 550 ml/hr during the procedure (144). Interestingly, these same investigators reported 1 year earlier that dehydration was *not* a risk factor for renal dysfunction. Furthermore, closer scrutiny of their previous study did not reveal aggressive hydration to the degree noted previously. Furthermore, in dehydrated states, both the renal blood flow and glomerular filtration rates are decreased; therefore, overall duration of tubular exposure to radiocontrast medium will be increased and hence increase the probability of tubular injury (18,20). Thus, although in some prospective studies dehydration has not been found to be a risk factor for contrast nephropathy, the majority of studies, prospective as well as retrospective, support its candidacy as a risk factor.

A number of studies have evaluated the effects of furosemide as well as mannitol at various time periods before, during, and after angiographic studies. Mannitol has been shown to prevent ischemic renal failure in the dog and maintains glomerular filtration rate during controlled renal hypoperfusion studies in rat models (145,146). In a study of Old et al. (142), an infusion of 500 ml of 5% mannitol prevented contrast-induced declines in renal function in six patients with renal insufficiency (mean baseline serum creatinine 2.5 mg/dl). A comparable group of five patients not receiving mannitol experienced a significant increase in serum creatinine from 2.3 to 3.7 mg/dl following exposure to the ionic radiocontrast agent. In the largest study published to date, 37 patients all with chronic renal insufficiency were given 1,500 ml of one-half normal saline and then 250 ml of 20% mannitol within 60 min of the procedure (125). Eight of the 37 patients had significant increases in serum creatinine. The authors concluded that mannitol offered protection because a similar group of 40 patients who did not receive this therapy experienced a 70% incidence of renal failure. Similar studies by Shafi et al. (129) demonstrate similar findings. These and other studies support the notion that mannitol is useful in preventing acute renal failure following radiocontrast medium administration.

This questionable renal per serving effect of mannitol may be related to systemic increases in atrial natriuretic peptide. A recent study in patients documents significant increases in plasma atrial natriuretic peptide levels during mannitol infusion. This increase correlated with an increase in renal blood flow (143). Unfortunately, an inhibitor of atrial peptide was not given to fully assess this possible mechanism on renal function.

A problem may develop, however, with the use of mannitol for this prophylactic indication if not closely monitored. Mannitol is generally given prior to a radiographic procedure; however, if the procedure is delayed and mannitol infusion not stopped, a diuresis would ensue prior to angiographic study and the patient could conceivably be relatively dehydrated at the start of the procedure. Hence, the patient's risk for nephropathy may potentially be increased secondary to dehydration.

Thus, it is my feeling, based on these studies, that mannitol is a useful prophylactic agent if used appropriately and the timing is carefully scrutinized so that the radiocontrast medium is given at the time of maximal sustained diuresis.

A number of studies have used intravenous furosemide alone and in combination with mannitol for prophylaxis against radiocontrast induced nephropathy. Porush et al. (140) evaluated 17 patients with an average serum creatinine of 3.8 who were to receive intravenous radiocontrast studies. These patients received intravenous furosemide in a milligram dose that was equal to 4,000 divided by the creatinine clearance. Furosemide was administered 1 hr prior to the intravenous contrast procedure. Urine output was replaced for 20 hr with half normal saline during this study. Another study by Beroniade (2) using furosemide to initiate and maintain diuresis of 300 cc per hr with replacement of urine with half normal saline and 20 mEq of potassium chloride also showed a significant decrease in the incidence of contrast-induced renal injury. In a small, prospective, randomized study 15 patients were given either furosemide with hydration, using a similar dosing formula to that of Porush and colleagues, or hydration alone prior to ionic radiocontrast medium administration. Data from these patients support prior observations that furosemide administration results in a significant attenuation in the rise of serum creatinine following angiographic studies (unpublished observations). Thus, furosemide with maintenance of good urine output clearly has a role as a prophylactic agent when given prior to injection of radiocontrast medium.

Recently, two separate clinical studies evaluating the prophylactic effects of calcium antagonists on radiocontrast-induced decreases in renal function were performed. These studies were based on the initial observation made in 1985 that calcium antagonists obliterate decreases in renal blood flow and glomerular filtration rate following intrarenal radiocontrast medium administration (39). In one study by Russo et al. (149) 30 male patients undergoing intravenous pyelography for hematuria and proteinuria were investigated. This study evaluated not only the possible prophylactic effects of calcium antagonists but also compared high- versus low-osmotic radiocontrast media. Radiocontrast medium was infused and the calcium antagonist nifedipine was chosen for use only in the group that received a hyperosmolar radiocontrast agent. Ten patients received nifedipine along with the hyperosmolar radiocontrast medium, diatrizoate meglumine. Nifedipine, 10 mg, was given sublingually 5 min before the hyperosmolar radiocontrast agent was injected. The results demonstrate that nifedipine significantly increased glomerular filtration rate and renal plasma flow as early as 1 hr following the procedure. These increases in renal hemodynamics were statistically significant when compared with controls. Unfortunately, this study did not follow patients long-term, i.e., 24 to 48 hr following the procedure to evaluate if any longer-term changes had occurred.

Neumayer et al. (150), in a separate study, also demonstrated a prophylactic effect of the calcium antagonist nitrendipine. These investigators in a prospective, randomized, double-blind clinical trial investigated 35 patients after various intravascular radiocontrast studies including renal arteriography, intravenous pyelography, etc. They evaluated the effect of nitrendipine on renal hemodynamics as well as the nonionic radiocontrast medium iopamidol. These investigators followed patients for 48 hr and evaluated urinary enzyme activity as well as renal hemodynamics. The results demonstrate a clear attenuation in the fall of glomerular filtration rate in the nitrendipine group with a return to baseline glomerular filtration rate after 48 hr; this was not true in the control group, which had a persistent 20% decline in glomerular filtration rate in the 48 hr following radiocontrast administration. Interestingly, urinary protein excretion also increased in the control group receiving radiocontrast medium and did not increase in the nitrendipine group. However, the baseline levels of urinary protein excretion in the nitrendipine group were roughly 2½ times that of the control group. This is in keeping with previous studies documenting that the dihydropyridine compounds increase proteinuria in various pathophysiological states such as diabetes (153). Thus, calcium antagonists may have an important role in attenuating declines in renal hemodynamics following either high- or low-osmolar radiocontrast media.

A number of low-osmolar radiocontrast media are available for clinical use, all with variable effects on renal hemodynamics and function, depending upon the study reviewed. The majority of prospective studies regarding the cardiac effects of low-osmolar radiocontrast media, however, suggest that they are clearly beneficial, as they result in fewer arrhythmias, less hypotension, and less interaction with calcium antagonists (154–159).

The available data on the relative renal toxic effects of these agents, however, are disparate. The majority of clinical studies, as reported earlier in this chapter, do not support a less-toxic effect of the low-osmolar agents for reducing the risk of renal failure in high-risk populations, e.g., diabetic patients with renal insufficiency. In fact, recent studies in high-risk populations that carefully examine glomerular filtration rate clearly show similar decreases with both low- and high-osmolar radiocontrast agents (100–102,104,150). Furthermore, an evaluation of the cost-benefit ratio between low- and high-osmolar agents does not appear to justify the increased cost in the population at high risk for renal dysfunction (160).

Patients with severe renal dysfunction should have an adjustment in the dose of radiocontrast medium administered. A recent paper by Cigarroa and coworkers (161) provides guidelines for dosing of radiocontrast media to reduce the risk of contrast nephropathy in patients with renal disease. These investigators clearly show, in a group of diabetic patients, that appropriate dose reductions of radiocontrast medium can certainly prevent significant increases in radiocontrast-induced renal dysfunction. The formula suggested is as follows:

$$\text{Radiocontrast medium limit} = \frac{\text{5 ml contrast/kg (max = 300 ml)}}{\text{serum creatinine (mg/dl)}}$$

A summary of all recommended prophylactic procedures for prevention of renal function following radiocontrast medium injection are noted in Table 3.

TABLE 3. *Summary of recommended prophylaxis for intervention against radiocontrast medium–induced renal dysfunction*[a]

Hydration (9,126,140,147,148)
Furosemide (2,84,138)
Mannitol (124,128,139,141,142)
Calcium antagonists (145,146)
Nonionic contrast medium (101,102,104,111,137)

[a]Note also that use of minimal contrast volume, avoidance of repeated contrast injections, and discontinuance of prostaglandin antagonists, all have at least theoretical rationale for minimizing exacerbation of preexisting renal dysfunction following radiocontrast injections (84).

SUMMARY

Patients with preexisting renal insufficiency and diabetes, heart failure, or other conditions affecting renal hemodynamics are clearly at very high risk for radiocontrast-induced renal dysfunction. Furthermore, there is no single study that shows total protection from radiocontrast-induced renal dysfunction regardless of the osmotic concentration of the radiocontrast medium used or other prophylactic interventions employed. However, a number of studies in these high-risk patients support the concept that adequate hydration along with either a calcium antagonist and/or furosemide attenuate the rise in serum creatinine and in this way eliminate the need for dialysis in a very large group of these high-risk patients. At this writing, I do not feel there are enough data to support the use of the very expensive low-osmolar agents to preserve renal function alone (159). However, in these high-risk patients, if prevention of cardiac arrhythmias and/or dysfunction (clearly associated with high-osmolar contrast media) is an issue, then clearly the lower-osmotic agents should be used (159).

ACKNOWLEDGMENT

We would like to thank Mrs. Peggy Bourque for her excellent and diligent work on this chapter.

REFERENCES

1. Hou SH, Bushinsky DA, Wish JB, et al. Hospital-acquired renal insufficiency: a prospective study. *Am J Med* 1983;74:243–256.
2. Beroniade VC. Prevention of acute renal failure secondary to radiocontrast agents. In: *Abstracts to the Eighth International Congress of Nephrology*. Athens: University Studio Publishing, 1981;380.
3. Osborne ED, Sutherland CG, Scholl AJ, et al. Roentgenography or urinary tract during excretion of sodium iodide. *JAMA* 1923;80:368–372.
4. Silpananta P, Illescas FF, Sheldon H. Multiple malignant neoplasms 40 years after angiography with Thorotrast. *Can Med Assoc J* 1983;128:289–294.

5. Sutton D. Arteriography and therapeutic angiography. In: Sutton D, ed. *Textbook of radiology and imaging*, 4th ed, vol 2. Edinburgh: Churchill-Livingstone, 1987;692–699.
6. Alexander RD, Berkes SL, Abuelo G. Contrast media induced oliguric renal failure. *Arch Intern Med* 1978;138:381–384.
7. Ansari Z, Baldwin DS. Acute renal failure due to radiocontrast agents. *Nephron* 1976;17:28–40.
8. Bartley O, Bengtsson U, Cedarbon G. Renal function before and after angiography with large doses of contrast media. *Acta Radiol* 1969;8:9–12.
9. Byrd L, Sherman RL. Radiocontrast-induced acute renal failure: a clinical and pathophysiologic review. *Medicine* 1979;58:270–278.
10. Diaz-Buxo JA, Wagoner RD, Hattery RR, et al. Acute renal failure after excretory urography in diabetic patients. *Ann Intern Med* 1975;83:155–161.
11. Krumlovsky FA, Simon N, Santhanam S, delGreco F, Roxe D, Pomaranc MM. Acute renal failure: association with administration of radiographic contrast material. *JAMA* 1978;239:125–127.
12. Spataro RF. Newer contrast agents for urology. *Radiol Clin North Am* 1984;22:365–379.
13. Bettmann MA. Angiographic contrast agents: conventional and new media compared. *Am J Radiol* 1982;139:787–794.
14. Mudge GH. Nephrotoxicity of urographic radiocontrast drugs. *Kidney Int* 1980;18:540–552.
15. Schiantarelli P, Peroni F, Tirone P, et al. Effects of iodinated contrast media on erthrocytes. *Invest Radiol* 1973;8:199–203.
16. Talner LB. Urographic contrast media in uremia, physiology, and pharmacology. *Radiol Clin North Am* 1972;10:421–432.
17. Sage MR. Kinetics of water soluble contrast media in the central nervous system. *Am J Roentgenol* 1983;141:815–824.
18. Morris TW, Fischer HW. The pharmacology of intravascular radiocontrast media. *Annu Rev Pharmacol Toxicol* 1986;26:143–160.
19. Dean PB, Kivisaari L, Kormano M. The diagnostic potential of contrast enhancement pharmacokinetics. *Invest Radiol* 1978;13:533–540.
20. Burgener FA, Hamlin DJ. Contrast enhancement in abdominal CT: bolus versus infusion. *Am J Roentgenol* 1982;137:351–358.
21. Mudge GH. The maximal urinary concentration of diatrizoate. *Invest Radiol* 1980;15(suppl):S67–S78.
22. Spataro RF, Fischer HW, Boglan L. Urography with low osmolality contrast media: comparative urinary excretion of iopamidol, hexabrix and diatrizoate. *Invest Radiol* 1982;14:494–500.
23. Katzberg RW, Pabico RC, Morris TW, Hayakawa K, McKenna BA, Panner BJ, et al. Effects of contrast media on renal function and subcellular morphology in the dog. *Invest Radiol* 1986;21:64–70.
24. Benness GT. Urographic contrast agents: a comparison of sodium and methylglucamine salts. *Clin Radiol* 1970;21:150–157.
25. Cattel WR, Fry IK, Spencer AG, et al. Excretion urography. *Br J Radiol* 1967;40:561–565.
26. Bahlmann J, Krüskemper HL. Elimination of iodine-containing contrast media by hemodialysis. *Nephron* 1973;19:250–255.
27. Von Baars HG, Schabel J, Weiss M. Kontrastmitted-elimination durch Hämodialyze. *Urol Nephrol* 1984;77:473–481.
28. Ackrill P, McIntosh CS, Nimmon C, et al. A comparison of the clearance of urographic contrast medium (sodium diatrizoate) by peritoneal and hemodialysis. *Clin Sci* 1976;50:69–74.
29. Milman N, Christensen E. Elimination of diatrizoate by peritoneal dialysis in renal failure. *Acta Radiol* 1974;15:265–272.
30. Waaler A, Svaland M, Fairchald P, Jakobsen JA, Kolmannskog F, Berg KJ. Elimination of Iohexol, a low osmolar non-ionic contrast medium by hemodialysis in patients with chronic renal failure. *Nephron* 1990;56:81–85.
31. Morris TW, Katzberg RW, Fischer HW. A comparison of the hemodynamic responses to metrizamide and meglumine/sodium dia-trizoate in canine renal angiography. *Invest Radiol* 1978; 13:74–81.
32. Norby LH, DiBona GF. The renal vascular effects of meglumine diatrizoate. *J Pharmacol Exp Ther* 1975;193:932–938.
33. Talner LB, Davidson AJ. Renal hemodynamic effects of contrast media. *Invest Radiol* 1968;3: 301–306.

34. Caldicot WJH, Hollenberg NK, Abrams HL. Characteristics of response of renal vascular bed to contrast media. *Invest Radiol* 1970;5:539–547.
35. Harvey RB. Vascular resistance changes produced by hyperosmotic solutions. *Am J Physiol* 1960; 199:31–34.
36. Katzberg RW, Schulman G, Meggs LG, Caldicott WJH, Damiano MM, Hollenberg NK. Mechanism of the renal response to contrast medium in dogs: decrease in renal function due to hypertoxicity. *Invest Radiol* 1983;18:74–80.
37. Larson TS, Hudson K, Mertz JI, Romero JC, Knox FG. Renal vasoconstrictive response to contrast medium. *J Lab Clin Med* 1983;101:385–391.
38. Arend LJ, Bakris GL, Burnett JC Jr, Megerian C, Spielmann WS. Role of intrarenal adenosine in the renal hemodynamic response to contrast media. *J Lab Clin Med* 1987;110:406–411.
39. Bakris GL, Burnett JC Jr. A role for calcium in radiocontrast-induced reduction in renal hemodynamics. *Kidney Int* 1985;27:465–468.
40. Deray G, Martinez F, Cacoub P, Baumelou B, Baumelou A, Jacobs C. A role for adenosine, calcium and ischemia in radiocontrast-induced intrarenal vasoconstriction. *Am J Nephrol* 1990;10: 316–322.
41. Bakris GL, Lass NA, Gaber CA, Jones JD, Burnett JC Jr. Radiocontrast medium-induced declines in renal function: a role for oxygen free radicals. *Am J Physiol* 1990;258:F115–F120.
42. Margulies KB, McKinley LJ, Cavero PG, Burnett JC Jr. Induction and prevention of radiocontrast-induced nephropathy in dogs with heart failure. *Kidney Int* 1990;38:1101–1108.
43. Mudge GH, Meier FA, Ward KK. Pathogenesis of renal impairment induced by radiocontrast drugs. In: Solez K, Whelton A, eds. *Acute renal failure*. New York: Marcel Dekker, 1984;361–388.
44. Gerber JG, Branch RA, Nies AS, Hollifield JW, Gerkens JF. Influence of hypertonic saline on canine renal blood flow and renin release. *Am J Physiol* 1979;237:F441–F446.
45. Katzberg, RW, Morris TW, Burgerer FA. Renal renin and hemodynamic responses to selective renal artery catherization and angiography. *Invest Radiol* 1977;12:381–386.
46. Humes HD, Hunt DA, White MD. Direct toxic effect of the radiocontrast agent diatrizoate on renal proximal tubule cells. *Am J Physiol* 1987;252:F246–F255.
47. Ziegler TW, Ludens JH, Fanestil DD, Talner LB. Inhibition of active sodium transport by radiographic contrast media. *Kidney Int* 1975;7:68–76.
48. Messana JM, Gieslinski DA, Nguyen VD, Humes HD. Comparison of the toxicity of the radiocontrast agents, iopanidol and diatrizoate to rabbit renal proximal tubule cells in vitro. *J Pharmacol Exp Ther* 1988;244:1139–1144.
49. Navar LG, Champion WJ, Thomas CE. Effects of calcium channel blockade on renal vascular resistance responses to changes in perfusion pressure and angiotensin converting enzyme inhibition in dogs. *Circ Res* 1986;58:874–881.
50. Baer PG, Navar LG. Renal vasodilatation and uncoupling of blood flow and filtration rate autoregulation. *Kidney Int* 1973;4:12–21.
51. Müller-Suur R, Gutsche HU, Schurek HJ. Acute reversible inhibition of tubuloglomerular feedback mediated afferent vasoconstriction by the calcium antagonist verapamil. *Curr Probl Clin Biochem* 1976;6:291–298.
52. Osswald H, Spielman WS, Knox FG. Mechanism of adenosine-mediated decreases in glomerular filtration rate. *Circ Res* 1978;43:465–469.
53. Tagawa Hand Vander AJ. EFfects of adenosine compounds on renal function and renin secretion in dogs. *Circ Res* 1970;26:327–338.
54. Hall JE, Granger JP, Hester RI. Interactions between adenosine and angiotensin II in controlling glomerular filtration. *Am J Physiol* 1985;248:F340–F346.
55. Spielman WS, Thompson CI. A proposed role for adenosine in the regulation of renal hemodynamics and renin release. *Am J Physiol* 1982;242:F423–F435.
56. Baud L, Ardaillou R. Reactive oxygen species: production and role in the kidney. *Am J Physiol* 1986;251:F765–F776.
57. Cross CE, Halliwell B, Borish ET, Pryor WA, Awes BN, Saul RL, McCord JM, Harman D. Oxygen radicals and human disease. *Ann Intern Med* 1987;107:526–545.
58. Shah SV. Role of active oxygen metabolites in experimental glomerular disease. *Kidney Int* 1989; 35:1093–1106.
59. Baud L, Hagege J, Sraer J, Rondeau E, Perez J, Ardaillon R. Reactive oxygen production by

cultured rat glomerular mesangial cells during phagocytosis is associated with stimulation of lipoxygenase activity. *J Exp Med* 1983;158:1836–1852.
60. Messana JM, Cieslinski DA, O'Connor RP, Humes HD. Glutathione protects against exogenous oxidant injury to rabbit renal proximal tubule. *Am J Physiol* 1988;255:F874–F884.
61. Scaduto RC Jr, Gattone VH, Grotyohann LW, Wertz J, Martin LF. Effect of an altered glutathione content on renal ischemic injury. *Am J Physiol* 1988;255:F911–F921.
62. Yoshioka T, Fogo A, Beckman JK. Reduced activity of antioxidant enzymes underlies contrast media-induced renal injury in volume depletion. *Kidney Int* 1992;41(4):1008–1015.
63. Hoyer Jr, Seiler MW. Pathophysiology of Tamm-Horsfall protein. *Kidney Int* 1987;16:279–289.
64. Patel R, McKenzie JK, McQueen EG. Tamm-Horsfall urinary microprotein and tubular obstruction by casts in acute renal failure. *Lancet* 1964;1:41–46.
65. Schwartz RH, Berdon WE, Wagner J, Becker J, Baker DH. Tamm-Horsfall urinary microprotein precipitation by urographic contrast agents: in vitro studies. *Am J Roentgenol* 1970;108:698–702.
66. Berdon WE, Schwartz RH, Becker J, Baker DH. Tamm-Horsfall proteinuria: its relationship to prolonged nephrograms in infants and children and to renal failure following intravenous urography in adults with multiple myeloma. *Radiology* 1969;92:714–720.
67. Bakris GL, Gaber AO, Jones JD. Oxygen free radical involvement in urinary Tamm-Horsfall protein excretion after intrarenal injection of contrast medium. *Radiology* 1990;175:51–60.
68. Nicot GS, Merle LJ, Charmes JP, Valette JP, Novaille YD, Lachatre GF, Robert CL. Transient proteinuria, enzymuria and glomerular nephrotoxic reaction induced by radiocontrast media. *JAMA* 1984;252:2432–2434.
69. Parvez Z, Ramamursthy S, Patel NB, Moncada R. Enzyme markers of contrast media-induced renal failure. *Invest Radiol* 1990;25:5133–5134.
70. Lang J, Lasser EC. Inhibition of adenosine triphosphate and carbonic anhydrase by contrast media. *Invest Radiol* 1975;10:314–316.
71. Lang JH, Lasser EC. Nonspecific inhibition of enzymes by organic contrast media. *J Med Chem* 1971;14:233–238.
72. Lasser EC, Lang JH, Hamblin AE, Rosen L. Contrast and electrolyte dynamics of the intravenous pyelogram. I. Urinary pH and electrolyte changes in the canine IVP. *Invest Radiol* 1975;10:300–306.
73. Talner LB, Rushmer HN, Coel MN. The effect of renal artery injection of contrast material on urinary enzyme excretion. *Invest Radiol* 1972;7:311–322.
74. DeRubertis FR, Craven PA. Effects of osmolality and oxygen availability on soluble cyclic AMP dependent protein kinase activity of rat renal inner medulla. *J Clin Invest* 1978;62:1210–1221.
75. Kim Ms, Akera T. O_2 free radicals: cause of ischemia-reperfusion injury to cardiac Na/K/ATPase. *Am J Physiol* 1987;252:H252–H257.
76. Kato K, Kato M, Matsuoka T, Mustapha A. Depression of membrane bound Na/K/ATPase activity induced by free radicals and by ischemia of kidney. *Am J Physiol* 1988;254:C330–C337.
77. Brezis M, Rosen SN, Epstei FH. The pathophysiologic implications of medullary hypoxia. *Am J Kidney Dis* 1989;13:253–258.
78. Lear S, Silva P, Kelley VE, Epstein FH. Prostaglandin E_2 inhibits oxygen consumption in rabbit medullary thick ascending limb. *Am J Physiol* 1990;258:F1372–F1378.
79. Heyman S, Brezis M, Greenfeld J, et al. Protective role of furosemide and saline in radiocontrast induced acute renal failure. *Clin Res* 1988;36:520A.
80. Heyman SN, Brezis M, Reubinoff CA, et al. Acute renal failure with selective medullary injury in the rat. *J Clin Invest* 1988;82:401–412.
81. Vari RC, Natarajan LA, Whitescarver SA, Jackson BA, Ott CE. Induction, prevention and mechanisms of contrast medium-induced acute renal failure. *Kidney Int* 1988;33:699–707.
82. Lund G, Einzig S, Rysany J, Salomonointz E, Castaneda-Zuniga W, Amplatz K. Effect of prostaglandin inhibition on the renal vascular response to ionic and nonionic contrast media in the dog. *Acta Radiol Diagn* 1984;25:407–410.
83. Workman RJ, Schaff MI, Jackson RV, Diggs J, Frazer MG, Briscoe C. Relationship of renal hemodynamics and functional changes following intravascular contrast to the renin-angiotensin system and renal prostacycline in the dog. *Invest Radiol* 1983;18:160–166.
84. Margulies KB, McKinley LJ, Allgren R, Stanson AW, Burnett JC Jr. Intraarterial atrial natriuretic factor attenuates radiocontrast-induced nephropathy in humans. *J Am Soc Nephrol* 1991;2(3):666 (abstract).

85. Berns AS. Nephrotoxicity of contrast media. *Kidney Int* 1989;36:730–740.
86. Eisenberg RL, Bank WD, Hedgcock MW. Renal failure after major angiography, *Am J Med* 1980;68:43–48.
87. Kumar S, Hull JD, Lathi S, Cohen AJ, Pletka PG. Incidence of renal failure after angiography. *Arch Intern Med* 1981;141:1268–1272.
88. Miller GM, Willie EJ, Hinman F. Renal complications from aortography. *Surgery* 1954;35:885–891.
89. Larsson H, Palmlov A. Abdominal aortography with special reference to its complications. *Acta Radiol* 1954;38:111–116.
90. Barnes BA, Shaw AS, Leaf A, Linton RR. Oliguria following diagnostic translumbar aortography. *N Engl J Med* 1955;252:113–117.
91. Edling NPG, Edvall CA, Helander CG. On renal damage due to aortography and its prevention by renal tests. *Acta Radiol* 1957;47:473–479.
92. Stark FR, Coburn JW. Renal failure following methylglucamine diatrizoate (Renografin) aortography. Report of a case with unilateral renal artery stenosis. *J Urol* 1966;96:845–851.
93. Port KF, Wagoner RD, Fulton RE. Acute renal failure after angiography. *Am J Roentgenol* 1974;121:544–550.
94. D'Elia JA, Gleason RE, Arday M, Malarick C, Godfrey K, Warran J, Kaldany A, Weinrauch LA. Nephrotoxicity from angiographic contrast material. A prospective study. *Am J Med* 1982;72:719–725.
95. Mason RA, Arbeit LA, Giron F. Renal dysfunction after arteriography. *JAMA* 1985;253:1001–1004.
96. Cochran ST, Wong WS, Roe DJ. Predicting angiography induced acute renal function impairment: clinical risk model. *Am J Roentgenol* 1983;14:1027–1033.
97. Weinrauch LA, Healy RW, Leland OS, Goldstein HH, Kassissieh SD, Libertino JA, Takacs FJ, D'Elia JA. Coronary angiography and acute renal failure in azotemic diabetic nephropathy. *Ann Intern Med* 1977;86:56–59.
98. Taliercio CP, Vliestra RE, Fisher LD, Burnett JC. Risks for renal dysfunction with coronary angiography. *Ann Intern Med* 1986;104:501–504.
99. Swartz RD, Rubin JE, Leeming BW, Silva P. Renal failure following major angiography. *Am J Med* 1978;65:31–37.
100. Parfrey PS, Griffiths SM, Barrett BJ, Paul DM, Genge M, Withers J, Farid N, McManomon P. Contrast material-induced renal failure in patients with diabetes mellitus, renal insufficiency or both. *N Engl J Med* 1989;320:143–149.
101. Schwab SJ, Hlatky MA, Pieper KS, et al. Contrast nephropathy: a randomized controlled trial of nonionic and ionic radiographic contrast agents. *N Engl J Med* 1989;320:149–153.
102. Davidson CJ, Hlatky M. Morris KG, Pieper K. Skelton TN, Schwab SJ, Bashore TM. Cardiovascular and renal toxicity of a nonionic radiographic contrast agent after cardiac catheterization. A prospective trial. *Ann Intern Med* 1989;110:119–124.
103. Kinnison ML, Powe NR, Steinberg EP. Results of randomized controlled trails of low versus high osmolality contrast media. *Radiology* 1989;170:381–389.
104. Gomes AS, Lois JF, Baker JD, McGlade CT, Bunnell DH, Hartzman S. Acute renal dysfunction in high risk patients after angiography: comparison of ionic and nonionic contrast media. *Radiology* 1989;170:65–68.
105. Albrechtsson U, Hultberg B, Larusdotir H, et al. Nephrotoxicity of ionic and nonionic contrast media in aortofemoral angiography. *Acta Radiol Diagn* 1985;26:615–618.
106. Tornquist C, Holtas S. Renal angiography with iohexol and metrizoate. *Radiology* 1984;150:331–334.
107. Bird CR, Drayer BP, Velja R, et al. Safety of contrast media in cerebral angiography; iopamidol vs. methylglucamine iothalamate. *AJNR* 1984;5:801–803.
108. Bryan RN, Miller SL, Roehm JO, et al. Neuroangiography with iohexol. *AJNR* 1983;4:344–346.
109. Sacks BA, Ellison HP, Bartek S, et al. A comparison of Hexabrix and Renografin 60 in peripheral arteriography. *AJR* 1983;140:975–977.
110. Skjennald A, Heldaas, J, Hoiseth A. Comparison of iohexol and meglumine-Na-Ca metrizoate in visceral angiography. *Acta Radiol Suppl (Stockh)* 1983;366:158–163.
111. Wolf GL. Adult peripheral angiography: results from four North American randomized clinical trials of ionic media versus iohexol. *Acta Radiol Suppl (Stockh)* 1983;366:166–170.
112. Barth KH, Mertens MA. A double-blind comparative study of Hexabrix and Renografin-76 in aortography and visceral arteriography. *Invest Radiol* 1984;19(suppl):S323–S325.

113. Roy P, Robillard P, L'Homme C, et al. Iohexol: a new nonionic agent in adult peripheral arteriography. *J Can Assoc Radiol* 1985;36:113–117.
114. Pathria M, Somers S, Gill G. Pain during angiography: a randomized double-blind trial comparing ioxaglate and diatrizoate. *J Can Assoc Radiol* 1987;38:32–34.
115. Gale MN, Robbins AH, Hamburger RJ, et al. Renal toxicity of contrast agents: iopamidol, iothalamate, and diatrizoate. *AJR* 1984;142:333–335.
116. Khoury GA, Hopper JC, Varghese Z, et al. Nephrotoxicity of ionic and non-ionic contrast material in vascular imaging and selective renal arteriography. *Br J Radiol* 1983;56:631–635.
117. Harkonen S, Kjellstrand CM. Exacerbation of diabetic renal failure following intravenous pyelography. *Am J Med* 1977;63:939–946.
118. Van Zee BE, Hoy WE, Talley TE, Jaenike JR. Renal injury associated with intravenous pyelography in nondiabetic and diabetic patients. *Ann Intern Med* 1978;89:51–54.
119. Peltz D, Fox AJ, Vinuela F. Clinical trial of iohexol vs. Conray 60 for cerebral angiography. *AJNR* 1984;5:565–568.
120. Gordon IJ, Skolbar RS, Chicatelli PD, et al. A comparative investigation with meglumine metrizoate. *Acta Radiol Suppl (Stockh)*, 1983;366:65–69.
121. Pendergrass EP, Hodges PJ, Trondreau RJ, Powell CC, Burdick ED. Further consideration of deaths and unfavorable sequelae following administration of contrast media in urography in the United States. *Am J Roentgenol* 1955;74:262–287.
122. Fischermann K, Ostenfeld J. Death following intravenous urography. *Nord Med* 1951;45:240–248.
123. Kamdar A, Weidman P, Makoff DL, Massry SG. Acute renal failure following intravenous use of radiographic contrast dyes in patients with diabetes mellitus. *Diabetes* 1977;26:643–649.
124. Pillay VK, Robbins PC, Schwartz FD, Kark RK. Acute renal failure following intravenous urography in patients with long-standing diabetes mellitus and azotemia. *Radiology* 1975;145:633–636.
125. Anto HR, Chou SY, Porush JG, Shapiro WB. Infusion intravenous pyelography and renal function. Effects of hypertonic mannitol in patients with chronic renal insufficiency. *Arch Intern Med* 1981;141:1652–1656.
126. Harkonen S, Kjellstrand CM. Intravenous pyelography in nonuremic diabetic patients. *Nephron* 1979;24:268–270.
127. Carvallo A, Rakowski TA, Argy WP, Schriender GE. Acute renal failure following drip infusion pyelography. *Am J Med* 1975;65:38–45.
128. Ortuno J. Renal function impairment caused by intravenous urography. *Arch Intern Med* 1981; 141:1271–1274.
129. Shafi T, Shyan-Yik C, Porush JG, Shapiro WB. Infusion intravenous pyelography and renal function. Effects in patients with chronic renal insufficiency. *Arch Intern Med* 1978;138:1218–1221.
130. Witter DM, Friedman EA. Low risk of contrast media-induced acute renal failure in nonazotemic type-2 diabetes mellitus. *Kidney Int* 1982;21:739–743.
131. Bergman AL, Ellison MR, Dunea G. Acute renal failure after drip infusion pyelography. *N Engl J Med* 1978;279:1277–1282.
132. Harkonen S, Kjellstrand C. Contrast nephropathy. *Am J Nephrol* 1981;7:69–77.
133. Diaz-Buxo JA, Wagoner RD, Hattery RR, Palumbo PJ. Acute renal failure after excretory urography in diabetic patients. *Ann Intern Med* 1975;83:155–158.
134. MacEwan DW, Dunbar JS. Intravenous pyelography in children with renal insufficiency. *Radiology* 1962;78:893–898.
135. Schwartz WB, Hurwit A, Ettinger A. Intravenous urography in the patient with renal insufficiency. *N Engl J Med* 1963;269:277–283.
136. Cramer BC, Porfrey PS, Hutchinson TA, Baran D, Melanson DM, Ethier RE, Seely JF. Renal function following infusion of radiologic contrast material. A prospective controlled study. *Arch Intern Med* 1985;145:87–89.
137. Sunnegardh O, Hietala SO, Wirell S, Ekelund L. Systemic, pulmonary and renal hemodynamic effects of intravenously infused iopentol. *Acta Radiol* 1990;31:395–399.
138. Berg KJ, Kolmannskog F, Lillevold PE, Nordal KP, Ressem L, Rootwelt K, Svaland MG. Iopentol in patients with chronic renal failure: its effects on renal function and its use as glomerular filtration rate parameter. *Scan J Clin Lab Invest* 1992;52:27–33.
139. Barrett BJ, Parfrey PS, Vavasour HM, McDonald J, Kent G. Contrast nephropathy in patients with impaired renal function: High versus low osmolar media. *Kidney Int* 1992;41(5):1274–1279.
140. Donadio C, Tramonti G, Giordani R, Lucchett A, et al. Effects on renal hemodynamics and tubular function of the contrast medium iohexol in renal patients. *Ren Fail* 1990;12(3):141–146.

141. Porush JG, Chou SY, Anto HR, Oguagha C, Shapiro WB, Faubert PF. Infusion intravenous pyelography and renal function: effects of hypertonic mannitol and furosemide in patients with chronic renal insufficiency. In: Eliahou HE, ed. *Acute renal failure*. London: John Libbey, 1982; 161–167.
142. Old CW, Duarte CM, Lehrner LM, et al. A prospective evaluation of mannitol in the prevention of radiocontrast acute renal failure. *Clin Res* 1981;29:472 (abstract).
143. Kurnik BRC, Weisberg LS, Cuttler IM, Kurnik PB. Effects of atrial natriuretic peptide versus mannitol on renal blood flow during radiocontrast infusion in chronic renal failure. *J Lab Clin Med* 1990;116:27–35.
144. Eisenberg RL, Bank WO, Hedgcock MW. Renal failure after major angiography can be avoided with hydration. *Am J Roentgenol* 1981;136:859–861.
145. Cronin RE, Erickson AB, DeTorrente A, McDonald KM, Schrier RW. Norepinephrine-induced acute renal failure: a reversible ischemic model of acute renal failure. *Kidney Int* 1978;14:187–193.
146. Morris CR, Alexander EA, Bruns F, Levinsky N. Restoration and maintenance of glomerular filtration by mannitol during hypoperfusion of the kidney. *J Clin Invest* 1972;51:1555–1564.
147. Berkseth RO, Kjellstrand CM. Radiologic contrast induced nephropathy. *Med Clin North Am* 1984; 68:351–371.
148. Golman K, Cederholm C. Contrast medium-induced acute renal failure: can it be prevented? *Invest Radiol* 1990;25:S127–S128.
149. Russo D, Testa A, Della Volpe L, Sansone G. Randomized prospective study on renal effects of two different contrast media in humans: protective role of a calcium channel blocker. *Nephron* 1990;55:254–257.
150. Neumayer HH, Junge W, Küfner A, Wenning A. Prevention of radiocontrast media-induced nephrotoxicity by the calcium channel blocker nitrendipine: a prospective randomized clinical trial. *Nephrol Dial Transplant* 1989;4:1030–1036.
151. Danford RO, Davidson AJ, Goldman RL. Drip infusion pyelography. *N Engl J Med* 1969;280: 1022–1026.
152. Dudzinski PJ, Petrone AF, Persoff M, et al. Acute renal failure following high dose excretory urography in dehydrated patients. *J Urol* 1971;106:619–628.
153. Demarie BK. Bakris GL. Effects of different calcium antagonists of proteinuria associated with diabetes mellitus. *Ann Intern Med* 1990;113:987–988.
154. Aron NB, Feinfeld DA, Peters AT, Lynn RI. Acute renal failure associated with ioxaglate, a low osmolality radiocontrast agent. *Am J Kidney Dis* 1989;13:189–193.
155. Higgins CB, Kuber M, Slutsky RA. Interaction between verapamil and contrast media in coronary arteriography: comparison of standard ionic and new nonionic media. *Circulation* 1983;68:628–635.
156. Gerber KH, Higgins CB, Yuh YS, Koziol JA. Regional myocardial hemodynamic and metabolic effects of ionic and nonionic contrast media in normal and ischemic states. *Circulation* 1982;65: 1307–1314.
157. Lund G, Einzigs, Rysavy J, Borgwardt B, et al. Role of ischemia in contrast-induced renal damage: an experimental study. *Circulation* 1984;69:783–789.
158. Morris DL, Wisenski JA, Gertz EW, et al. Potentiation by nifedipine and diltiazem of the hypotensive response after contrast angiography. *J Am Coll Cardiol* 1985;6:785–791.
159. Steinberg EP, Moore RD, Powe NR, Gopalan R, Davidoff AJ, Litt M, Graziano S, Brinker JA. Safety and cost effectiveness of high osmolality as compared with low osmolality contrast material in patients undergoing cardiac angiography. *N Engl J Med* 1992;326:425–430.
160. Fischer HW, Spataro RF, Rosenberg RM. Medical and economic considerations in using a new contrast medium. *Arch Intern Med* 1988;146:1717–1722.
161. Cigarroa RG, Lange RA, Williams RH, Willis LD. Dosing of contrast material to prevent contrast nephropathy in patients with renal disease. *Am J Med* 1989;86:649–652.

Toxicology of the Kidney, Second Edition,
edited by Jerry B. Hook and Robin S. Goldstein.
Raven Press, Ltd., New York © 1993.

14

Aliphatic Halogenated Hydrocarbons

Adnan A. Elfarra

Department of Comparative Biosciences, University of Wisconsin, School of Veterinary Medicine, Madison, Wisconsin 53706

Aliphatic halogenated hydrocarbons are used extensively as industrial solvents, pesticides, and chemical intermediates in the production of other chemicals. Many haloalkanes, haloalkenes, and haloalkynes are released into the environment and have been detected in drinking water. Acute, subchronic, or chronic exposure to these chemicals by humans and animals has been associated with the induction of a wide variety of toxicological effects, including nephrotoxicity (Table 1), hepatotoxicity, mutagenicity, and carcinogenicity. Current evidence indicates that the target organ selectivity and nephrotoxic potency of these chemicals are largely dependent on the halogenated hydrocarbon used and the species studied. This chapter reviews current knowledge of the mechanisms of activation of aliphatic halogenated hydrocarbons, and gives selected examples. An attempt will also be made to discuss progress made on the molecular and cellular events associated with nephrotoxicity, to discuss the biochemical basis of target organ selectivity, and to correlate known species differences in activation with toxicity. Several aspects of halogenated hydrocarbon bioactivation and nephrotoxicity have been reviewed (49,57–68).

BIOACTIVATION MECHANISMS

Biotransformation of halogenated hydrocarbons to highly reactive electrophilic intermediates, free radicals, or stable but toxic metabolites has been implicated in their mechanisms of nephrotoxicity (49,67,68). Current evidence indicates that reactive electrophilic metabolites may cause cytotoxicity following covalent modifications of critical cellular macromolecules; free radical metabolites may result in the production of reactive oxygen species and/or the stimulation of peroxidative damage to cellular membranes; the stable, but toxic metabolites may directly inhibit critical cellular function(s).

The kidneys contain a wide variety of enzymes capable of catalyzing the metabolism of aliphatic halogenated hydrocarbons to chemically reactive metabolites (67, 69–75). Reactive metabolites with slightly longer half-lives may also be formed in

TABLE 1. *Aliphatic halogenated hydrocarbons that are shown to be nephrotoxic*

Chemical name (common name)	Reference(s)
I. Haloalkanes	
Chloromethane (methyl chloride)	1,2
Dichloromethane (methylene chloride)	3
Trichloromethane (chloroform)	4–6
Tetrachloromethane (carbon tetrachloride)	7–10
1,2-Dichloroethane (ethylene dichloride)	11
1,2-Dibromoethane (ethylene dibromide)	3,12,13
1,1,2-Trichloroethane	14,15
1,2-Dichloropropane	16
1,2-Dibromo-3-chloropropane	3,17–20
II. Haloalkenes	
1,1-Dichloroethylene (vinylidene chloride)	21–24
cis/trans 1,2-Dichloroethylene (dichloroethylene)	14
Trichloroethylene	25–27
Tetrachloroethylene (perchloroethylene)	28,29
Tetrafluoroethylene	30
1-Chloro-1,2,2-trifluoroethylene	31,32
1,1-Dichloro-2,2-difluoroethylene	33,34
1,3-Dichloro-1-propene	35,36
1,1,2-trichloro-3,3,3-trifluoro-1-propene	37
Hexafluoropropene	31
Hexachlorobutadiene	38–42
3-Chloro-1-propene (allyl chloride)	43,44
Chloroethylene (vinyl chloride)	45
III. Haloalkynes	
Dichloroacetylene	46–48
IV. Miscellaneous	
2,2-Dichloro-1,1-difluoro-1-methoxyethane (methoxyflurane)	49
3-Chloropropane 1,2-oxide (epichlorohydrin)	50
3-Chloro-1,2-propanediol (α-chlorohydrin)	50,51
3-Chlorolactate	52,53
tris(2,3-dibromopropyl)phosphate	54
2-Bromoethylamine	55,56

the liver and translocated to the kidneys via the circulation. With some chemicals, however, stable metabolites reaching the kidneys may be metabolized further by renal enzymes to generate chemically reactive forms (59,61–65). The enzyme systems most frequently associated with the bioactivation of aliphatic halogenated hydrocarbons are the cytochrome P-450–dependent monooxygenases and the glutathione *S*-transferases. Studies on the purification and characterization of these enzymes and the effects of various inducers and inhibitors on their enzymatic activities, have been reported (69,74–86). Immunohistochemical methods have shown that different cytochrome P-450–dependent monooxygenases have different localizations in the nephron (80). In the following sections, the role of metabolism by cytochrome P-450 and glutathione *S*-transferase in the nephrotoxicity of aliphatic halogenated hydrocarbons is discussed.

Cytochrome P-450–dependent Activation

Cytochrome P-450–dependent activation has been implicated in the nephrotoxicity of several haloalkanes, e.g., $CHCl_3$, CCl_4, and methoxyflurane, and haloalkenes, e.g., 1,1-dichloroethylene. The role of cytochrome P-450 in the activation of these chemicals to the three classes of metabolites, namely, the electrophilic metabolites, free radicals, and the stable but toxic metabolites in the nephrotoxicity of these chemicals will be discussed separately.

Metabolism to Highly Electrophilic Metabolites

The reaction of reactive electrophilic metabolites with nucleophilic groups on cellular proteins, lipids, and nucleic acids may result in covalent modifications of these macromolecules. These covalent modifications may lead to inhibition of critical cellular function leading to cytotoxicity and cell death. Although kidney cells have a high concentration of glutathione, which usually protects cellular macromolecules against covalent modifications by forming glutathione conjugates with the reactive species, cellular macromolecules may be alkylated after cellular glutathione concentrations are depleted.

Haloalkanes

Cytochrome P-450–dependent oxidation of haloalkanes usually proceeds by carbon oxidation at C-H bonds to yield *geminal*-halohydrins (Fig. 1), which are unstable and nonenzymatically undergo conversion to aldehydes or acyl halides (87,88). Alternatively, halogenated hydrocarbon radicals (Fig. 2) produced by cytochrome P-450–dependent reductive dehalogenation reactions may react with oxygen resulting in the formation of oxidation products (88). The metabolism of $CHCl_3$ (Fig. 1) and CCl_4 (Fig. 2) to phosgene, an electrophilic metabolite, are representative examples of these bioactivation reactions.

The potency of $CHCl_3$-induced nephrotoxicity varies with species; mice are more susceptible than rats, rabbits, or dogs (4–6,89,90). In mice, there are significant sex and strain differences; male ICR mice are susceptible, whereas female mice are resistant. Histopathological examination of renal tissues has shown that tubular swelling, necrosis, and casts are localized primarily in the proximal tubules. In addition, $CHCl_3$-induced nephrotoxicity is associated with proteinuria, glucosuria, and elevated blood urea nitrogen concentrations. *In vitro* uptake of organic acids and bases by renal cortical slices is also decreased by *in vivo* treatment with $CHCl_3$ (91).

Recent reports have shown a close correlation between the activities of renal cytochromes P-450 and $CHCl_3$-induced nephrotoxicity (89,92,93). More importantly, a close correlation between $CHCl_3$-induced nephrotoxicity and the metabolism of $CHCl_3$ by renal cytochrome P-450 has also been obtained (6,90,92). The

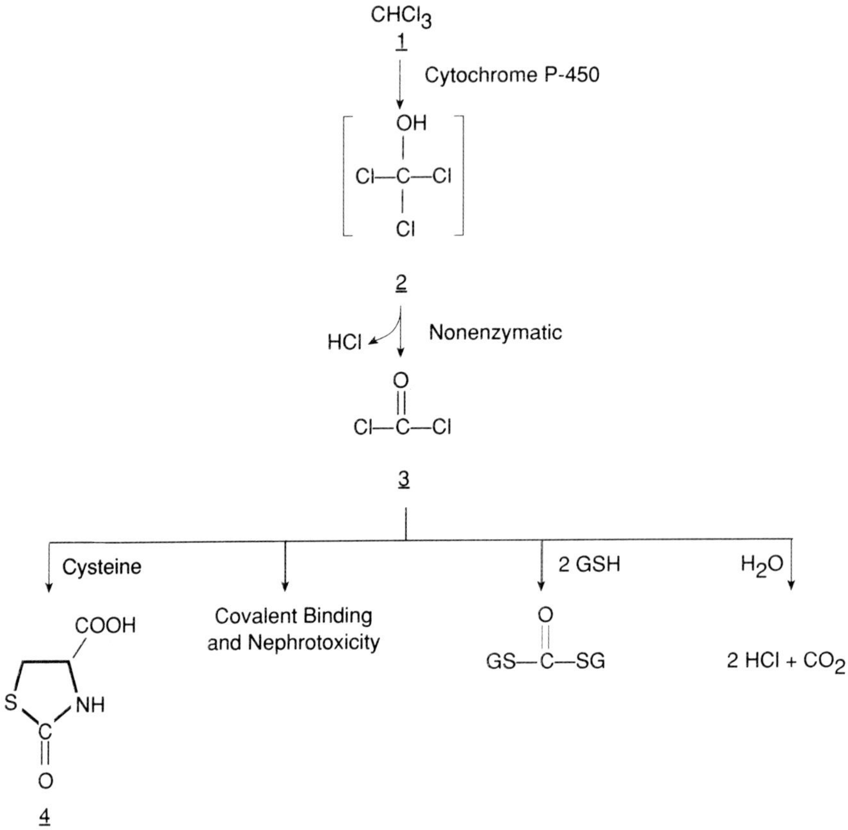

FIG. 1. Bioactivation of chloroform (*1*) to phosgene (*3*) by cytochrome P-450–dependent monooxygenases. *2*, Trichloromethanol (a *geminal* halohydrin); *4*, 2-oxothiazolidine-4-carboxylic acid.

covalent binding of $^{14}CHCl_3$-derived metabolites to renal macromolecules is greater in male mice than in female mice. *In vitro* studies have shown that male mice kidney homogenates metabolize $CHCl_3$ to phosgene, which reacts with cysteine to form 2-oxothizolidine-4-carboxylic acid (Fig. 1), a stable product. The renal metabolism of $CHCl_3$ to phosgene requires the presence of oxygen and NADPH and can be inhibited by carbon monoxide, indicating a role for renal cytochromes P-450 in the bioactivation of $CHCl_3$. Further evidence to support this hypothesis has been obtained by the finding that $CDCl_3$ is much less nephrotoxic than $CHCl_3$ to mice *in vivo* and to kidney slices *in vitro*. Thus, the renal bioactivation of $CHCl_3$ to phosgene (Fig. 1) and the subsequent reaction of phosgene with renal macromolecules play an important role in $CHCl_3$-induced nephrotoxicity. Future studies should identify the critical sites on renal macromolecules that are alkylated by phosgene, and

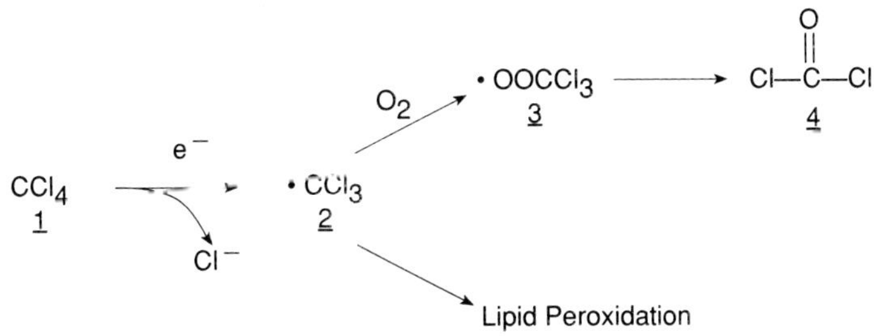

FIG. 2. Bioactivation of carbon tetrachloride (*1*) to trichloromethyl free radical (*2*), trichloromethyl peroxy free radical (*3*) and phosgene (*4*) by the cytochrome P-450–dependent reductive oxygenation pathway.

explain how renal macromolecule modifications may lead to renal tubular necrosis. In addition, since in some animal species $CHCl_3$ administration has also been associated with hepatotoxicity and carcinogenicity (5,94), further work is needed to clarify the biochemical basis for $CHCl_3$-induced target organ selectivity.

As indicated above, CCl_4 is both nephrotoxic and metabolized to phosgene (Fig. 2). The renal lesion produced by CCl_4, however, differs from that produced by $CHCl_3$ in that it is delayed in onset and is only associated with subtle morphological changes in the proximal tubular region of the nephron (57). Moreover, humans appear to be more sensitive to the acute nephrotoxic effects of CCl_4 than most laboratory animal species. In rats, $^{14}CCl_4$ administration results in covalent binding of the radiolabel to kidney and liver proteins and lipids (95). $^{14}CCl_4$ is also known to be metabolized by mouse kidney homogenates and rat kidney slices to yield $^{14}CHCl_3$ and $^{14}CO_2$, respectively (96,97), but the role of $CHCl_3$ or phosgene in CCl_4 nephrotoxicity remains unclear.

Haloalkenes

Cytochrome P-450–dependent oxidation of haloalkenes is known to result in the formation of electrophilic metabolites (87,98,99). The hepatic cytochrome P-450–dependent metabolism of chloroethylene yields 2-chloroethylene oxide, a highly electrophilic metabolite that nonenzymatically rearranges to 2-chloroacetaldehyde, a less reactive alkylating agent (98). The hepatic cytochrome P-450–dependent metabolism of 1,1-dichloroethylene yields the electrophilic metabolites 1,1-dichloroethylene oxide, 2-chloroacetylchloride, and 2,2-dichloroacetaldehyde (Fig. 3); 1,1-dichloroethylene oxide is not an obligate precursor to 2,2-dichloroacetaldehyde and 2-chloroacetyl chloride (99).

In rats, the nephrotoxicity of 1,1-dichloroethylene is associated with severe cortical tubular necrosis and increased kidney weights, plasma creatinine, and blood urea nitrogen concentrations (21–23). Treatment of mice with carbon disulfide in-

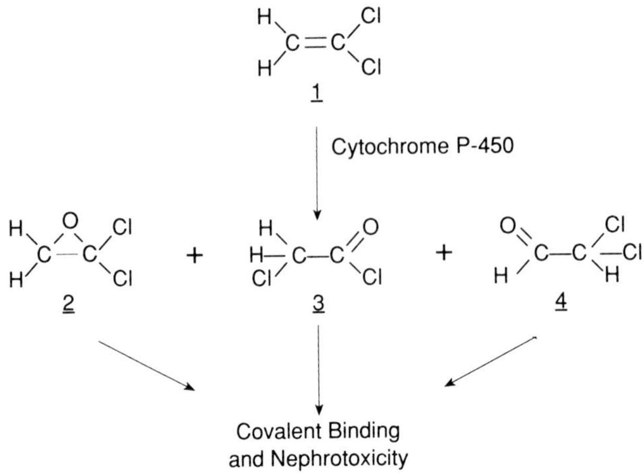

FIG. 3. Bioactivation of 1,1-dichloroethylene (*1*) to 1,1-dichloroethylene oxide (*2*), 2-chloroacetylchloride (*3*) and 2,2-dichloroacetaldehyde (*4*) by cytochrome P-450–dependent monooxygenases.

hibits hepatic and renal cytochrome P-450 activities and protects against renal and hepatic injury by 1,1-dichloroethylene (100). In rats, however, pretreatment with polychlorinated biphenyl or phenobarbital, which induced or had no effect on the level of renal cytochrome P-450, protected against 1,1-dichloroethylene nephrotoxicity (23). Administration of [^{14}C]-1,1-dichloroethylene to mice resulted in the highest covalent binding in the kidneys (101), but renal microsomes could not bioactivate 1,1-dichloroethylene to electrophilic metabolites (102). Although it is possible that 1,1-dichloroethylene metabolites may be translocated from the liver to the kidneys to cause nephrotoxicity (102,103), more studies are needed to provide evidence for this hypothesis.

Metabolism to Free Radicals

Depending on their chemical reactivities, free radicals may abstract hydrogen atoms from lipids or proteins leading to toxicity. Abstraction of hydrogen atoms from lipids initiates lipid peroxidation, whereas abstraction of hydrogen atoms from protein thiols may lead to the formation of disulfides or mixed disulfides. Formation of glutathione disulfides may lead to the depletion of cellular glutathione and NADPH, which would shift the redox state of cellular constituents and cause oxidative stress (103–105). These reactions may have adverse effects on lipid and protein integrity and function leading to cytotoxicity and cell death (103–105). In addition, free radicals may bind covalently to critical cellular macromolecules leading to toxicity.

As indicated above, CCl_4 is metabolized by cytochrome P-450 to trichloromethyl radical (Fig. 2); other halogenated hydrocarbons may also be metabolized by cytochrome P-450 to free radicals (87,88). Whereas lipid peroxidation has been shown to play an important role in the hepatotoxicity of CCl_4 (106), the role of free radicals or lipid peroxidation in CCl_4-induced nephrotoxicity remains unclear.

Metabolism to Stable but Nephrotoxic Metabolites

The metabolism of a number of haloalkanes to stable but toxic metabolites, e.g., fluoride ion and oxalic acid (Fig. 4), has been suggested to play a role in the nephrotoxicity of these chemicals (49,107,108). For example, the cytochrome P-450–dependent metabolism of 2,2-dichloro-1,1-difluoro-1-methoxyethane yields both fluoride ion and oxalic acid (Fig. 4); oxalic acid is also a known metabolite of 1,2-dibromo-3-chloropropane.

Fluoride is known to inhibit many renal enzyme systems (109), whereas oxalic acid may precipitate as calcium oxalate crystals at the corticomedullary junction causing focal necrosis (50). The renal functional and morphological changes associated with oxalic acid nephrotoxicity were insufficient to explain the nephrotoxic effects of 2,2-dichloro-1,1-difluoro-1-methoxyethane and 1,2-dibromo-2-chloropropane (49,50,110). Several studies, however, implicate the metabolism of 2,2-dichloro-1,1-difluoro-1-methoxyethane to fluoride ion in the nephrotoxicity of this chemical (49). In rats, strain differences in the metabolism of 2,2-dichloro-1,1-difluoro-1-methoxyethane to fluoride ion, and in the susceptibility to the nephrotoxic effects of fluoride ion were correlated closely with the nephrotoxicity of 2,2-dichloro-1,1-difluoro-1-methoxyethane (49). Moreover, cytochrome P-450 inducers increased the defluorination rates and the nephrotoxicity of 2,2-dichloro-1,1-difluoro-1-methoxyethane, whereas inhibitors of cytochrome P-450 decreased the rates of defluorination and the nephrotoxicity. Collectively, these results provide evidence for the role of cytochrome P-450–dependent metabolism of 2,2-dichloro-1,1-difluoro-1-methoxyethane to fluoride ion in the nephrotoxicity of this chemical.

Glutathione *S*-Transferase–Dependent Activation

The glutathione *S*-transferases, which catalyze the first step in mercapturic acid biosynthesis (111), and other enzymes that catalyze mercapturic acid formation (112) have been associated with the detoxication of a variety of chemicals. Current evidence, however, has also implicated these enzymes in the bioactivation of halogenated hydrocarbons to nephrotoxic metabolites (Table 2). Two types of nephrotoxic glutathione and cysteine *S*-conjugates, namely, direct-acting through the formation of reactive episulfonium ions, and indirect-acting which require activation by cysteine conjugate β-lyase to generate reactive thiols, have been described (59).

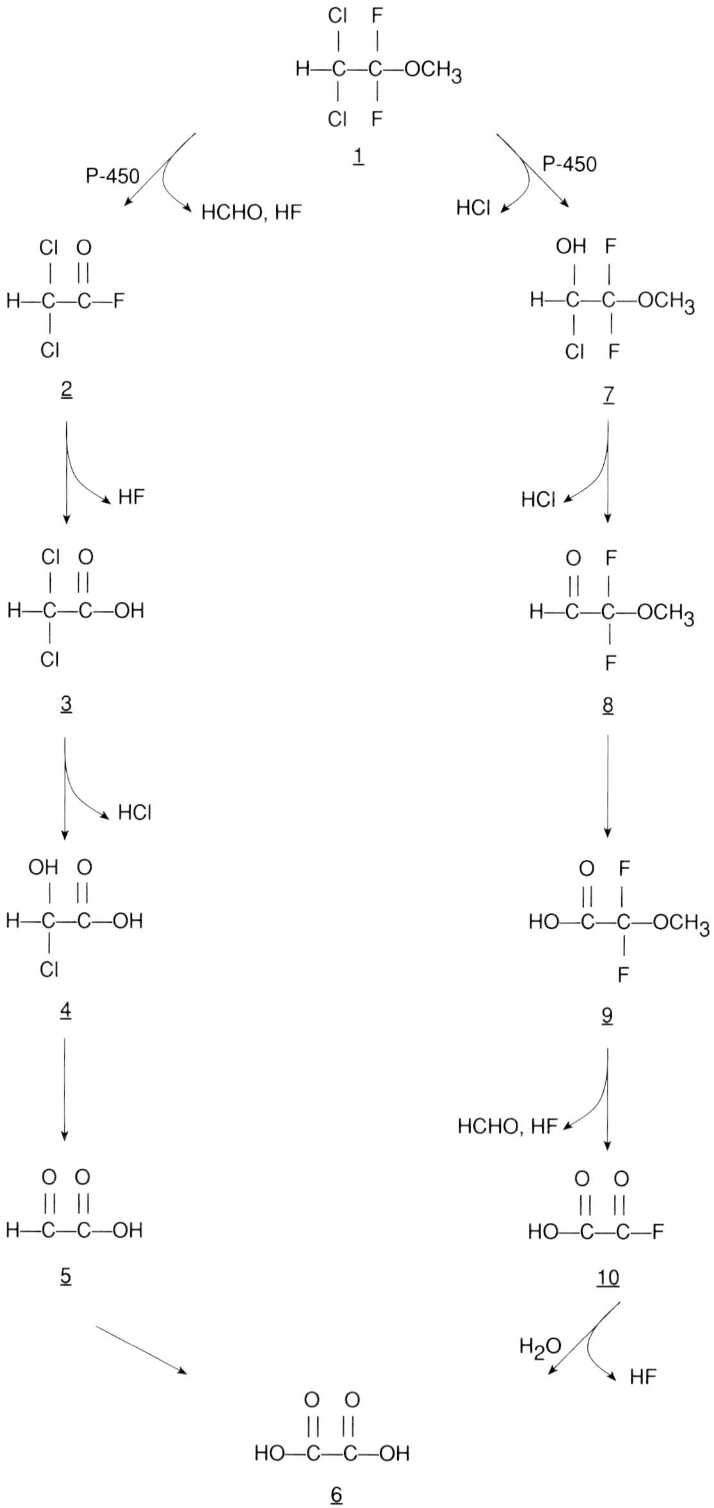

Role of Reactive Episulfonium Ions in Nephrotoxicity

Glutathione-dependent metabolism of 1,2-dichloroethane, 1,2-dibromoethane and 1,2-dibromo-3-chloropropane by the hepatic and renal cytosolic fractions of rats and mice has been reported (71,129). Direct evidence for the formation of *S*-(2-haloethyl)glutathione and *S*-(2-haloethyl)cysteine (Fig. 5) after 1,2-dichloroethane and 1,2-dibromoethane treatments, is not available, but cysteine conjugates that could arise from these metabolites have been isolated from the urine of rats given 1,2-dihaloethane (130). Recently, *S*-(2-chloroethyl)glutathione was identified as a metabolite of 1-bromo-2-chloroethane in the rat (131). Treatment of rats with *S*-(2-chloroethyl)cysteine or *S*-(2-chloroethyl)glutathione resulted in dose- and time-dependent increases in blood urea nitrogen and urine glucose concentrations (113, 114). These biochemical changes were associated with acute proximal tubular necrosis, most notably in the juxtaglomerular regions. In addition, no hepatic lesions were seen following the administration of either conjugate (113,114). *In vitro*, *S*-(2-chloroethyl)cysteine inhibited *p*-aminohippurate ion uptake in both brush border membrane and basolateral membrane vesicles, the activities of γ-glutamyl transpeptidase (a brush border membrane enzyme marker), Na^+K^+–ATPase (a basolateral membrane enzyme marker), and state 3 respiration in rat kidney mitochondria (72,132).

The biochemical basis of *S*-(2-chloroethyl)glutathione and *S*-(2-chloroethyl)cysteine target organ selectivity was investigated using probenecid and AT-125 [L-α-*S*,5*S*)-α-amino-3-chloro-4,5-dihydro-5-isoxazoleacetic acid], inhibitors of the organic acid transport system and γ-glutamyl transpeptidase, respectively (113,114, 132). Treatment of rats with probenecid protected against the nephrotoxicity of both conjugates. *In vitro*, pretreatment with probenecid protected against *S*-(2-chloroethyl)cysteine–induced inhibition of the γ-glutamyl transpeptidase activity in brush border membrane, but had no effect on the Na^+K^+–ATPase in basolateral membrane vesicles (132). These results suggest that renal transport mechanisms play an important role in determining the target organ of toxicity caused by these *S*-conjugates, possibly by allowing their accumulation in renal tubular cells. Pretreatment with AT-125 did not inhibit the nephrotoxicity of *S*-(2-chloroethyl)glutathione in rats (114) indicating that γ-glutamyl transpeptidase activity is not involved in *S*-(2-chloroethyl)glutathione-induced nephrotoxicity. This experiment, however, does not determine whether metabolism of *S*-(2-chloroethyl)glutathione by γ-glutamyl cyclotransferase, which is present inside the renal tubular cell (133), plays a role in *S*-(2-chloroethyl)glutathione–induced nephrotoxicity.

FIG. 4. Postulated pathways for the cytochrome P-450–dependent bioactivation of 2,2-dichloro-1,1-difluoro-1-methoxyethane (*1*) to oxalic acid (*6*) and fluoride ion. *2*, 2,2-dichloroacetylfluoride; *3*, dichloroacetic acid; *4*, hydroxychloroacetic acid; *5*, glyoxalic acid; *7*, 2-chloro-1,1-difluoro-2-hydroxy-1-methoxyethane; *8*, 2,2-difluoromethoxyacetaldehyde; *9*, 2,2-difluoromethoxy acetic acid; *10*, monooxalyl fluoride.

TABLE 2. *Aliphatic halogenated hydrocarbons whose glutathione or cysteine S-conjugates are shown to be nephrotoxic*

Chemical name (common name)	Reference(s)
I. Haloalkanes	
1,2-Dichloroethane (ethylene dichloride)	113,114
II. Haloalkenes	
Trichloroethylene	27,115–118
Tetrachloroethylene (perchloroethylene)	119,120
Tetrafluoroethylene	30,121
1-Chloro-1,2,2-trifluoroethylene	122–125
1,1-Dichloro-2,2-difluoroethylene	34,126
1,1-Dibromo-2,2-difluoroethylene	34,126
1,1,2-Trichloro-3,3,3-trifluoro-1-propene	37
Hexafluoropropene	119,127
Hexachlorobutadiene	41
III. Haloalkynes	
Dichloroacetylene	128

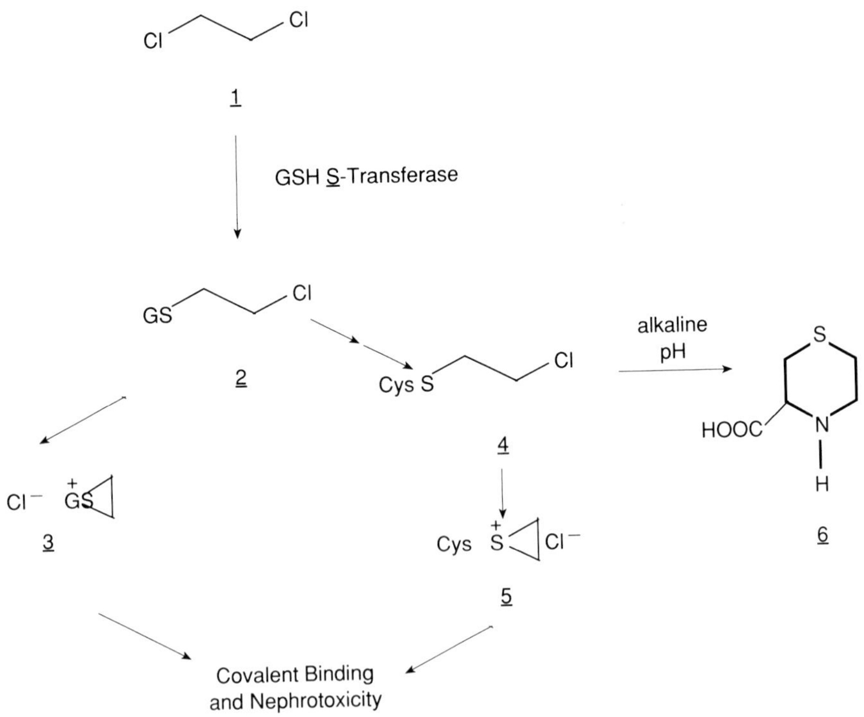

FIG. 5. Postulated mechanism for the glutathione-dependent bioactivation of 1,2-dichloroethane (*1*) to glutathione- and cysteine-derived episulfonium ions (*3,5*). (*2*), *S*-(2-chloroethyl)glutathione; *4*, *S*-(2-chloroethyl)cysteine; *6*, thiomorpholine-3-carboxylic acid.

The findings that *S*-(2-chloroethyl)cysteine is not a substrate for cysteine conjugate β-lyase, and that equimolar doses of analogues of *S*-(2-chloroethyl)cysteine, namely *S*-ethylcysteine, *S*-(2-hydroxyethyl)cysteine, and *S*-(3-chloropropyl)cysteine, failed to produce nephrotoxicity *in vivo* or cytotoxicity *in vitro* (113,134) provide evidence for the role of an episulfonium ion, formed by the intramolecular displacement of the chlorine atom by the sulfur atom (Fig. 5), in *S*-(2-chloroethyl) cysteine–induced nephrotoxicity. In the case of *S*-ethylcysteine, an episulfonium ion cannot occur; with *S*-(2-hydroxyethyl)cysteine, episulfonium ion formation is unlikely, because the hydroxyl group is not a good leaving group; with *S*-(3-chloropropyl)cysteine, formation of a 4-membered ring sulfonium ion is kinetically much less favored than formation of a 3-membered ring episulfonium ion.

Thiomorpholine-3-carboxylic acid (Fig. 5) is a chemically stable product formed by the internal displacement of the chlorine atom by the amino group under nonphysiological alkaline conditions (135). The finding that this chemical was much less toxic than *S*-(2-chloroethyl)cysteine (136), along with the fact that thiomorpholine-3-carboxylic acid was not detected under physiological pH or following exposure of rats to either 1,2-dichloroethane or *S*-(2-chloroethyl)cysteine, suggest that thiomorpholine-3-carboxylic acid is not likely to play a major role in either *S*-(2-chloroethyl)cysteine or 1,2-dichloroethane–induced nephrotoxicity. It is of interest to note that *S*-(2-chloroethyl)cysteine was a more efficient alkylating agent *in vitro* and a more potent nephrotoxin *in vivo* than *S*-(2-chloroethyl)glutathione (114,135, 137).

Collectively, these results suggest that hepatic and renal glutathione *S*-transferase–catalyzed reactions between 1,2-dichloroethane and glutathione may yield *S*-(2-chloroethyl)glutathione (Fig. 5). Hepatic *S*-(2-chloroethyl)glutathione may be translocated into kidney tubular cells via the circulation and a probenecid-sensitive organic acid transport system. An electrophilic episulfonium ion may form directly by the internal displacement of the second chlorine atom by the sulfur atom, or after metabolism of *S*-(2-chloroethyl)glutathione by γ-glutamyl cyclotransferase and peptidases to yield *S*-(2-chloroethyl)cysteine. Alkylation of critical renal macromolecules by episulfonium ions appears to initiate the cascade of events leading to cytotoxicity and cell death. Further studies, however, are needed to clarify these events and how they may relate to nephrotoxicity. In addition, although reactive episulfonium ions have been implicated in the bioactivation of 1,2-dibromoethane and 1,2-dibromo-3-chloropropane to mutagenic and cytotoxic metabolites (138, 139), the role of episulfonium ions in the nephrotoxicity of these chemicals remains unclear.

Role of Cysteine Conjugate β-Lyase–Dependent Activation in Nephrotoxicity

The second type of nephrotoxic glutathione *S*-conjugates is exemplified by the conjugates of haloalkenes (Table 2), such as trichloroethylene, chlorotrifluoroethylene, tetrafluoroethylene, 1,1,2-trichloro-3,3,3-trifluoro-1-propene, and hexachlorobutadiene. The nephrotoxicity of these conjugates requires cleavage of the corresponding cysteine conjugates by cysteine conjugate β-lyase to generate reactive thiols (Fig. 6) which are believed to be the proximate or ultimate toxic species (59).

Biosynthesis of Haloalkene Glutathione S-Conjugates

For several nephrotoxic haloalkenes, glutathione conjugate formation by glutathione *S*-transferases of rat and mouse liver and kidney has been demonstrated and the products characterized (30,37,120,127,140–145). It is of interest to note that, with several haloalkenes, hepatic microsomal glutathione *S*-transferase is more efficient in catalyzing glutathione conjugate formation than cytosolic glutathione *S*-transferases (140–142). In addition, depending on the structure of the haloalkene used, substitution and/or addition products are also formed. For example, with chlorotrifluoroethylene and tetrafluoroethylene, the addition products, *S*-(2-chloro-1,1,2-trifluoroethyl)glutathione and *S*-(1,1,2,2-tetrafluoroethyl)glutathione, respectively, are formed, whereas with hexachlorobutadiene and tetrachloroethylene, the substitution products, *S*-(1,1,2,3,4-pentachlorobutadiene)glutathione and *S*-(1,2,2-trichlorovinyl)glutathione, respectively, are formed. Both the addition and substitution products, *S*-(1,1,2,3,3,3-hexafluoropropyl)glutathione and *S*-(1,2,3,3,3-pentafluoropropenyl)glutathione, respectively, are formed when hexafluoropro-

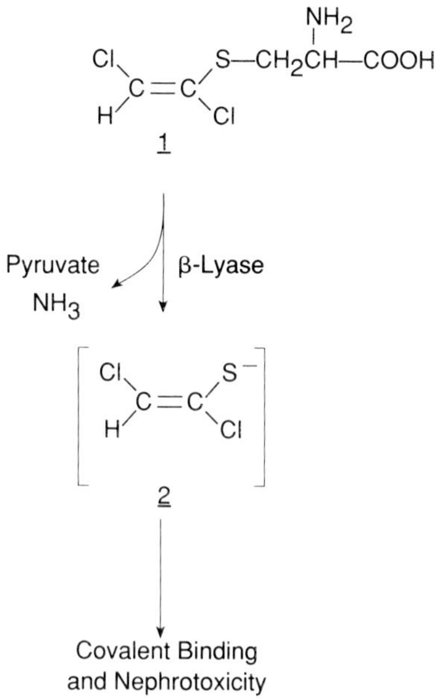

FIG. 6. Bioactivation of *S*-(1,2-dichlorovinyl)-L-cysteine (*1*) to a reactive thiol (*2*) by cysteine conjugate β-lyase.

pene is incubated with rat hepatic microsomes or cytosol in the presence of glutathione. Incubation of hexafluoropropene with rat kidney cytosol and glutathione, however, results in the exclusive formation of *S*-(1,1,2,3,3,3-hexafluoropropyl) glutathione, whereas no glutathione conjugates are detected in the presence of kidney microsomes (127).

Evidence for the glutathione conjugate pathway *in vivo* has been obtained by the identification of the glutathione, cysteinylglycine, cysteine, and *N*-acetylcysteine conjugates in bile and urine (26,27,30,37,41,127,143,145,146). Current evidence suggests that the fate of the biliary metabolites and their role in haloalkene-induced nephrotoxicity may depend on the haloalkene used. For example, rats fitted with a biliary cannula were significantly protected from the nephrotoxicity of hexachlorobutadiene, whereas nephrotoxicity was observed when rats were given bile containing hexachlorobutadiene metabolites (41). These results show that hepatic metabolites of hexachlorobutadiene are primarily responsible for the nephrotoxicity of hexachlorobutadiene. With hexafluoropropene, however, the only urinary metabolite detected was *N*-acetyl-*S*-(1,1,2,3,3,3-hexafluoropropyl)-L-cysteine; none of its precursors were detected in bile (127). The only biliary metabolite detected with hexafluoropropene was *S*-(1,2,3,3,3-pentafluoropropenyl)glutathione. These results suggest that the hexafluoropropene biliary glutathione conjugate metabolite was not translocated to the kidney and that intrarenal metabolism of hexafluoropropene may be responsible for the appearance of *N*-acetyl-*S*(1,1,2,3,3,3-hexafluoropropyl)-L-cysteine in urine, and for hexafluoropropene-induced nephrotoxicity.

Translocation of Plasma Glutathione and Cysteine S-*conjugates into the Kidney*

Renal tubular cells may be exposed to higher concentrations of glutathione and cysteine *S*-conjugates due to a variety of mechanisms (60,63). Metabolism of the glutathione conjugates by γ-glutamyl transpeptidase and aminopeptidase M, which may occur at both the brush border and basolateral membranes, is usually followed by uptake of cysteine conjugates by renal proximal tubular cells (116,147). Alternatively, plasma glutathione *S*-conjugates may be actively transported across the basolateral membrane by a sodium-dependent uptake mechanism that is inhibited by probenecid but not by cysteine *S*-conjugates (148). The glutathione *S*-conjugates that are transported into renal proximal tubular cells may undergo metabolism by γ-glutamyl cyclotransferase and peptidases to yield the corresponding cysteine *S*-conjugates (114,133).

The transport of nephrotoxic cysteine and *N*-acetylcysteine *S*-conjugates in freshly isolated rat renal proximal tubular cells, LLC-PK_1 kidney cell line, rat kidney cortex membrane vesicles, rat kidney proximal tubules, and rabbit renal cortical slices has been characterized (147–156). These studies provide evidence for the role of both the Na^+-dependent organic acid transport system and the Na^+-independent transport systems L and T in the renal uptake of cysteine conjugates; with *N*-acetylcysteine *S*-conjugates, the Na^+-dependent organic acid transport system appears to be the only transport system involved.

Renal Metabolism of Nephrotoxic Cysteine Conjugates by Cysteine Conjugate β-Lyase

As shown in Table 2, several haloalkene cysteine *S*-conjugates are selective nephrotoxins. Histopathological examination of renal tissues has shown that lesions appear to be localized in the straight portion of the proximal tubule, known as the S_3 segment. Current evidence suggests that metabolism of nephrotoxic cysteine conjugates, e.g., *S*-(1,2-dichlorovinyl)-L-cysteine (Fig. 6), by renal cysteine conjugate β-lyase yields reactive sulfur-containing fragments, which alkylate renal macromolecules leading to nephrotoxicity (59–68,72,116–118,157–161). This evidence is based on the following findings: (a) aminooxyacetic acid, an inhibitor of β-lyase, protects against cysteine *S*-conjugate nephrotoxicity; (b) α-methylcysteine conjugates, which cannot be metabolized by β-lyase, are not nephrotoxic; (c) α-keto acids enhance β-lyase activity and potentiate the cytotoxicity of cysteine *S*-conjugates; (d) homocysteine analogues of nephrotoxic cysteine *S*-conjugates, which are metabolized to reactive thiols similar to those produced from the cysteine conjugates, are also nephrotoxic; (e) kidney mitoplasts, which do not contain most of the mitochondrial β-lyase activity, are much less susceptible than mitochondria to the toxicity of cysteine *S*-conjugates; (f) species differences in β-lyase activity correlate with that of *S*-(1,2-dichlorovinyl)-L-cysteine–induced toxicity; (g) *in vivo* and *in vitro* β-lyase–dependent covalent binding of cysteine *S*-conjugates to renal macromolecules correlate with the nephrotoxicity of these conjugates.

The biochemical basis for the *in vivo* target organ selectivity of cysteine *S*-conjugates was investigated using *S*-(2-benzothiazolyl)-L-cysteine and *S*-(6-purinyl)-L-cysteine as models (159,162). These conjugates, in contrast to nephrotoxic cysteine conjugates, are metabolized by β-lyase to stable thiols (Figs. 7 and 8). Treatment of rats with *S*-(6-purinyl)-L-cysteine resulted in the detection of 6-mercaptopurine and its further metabolites, 6-methylthiopurine and 6-thiouric acid. Treatment of rats with *S*-(2-benzothiazolyl)-L-cysteine resulted in the detection of 2-mercaptobenzothiazole and its *S*-glucuronic acid. At 30 min after *S*-(6-purinyl)-L-cysteine treatment, renal concentrations of 6-mercaptopurine and its metabolites were nearly 90- and 2.5-fold higher than that of plasma and liver, respectively, whereas with *S*-(2-benzothiazolyl)-L-cysteine, kidney, liver, and plasma concentrations of 2-mercaptobenzothiazole and its glucuronic acid, were similar. Current evidence suggest, that the target organ selectivity of *S*-(6-purinyl)-L-cysteine may be at least in part due to differences in the rates of metabolism of this conjugate by hepatic and renal β-lyases since rates of *S*-(6-purinyl)-L-cysteine metabolism by renal β-lyases were much higher than those of liver β-lyases (185). With *S*-(2-benzothiazolyl)-L-cysteine, the lack of selectivity was attributed at least in part to the similar rates of metabolism of this conjugate by hepatic and renal β-lyases (159,162).

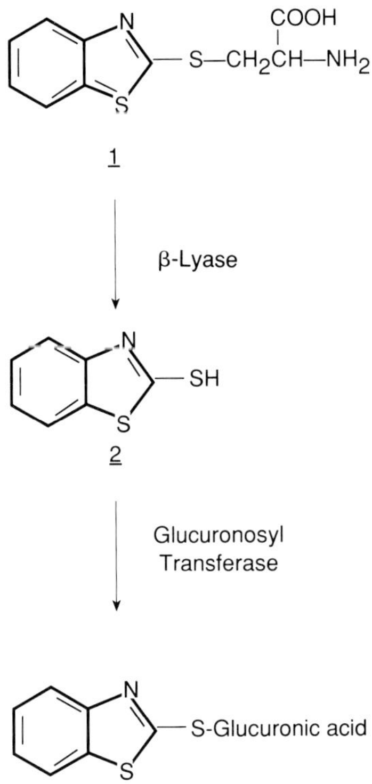

FIG. 7. Postulated pathways for the *in vivo* metabolism of *S*-(2-benzothiazolyl)-L-cysteine (*1*) to 2-mercaptobenzothiazole (*2*) and 2-mercaptobenzothiazole *S*-glucuronic acid (*3*).

Although the roles of renal β-lyase and renal transport mechanisms in the toxicity of haloalkene *S*-conjugates have been established, several findings remain to be clarified. For example, with isolated rat kidney cells, aminooxyacetic acid was a potent inhibitor of β-lyase activity, but did not completely protect the cells from the cytotoxicity of *S*-(1,2-dichlorovinyl)-L-cysteine (160); in rabbits, *S*-(1,2-dichlorovinyl)-D-cysteine, which is not a substrate for β-lyase, was shown to be as equally nephrotoxic as the optical isomer, *S*-(1,2-dichlorovinyl)-L-cysteine (163); the distribution of the cytosolic β-lyase within the proximal tubule, as determined by immunocytochemistry, is inconsistent with the hypothesis that a higher concentration of the enzyme in the S_3 segment may explain the segment sensitivity to nephrotoxic cysteine conjugates (164). These results clearly show that further studies are needed to fully understand the mechanisms of activation and toxicity of cysteine *S*-conjugates.

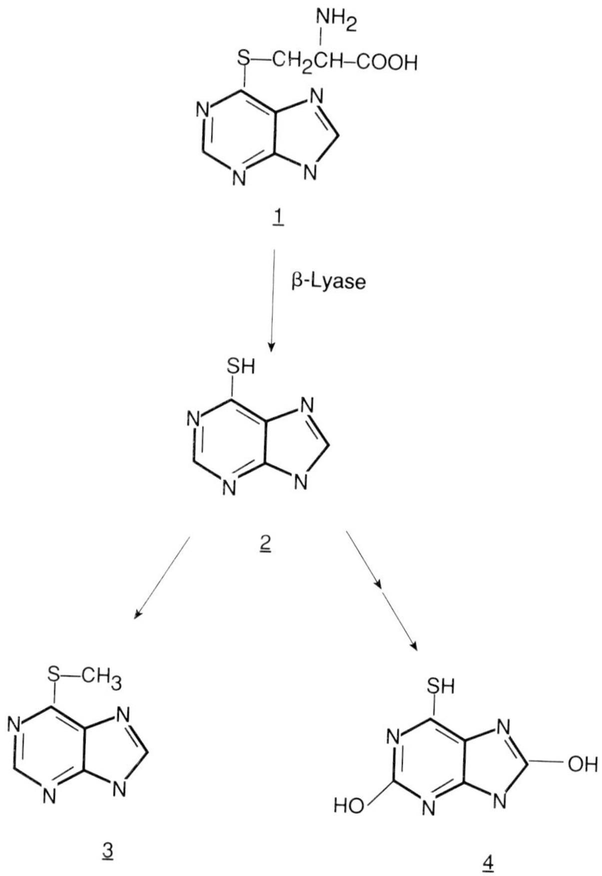

FIG. 8. Postulated pathways for the *in vivo* metabolism of *S*-(6-purinyl)-L-cysteine (*1*) to 6-mercaptopurine (*2*), 6-methylthiopurine (*3*), and 6-thiouric acid (*4*).

Regulation of In Vivo *Conjugate β-Lyase Activity*

As indicated above, *in vitro* experiments have shown that cysteine conjugate β-lyase activity is regulated by the inclusion of α-keto acids (157,165). However, the extent to which such a regulation may play a role in the target organ and segment selectivity of cysteine conjugate toxicity is unclear. Moreover, current evidence suggests that nephrotoxic cysteine *S*-conjugates that are transported into renal proximal tubular cells may undergo metabolism by a variety of enzymes (Fig. 9), including cysteine conjugate *N*-acetyltransferase, cysteine conjugate β-lyase, cysteine conjugate *S*-oxidase, cysteine conjugate transaminases, and L-amino acid oxidase (72,73,112,117,165–168). Evidence has been provided that the relative contributions of these enzymatic reactions determine the *in vivo* β-lyase activity and affect

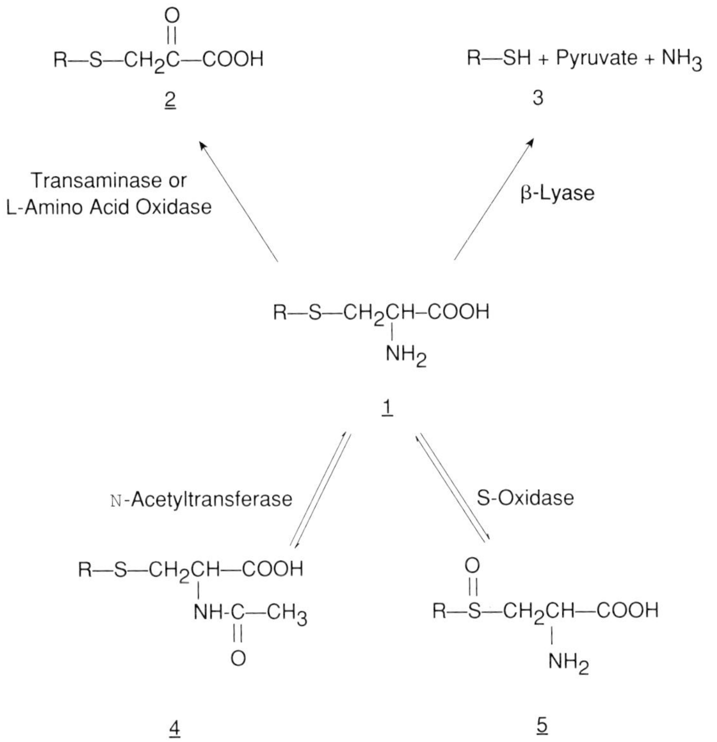

FIG. 9. Pathways for the *in vivo* metabolism of cysteine *S*-conjugates (*1*) to α-keto acids (*2*), thiols (*3*), mercapturic acids (*4*), and sulfoxides (*5*).

the toxicity of cysteine *S*-conjugates. For example, the higher *in vivo* β-lyase activity of guinea pigs, compared to rats, mice, and hamsters, is attributed to a lower cysteine conjugate *N*-acetyltransferase activity in the guinea pig compared to the other species rather than a difference in rates of metabolism by β-lyase (159). In addition, guinea pigs and calves, which have lower cysteine *S*-conjugate *N*-acetyltransferase activities than rats are much more sensitive to *S*-(1,2-dichlorovinyl)-L-cysteine-induced toxicity (159,169).

Although mercapturic acids can be deacetylated to regenerate the cysteine conjugates, deacetylation reactions may occur at slower rates compared with the rates of excretion of mercapturic acid into urine, or the rates of metabolism by β-lyase. Consistent with this hypothesis, is the finding that *in vitro* and *in vivo* toxicity and covalent binding of nephrotoxic cysteine *S*-conjugates are higher than that of the corresponding mercapturic acids (117,121,126,153). Although these results indicate that acetylation/deacetylation reactions play a role in the toxicity of cysteine *S*-conjugates, the finding that rabbit renal cortical slices incubated with either *S*-(1,2-dichlorovinyl)-L-cysteine or its mercapturic acid exhibited similar S_3 segment specificity (154), suggests that these reactions do not play an important role in the segment specificity of nephrotoxic cysteine *S*-conjugates.

Metabolism of nephrotoxic cysteine *S*-conjugates by L-amino acid oxidases or transaminases may produce the corresponding α-keto acids (166,167). Although metabolism of nephrotoxic cysteine *S*-conjugates by these enzymes may not contribute directly to *S*-conjugate covalent binding to renal macromolecules, further studies are needed to clarify the role of these enzymes in *S*-conjugate–induced toxicity.

Sulfoxidation of cysteine *S*-conjugates is a major metabolic pathway *in vivo*, but not until recently have the nature of the enzymes involved and their role in the metabolism and toxicity of *S*-conjugates been investigated (73). Current evidence indicates that sulfoxidation of cysteine *S*-conjugates is catalyzed by flavin-containing monooxygenases rather than by cytochrome P-450–dependent monooxygenases or peroxidases. Preliminary results indicate that the formation of *S*-conjugate sulfoxides may be of toxicological significance. For example, *S*-(1,2-dichlorovinyl)-L-cysteine sulfoxide, a putative metabolite of *S*-(1,2-dichlorovinyl)-L-cysteine, was found to be a much more potent nephrotoxin than *S*-(1,2-dichlorovinyl)-L-cysteine (170). The sulfoxidation of *S*-(1,2-dichlorovinyl)-L-cysteine allows the molecule to act as a Michael acceptor in its reactions with biological nucleophiles leading to depletion of glutathione and toxicity (171). Hence, sulfoxidation of cysteine *S*-conjugates may alter the metabolism and disposition of cysteine *S*-conjugates, and may represent a novel mechanism of activation of *S*-conjugates.

In summary, the *in vivo* metabolism of nephrotoxic cysteine *S*-conjugates is a complicated process. Evidence has been presented for the metabolism of cysteine *S*-conjugates by β-lyase, *N*-acetyltransferase, transaminase, L-amino acid oxidase, and *S*-oxidase. However, the role of each pathway in the nephrotoxicity of *S*-conjugates is not well understood. Therefore, additional studies are needed to fully understand the role of the various metabolic pathways and how they may relate to the target organ and segment selectivity of nephrotoxic cysteine *S*-conjugates.

CYTOTOXICITY OF CYSTEINE *S*-CONJUGATES

The cytotoxicity of haloalkene cysteine *S*-conjugates in isolated rat renal epithelial cells, LLC-PK_1 cell line, and primary cultures of human proximal tubular cells has been characterized (126,147,150,156,157,160,172–175). These studies provided further evidence for the role of renal transport systems and metabolism by β-lyase in the toxicity of these conjugates. These studies have also shown that mitochondria may be the primary targets of nephrotoxic cysteine *S*-conjugates, since alterations in mitochondrial function were strongly correlated with decreases in cell viability (160). Formation of plasma membrane blebs appeared to be associated with a loss of Ca^{2+} from the mitochondria and an elevation of cytosolic Ca^{2+} concentration (172,175). In LLC-PK_1 cells, depletion of nonprotein thiols and formation of lipid peroxidation products occurred prior to cell death (174).

The mechanism by which haloalkene cysteine *S*-conjugates produce toxicity in rat kidney mitochondria was studied (176–178). The results indicate that the inhibition of energy metabolism and the oxidation of glutathione are among the early events that lead to alterations in mitochondrial function and irreversible damage to mitochondrial structure. The finding that some of the mitochondrial covalent binding from ^{35}S-labeled conjugates was removed by treatment with dithiothreitol, suggests that mixed disulfides may have been formed by the reaction of the reactive sulfur metabolites generated from *S*-conjugates and the sulfhydryl groups of cellular protein. In LLC-PK_1 cells, dithiothreitol blocked lipid peroxidation and toxicity at a step beyond the depletion of nonprotein thiols and covalent binding (174). *N,N'*-diphenyl-*p*-phenylenediamine, an antioxidant, inhibited the cytotoxicity of *S*-(1,2-dichlorovinyl)-L-cysteine in both LLC-PK_1 cells and isolated rat kidney proximal tubular cells at *S*-(1,2-dichlorovinyl)-L-cysteine concentrations of 250 to 500 and 25 to 50 μM, respectively. The inability of the antioxidants to protect isolated kidney cells against the cytotoxicity of *S*-(1,2-dichlorovinyl)-L-cysteine at concentrations higher than 50 μM suggests that a nonperoxidative mechanism, e.g., extensive covalent modifications, may become the primary mechanism involved in cell death at high *S*-conjugate concentrations. Consistent with this hypothesis is the finding that freshly isolated cells exhibit higher bioactivation rates than the LLC-PK_1 cells (174). Nevertheless, it does appear that mitochondrial and/or cellular lipid peroxidation events play a significant role in the mechanism of cysteine *S*-conjugate–induced cytotoxicity.

Evidence for the role of lipid peroxidation in the *in vivo* nephrotoxicity of haloalkene cysteine *S*-conjugates is indicated by the recent report that *S*-(1,2-dichlorovinyl)-L-cysteine depletes kidney glutathione concentrations and initiates lipid peroxidation *in vivo* (179). It is of interest to note that *in vivo* treatment of rats with hexachlorobutadiene inhibited the glutathione reductase activity in the renal cortex prior to the development of marked morphological damage (180). Recent results have also indicated that methimazole, an antioxidant, protects against the *in vivo* nephrotoxicity of *S*-(1,2-dichlorovinyl)-L-cysteine (181,182).

CONCLUDING REMARKS

Significant progress has been made in the past 10 years with regard to the mechanisms of activation of halogenated hydrocarbons, the biochemical basis for species and target organ selectivity, and the critical cellular events that lead to the expression of nephrotoxicity. In addition, the role of β-lyase in the mechanisms of cytotoxicity of nephrotoxic cysteine *S*-conjugates was validated with primary cultures of human proximal tubular cells (173). Furthermore, the human kidney enzymes believed to be involved in aliphatic halogenated hydrocarbon-induced nephrotoxicity have been isolated and characterized (77,80,183). It is clear, however, that the mechanisms of aliphatic halogenated hydrocarbon-induced nephrotoxicity are more complex than previously anticipated. In addition, the recent report that mice fetal kidneys during late gestation were able to activate *S*-(1,2-dichlorovinyl)-L-cysteine poses new questions with regard to the potential toxicity of *S*-conjugates in fetal kidneys (184). Future studies should provide detailed information with regard to the bioactivation of halogenated hydrocarbons, the biochemical basis of its target organ and segment specificity, and the roles of cysteine conjugate *S*-oxidase and lipid peroxidation in the nephrotoxicity of cysteine *S*-conjugates. Studies aimed at evaluation of human risk based on cell culture or animal models are also warranted.

ACKNOWLEDGMENTS

Studies conducted in the author's laboratory were supported by National Institute of Environmental Health Sciences Institutional Grant T32 ES07015, a Biomedical Research Support grant from the University of Wisconsin–Madison, and Grant IN-35-31-21 from the American Cancer Society.

REFERENCES

1. Morgan KT, Swenberg JA, Hamm TE Jr, Wokowski-Tyl R, Phelps M. Histopathology of acute toxic response in rats and mice exposed to methylene chloride by inhalation. *Fundam Appl Toxicol* 1982;2:293–299.
2. Chellman GJ, White RD, Norton RM, Bus JS. Inhibition of the acute toxicity of methylene chloride in male B6C3F1 mice by glutathione depletion. *Toxicol Appl Pharmacol* 1986;86:93–104.
3. Kluwe WM, Harrington FW, Cooper SE. Toxic effects of organohalide compounds on renal tubular cells *in vivo* and *in vitro*. *J Pharmacol Exp Ther* 1982;220:597–603.
4. Eschenbrenner AB, Miller E. Sex differences in kidney morphology and chloroform necrosis. *Science* 1945;102:302–303.
5. Torkelson TE, Oyen F, Rowe VK. The toxicology of chloroform as determined by single and repeated exposure of laboratory animals. *Am Ind Hyg Assoc J* 1976;37:697–705.
6. Smith JH, Maita K, Sleight SD, Hook JB. Mechanism of cholorform toxicity. I. Time course of chloroform toxicity in male and female mice. *Toxicol Appl Pharmacol* 1983;70:467–479.
7. Sirota J. Carbon tetrachloride poisoning in man. I. The mechanisms of renal failure and recovery. *J Clin Invest* 1949;28:1412–1422.
8. Guild WR, Young JV, Merril JP. Anuria due to carbon tetrachloride intoxication. *Am J Pathol* 1958;48:1221–1227.
9. Cornish HH, Ryan RC. A study of carbon tetrachloride. VI. Aminoaciduria in response to carbon tetrachloride inhalation. *Toxicol Appl Pharmacol* 1964;6:96–102.
10. Alston WC. Hepatic and renal complications arising from accidental carbon tetrachloride poisoning in the human subject. *J Clin Pathol* 1970;23:249–253.
11. Spencer HC, Rowe VK, Adams EM, McCollister DD, Irish DD. Vapor toxicity of ethylene dichloride determined by experiments on laboratory animals. *Arch Ind Hyg Occup Med* 1951;4:482–493.
12. Rowe VK, Spencer JC, McCollister DD, Hollingsworth RL, Adams EM. Toxicity of ethylene dibromide determined on experimental animals. *Arch Ind Hyg Occup Med* 1952;6:158–173.
13. Olmstead EV. Pathological changes in ethylene dibromide poisoning. *Arch Ind Health* 1960;21: 525–529.
14. Plaa GL, Larson RE. Relative nephrotoxic properties of chlorinated methane, ethane, and ethylene derivatives in mice. *Toxicol Appl Pharmacol* 1965;7:37–44.
15. Klaassen CD, Plaa GL. Relative effects of various chlorinated hydrocarbons on liver and kidney function in mice. *Toxicol Appl Pharmacol* 1966;8:139–151.
16. Jones AR, Porter K, Stevenson D. The renal toxicity of some halogenated derivatives of propane in the rat. *Naturwissenschaften* 1981;68:98–99.
17. Kluwe WM, McNish R, Hook JB. Acute nephrotoxicities and hepatotoxicities of 1,2-dibromo-3-chloropropane and 1,2-dibromoethane in male and female F344 rats. *Toxicol Lett* 1981;8:317–321.

18. Kluwe WM. Acute toxocity of 1,2-dibromo-3-chloropropane in the F344 male rats. I. Dose-response relationships and differences in routes of exposures. *Toxicol Appl Pharmacol* 1981;59:71–83.
19. Omichinski JG, Brunborg G, Soderlund EJ, et al. Renal necrosis and DNA damage caused by selectively deuterated and methylated analogs of 1,2-dibromo-3-chloropropane in the rat. *Toxicol Appl Pharmacol* 1987;91:358–370.
20. Soderlund EJ, Lag M, Holme JA, et al. Species differences in kidney necrosis and DNA damage, distribution and glutathione-dependent metabolism of 1,2-dibromo-3-chloropropane. *Pharmacol Toxicol* 1990;66:287–293.
21. Pendergast JA, Jones RA, Jenkins LJ, Siegal J. Effects on experimental animals of long term inhalation of trichloroethylene, carbon tetrachloride, 1,1,1-trichloroethane, dichloro-difluoromethane and 1,1-dichloroethylene. *Toxicol Appl Pharmacol* 1967;10:270–289.
22. Jenkins LJ, Andersen ME. 1,1-Dichloroethylene nephrotoxicity in the rat. *Toxicol Appl Pharmacol* 1978;46:131–141.
23. Jackson NM, Conolly RB. Acute nephrotoxicity of 1,1-dichloroethylene in the rat after inhalation exposure. *Toxicol Lett* 1985;29:191–199.
24. E.P.A. Vinylidine chloride: health and environmental impacts. *EPA Office of Toxic Substances* 1976;560/6-76-023.
25. National Toxicology Program. Toxicology and carcinogenesis studies of trichloroethylene in F344/N rats and B6C3F1 mice (gavage). Pub. No. (NH) 1982;83-1799.
26. Dekant W, Metzler M, Henschler D. Identification of *S*-(1,2-dichlorovinyl)-*N*-acetyl cysteine as a urinary metabolite of trichloroethylene: a possible explanation for its nephrocarcinogenicity in male rats. *Biochem Pharmacol* 1986;35:2455–2458.
27. Dekant W, Koob M, Henschler D. Metabolism of trichloroethene—*in vivo* and *in vitro* evidence for activation by glutathione conjugation. *Chem Biol Interact* 1990;73:89–101.
28. Current Intelligence Bulletin, No. 20. *Tetrachloroethylene (perchloroethylene)*. U.S. Dept. of Health, Education and Welfare, PHS, NIOSH, January, 1978.
29. National Toxicolgy Program NTP TR 311. United States Dept. of Health, Education and Welfare, United States Public Health Service, Washington, DC, 1986.
30. Odum J, Green T. The metabolism and nephrotoxicity of tetrafluoroethylene in the rat. *Toxicol Appl Pharmacol* 1984;76:306–318.
31. Potter CL, Gandolfi AJ, Nagle R, Clayton JW. Effects of inhaled chlorotrifluoroethylene and hexafluoropropene on the rat kidney. *Toxicol Appl Pharmacol* 1981;59:431–440.
32. Buckley LA, Clayton JW, Nagle RB, Gandolfi AJ. Chlorotrifluoroethylene nephrotoxicity in rats: a subacute study. *Fundam Appl Toxicol* 1982;2:181–186.
33. Commandeur JNM, Oosterdorp RAJ, Schoofs PR, Xu B, Vermeulen NPE. Nephrotoxicity and hepatotoxicity of 1,1-dichloro-2,2-difluoroethylene in the rat. Implications for the differential mechanisms of bioactivation. *Biochem Pharmacol* 1987;36:4229–4237.
34. Commandeur JNM, Brakenhoff JPG, DeKanter FJJ, Vermeulen NPE. Nephrotoxicity of mercapturic acids of three structurally related 2,2-difluoroethylenes in the rat. Implications for different bioactivation mechanisms. *Biochem Pharmacol* 1988;37:4495–4504.
35. Torkelson TR, Oyen F. The toxicity of 1,3-dichloropropene as determined by repeated exposure of laboratory animals. *Am Ind Hyg Assoc J* 1977;38:217–223.
36. Osterloh J, Xiwen H. Effects of 1,3-dichloropropene on the kidney of Fischer 344 rats after pretreatment with diethylmaleate, buthionine sulfoximine, and aminooxyacetic acid. *J Toxicol Environ Health* 1990;28:247–255.
37. Vamvakas S, Kremling E, Dekant W. Metabolic activation of the nephrotoxic haloalkene 1,1,2-trichloro-3,3,3-trifluoro-1-propene by glutathione conjugation. *Biochem Pharmacol* 1989;38: 2297–2304.
38. Berndt WO, Mehendale HM. Effects of hexachlorobutadiene on renal function and renal organic ion transport in the rat. *Toxicology* 1979;14:55–65.
39. Lock EA, Ishmael J. The acute toxic effects of hexachlorobutadiene on rat kidney. *Arch Toxicol* 1979;43:47–57.
40. Hook JB, Ishmael J, Lock EA. Nephrotoxicity of hexachloro-1,3-butadiene in the rat: the effect of age, sex and strain. *Toxicol Appl Pharmacol* 1983;67:122–131.
41. Nash JA, King LJ, Lock EA, Green T. The metabolism and disposition of hexachloro-1,3-butadiene in the rat and its relevance to nephrotoxicity. *Toxicol Appl Pharmacol* 1984;73:124–137.
42. Lock EA, Ishmael J, Hook JB. Nephrotoxicity of hexachloro-1,3-butadiene in the mouse: the

effects of age, sex, strain, monooxygenase modifiers, and the role of glutathione. *Toxicol Appl Pharmacol* 1984;72:484–494.
43. Adams EM, Spencer HC, Irish DD. The acute vapor toxicity of allyl chloride. *J Ind Hyg Toxicol* 1940;22:79–86.
44. Torkelson TR, Wolf MA, Oyen F, Rowe VK. Vapor toxicity of allyl chloride as determined on laboratory animals. *Am Ind Hyg Assoc J* 1959;20:212–223.
45. Torkelson TR, Oyen F, Rowe VK. The toxicity of vinyl chloride as determined by repeated exposure of laboratory animals. *Am Ind Hyg Assoc J* 1961;22:354–361.
46. Reichert D, Ewald D, Henschler D. Generation and inhalation toxicity of dichloroacetylene. *Fd Cosmet Toxicol* 1975;13:511–515.
47. Reichert D, Henschler D. Nephrotoxic and hepatotoxic effects of dichloroacetylene. *Fd Cosmet Toxicol* 1978;16:227–235.
48. Reichert D, Spengler U, Romen W, Henschler D. Carcinogenicity of dichloroacetylene: an inhalation study. *Carcinogenesis* 1984;5:1411–1420.
49. Mazze RI. Methoxyflurane nephropathy. In: Hook JB, ed. *Toxicology of the kidney*. New York: Raven Press, 1981;135–149.
50. Kluwe WM, Gupta BN, Lamb JC. The comparative effects of 1,2-dibromo-3-chloropropane and its metabolites, 3-chloro-1,2-propane-oxide (epichlorohydrin), 3-chloro-1,2-propanediol (α-chlorohydrin), and oxalic acid, on the urogenital system of male rats. *Toxicol Appl Pharmacol* 1983;70:67–86.
51. Jones AR, Gadiel P, Murcott C. The renal toxicity of the rodenticide α-chlorohydrin in the rat. *Naturwissenschaften* 1979;66:425.
52. Porter KE, Jones AR. The renal toxicity of (R)-3-chloroacetate in the rat. *Chem Biol Interact* 1987;62:157–166.
53. Dobbie MS, Porter KE, Jones AR. Is the nephrotoxicity of (R)-3-chlorolacetate in the rat caused by 3-chloropyruvate? *Xenobiotica* 1988;18:1389–1399.
54. Soderlund EJ, Dybing E, Nelson SD. Nephrotoxicity and hepatotoxicity of tris(2,3-dibromopropyl)phosphate in the rat. *Toxicol Appl Pharmacol* 1980;56:171–186.
55. Davies DJ. The structural changes in the kidney and urinary tract caused by ethyleneimine. *J Pathol* 1969;97;695–703.
56. Powell CJ, Tyobeka T, Bach PH. Bridges JW. The nephrotoxicity of structural analogues of 2-bromoethaneamine. In: Bach PH, Lock EA, eds. *Renal heterogeneity and target cell toxicity*. Chichester: Wiley, 1985;195–198.
57. Kluwe WM. The nephrotoxicity of low molecular weight halogenated alkane solvents, pesticides, and chemical intermediates. In: Hook JB, ed. *Toxicology of the kidney*. New York: Raven Press, 1981;179–226.
58. Rush GF, Smith JH, Newton JF, Hook JB. Chemically induced nephrotoxicity. Role of metabolic activation. *CRC Crit Rev Toxicol* 1984;13:99–160.
59. Elfarra AA, Anders MW. Renal processing of glutathione conjugates. Role in nephrotoxicity. *Biochem Pharmacol* 1984;33:3729–3732.
60. Monks TJ, Lau SS. Renal transport processes and glutathione conjugate-mediated nephrotoxicity. *Drug Metab Dispos* 1987;15:437–441.
61. Lock EA. The nephrotoxicity of haloalkane and haloalkene glutathione conjugates. In: de Matteis F, Lock EA, eds. *Selectivity and molecular mechanisms of toxicity*. London: Macmillan, 1987;59–83.
62. Anders MW, Elfarra AA, Lash LH. Cellular effects of reactive intermediates: nephrotoxicity of *S*-conjugates of amino acids. *Arch Toxicol* 1987;60:103–108.
63. Anders MW, Lash LH, Dekant W, Elfarra AA, Dohn DR. Biosynthesis and biotransformation of glutathione *S*-conjugates to toxic metabolites. *CRC Crit Rev Toxicol* 1988;18:311–341.
64. Lock EA. Studies on the mechanism of nephrotoxicity and nephrocarcinogenicity of halogenated alkenes. *CRC Crit Rev Toxicol* 1988;19:23–42.
65. Dekant W, Vamvakas S, Anders MW Bioactivation of nephrotoxic haloalkenes by glutathione conjugation: formation of toxic and mutagenic intermediates by cysteine conjugate β-lyase. *Drug Metab Rev* 1989;20:43–83.
66. Commandeur JNM, Vermeulen NPE. Molecular and biochemical mechanisms of chemically induced nephrotoxicity: a review. *CRC Crit Rev Toxicol* 1990;3:171–194.
67. Tarloff JB, Goldstein RS, Hook JB. Xenobiotic biotransformation by the kidney. Pharmacological and toxicological aspects. In: Gibson GG, ed. *Progress in drug metabolism*, vol 12. New York: Taylor & Francis, 1990;1–39.

68. Monks TJ, Anders MW, Dekant W, Stevens JL, Lau SS, Van Bladesen PJ. Glutathione conjugate mediated toxicities. *Toxicol Appl Pharmacol* 1990;106:1–19.
69. Jones DP, Orrenius S, Jackson SW. Cytochrome P-450-linked monooxygenase systems in the kidney. In: Gram TE, ed. *Extrahepatic metabolism of drugs and other foreign compounds*. New York: Spectrum, 1980;123–158.
70. Anders MW. Metabolism of drugs by the kidneys. *Kidney Int* 1980;18:636–647.
71. MacFarland RT, Gandolfi AJ, Sipes IG. Extrahepatic GSH-dependent metabolism of 1,2-dibromoethane and 1,2-dibromo-3-chloropropane in the rat and mouse. *Drug Chem Toxicol* 1984; 7:213–227.
72. Lash LH, Elfarra AA, Anders MW. Renal cysteine conjugate β-lyase. Bioactivation of nephrotoxic cysteine *S*-conjugates in mitochondrial outer membrane. *J Biol Chem* 1986;261:5930–5935.
73. Sausen PJ, Elfarra AA. Cysteine conjugate *S*-oxidase. Characterization of a novel enzymatic activity in rat hepatic and renal microsomes. *J Biol Chem* 1990;265:6139–6145.
74. Black SD, Coon MJ. Comparative structures of P-450 cytochromes. In: Ortiz de Montellano PR, ed. *Cytochrome P-450. Structure, mechanism, and biochemistry*. New York: Plenum Press, 1986;161–216.
75. Masters BSS, Muerhoff AS, Okita RT. Enzymology of extrahepatic cytochromes P-450. In: Guengerich FP, ed. *Mammalian cytochromes P-450*, vol 1. Boca Raton: CRC Press, 1987;108–133.
76. Chasseaud LF. Extrahepatic conjugation with glutathione. In: Gram TE, ed. *Extrahepatic metabolism of drugs and other foreign compounds*. New York: Spectrum, 1980;427–452.
77. Baars AJ, Mukhtar H, Zoetemelk CEM, Jansen M, Brelimer DD. Glutathione *S*-transferase activity in the rat and human tissues and organs. *Comp Biochem Physiol* 1981;70C:285–288.
78. Hook JB, Elcombe CR, Rose MS, Lock EA. Characterization of the effects of known hepatic monooxygenase inducers on male and female rat and mouse kidneys. *Life Sci* 1982;31:1077–1084.
79. Rush GF, Wilson DM, Hook JB. Selective induction and inhibition of renal mixed function oxidases in the rat and rabbit. *Fundam Appl Toxicol* 1983;3:161–168.
80. Baron J, Kawabata TT, Redick JA, et al. Localization of carcinogen-metabolizing enzymes in human and animal tissues. In: Rydstrom J, Montelius, J, Bengtsson M, eds. *Extrahepatic drug metabolism and chemical carcinogenesis*. Amsterdam: Elsevier, 1983;73–88.
81. Mohandas J, Marshall JJ, Duggin GG, Horvath JS, Tiller DJ. Differential distribution of glutathione and glutathione-related enzymes in rabbit kidney. *Biochem Pharmacol* 1984;33:1801–1807.
82. Guthenberg C, Jensson H, Nystrom E, Tahin MK, Mannervik B. Isoenzymes of glutathione transferase in rat kidney cytosol. *Biochem J* 1985;230:609–615.
83. Yoshimota M, Kusunose E, Yamamoto S, Maekawa M, Kusunose M. Purification and characterization of two forms of cytochrome-P-450 from rat kidney cortex microsomes. *Biochem International* 1986;13:749–755.
84. Trakshel GM, Maines MD. Characterization of glutathione *S*-transferases in rat kidney. *Biochem J* 1988;252:127–136.
85. Waziens ID, Cugnenc PH, Yang CS, Leroux JP, Beaune PH. Cytochrome P-450 isoenzymes, epoxide hydrolase and glutathione transferases in rat and human hepatic and extrahepatic tissues. *J Pharmacol Exp Ther* 1990;253:387–394.
86. Vos RME, Van Bladeren PJ. Glutathione *S*-transferases in relation to their role in the biotransformation of xenobiotics. *Chem Biol Interact* 1990;75:241–265.
87. MacDonald TL. Chemical mechanisms of halocarbon metabolism. *CRC Crit Rev Toxicol* 1983; 11:85–120.
88. Anders MW, Pohl LR. Halogenated alkanes. In: Anders MW, ed. *Bioactivation of foreign compounds*. Orlando, FL: Academic Press, 1985;283–315.
89. Smith JH, Maita K, Sleight SD, Hook JB. Effect of sex hormone status on chloroform nephrotoxicity and renal mixed function oxidases in mice. *Toxicology* 1984;30:305–316.
90. Pohl LR, George JW, Satoh H. Strain differences in chloroform-induced nephrotoxicity: different rates of metabolism of chloroform to phosgene by the mouse kidney. *Drug Metab Dispos* 1984; 12:304–308.
91. Kluwe WM, Hook JB. Polybrominated biphenyl-induced potentiation of chloroform toxicity. *Toxicol Appl Pharmacol* 1978;45:861–869.
92. Smith JH. Role of renal metabolism in chloroform nephrotoxicity. *Comments Toxicol* 1986;1: 125–144.
93. Bailie MB, Smith JH, Newton JF, Hook JB. Mechanism of chloroform nephrotoxicity. IV. Pheno-

barbital potentiation of *in vitro* chloroform metabolism and toxicity in rabbit kidneys. *Toxicol Appl Pharmacol* 1984;74:285–292.

94. Pohl LR. Biochemical toxicology of chloroform. *Rev Biochem Toxicol* 1979;1:79–107.
95. Villarruel MC, de Toranzo EG, Castro JA. Carbon tetrachloride activation, lipid peroxidation and the mixed function oxygenase activity of various rat tissues. *Toxicol Appl Pharmacol* 1977; 41:337–344.
96. Butler TC. Reduction of carbon tetrachloride *in vivo* and reduction of carbon tetrachloride and chloroform *in vitro* by tissue and tissue constituents. *J Pharmacol Exp Ther* 1961;134:311–319.
97. Paul BB, Rubinstein D. Metabolism of carbon tetrachloride and chloroform by the rat. *J Pharmacol Exp Ther* 1963;141:141–148.
98. Guengerich FP, Crawford WM Jr, Watanabe PG. Activation of vinyl chloride to covalently bound metabolites. Roles of 2-chloroethylene oxide and 2-chloroacetaldehyde. *Biochemistry* 1979;18: 5177–5182.
99. Liebler DC, Guengerich FP. Olefin oxidation by cytochrome P-450. Evidence for group migration in catalytic intermediates formed with vinylidene chloride and trans-1-phenyl-1-butene. *Biochemistry* 1983;225:5482–5489.
100. Masuda Y, Nakayama N. Protective action of diethyldithiocarbamate and carbon disulfide against acute toxicities induced by 1,1-dichloroethylene in mice. *Toxicol Appl Pharmacol* 1983;71:42–53.
101. Okine LK, Gochee JM, Gram TE. Studies on the distribution and covalent binding of 1,1-dichloroethylene in the mouse. *Biochem Pharmacol* 1985;34:4051–4057.
102. Okine LK, Gram TE. *In vitro* studies on the metabolism and covalent binding of [^{14}C]-1,1-dichloroethylene by mouse liver, kidney and lung. *Biochem Pharmacol* 1986;35:2789–2795.
103. Nelson SD, Pearson PG. Covalent and noncovalent interactions in acute lethal cell injury by chemicals. *Annu Rev Pharmacol Toxicol* 1990;30:169–195.
104. Ziegler DM. Role of reversible oxidant-reduction of enzyme thiols-disulfides in metabolic regulation. *Annu Rev Biochem* 1985;54:305–329.
105. Reed DJ. Glutathione: toxicological implications. *Annu Rev Pharmacol Toxicol* 1990;30:603–631.
106. Recknagel RO. Carbon tetrachloride hepatotoxicity: status quo and future prospects. *Trends Pharm Sci* 1983;4:129–131.
107. Jones AR, Milton DH, Murcott C. The oxidative metabolism of α-chlorohydrin in the male rat and the formation of spermatocoeles. *Xenobiotica* 1978;8:573–582.
108. Jones AR, Fakhouri G, Gadiel P. The metabolism of the soil fumigant 1,2-dibromo-3-chloropropane in the rat. *Experientia* 1979;35:1432–1434.
109. Wiseman A. Effect of inorganic fluoride on enzymes. In: Smith FA, ed. *Handbook of experimental pharmacology, pharmacology of fluorides*. New York: Springer-Verlag, 1970;48–93.
110. Lag M, Omichinski JG, Solderlund EJ, et al. Role of P-450 activity and glutathione levels in 1,2-dibromo-3-chloropropane tissue distribution, renal necrosis and *in vivo* DNA damage. *Toxicology* 1989;56:273–288.
111. Sies H, Ketterer B, eds. *Glutathione conjugation. Mechanisms and biological significance*. New York: Academic Press, 1988.
112. Jakoby W, Stevens J, Duffel M, Weisiger R. The terminal enzymes of mercapturate formation and the thiomethyl shunt. *Rev Biochem Toxicol* 1984;6:97–115.
113. Elfarra A, Baggs R, Anders M. Structure-nephrotoxicity relationships of *S*-(2-chloroethyl)-DL-cysteine and analogs. Role for an episulfonium ion. *J Pharmacol Exp Ther* 1985;233:512–516.
114. Kramer RA, Fouremen G, Greene KE, Reed DJ. Nephrotoxicity of *S*-(2-chloroethyl)glutathione in the Fischer rat. Evidence for γ-glutamyltranspeptidase-independent uptake by the kidney. *J Pharmacol Exp Ther* 1987;242:741–748.
115. Terracini B, Parker VH. A pathological study on the toxicity of *S*-dichlorovinyl-L-cysteine. *Fd Cosmet Toxicol* 1965;3:67–74.
116. Elfarra A, Jakobson I, Anders M. Mechanism of *S*-(1,2-dichlorovinyl)glutathione-induced nephrotoxicity. *Biochem Pharmacol* 1986;35:283–288.
117. Elfarra A, Lash L, Anders M. Metabolic activation and detoxication of nephrotoxic cysteine and homocysteine *S*-conjugates. *Proc Natl Acad Sci USA* 1986;83:2667–2671.
118. Darnerud PO, Brandt I, Feil VJ, Bakke JE. *S*-(1,2-dichloro-[^{14}C] vinyl)-L-cysteine in the mouse kidney: correlation between tissue binding and toxicity. *Toxicol Appl Pharmacol* 1988;95:423–434.
119. Green T, Odum J. Structure/activity studies of the nephrotoxic and mutagenic action of cysteine conjugates of chloro- and fluroralkenes. *Chem Biol Interact* 1985;54:15–31.

120. Dekant W, Martens G, Vamvakas S, Metzler M, Henschler D. Bioactivation of tetrachloroethylene. Role of glutathione *S*-transferase-catalyzed conjugation *versus* cytochrome P-450-dependent phospholipid alkylation. *Drug Metab Dispos* 1987;15:702–709.
121. Commandeur JNM, DeKanter FJJ, Vermeulen NPE. Bioactivation of the cysteine *S*-conjugate and mercapturic acid of tetrafluoroethylene to acylating reactive intermediates in the rat. Dependence of activation and deactivation activities on acetyl coenzyme A availability. *Mol Pharmacol* 1989; 36:654–663.
122. Hassall CD, Gandolfi AJ, Duhamel RC, Brendel K. The formation and biotransformation of cysteine conjugates of halogenated ethylenes by rabbit renal tubules. *Chem Biol Interact* 1984;49:283–297.
123. Dohn DR, Leininger JR, Lash LH, Quebbemann AJ, Anders MW. Nephrotoxicity of *S*-(2-chloro-1,1,2-trifluoroethyl)glutathione and *S*-(2-chloro-1,1,2-trifluoroethyl)-L-cysteine, the glutathione and cysteine conjugates of chlorotrifluoroethene. *J Pharmacol Exp Ther* 1985;235:851–857.
124. Banki K, Elfarra AA, Lash LH, Anders MW. Metabolism of *S*-(2-chloro-1,1,2-trifluoroethyl)-L-cysteine to hydrogen sulfide and the role of hydrogen sulfide in *S*-(2-chloro-1,1,2-trifluoroethyl)-L-cysteine-induced mitochondrial toxicity. *Biochem Biophys Res Commun* 1986;138:707–713.
125. Dekant W, Lash LH, Anders MW. Bioactivation mechanism of the cytotoxic and nephrotoxic *S*-conjugate *S*-(2-chloro-1,1,2-trifluoroethyl)-L-cysteine. *Proc Natl Acad Sci USA* 1987;84:7443–7447.
126. Boogaard PJ, Commandeur JNM, Mulder GJ, Vermeulen NPE, Nagelkerke JF. Toxicity of the cysteine *S*-conjugates and mercapturic acids of four structurally related difluoroethylenes in isolated proximal tubular cells from rat kidney. *Biochem Pharmacol* 1989;38:3731–3741.
127. Koob M, Dekant W. Metabolism of hexafluoropropene. Evidence for bioactivation by glutathione conjugate formation in the kidney. *Drug Metab Dispos* 1990;18:911–916.
128. Karhai W, Dekant W, Henschler D. Metabolism of the nephrotoxin dichloroacetylene by glutathione conjugation. *Chem Res Toxicol* 1989;2:51–56.
129. Guengerich FR, Crawford WM, Domoradski JY, MacDinald TL, Watanabe PG. *In vitro* activation of 1,2-dichloroethane by microsomal and cytosolic enzymes. *Toxicol Appl Pharmacol* 1980;55: 303–317.
130. Anders MW, Livesey JC. Metabolism of 1,2-dihaloethanes. *Banbury Report 5:Ethylene dichloride: a potential health risk. Cold Spring Harbor Laboratory* 1980;331–341.
131. Marchard DH, Reed DJ. Identification of the reactive glutathione conjugate *S*-(2-chloroethyl) glutathione in the bile of 1-bromo-2-chloroethane-treated rats by high pressure liquid chromatography and precolumn derivatization with *o*-phthaldehyde. *Chem Res Toxicol* 1989;2:449–454.
132. Guo W, Chakrabarti S, Malick MA, Cote MG. Effect of *S*-(2-chloroethyl)-DL-cysteine on the transport of *p*-aminohippurate ion in renal plasma membrane vesicles. *Arch Biochem Biophys* 1990;283:206–209.
133. Drieman JC, Thijssen HH, Struyker-Boudier HA. Renal selective N-acetyl-γ-glutamyl prodrugs. II. Carrier-mediated transport and intracellular conversion as determinants in the renal selectivity of N-acetyl-γ-glutamyl sulfamethoxazole. *J Pharmacol Exp Ther* 1990;252:1255–1260.
134. Webb WW, Elfarra AA, Webster KD, Thorm RE, Anders MW. Role for an episulfonium ion: *S*-(2-chloroethyl)-DL-cysteine-induced cytotoxicity and its reaction with glutathione. *Biochemistry* 1987;26:3017–3023.
135. Schasteen CS, Reed DJ. The hydrolysis and alkylation activities of *S*-(2-haloethyl)-L-cysteine analogs. Evidence for extended half-life. *Toxicol Appl Pharmacol* 1983;70:423–432.
136. Webster KD, Anders MW. Bioactivation mechanism of α-thiomorpholine-3-carboxylic acid. *Arch Biochem Biophys* 1989;273:562–571.
137. Reed DJ, Foureman GL. A comparison of the alkylating capabilities of the cysteinyl and glutathionyl conjugates of 1,2-dichloroethane. *Adv Exp Med Biol* 1986;197:469–475.
138. Peterson LA, Harris TM, Guengerich FP. Evidence for an episulfonium ion in the formation of *S*-[2-N^7-guanyl)ethyl]glutathione in DNA. *J Am Chem Soc* 1988;110:3284–3291.
139. Pearson PG, Soderlund EJ, Dybing E, Nelson SD. Metabolic activation of 1,2-dibromo-3-chloropropane: evidence for the formation of reactive episulfonium ion intermediates. *Biochemistry* 1990; 29:4971–4981.
140. Dohn DR, Anders MW. The enzymatic reaction of chlorotrifluoroethylene with glutathione. *Biochem Biophys Res Commun* 1982;109:1339–1345.
141. Dohn DR, Quebbemann AJ, Borch RF, Anders MW. Enzymatic reaction of chlorotrifluoroethyl-

ene with glutathione. ^{19}F NMR evidence for stereochemical control of the reaction. *Biochemistry* 1985;24:5137–5143.
142. Wolf CR, Berry PN, Nash JA, Green T, Lock EA. Role of microsomal and cytosolic glutathione *S*-transferases in the conjugation of hexachloro-1,3-butadiene and its possible relevance to toxicity. *J Pharmacol Exp Ther* 1984;228:202–208.
143. Jones TW, Gerdes RG, Ormstad K, Orrenius S. The formation of both a mono- and a bis-substituted glutathione conjugate of hexachlorobutadiene by isolated hepatocytes and following *in vivo* adminstration to the rat. *Chem Biol Interact* 1985;56:251–267.
144. Dekant W, Vamvakas S, Henschler D, Anders MW. Enzymatic conjugation of hexachloro-1,3-butadiene with glutathione. Formation of 1-(glutathion-*S*-yl)-1,2,3,4,4-pentachlorobuta-1,3-diene and 1,4-(bis)-(glutathion-*S*-yl)-1,2,3,4-tetrachlorobuta-1,3-diene. *Drug Metab Dispos* 1988; 16:701–706.
145. Dekant W, Schrenk D, Vamvakas S, Henschler D. Metabolism of hexachloro-1,3-butadiene in mice: *in vivo* and *in vitro* evidence for activation by glutathione conjugation. *Xenobiotica* 1988;18: 803–816.
146. Commandeur JNM, Vermeulen NPE. Identification of *N*-acetyl(1,2-dichlorovinyl)-L-cysteine as two regioisomeric mercapturic acids of trichloroethylene in the rat. *Chem Res Toxicol* 1990;3:212–218.
147. Mertens JJWM, Weijen JGJ, Van Doorn WJ, Spenkelink B, Temmink JHM, Van Bladeren PJV. Differential toxicity as a result of apical and basolateral treatment of LLC-PK1 monolayers with *S*-(1,2,3,4,4-pentachlorobutadienyl)glutathione and *N*-acetyl-*S*-(1,2,3,4,4-pentachlorobutadienyl)-L-cysteine. *Chem Biol Interact* 1988;65:282–293.
148. Lash LH, Jones DP. Uptake of the glutathione conjugate *S*-(1,2-dichlorovinyl) glutathione by renal basal-lateral membrane vesicles and isolated kidney cells. *Mol Pharmacol* 1985;28:278–282.
149. Lash LH, Anders MW. Uptake of nephrotoxic *S*-conjugates by isolated rat renal proximal tubular cells. *J Pharmacol Exp Ther* 1989;248:531–537.
150. Schaeffer VH, Stevens JL. The transport of cysteine conjugates in LLC-PK1 cells and its role in toxicity. *Mol Pharmacol* 1987;31:506–512.
151. Schaeffer VH, Stevens JL. Mechanism of transport for toxic cysteine conjugates in rat kidney cortex membrane vesicles. *Mol Pharmacol* 1987;32:293–298.
152. Lock EA, Odum J, Ormond P. Transport of *N*-acetyl-*S*-pentachloro-1,3-butadienylcysteine by rat renal cortex. *Arch Toxicol* 1986;59:12–15.
153. Zhang G, Stevens JL. Transport and activation of *S*-(1,2-dichlorovinyl)-L-cysteine and *N*-acetyl-*S*-(1,2-dichlorovinyl)-L-cysteine in rat kidney proximal tubules. *Toxicol Appl Pharmacol* 1989; 100:51–61.
154. Wolfgang GHI, Gandolfi AJ, Stevens JL, Brendel K. *N*-acetyl-*S*-(1,2-dichlorovinyl)-L-cysteine produces a similar toxicity to *S*-(1,2-dichlorovinyl)-L-cysteine in rabbit renal slices: differential transport and metabolism. *Toxicol Appl Pharmacol* 1989;101:205–219.
155. Wolfgang GH, Gandolfi AJ, Nagle RB, Brendel K, Stevens JL. Assessment of *S*-(1,2-dichlorovinyl)-L-cysteine induced toxic events in rabbit renal cortical slices. Biochemical and histological evaluation of uptake, covalent binding, and toxicity. *Chem Biol Interact* 1990;75:153–170.
156. Mertens JJWM, Keukens EAJ, Appel M, Spenkelink B, Temmink JHM, Van Bladeren PJ. Cytotoxicity of *S*-(1,2,3,4,4-pentachlorobutadienyl)-L-cysteine after apical and basolateral exposure of LLC-PK1 monolayers. Involvement of an amino acid transport system. *Chem Biol Interact* 1990; 75:119–130.
157. Elfarra AA, Lash LH, Anders MW. α-Keto acids stimulate rat renal cysteine conjugate β-lyase activity and potentiate the cytotoxicity of *S*-(1,2-dichlorovinyl)-L-cysteine. *Mol Pharmacol* 1987; 31:208–212.
158. Lash LH, Elfarra AA, Rakiewicz-Nemeth D, Anders MW. Bioactivation mechanism of cytotoxic homocysteine *S*-conjugates. *Arch Biochem Biophys* 1990;276:322–330.
159. Elfarra AA, Hwang IY. *In vivo* metabolites of *S*-(2-benzothiazolyl)-L-cysteine as markers of *in vivo* cysteine conjugate β-lyase and thiol glucuronosyl transferase activities. *Drug Metab Dispos* 1990;18:917–922.
160. Lash LH, Anders MW. Cytotoxicity of *S*-(1,2-dichlorovinyl)glutathione and *S*-(1,2-dichlorovinyl)cysteine in isolated rat kidney cells. *J Biol Chem* 1986;261:13076–13081.
161. Darnerud PO, Brandt I, Feil VJ, Bakke JE. Dichlorovinyl cysteine in the mouse kidney: tissue-binding and toxicity after glutathione depletion and probenecid treatment. *Arch Toxicol* 1989; 63:345–350.
162. Hwang IY, Elfarra AA. Cysteine *S*-conjugates may act as kidney selective prodrugs. Formation of

6-mercaptopurine by the renal metabolism of *S*-(6-purinyl)-L-cysteine. *J Pharmacol Exp Ther* 1989;251:448–454.
163. Wolfgang GHI, Gandolfi AJ, Stevens JL, Brendel K. *In vitro* and *in vivo* nephrotoxicity of the L and D isomers of *S*-(1,2-dichlorovinyl)cysteine. *Toxicology* 1989;58:33–42.
164. Jones T, Qin C, Schaeffer V, Stevens J. Immunohistochemical localization of glutamine transaminase K, a rat kidney cysteine conjugate β-lyase, and the relationship to the segment specificity of cysteine conjugate nephrotoxicity. *Mol Pharmacol* 1988;34:621–627.
165. Stevens JL, Robbins JD, Byrd RA. A purified cysteine conjugate β lyase from rat kidney cytosol. Requirement for an α-keto acid or an amino acid oxidase for activity and identity with soluble glutamine transaminase K. *J Biol Chem* 1986;261:15529–15537.
166. Stevens JL, Hatzinger PB, Hayden PJ. Quantitation of multiple pathways for the metabolism of nephrotoxic cysteine conjugates using selective inhibitors of L-α-hydroxy acid oxidase and cysteine conjugate β-lyase. *Drug Metab Dispos* 1989;17:297–303.
167. Tomisawa H, Ichimato N, Takanhashi Y, Ichihara S, Fukazawa H, Tateishi M. Purification and characterization of cysteine conjugate transaminases from rat liver. *Xenobiotica* 1988;18:1015–1028.
168. Pratt IS, Lock EA. Deacetylation and further metabolism of the mercapturic acid of hexachloro-1,3-butadiene by rat kidney cytosol *in vitro*. *Arch Toxicol* 1988;52:341–345.
169. Bakke JE, Davison KL, Larsen GL. Evidence for the absence of cysteine *S*-conjugate *N*-acetyltransferase activity in the metabolism of propachlor, naphthalene, and dichlobanil in calves. *Xenobiotica* 1990;20:801–807.
170. Sausen PJ, Elfarra AA. *S*-(1,2-dichlorovinyl)-L-cysteine sulfoxide, a putative metabolite of *S*-(1,2-dichlorovinyl)-L-cysteine, is a potent nephrotoxin. *Toxicologist* 1990;10:267.
171. Sausen PJ, Elfarra AA. Reactivity of cysteine conjugate sulfoxides: formation of *S*-[1-chloro-2-(*S*-glutathionyl)vinyl]-L-cysteine sulfoxide by the reaction of *S*-(1,2-dichlorovinyl)-L-cysteine sulfoxide with glutathione. *Chem Res Toxicol* 1991;4:655–660.
172. Jones TW, Wallin A, Thor H, Gerdes RG, Ormstad K, Orrenius S. The mechanism of pentachlorobutadienyl-glutathione nephrotoxicity studied with isolated rat renal epithelial cells. *Arch Biochem Biophys* 1986;251:504–513.
173. Chen JC, Stevens JL, Trifillis AL, Jones TW. Renal cysteine conjugate β-lyase-mediated toxicity studied with primary cultures of human proximal tubular cells. *Toxicol Appl Pharmacol* 1990; 103:463–473.
174. Chen Q, Jones TW, Brown PC, Stevens JL. The mechanism of cysteine conjugate cytotoxicity in renal epithelial cells. Covalent binding leads to thiol depletion and lipid peroxidation. *J Biol Chem* 1990;265:21603–21611.
175. Vamvakas S, Sharma VK, Shen S, Anders MW. Perturbations of intracellular calcium distribution in kidney cells by nephrotoxic haloalkenyl cysteine *S*-conjugates. *Mol Pharmacol* 1990;38:455–461.
176. Lash LH, Anders MW. Mechanism of *S*-(1,2-dichlorovinyl)-L-cysteine- and *S*-(1,2-dichlorovinyl)-L-homocysteine-induced renal mitochondrial toxicity. *Mol Pharmacol* 1987;32:549–556.
177. Banki K, Anders MW. Inhibition of rat kidney mitochondrial DNA, RNA and protein synthesis by halogenated cysteine *S*-conjugates. *Carcinogenesis* 1989;10:767–772.
178. Hayden PJ, Stevens JL. Cysteine conjugate toxicity, metabolism, and binding to macromolecules in isolated rat kidney mitochondria. *Mol Pharmacol* 1990;37:468–476.
179. Beuter W, Cojocel C, Muller H, Donnaubauer HH, Mayer D. Peroxidative damage and nephrotoxicity of dichlorovinylcysteine in mice. *J Appl Toxicol* 1989;9:181–186.
180. Lock EA, Schnellmann RG. The effect of haloalkene cysteine conjugates on rat renal glutathione reductase and lipoyl dehydrogenase activities. *Toxicol Appl Pharmacol* 1990;104:180–190.
181. Elfarra AA, Sausen PJ, Quinones C. Protection of rats from *S*-(1,2-dichlorovinyl)-L-cysteine and cephaloridine-induced nephrotoxicity by methimazole. *Toxicologist* 1990;10:267.
182. Sausen PJ, Elfarra AA, Cooley A. Methimazole protection of rats against chemically induced kidney damage *in vivo*. *J Pharmacol Exp Ther* 1992;260:393–401.
183. Lash LH, Nelson RM, Van Dyke RA, Anders MW. Purification and characterization of human kidney cytosolic cysteine conjugate β-lyase activity. *Drug Metab Dispos* 1990;18:50–54.
184. Darnerud PO, Olsson L. Transplacental passage and fetal kidney binding of ^{14}C-dichlorovinyl cysteine in mice. *Toxicol Lett* 1990;52:63–72.
185. Hwang IY, Elfarra AA. Kidney selective prodrugs of 6-mercaptopurine: biochemical basis of the kidney selectivity of *S*-(6-purinyl)-L-cysteine. *J Pharmacol Exp Ther* 1991;258:171–177.

Toxicology of the Kidney, Second Edition,
edited by Jerry B. Hook and Robin S. Goldstein.
Raven Press, Ltd., New York © 1993.

15

Nephrotoxicity of Bromobenzene: The Role of Quinone-Thioethers

Serrine S. Lau and Terrence J. Monks

*Division of Pharmacology and Toxicology, College of Pharmacy,
The University of Texas at Austin, Austin, Texas 78712*

Bromobenzene causes a number of adverse toxic effects when administered to various experimental animals, including severe hepatic centrilobular necrosis, pulmonary necrosis, and renal proximal tubular necrosis. Much of the early mechanistic work on bromobenzene-mediated toxicities focused upon its effects in the liver. It was clearly established that in order for bromobenzene to produce hepatotoxicity, it was necessary for the compound to undergo cytochrome(s) P-450–mediated metabolism to a reactive metabolite. The reactive metabolite(s) was capable of binding covalently to tissue macromolecules, and the extent of this binding correlated with the extent of liver damage. The exact role of this covalent binding in the development of hepatic toxicity caused by bromobenzene remains a contentious issue (1). Thus, although several studies demonstrated that the covalent binding of bromobenzene could be dissociated from cell death, none has yet been able to demonstrate cell death in the absence of covalent binding. The manipulations that therefore dissociate covalent binding and toxicity probably do so by influencing events subsequent to the covalent binding of reactive metabolites to tissue macromolecules. That is, they influence the consequences and progression of the initial toxic insult. Covalent binding can therefore be regarded as a necessary but insufficient step in the toxic process.

In contrast to bromobenzene-mediated hepatotoxicity, the mechanism of bromobenzene-mediated nephrotoxicity remained unclear. The work of Reid (2) suggested that bromobenzene nephrotoxicity might be caused by a metabolite formed in the liver and subsequently transported to the kidney. The nature of this liver-derived circulating metabolite was unclear. A prime candidate was bromobenzene-3,4-oxide, the putative hepatotoxic metabolite, which might be sufficiently stable to escape the liver and produce toxicity at extrahepatic sites. It was subsequently demonstrated that the 3,4-epoxide was indeed capable of diffusing out of hepatocytes and that as much as 35% of this metabolite was capable of leaving the cells in which it was formed (3,4). Moreover, bromobenzene-3,4-oxide could be demonstrated in retro-orbital sinus blood of rats treated with bromobenzene (5). However, the inability of the kidney to catalyze the formation of the 3,4-epoxide, in conjunction with the relatively high renal activity of the glutathione (GSH) *S*-transferase required for detoxication of the 3,4-epoxide (6) suggested that any of the epoxide reaching the kidney from the liver could be efficiently detoxified there.

THE ROLE OF PHENOLIC BROMOBENZENE METABOLITES

The focus of research therefore shifted to examining the possible roles played by the primary phenolic metabolites of bromobenzene in the development of the nephrotoxicity. Rush et al. (7) demonstrated that *ortho*-bromophenol, *meta*-bromophenol, *para*-bromophenol, and 4-bromocatechol were all capable of producing renal damage when administered by tail-vein injection to ICR mice at a dose of 0.56 mmol/kg. Of these phenolic bromobenzene metabolites, 4-bromocatechol was the most potent, both *in vivo*, as evidenced by elevations in blood urea nitrogen (BUN) concentrations, and *in vitro*, as evidenced by a decrease in the ability of renal cortical slices to accumulate either organic anions (*para*-aminohippurate) or organic cations (tetraethylammonium). Moreover, the renal damage produced by 4-bromocatechol could not be distinguished morphologically from that produced by bromobenzene. In contrast, intraperitoneal administration of 4-bromocatechol to male Sprague-Dawley rats, at a dose of 2.55 mmol/kg (i.e., approximately five times the dose required to produce substantial elevations in BUN in mice), caused no apparent histological alterations to the kidneys and BUN concentrations remained in the normal range (8). Mice are known to be more sensitive to the nephrotoxic effects of bromobenzene (2) and species differences exist in bromobenzene metabolism (9). However, the basis for the differences seen in the susceptibility of mice and rats to 4-bromocatechol–mediated nephrotoxicity, and the basis for the tissue selectivity of 4-bromocatechol in mice, remain to be determined.

The finding that *ortho*-bromophenol was capable of causing severe GSH depletion in isolated hepatocytes (10) prompted an investigation of the *in vivo* effects of this metabolite. In contrast to its effects *in vitro, ortho*-bromophenol was not hepatotoxic *in vivo*. However, *ortho*-bromophenol caused GSH depletion in both the liver and kidney and was capable of reproducing the nephrotoxicity caused by bromobenzene, but at much lower doses (11). The data also indicated that the toxicity was caused by a metabolite of *ortho*-bromophenol, formed in the liver and transported by the circulation to the kidney. Thus, the *in vivo* covalent binding of *ortho*-bromo[^{14}C]-phenol was greater to renal tissue than to liver tissue. Indeed, in phenobarbital pretreated animals, covalent binding was ten-fold greater in the kidney than in the liver (Table 1). In contrast, whereas liver microsomes effectively catalyzed the metabolism of *ortho*-bromo-[^{14}C]-phenol to covalently bound material (K_m, 27 μM; V_{max} 0.5 nmol/mg/min) covalent binding could not be identified in microsomes prepared from rat kidney (Table 2).

TABLE 1. *Covalent binding of* ortho-*bromo-[¹⁴C]-phenol to rat liver and kidney proteins* in vivo

	Pretreatment	
	Noninduced	Phenobarbital
Liver	0.35 ± 0.07[a]	0.49 ± 0.07
Kidney	1.35 ± 0.63	1.71 ± 1.53

[a]Data represent the mean ± S.D. (n = 5–8) and are expressed as nmol covalently bound material per mg protein. (Data adapted from Lau et al., ref. 11.)

THE ROLE OF 2-BROMOHYDROQUINONE

Subsequently, 2-bromohydroquinone (2-BrHQ) was identified as a major *in vivo* and *in vitro* metabolite of both bromobenzene and *ortho*-bromophenol in male Sprague-Dawley rats (12). In addition, pretreatment of rats with piperonyl butoxide protected them against the nephrotoxicity of *ortho*-bromophenol, suggesting that 2-BrHQ was a cytochrome(s) P-450–catalyzed metabolite of *ortho*-bromophenol (11). Administration of 2-BrHQ (0.8 mmol/kg ip) caused severe renal proximal tubular necrosis and elevations in BUN concentrations. Interestingly, however, 2-BrHQ formation from *ortho*-bromophenol was 50-fold higher in liver microsomes than in kidney microsomes (Table 2) yet 2-BrHQ had no discernible effect on liver histology *in vivo*. Thus, although 2-BrHQ appeared to be selectively synthesized from *ortho*-bromophenol in the liver, it was selectively nephrotoxic. *This raised the question of how and in what form was 2-BrHQ delivered to the kidney?* A clue to the answer of this question was provided by the finding that following administration of 2-BrHQ to rats, both hepatic and renal GSH concentrations decreased. In addition, GSH inhibited the *in vitro* covalent biding of *ortho*-bromo-[^{14}C]-phenol to rat liver microsomal protein with the concomitant formation of water-soluble metabolites (12). By using either *ortho*-bromo-[^{14}C]-phenol or [^{35}S]-GSH in the microsomal reaction mixtures, several radioactive containing peaks were eluted upon high-performance liquid chromatographic (HPLC) analysis of the aqueous metabolites. The relative amounts of [^{14}C] and [^{35}S] in these peaks indicated the formation

TABLE 2. In vitro *covalent binding and 2-bromohydroquinone formation from* ortho-*bromo-[¹⁴C]-phenol in rat liver and kidney microsomes*

	Covalent binding	2-Bromohydroquinone
Liver	8.45 ± 0.71[a]	55.96 ± 0.80
Kidney	0.07 ± 0.01	1.09 ± 0.41

[a]Data represent the mean ± S.D. (n = 3) and are expressed as nmol covalently bound material per mg protein per 15 min. (Data adapted from Lau et al., ref. 12.)

of both monosubstituted GSH conjugates and disubstituted GSH conjugates (13). Moreover, chemical oxidation of 2-BrHQ, to give the corresponding 1,4-quinone, followed by addition of GSH, gave rise, upon analysis of the reaction mixture by HPLC, to a similar spectrum of ultraviolet (UV)-absorbing products as that seen in the microsomal system. Purification of the synthetic compounds and analysis by nuclear magnetic resonance spectroscopy, revealed the formation of 2-Br-3-(glutathion-*S*-yl) hydroquinone, 2-Br-5-(glutathion-*S*-yl)hydroquinone, 2-Br-6-(glutathion-*S*-yl)hydroquinone, and 2-Br-3,5 or 6-(diglutathion-*S*-yl)-hydroquinone (13).

The enzyme(s) responsible for the oxidation of 2-BrHQ *in vivo* remains unclear. However, neither cytochromes P-450 nor prostaglandin H synthase (PES) appears to play a major role in this oxidation since pretreatment of rats with piperonyl butoxide, which protected the animals from *ortho*-bromophenol–induced nephrotoxicity, failed to protect them against 2-BrHQ–mediated nephrotoxicity (13). Moreover, although rat renal papillary PES effectively catalyzed the *in vitro* co-oxidation of 2-BrHQ, and the subsequent formation of GSH conjugates (14) pretreatment of rats with either indomethacin or aspirin, inhibitors of the cyclooxygenase component of PES, did not protect the animals from 2-BrHQ–induced nephrotoxicity (Table 3) even though this protocol significantly inhibited prostaglandin biosynthesis (unpublished data). Schnellman and Mandel (15) have also shown that neither cytochromes P-450 nor PES plays a role in 2-BrHQ–induced cytotoxicity to isolated rabbit renal proximal tubules.

THE ROLE OF QUINONE-THIOETHERS

Administration of chemically synthesized 2-Br-(diglutathion-*S*-yl)HQ to rats by intravenous injection caused elevations in BUN at doses of 15 to 30 μmol/kg (13) and proteinuria, enzymuria, and glucosuria at 10 μmol/kg (16). In addition, the

TABLE 3. *The effect of aspirin, indomethacin, and piperonyl butoxide on the* in vivo *nephrotoxicity of 2-BrHQ*

Treatments	Blood urea nitrogen (mg/100 ml) Before 2-BrHQ	After 2-BrHQ
Untreated	15.8 ± 1.9 (*n* = 9)	125.4 ± 19.2 (*n* = 6)
Aspirin	13.6 ± 1.8 (*n* = 10)	128.0 ± 18.7 (*n* = 5)
Indomethacin	14.3 ± 1.2 (*n* = 10)	125.2 ± 23.4 (*n* = 7)
Piperonyl butoxide	15.0 ± 1.6 (*n* = 6)	127.3 ± 4.3 (*n* = 6)

Groups of rats were treated with ip injections of aspirin (50 mg/kg) or indomethacin (1.5 mg/kg) on the first and second day at 8:00 A.M. and 5:00 P.M., and on the third day at 8:00 A.M. 2-BrHQ (0.8 mmol/kg) was administered 2 hr after the last dose of aspirin or indomethacin. Piperonyl butoxide (1,600 mg/kg SC) was given 30 min prior to 2-BrHQ administration. Blood samples were taken from the retro-orbital sinus immediately prior to and 24 hr after 2-BrHQ administration and BUN levels determined. Figures represent the mean ± S.D.

histopathological alterations exhibited by the kidney were indistinguishable from those observed following either bromobenzene (9.3 mmol/kg), *ortho*-bromophenol (1.9 mmol/kg), or 2-BrHQ (0.83 mmol/kg) administration. Thus, the dose of 2-Br-(diglutathion-*S*-yl)HQ required to produce renal proximal tubular necrosis in the rat was approximately one one-thousandth of that of the parent compound, bromobenzene. 2-Br-(diglutathion-*S*-yl)HQ is therefore a relatively potent and specific nephrotoxicant. The proposed pathway of bromobenzene metabolism that leads to renal proximal tubular necrosis in male Sprague-Dawley rats is illustrated in Fig. 1. Interestingly, each of the mono-GSH substituted conjugates also caused increases in BUN when administered to rats (50 μmol/kg) but the magnitude of this elevation was less than that caused by 2-Br-(diglutathion-*S*-yl)HQ. These studies raised two important questions. *What are the bases for the target organ toxicity of the GSH conjugates of 2-BrHQ, and what are the reasons underlying the differential toxicity of the mono and disubstituted GSH conjugates?*

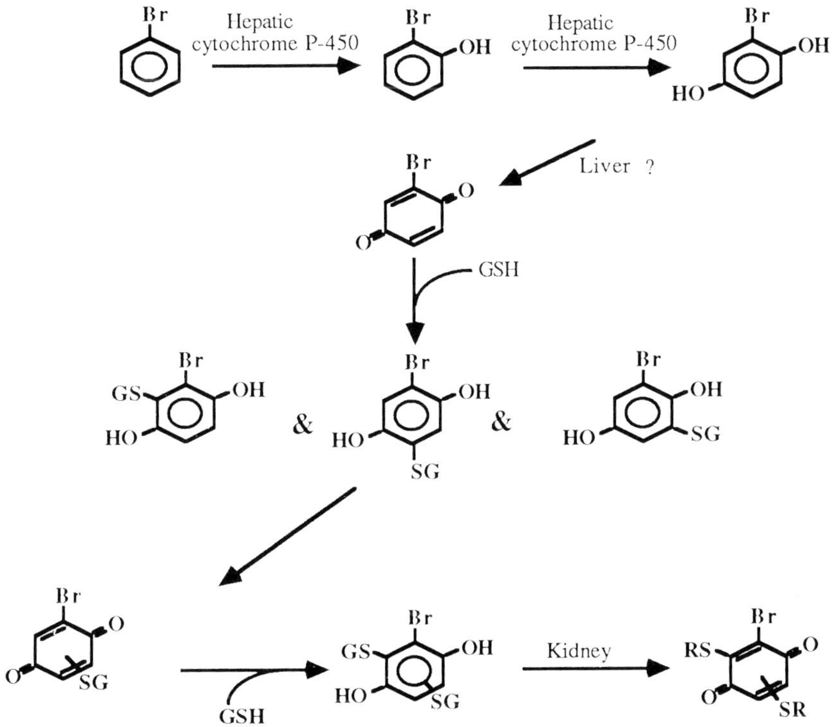

FIG. 1. Proposed pathway of bromobenzene metabolism to nephrotoxic metabolites in the male Sprague Dawley rat. The first two hydroxylations are catalyzed by cytochrome(s) P-450 within the liver. The mechanism and site of oxidation of 2-BrHQ and its thioethers are unclear at present. The evidence suggests that the final oxidation occurs within the kidney, although the nature of the ultimate reactive species remains to be determined. (Extended from Monks et al., ref. 13.)

THE ROLE OF γ-GLUTAMYL TRANSPEPTIDASE AND RENAL TRANSPORT MECHANISMS

The first step in the metabolism of GSH and its *S*-conjugates involves either hydrolysis or transpeptidation by γ-glutamyl transpeptidase (γ-GT) and transfer of the γ-glutamyl group to an appropriate acceptor (water for hydrolysis, an amino acid for transpeptidation). γ-GT is an ubiquitous enzyme, it is membrane bound, and its active site is oriented on the outer surface of cell membranes. In the kidney, γ-GT is found in high concentrations within the brush border membrane of renal proximal tubular cells (the active site being exposed to the tubular lumen) and at lower concentrations in the basal-lateral membrane. Although experimental evidence exists to the contrary, it is generally accepted that the majority of GSH and its *S*-conjugates require metabolism by γ-GT to facilitate transport across cellular membranes into the cytosol. In contrast, a fraction (the exact amount of which remains debatable) of extracellular GSH and its *S*-conjugates may be transported intact across cellular membranes by a sodium-dependent, probenecid-sensitive, transport system (17). The relative contribution of γ-GT–dependent and γ-GT–independent GSH transport within the kidney therefore remains equivocal (18). A role for differences in renal transport contributing to the differential toxicity of 2-Br-(diglutathion-*S*-yl)HQ and the 2-Br-mono-(glutathion-*S*-yl)HQ conjugates was obtained from studies using renal cortical slices. Thus, the rate of uptake of 2-Br-(diglutathion-*S*-yl)HQ by renal slices was between two- and seven-fold greater than that of the 2-Br-mono-(glutathion-*S*-yl)HQ conjugates (19). However, studies on the kinetics of the γ-GT–mediated metabolism of 2-Br-(glutathion-*S*-yl)HQ conjugates indicated that this step probably does not contribute to the observed differences in the toxicity of the various isomers (20). Thus, 2-Br-(diglutathion-*S*-yl)HQ exhibited the lowest affinity for γ-GT (i.e., the highest K_m) and the lowest V_{max}. However, the absolute amount of this enzyme within the kidney is more than sufficient to rapidly process the dose of 2-Br-(diglutathion-*S*-yl)HQ (10 to 30 μmol/kg) required to produce toxicity (20). Thus, factors contributing to the differential nephrotoxicity of the various GSH conjugates are probably located downstream from γ-GT.

Further evidence implicating a role for γ-GT in the nephrotoxicity of 2-BrHQ and 2-Br-(diglutathion-*S*-yl)HQ was obtained from studies using L-(α-5S)-α-amino-*S*-chloro-4,5-dihydro-5-isoxazoleacetic acid (AT-125; Acivicin) an inhibitor of γ-GT (21–24). Pretreatment of rats with AT-125 (10 mg/kg ip) 1 hr prior to administration of 2-BrHQ (0.83 mmol/kg) significantly inhibited renal γ-GT activity and protected the animals from the nephrotoxicity (13). This data strongly suggested that GSH conjugates of 2-BrHQ, rather than 2-BrHQ itself, were responsible for the toxicity. Similar data were obtained when AT-125 was used to protect against 2-Br-(diglutathion-*S*-yl)HQ–mediated nephrotoxicity (16). In addition, the data also indicated that metabolism of 2-Br-(diglutathion-*S*-yl)HQ was probably required in order to produce toxicity.

Alternatively, probenecid, which inhibits the organic anion transporter in renal proximal tubules (25), blocks both the uptake and nephrotoxicity of several haloalkenal and haloalkanal *S*-conjugates that are activated by the cysteine conjugate β-lyase pathway (26–28). However, pretreatment of rats with probenecid failed to protect them from either 2-Br-(diglutathion-*S*-yl)HQ–mediated renal necrosis (16) or from the *in vivo* nephrotoxicity of 2-Br-(dicystein-*S*-yl)HQ (29). Probenecid pretreatment did protect animals from both 2-Br-(di-*N*-acetylcystein-*S*-yl)HQ and to a lesser extent, 2-Br-6-(*N*-acetylcystein-*S*-yl)HQ mediated nephrotoxicity. It has been suggested that the renal sulfate transporter may be responsible for the uptake of 2-Br-3-(*N*-acetylcystein-*S*-yl)HQ into renal proximal tubular cells (30).

Possible Mechanisms of 2-Br-(diglutathion-*S*-yl)HQ–Mediated Nephrotoxicity

Are GSH conjugates formed as in vivo *metabolites of 2-BrHQ?* Studies on the *in vivo* disposition of 2-Br-[^{14}C]-HQ in rats demonstrated that each of the 2-Br-mono-(GSyl)HQ conjugates and 2-Br-(diglutathion-*S*-yl)HQ could be identified as urinary metabolites (31). This study also provided evidence for the mechanism by which AT-125 offered protection against 2-BrHQ–mediated nephrotoxicity. Thus, AT-125 inhibited renal γ-GT, after 24 hr, by 76%, renal covalent binding by 73%, and 2-BrHQ–mediated nephrotoxicity, as assessed by elevations in BUN, by 70%. These alterations were accompanied by an increase in the urinary excretion of each of the GSH conjugates, an increase in the fecal excretion of radioactivity, and a decrease in plasma radioactivity at 24 hr. The data were therefore consistent with the view that 2-BrHQ is metabolized *in vivo* to nephrotoxic GSH conjugates and that AT-125 inhibits nephrotoxicity by decreasing the γ-GT–mediated proximal tubular accumulation of the toxic metabolite(s) thereby facilitating their excretion into urine. Interestingly however, neither the corresponding cysteine nor *N*-acetylcysteine conjugates of 2-BrHQ could be identified as major *in vivo* metabolites (31).

The biochemical basis for the renal specific toxicity of 2-Br-(diglutathion-*S*-yl)HQ remains unclear. However, GSH and cysteine conjugates of a variety of aliphatic compounds, particularly those of the halogenated alkanes and alkenes, have also been shown to be nephrotoxic (32–38). In addition, conjugation with GSH has been implicated in the activation of a number of chemicals to metabolites that form adducts with DNA (39–46) and to metabolites that are both mutagenic and carcinogenic (47–55). It is likely that GSH-dependent metabolic activation within the kidney probably has greater toxicological significance than that mediated by the cytochrome P-450–dependent monooxygenases, a consequence of the relatively low activity of renal P-450, the high activity of GSH-related enzymes, and the rapid turnover of GSH within the kidney (56–59). For example, the nephrotoxicity of both trichloroethylene and hexachloro-1,3-butadiene, is dependent upon both GSH conjugate formation and the subsequent processing of the resulting conjugates by the enzymes of the β-lyase pathway (60–63). Convincing evidence for the involvement of this pathway in haloalkane and haloalkenal nephrotoxicity stems from a number of *in vivo* and *in vitro* studies (32–38).

EVIDENCE AGAINST THE INVOLVEMENT OF CYSTEINE CONJUGATE β-LYASE

In contrast to the nephrotoxicity of the haloalkanes and haloalkenes, the nephrotoxicity of 2-Br-(diglutathion-*S*-yl)HQ does not appear to involve the β-lyase pathway. Several lines of evidence support this contention. 6-Br-2,5-dihydroxythiophenol was synthesized as a putative β-lyase–catalyzed metabolite of 2-Br-3-(glutathion-*S*-yl)HQ (58). Administration of this compound to rats (0.27 mmol/kg ip) did cause elevations in BUN and renal proximal tubular necrosis without any apparent adverse effects to the liver. However, when a series of isomeric bromothiophenols were administered to rats (0.2 to 0.8 mmol/kg ip) no apparent histological alterations were seen in the kidney and no dose-related increases in BUN were seen. These findings suggested that the quinone function of 6-Br-2,5-dihydroxythiophenol, rather than the thiol function, was necessary for the expression of toxicity. The kidney-specific toxicity of 2-Br-(diglutathion-*S*-yl)HQ was rationalized upon the high specific activity of brush border γ-GT, which permitted the selective accumulation of this conjugate into proximal tubular cells. Such a mechanism appears inadequate to explain the kidney-specific toxicity of 6-Br-2,5-dihydroxythiophenol. However, pretreatment of rats with AT-125 decreased the nephrotoxicity of 6-Br-2,5-dihydroxythiophenol (Fig. 2) and it is probable that the thiophenol forms either a mixed disulfide or a conjugate with GSH *in vivo* and that it is these products that are targeted by γ-GT to renal proximal tubule cells. Although *in vivo* evidence for such a pathway is lacking, 6-Br-2,5-dihydroxythiophenol readily undergoes disulfide formation in the presence of oxygen (64).

Further evidence against the involvement of β-lyase in 2-Br-(diglutathion-*S*-yl)HQ nephrotoxicity was obtained in studies utilizing aminooxyacetic acid, a general inhibitor of pyridoxal phosphate–dependent enzymes and thus of β-lyase. Pretreatment of rats with aminooxyacetic acid (55 mg/kg ip) 1 hr prior to 2-Br-(diglutathion-*S*-yl)HQ (10 μmol/kg iv) administration had little effect on 2-Br-(diglutathion-*S*-yl)HQ–induced glucosuria, proteinuria, and enzymuria, and on eleva-

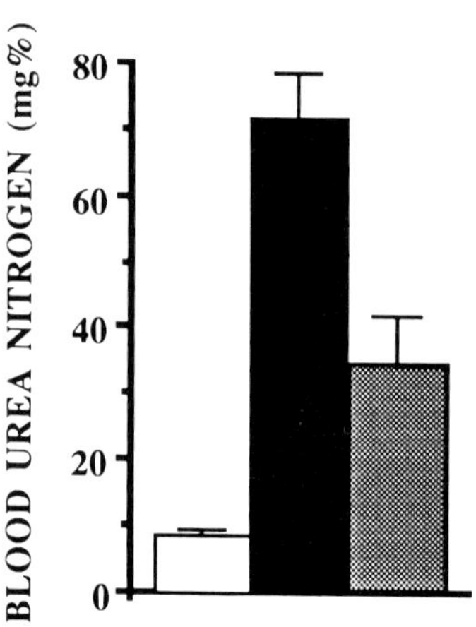

FIG. 2. Inhibition of 6-bromo-2,5-dihydroxythiophenol nephrotoxicity by AT-125. Animals were treated with AT-125 (10 mg/kg) 1 hr prior to the administration of 6-bromo-2,5-dihydroxythiophenol (0.27 mmol/kg ip), euthanized 24 hr later, and blood urea nitrogen concentrations determined. Values represent the mean ± S.E. (*n* = 6). □, Control; ■, 6-bromo-2,5-dihydroxythiophenol (0.27 mmol/kg ip); ▨, 6-bromo-2,5-dihydroxythiophenol (0.27 mmol/kg ip) plus AT-125 (10 mg/kg).

tions of BUN (12). A similar lack of protection with aminooxyacetic acid was seen in the nephrotoxicity caused by 2,3,5-(triglutathion-*S*-yl)hydroquinone (20 μmol/kg iv) (65). Aminooxyacetic acid (0.1 mM) also had minor effects on the *in vitro* covalent binding of 2-Br-(glutathion-[^{35}S]-yl)HQ conjugates to rat kidney homogenates (16). Finally, as stated above, neither cysteine nor *N*-acetylcysteine conjugates appear to be excreted as major urinary metabolites of 2-BrHQ, despite the formation of the corresponding GSH conjugates. Although the inability to identify these metabolites in urine does not preclude their formation *in situ*, the data taken together argue against a major role for β-lyase in 2-Br-(diglutathion-*S*-yl)HQ–mediated nephrotoxicity.

γ-GLUTAMYL TRANSPEPTIDASE AND THE REGULATION OF QUINOL-THIOETHER OXIDATION

If processing of 2-Br-(diglutathion-*S*-yl)HQ to a reactive thiol by β-lyase is not involved in the nephrotoxicity, then presumably the quinone function of the molecule must be important. In contrast to the effects of AT-125 and aminooxyacetic acid on the *in vitro* covalent binding of 2-Br-(glutathion-[^{35}S]-yl)HQ conjugates to rat kidney homogenates (see above) ascorbic acid (1mM) inhibited binding of the 2-Br-mono-(glutathion-[^{35}S]-yl)HQ conjugates by 62% to 87% (16). However, the amount of 2-Br-(diglutathion-[^{35}S]-yl)HQ binding to rat kidney homogenates was substantially lower than that of the 2-Br-mono-(glutathion-[^{35}S]-yl)HQ conjugates, and this binding was only partially inhibited (28%) by ascorbic acid (16).

The reason for the differential effect of ascorbic acid on the *in vitro* covalent binding of 2-Br-(glutathion-[^{35}S]-yl)HQ conjugates to rat kidney homogenates may be related to the ease of oxidation of these conjugates. Thus, at pH 7.4, the oxidation potential ($E_{1/2}$, as determined by hydrodynamic voltammetry with amperometric detection) of 2-Br-(diglutathion-*S*-yl)HQ was substantially higher than either of the 2-Br-mono-(glutathion-*S*-yl)HQ conjugates (66). This means that 2-Br-(diglutathion-*S*-yl)HQ is far more difficult to oxidize than the 2-Br-mono-(glutathion-*S*-yl)HQ conjugates and may also explain why the covalent binding of 2-Br-(diglutathion-[^{35}S]-yl)HQ to kidney homogenates was two- to threefold less than that of the 2-Br-mono-(glutathion-[^{35}S]-yl)HQ conjugates. The ability of ascorbic acid to inhibit the covalent binding of the conjugates correlated with their oxidation potentials, as determined by cyclic voltammetry at pH 4.0 (16).

Although 2-Br-(diglutathion-*S*-yl)HQ is more difficult to oxidize than either of the 2-Br-mono-(glutathion-*S*-yl)HQ conjugates, and although oxidation to the quinone appears necessary for covalent binding, 2-Br-(diglutathion-*S*-yl)HQ is a more potent nephrotoxicant than the 2-Br-mono-(glutathion-*S*-yl)HQ conjugates. This apparent paradox was resolved when the effects of γ-GT and metabolism through the mercapturic acid pathway on the ease of oxidation of the various intermediates was investigated. Interestingly, although 2-Br-(diglutathion-*S*-yl)HQ was more difficult to oxidize than the 2-Br-mono-(glutathion-*S*-yl)HQ conjugates, 2-Br-(dicystein-*S*-yl)HQ had a far lower oxidation potential than 2-Br-(diglutathion-*S*-yl)HQ and was easier to oxidize than any of the 2-Br-mono-(cystein-*S*-yl)HQ conjugates. Thus, it appears that γ-GT serves at least two functions in the nephrotoxicity of 2-Br-(diglutathion-*S*-yl)HQ. First, it serves a transport function, in that metabolism to the cysteinylglycine and/or cysteine conjugate may be a prerequisite for transport across the apical (luminal) and/or basal-lateral membranes. Second, it serves to convert the relatively stable 2-Br-(diglutathion-*S*-yl)HQ into a readily oxidizable, and therefore potentially more reactive, metabolite, namely 2-Br-(dicystein-*S*-yl)HQ.

Based upon the ability of quinones to arylate tissue macromolecules and/or undergo redox cycling, with the concomitant generation of reactive oxygen species, 2-Br-(diglutathion-*S*-yl)HQ–mediated nephrotoxicity could be initiated by either, or both, of these reactions. However, at present there is little evidence to suggest that 2-Br-(diglutathion-*S*-yl)HQ undergoes redox cycling with the generation of reactive oxygen species. For example, whereas 2-Br-(diglutathion-*S*-yl)HQ does not stimulate NADPH consumption in microsomal incubations (unpublished data), the extent of the *in vivo* covalent binding of 2-Br-[^{14}C]-HQ to renal tissue correlated with the degree of nephrotoxicity, as monitored by increases in BUN (31). Schnellman et al. (67,68) also concluded that the toxicity of 2-BrHQ to rabbit renal proximal tubule suspensions was more likely a consequence of covalent binding (67) rather than of oxidative stress (68). Thus, 2-BrHQ neither increased oxidized GSH (GSSG) content nor initiated lipid peroxidation; the antioxidant butylated hydroxytoluene did not protect against 2-BrHQ–induced mitochondrial dysfunction; and inhibition of GSH reductase neither increased GSSG content nor potentiated 2-BrHQ–induced mitochondrial dysfunction and cell death (68). In addition, although 2-Br-3-(*N*-acetylcystein-*S*-yl)HQ rapidly depleted cellular GSH concentrations to less than 5% of controls within 5 min of application to suspensions of rat renal tubular epithelial cells, there was no concomitant oxidation of GSH to GSSG (69).

In contrast to 2-BrHQ and 2-Br-(diglutathion-*S*-yl)HQ, both the GSH and mercapturic acid conjugates of 2-methyl-1,4-naphthoquinone (menadione) undergo redox cycling with the concomitant generation of reactive oxygen species (70,71). In addition, 2-methyl-3-(*N*-acetylcystein-*S*-yl)-1,4-naphthoquinone (50 to 250 μM) was toxic when incubated with isolated rat renal epithelial cells and inhibition of GSH reductase with *N*,*N*-bis(2-chloroethyl)-*N*-nitrosourea potentiated the toxicity (71). These data suggest that redox cycling may play a role in the *in vitro* toxicity of 2-methyl-3-(*N*-acetylcystein-*S*-yl)-1,4-naphthoquinone (71). 2-Methyl-3-(*N*-acetylcystein-*S*-yl)-1,4-naphthoquinone also caused renal proximal tubular necrosis following administration (50 to 200 μmol/kg iv) to rats (72). Whether redox cycling plays a role in the *in vivo* nephrotoxicity of 2-methyl-3-(*N*-acetylcystein-*S*-yl)-1,4-naphthoquinone however, remains to be determined. In contrast, although 2-methyl-3-(glutathion-*S*-yl)-1,4-naphthoquinone (600 μM) produced toxicity in the isolated perfused rat kidney (73), it was not nephrotoxic when administered *in vivo* (200 μmol/kg iv) (72) nor when incubated with isolated rat renal epithelial cells (250 μM) (71). Apart from the obvious differences in the doses used, an explanation for the different results remains to be established.

OXIDATIVE CYCLIZATION AND 1,4-BENZOTHIAZINE FORMATION

Since the further metabolism of the GSH conjugates by γ-GT was required for the expression of toxicity, the fate of 2-Br-3-(glutathion-*S*-yl)HQ was examined in more detail (74). Initial attempts to synthesize the cystein-*S*-yl conjugates of 2-BrHQ resulted in the formation and deposition of an insoluble black precipitate, the nature of which was unclear. The same insoluble material was formed as the end product of the reaction of γ-GT with 2-Br-3-(glutathion-*S*-yl)HQ. When the precipitate was dissolved in either strong acid or base it gave rise to either a violet or red solution, respectively. The product(s) therefore exhibited properties of a pH indicator. When the amount of γ-GT used to catalyze this reaction was substantially decreased, and the reaction terminated at various times by freezing in a dry ice/acetone bath prior to the deposition of the insoluble pigment, intermediate products of the reaction could be identified by HPLC analysis. Isolation and purification of the first major intermediate of the reaction and analysis by both nuclear magnetic resonance (NMR), and mass spectroscopy revealed the formation of a 1,4-benzothiazine derivative, namely 2*H*-(3-glycinyl)-7-hydroxy-8-bromo-1,4-benzothiazine (74). This product arises via the oxidative cyclization of 2-Br-3-(cystein-*S*-ylglycyl) HQ (Fig. 3, reactions 6–9). Removal of the γ-glutamate moiety releases the cysteinyl amino group from the peptide bond and results in formation of a free α-amino group. Oxidation of the hydroquinone function in the conjugate permits condensation of the free α-amino group with the quinone carbonyl, elimination of water, and 1,4-benzothiazine formation. The subsequent acid-catalyzed elimination of glycine initiates the formation of dimeric and possibly polymeric products that eventually constitute the final insoluble product of these reactions. The pH indicator properties of the pigment(s) arising from these reactions are similar to those of the trichochrome polymers that are formed during phaeomelanin biosynthesis from *S*-(3,4-dihydroxyphenylalanine)-L-cysteine (75). The elucidation of this pathway also offered a possible explanation for the inability to identify either cystein-*S*-yl or *N*-acetylcystein-*S*-yl conjugates as major metabolites in the urine of rats treated with 2-Br-[^{14}C]-HQ (31). Moreover, it provided additional support to discount a major role for β-lyase in the development of the nephrotoxicity. Oxidative cyclization of the cystein-*S*-ylglycine conjugates (and possibly of the cystein-*S*-yl conjugate) diverts the products of the γ-GT catalyzed reaction away from the classic mercapturic acid pathway enzymes. Thus, little, if any, free 2-Br-(cystein-*S*-yl)HQ conjugates will be available for metabolism to reactive thiols by β-lyase. Consequently, inhibition of this enzyme with aminooxyacetic acid has little effect on the *in vivo* toxicity of 2-Br-(diglutathion-*S*-yl)HQ.

What, if any, are the toxicological consequences of these reactions? It seemed possible that the deposition of insoluble polymers within renal proximal tubules might contribute to the nephrotoxicity of the 2-Br-(glutathion-*S*-yl)HQ conjugates. This possibility was investigated by synthesizing the homocysteine conjugates of 2-BrHQ and determining their *in vivo* activity (76). The additional methylene group in homocysteine should effectively preclude cyclization of the α-amino group.

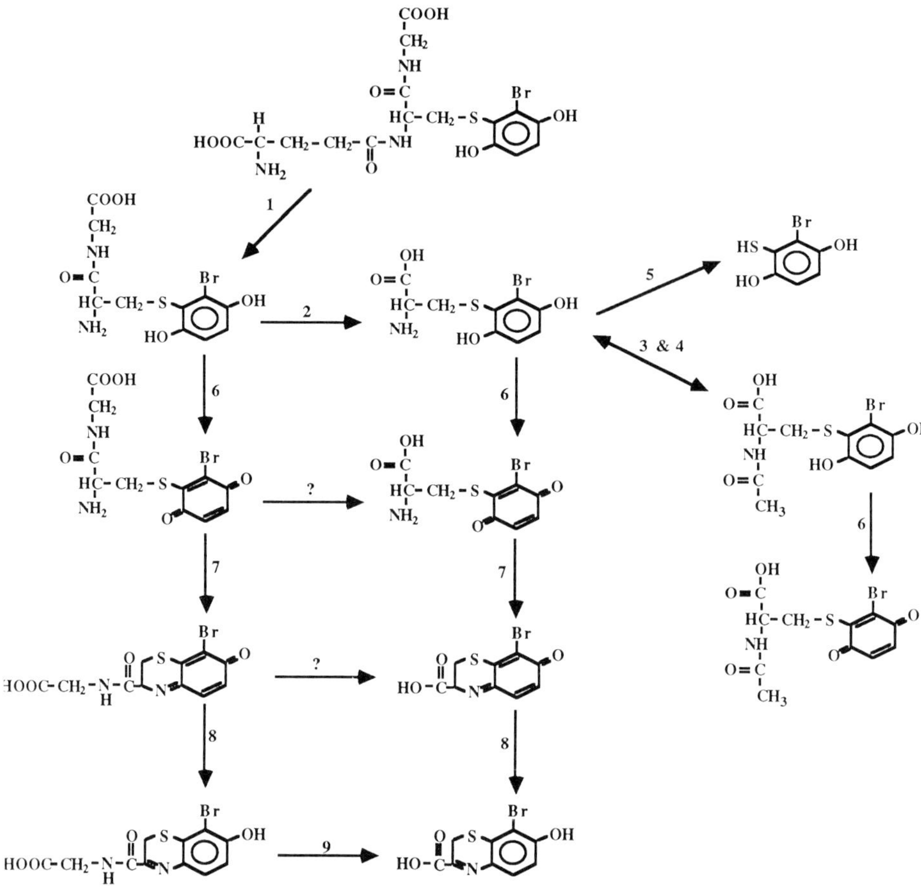

FIG. 3. Potential metabolic pathways of 2-bromo-3-(glutathion-*S*-yl)hydroquinone. (*1*) γ-Glutamyl transpeptidase; (*2*) cysteinylglycine dipeptidase/aminopeptidase M; (*3*) cysteine conjugate *N*-acetyltransferase; (*4*) *N*-acetylcysteine conjugate deacetylase; (*5*) cysteine conjugate β-lyase; (*6*) thioether oxidation; (*7*) intramolecular cyclization (via elimination of water); (*8*) 1,4-benzothiazine formation (via hydrogen shift) (*9* and *?*) elimination of glycine. Reactions *1* to *5* represent the mercapturic acid pathway and the thioether shunt. The products of reaction *6* all have the potential to arylate tissue macromolecules. Reactions *7* to *9* constitute a detoxication pathway via removal of the reactive quinone function, achieved by intramolecular cyclization and 1,4-benzothiazine formation. The products of reaction *8* can undergo further spontaneous reaction to dimeric and polymeric melanin-like pigments.

Thus, if oxidative cyclization and 1,4-benzothiazine formation are prerequisites for the development of nephrotoxicity, the homocysteine analogues should be without effect. However, administration of a mixture of isomeric 2-Br-(homocystein-*S*-yl)HQ conjugates to male Sprague-Dawley rats caused significant increases in BUN and renal proximal tubular necrosis, as observed histologically (76). Thus, at least for the 2-Br-(glutathion-*S*-yl)HQ conjugates, 1,4-benzothiazine formation appears to constitute an intramolecular detoxication reaction by eliminating the reactive quinone function from the molecule.

NEPHROTOXICITY OF 2-BROMO-(CYSTEIN-*S*-YL)HQ AND 2-BROMO-(*N*-ACETYLCYSTEIN-*S*-YL)HQ CONJUGATES

Although neither cystein-*S*-yl nor *N*-acetylcystein-*S*-yl conjugates appear to be excreted as major urinary metabolites of 2-BrHQ (31) this did not preclude the possibility that they may contribute to the nephrotoxicity observed following either 2-BrHQ or 2-Br-(diglutathion-*S*-yl)HQ administration to rats. The cystein-*S*-yl and *N*-acetylcystein-*S*-yl conjugates of 2-BrHQ were therefore synthesized and the *in vivo* toxicity of the resulting isomers examined. Consistent with the results found with the GSH conjugates, both 2-Br-(dicystein-*S*-yl)HQ and 2-Br-(di-*N*-acetylcystein-*S*-yl)HQ were more potent nephrotoxicants than their corresponding mono-substituted analogues (29). In addition, the cysteine conjugates were more toxic, on a per dose basis, than the *N*-acetylcysteine conjugates and substantial differences were observed in the relative toxicity caused by the 2-Br-mono-(*N*-acetylcystein-*S*-yl)HQ conjugates (29,77). Thus, the position of thiol addition significantly influenced the nephrotoxicity of the mercapturates; 2-Br-6-(*N*-acetylcystein-*S*-yl)HQ was a more potent nephrotoxicant than 2-Br-5-(*N*-acetylcystein-*S*-yl)HQ, whereas 2-Br-3-(*N*-acetylcystein-*S*-yl)HQ (200 μmol/kg iv) was essentially without effect. The reasons for these differences are unclear but it is likely that several factors contribute not only to the variation in isomeric potency, but also to the differences seen between the cysteine and *N*-acetylcysteine conjugates. For example, differences in oxidation potentials, in renal transport, and in the relative rates of *N*-acetylation and deacetylation may all play a role in determining the relative toxicity of each isomer. For example, 2-Br-6-(*N*-acetylcystein-*S*-yl)HQ was the most toxic of the mono-*N*-acetylcysteine conjugates and was the most rapidly deacetylated (78). This is an important correlation because the cystein-*S*-yl conjugates are easier to oxidize than the mercapturates (66,76). Consequently, deacetylation of the mercapturic acid may be necessary for the oxidation of the hydroquinone moiety and the formation of reactive quinones.

Although 2-Br-(di-*N*-acetylcystein-*S*-yl)HQ is nephrotoxic, its contribution to the nephrotoxicity of 2-Br-(diglutathion-*S*-yl)HQ *in vivo* is probably minor. In support of this view, both aminooxyacetic acid and probenecid almost completely inhibited the nephrotoxicity of 2-Br-(di-*N*-acetylcystein-*S*-yl)HQ. Since neither of these agents inhibited the nephrotoxicity of 2-Br-(diglutathion-*S*-yl)HQ it seems reasonable to assume that either 2-Br-(di-*N*-acetylcystein-*S*-yl)HQ is not formed as a major metabolite of the GSH conjugate *in vivo*, or the disposition of the mercapturate is different when it is formed from the GSH conjugate *in vivo*, compared to its disposition when it is administered systemically. Based upon prior observations on the *in vivo* disposition of 2-Br-[^{14}C]-HQ (31), the former explanation appears more likely. The ability of aminooxyacetic acid to inhibit the toxicity of 2-Br-(di-*N*-acetylcystein-*S*-yl)HQ also implies that deacetylation is a prerequisite for the toxicity of the mercapturate, since *N*-acetylcysteine conjugates are not substrates for β-lyase.

Additional studies support the contention that the disposition of the metabolites arising from the γ-GT catalyzed metabolism of the GSH conjugates *in vivo* is different from their disposition when administered systemically. In support of this view, aminooxyacetic acid almost completely inhibited the nephrotoxicity of 2-Br-6- (*N*-acetylcystein-*S*-yl)HQ and 2-Br-(di-*N*-acetylcystein-*S*-yl)HQ, yet only partially inhibited that of 2-Br-5&6-(cystein-*S*-yl)HQ and had no effect on 2-Br-(dicystein-*S*-yl)HQ nephrotoxicity (29). Thus, when the cysteine conjugates are generated intracellularly via deacetylation of the *N*-acetylcysteine conjugates, inhibition of β-lyase effectively prevents cytotoxicity. In contrast, when the cysteine conjugate was presented to renal proximal tubular cells extracellularly, either via the activity of γ-GT and dipeptidases on the GSH conjugates, or via systemic administration of the cysteine conjugates, the inhibition of β-lyase was less effective at reducing the ensuing toxicity. This also suggests that the target of the ultimate nephrotoxic metabolite(s) (perhaps the quinone form of the cysteine conjugates) generated from 2-Br-(diglutathion-*S*-yl)HQ *in vivo* may be the cell membrane (see below).

Although 2-Br-3-(*N*-acetylcystein-*S*-yl)HQ is essentially inactive as a renal toxicant *in vivo* (see above) concentrations of 25 to 50 μM did cause cytotoxicity when incubated with rat renal tubular epithelial cells *in vitro* (69). Moreover, the cytotoxicity was not prevented by aminooxyacetic acid but was inhibited by 1 mM probenecid (69). The reasons for the discrepancy between the *in vivo* and *in vitro* data are presently unclear but serve to highlight the problems involved with extrapolating *in vitro* data to the more complex system that exists *in vivo*.

SUBCELLULAR TARGETS OF QUINONE-THIOETHERS

Several important questions arise with respect to the *in vivo* fate of the products of the γ-GT catalyzed metabolism of 2-Br-(glutathion-*S*-yl)HQ conjugates. For example, *Does oxidative cyclization and 1,4-benzothiazine formation occur* in vivo? *If so, does this occur before or after the cysteine and/or cysteinylglycine conjugates are transported into the proximal tubular cells?* The answer to these questions have important implications with regard to the possible cellular targets for these conjugates and their mechanism of cytotoxicity. Since the cysteine conjugates, and probably the cysteinylglycine conjugates, are readily oxidized, it is possible that the resulting quinones interact with nucleophilic targets close to their site of formation, that is the brush border membrane of renal proximal tubular cells. The appearance of γ-GT in the urine of animals treated with 2-Br-(diglutathion-*S*-yl)HQ, and other quinone-thioethers, is an extremely sensitive indicator of the damage to proximal tubular cells (16,65,72). However, *Is the urinary excretion of γ-GT merely a consequence of cell damage or is the alteration of the brush border membrane, which permits the release of γ-GT into tubular fluid, an initiating event in cell damage?* We cannot answer this question at present but suffice it to say that increases in the urinary excretion of γ-GT occur at doses much lower than those required to cause elevations in BUN and other overt signs of proximal tubular necrosis, and at very early time points (within 1 to 2 hr) following administration of the quinone-thioethers. The question will probably best be answered by studying the time course of the biochemical and pathological changes that occur immediately following administration of 2-Br-(diglutathion-*S*-yl)HQ to rats and by comparing these changes to the onset of overt toxicity.

If the cysteine and/or cysteinylglycine conjugates are transported into proximal tubular cells *prior* to oxidation, then the resulting quinones will have the potential to interact with intracellular macromolecules. Mitochondria have been identified as the primary subcellular target for nephrotoxic aliphatic GSH and cysteine conjugates (79–81) and mitochondrial function is inhibited in *in vitro* incubations of 2-BrHQ with isolated rabbit renal proximal tubules (82). Whether or not mitochondria are *in vivo* targets for 2-Br-(diglutathion-*S*-yl)HQ remains to be determined but some of our preliminary work in this area (83) shows that 24 hr after administration of 2-BrHQ to rats, a time at which BUN concentrations are significantly increased, mitochondrial respiratory function, as assessed by a determination of the respiratory control ratio, appears unaffected. More detailed work is clearly required before a role for altered mitochondrial function in the development of 2-Br-(diglutathion-*S*-yl)HQ–mediated nephrotoxicity can be established.

SPECIES DIFFERENCES IN SUSCEPTIBILITY TO 2-BROMO-(DIGLUTATHION-*S*-YL)HQ–MEDIATED NEPHROTOXICITY

From the preceding discussion it is evident that although the activity of γ-GT is a prerequisite for 2-Br-(diglutathion-*S*-yl)HQ–mediated nephrotoxicity, factors other than γ-GT contribute significantly to the *modulation* of the toxicity. This brings the discussion full circle, because although rats (both Sprague-Dawley and Fischer 344) exhibit the highest level of renal γ-GT and are the most susceptible rodent species to 2-Br-(diglutathion-*S*-yl)HQ (20 μmol/kg iv)–induced nephrotoxicity, species differences in renal γ-GT did not correlate to susceptibility in the other species examined (84). The guinea pig, which exhibited the lowest activity of renal γ-GT of the species examined (8% of the rat) was the only other species found to be susceptible to 2-Br-(diglutathion-*S*-yl)HQ (200 μmol/kg intracardiac) although it required a dose ten times higher than that required to produce toxicity in rats. Thus, factors other than γ-GT probably play an important role in *modulating* species susceptibility to 2-Br-(diglutathion-*S*-yl)HQ nephrotoxicity (84).

Species variations in the apparent molecular weight of γ-GT subunits have been reported (85) and shown to be a consequence of differences in protein glycosylation (86). Recent work on the molecular biology of γ-GT (87–91) also suggest that differences exist not only between species but possibly also between tissues. Species differences also exist in the relative γ-glutamyl acceptor substrate specificity of renal γ-GT (85,92,93). Perhaps species differences in the proximal tubular luminal concentration of γ-glutamyl acceptors might contribute to differences in the regulation of γ-GT activity and susceptibility to 2-Br-(diglutathion-*S*-yl)HQ nephrotoxicity. Thus, although differences in the specific activity of renal γ-GT exist between species, differences in the structure and regulation of the enzyme may also contribute to its role in mediating the toxicity of 2-Br-(diglutathion-*S*-yl)HQ *in vivo*.

γ-GT catalyzes the first step of a series of reactions that result in mercapturic acid biosynthesis (Fig. 3, reactions 1–3). The final step in mercapturic acid synthesis involves the transfer of an acetyl group from acetyl coenzyme A to the cystein-*S*-yl amino group, catalyzed by thioether *N*-acetyltransferase. It has been suggested that the relative inability of guinea pigs to excrete mercapturic acids was a consequence of their inability to *N*-acetylate cysteine conjugates (94). However, in addition, the low activity of renal γ-GT in this species may also contribute to the relatively low rate of mercapturic acid synthesis. Renal γ-GT activity in the guinea pig may still be sufficient to allow considerable processing of GSH conjugates. In addition, metabolism of GSH conjugates by biliary and intestinal enzymes might also contribute to mercapturic acid formation in the guinea pig. The activity of the corresponding *N*-deacetylase in the guinea pig, compared to other species, is very high (unpublished data) and this might provide the basis upon which to explain the susceptibility of this species to 2-Br-(diglutathion-*S*-yl)HQ nephrotoxicity. Thus, the concentration of the cysteine conjugate generated by each species will depend not only upon the activity of γ-GT, but also upon the relative activities of the *N*-acetyltransferase and *N*-deacetylase enzymes (differences in the rate of transport of the cysteine and *N*-acetylcysteine conjugates both into and out of renal proximal tubular cells will also be important). Since the cystein-*S*-yl conjugates are easier to oxidize than the *N*-acetylcystein-*S*-yl conjugates (61), conditions favoring formation of the former will most likely increase the chances of initiating toxicity. In the guinea pig, the balance of these activities favors the formation of high cysteine conjugate concentrations.

Finally, since oxidation is important in the toxicity of these conjugates, species differences in the balance between those factors that contribute to quinone-thioether oxidation and quinone-thioether reduction, will also influence species susceptibility to nephrotoxicity. Such factors might include the availability of reducing equivalents such as NAD(P)H and GSH and enzymatic determinants such as the specific activity of NAD(P)H quinone oxidoreductase (Enzyme Commission [EC] 1.6.99.2). Quinone-GSH conjugates have been shown to be substrates for this enzyme (95). However, inhibition of rat renal NAD(P)H:quinone oxidoreductase with dicumarol did not significantly affect the nephrotoxicity of either 2-Br-mono-(glutathion-*S*-yl)HQ conjugates (100 μmol/kg iv) or of 2-Br-(diglutathion-*S*-yl)HQ (10 μmol/kg iv) (70). Although the mechanism of 2-BrHQ–thioether oxidation remains unclear, it seems logical that differences in the ability of each species to catalyze this oxidation will also determine susceptibility to nephrotoxicity.

SIGNIFICANCE AND OPPORTUNITIES

The National Toxicology Program recently determined, under the conditions of 2-year gavage experiments, that hydroquinone demonstrated "*evidence of carcinogenic activity*" in male F344/N rats, as shown by marked increases in tubular cell adenomas of the kidneys (96). The mechanism of hydroquinone-mediated nephrocarcinogenicity in male F344/N rats is not known. However, GSH conjugates of hydroquinone, in particular, 2,3,5-(triglutathion-*S*-yl)hydroquinone, are renal proximal tubular toxicants in male Sprague-Dawley rats (59). Whether these conjugates play a role in hydroquinone-mediated nephrocarcinogenicity remains to be determined.

Although this book focuses on renal toxicology, the relationships uncovered during studies of bromobenzene-mediated nephrotoxicity, specifically those relating to the biochemical basis of its target organ selectivity, have implications beyond renal toxicology and warrant a brief discussion. The renal specific toxicity of 2-Br-(diglutathion-*S*-yl)HQ is at least partially mediated by γ-GT. However, cells other than those of the epithelial cells of renal proximal tubules, such as pancreatic acinar and ductile epithelial cells and the epithelial cells of the jejunum, bile duct, epididymis, seminal vesicles, bronchioles, thyroid follicles, choroid plexus, ciliary body, and retinal pigment epithelium, which also express relatively high γ-GT activity, may also be exposed to higher concentrations of potentially toxic quinone-thioethers than other tissues (31,61). However, as noted above for the species differences, the toxicity of quinone-thioethers to γ-GT–containing cells will also be modulated by a variety of other factors. These factors may protect certain γ-GT containing tissues from the toxic effects of quinone-thioethers. The relative activities of cysteine conjugate *N*-acetyltransferase and the corresponding *N*-deacetylase probably contribute to both the species and tissue susceptibility of γ-GT–containing cells to the toxicity of quinone-thioethers. There is also increasing evidence indicating that a number of quinone-thioethers exhibit a variety of toxicological activity (97). Little is known of the mechanisms by which these compounds exert their toxicological actions nor of the factors that might regulate this activity. Quinone-thioether toxicology might therefore prove a fruitful area for future research.

Investigations with bromobenzene have therefore contributed substantially to our present understanding (or confusion) of the mechanisms by which chemicals cause toxicity (98). Indeed, it was in 1879 that two groups independently published the first identification of mercapturic acids in urine following the treatment of animals with bromobenzene (99,100). It is interesting to note that the spirit of scientific competition as evidenced by the desire to achieve precedence in publication, was alive and well 110 years ago! More recently, particularly over the past 20 years, several groups have continued to unravel the complex interrelationships that exist between the metabolism of bromobenzene and the development of toxicity. Indeed, the knowledge gained from these prior studies provided the firm foundation from which we have been able to proceed with our own studies.

ACKNOWLEDGMENTS

Portions of the work described in this chapter were supported by awards from the United States Public Health Service (ES 04662, GM 39338). Serrine S. Lau was the recipient of a Pharmaceutical Manufacturers Association Foundation Faculty Development Award. In addition, we would like to extend our appreciation to Barbara Hill (supported by a Pharmaceutical Manufacturers Association Foundation Pre-Doctoral Fellowship), Maria Rivera (supported by GM 13270), Rowena Sioco, Heather Kleiner, and Dr. Stony Lo for their constant hard work. Thanks are also due to many of our colleagues and collaborators. In particular, special thanks go to Dr. Jim Gillette for his constant encouragement and invaluable and insightful comments during the initial development of this work. In addition, Drs. Robert J. Highet, Thomas W. Jones, Rick G. Schnellman, and Jim Stevens have provided invaluable assistance with various aspects of the work described above. Finally, to the founding members of the RFC, "Bubba," Glenn, Jim, Jerry, Lois, and Ted, thanks for making research so much fun.

REFERENCES

1. Monks TJ, Lau SS. Reactive intermediates and their toxicological significance. *Toxicology* 1988;52:1–53.
2. Reid WD. Mechanism of renal necrosis induced by bromobenzene or chlorobenzene. *Exp Mol Pathol* 1973;19:197–214.
3. Monks TJ, Lau SS, Gillette JR. Diffusion of reactive metabolites out of hepatocytes: studies with bromobenzene. *J Pharmacol Exp Ther* 1984;228:393–399.
4. Gillette JR, Lau SS, Monks TJ. Intra and extracellular formation of metabolites from chemically reactive species. *Biochem Soc Trans* 1984;12:4–7.
5. Lau SS, Monks TJ, Greene KE, Gillette JR. Detection and half-life of bromobenzene-3,4-oxide in blood. *Xenobiotica* 1984;14:539–543.
6. Monks TJ, Lau SS. Activation and detoxification of bromobenzene in extrahepatic tissues. *Life Sci* 1984;35:561–568.
7. Rush GF, Newton JF, Maita K, Kuo C, Hook JB. Nephrotoxicity of phenolic bromobenzene metabolites in the mouse. *Toxicology* 1984;30:259–272.
8. Monks TJ, Lau SS, Highet RJ. Formation of non-toxic reactive metabolites of *para*-bromophenol: identification of a new glutathione conjugate. *Drug Metab Dispos* 1984;12:432–437.
9. Mitchell JR, Reid WD, Christie B, Moskowitz J, Krishna G, Brodie BB. Bromobenzene induced hepatic necrosis. Species differences and protection by SKF 525A. *Res Commun Chem Pathol Pharmacol* 1971;2:877–888.
10. Thor H, Svensson S, Hartzell P, Orrenius S. Biotransformation of bromobenzene to reactive metabolites by isolated hepatocytes. In: Snyder R, Parke DV, Kocsis JJ, Jollow DJ, Gibson GG, Witmer CM, eds. *Biological Reactive Intermediates*, Part A, vol 2. New York: Plenum Press, 1982;287–299.

11. Lau SS, Monks TJ, Greene KE, Gillette JR. The role of *ortho*-bromophenol in the nephrotoxicity of bromobenzene. *Toxicol Appl Pharmacol* 1984;72:539–549.
12. Lau SS, Monks TJ, Gillette JR. Identification of 2-bromohydroquinone as a metabolite of bromobenzene: implication for bromobenzene induced nephrotoxicity. *J Pharmacol Exp Ther* 1984; 230:360–366.
13. Monks TJ, Lau SS, Highet RJ, Gillette JR. Glutathione conjugates of 2-bromohydroquinone are nephrotoxic. *Drug Metab Dispos* 1985;13:553–559.
14. Lau SS, Monks TJ. Co-oxidation of 2-bromohydroquinone by renal prostaglandin synthase. Modulation of prostaglandin synthesis by 2-bromohydroquinone and glutathione. *Drug Metab Dispos* 1987;15:801–807.
15. Schnellman RG, Mandel LJ. Cellular toxicity of bromobenzene and bromobenzene metabolites to rabbit proximal tubules: the role and mechanism of 2-bromohydroquinone. *J Pharmacol Exp Ther* 1986;237:456–461.
16. Monks TJ, Highet RJ, Lau SS. 2-Bromo-(diglutathion-*S*-yl)hydroquinone nephrotoxicity: physiological, biochemical and electrochemical determinants. *Mol Pharmacol* 1988;34:492–500.
17. Lash LH, Jones DP. Renal glutathione transport. Characteristics of the sodium dependent system in the basal-lateral membrane. *J Biol Chem* 1983;259:14508–14514.
18. Monks TJ, Lau SS. Commentary: renal transport processes and glutathione conjugate mediated nephrotoxicity. *Drug Metab Dispos* 1987;15:437–441.
19. Lau SS, McMenamin MG, Monks TJ. Differential uptake of isomeric 2-bromohydroquinone-glutathione conjugates into kidney slices. *Biochem Biophys Res Commun* 1988;152:223–230.
20. Lo HH, Monks TJ, Lau SS. Kinetics of the γ-glutamyl transpeptidase catalysed hydrolysis and transpeptidation of isomeric 2-bromo-(glutathion-*S*-yl)hydroquinones. *Toxicologist* 1990;10:197.
21. Weber G. Biochemical strategy of cancer cells and the design of chemotherapy: G.H.A. Clowes Memorial Lecture. *Cancer Res* 1983;43:3466–3492.
22. Reed DJ, Ellis WW, Meck RA. The inhibition of γ-glutamyltranspeptidase and glutathione metabolism of isolated rat kidney cells by L-(αS,5S)-α-amino-3-chloro-4,5-dihydro-5-isoxazoleacetic acid (AT-125; NSC-163501). *Biochem Biophys Res Commun* 1980;94:1273–1277.
23. Allen L, Meck RA, Yunis A. The inhibition of γ-glutamyl transpeptidase from human pancreatic carcinoma cells by (αS,5S)-α-amino-3-chloro-4,5-dihydro-5-isoxazoleacetic acid (AT-125; NSC-163501). *Res Commun Chem Pathol Pharmacol* 1980;27:175–182.
24. Schasteen CS, Curthoys NP, Reed DJ. The binding mechanism of glutathione and the anti-tumor drug L-(αS,5S)-α-amino-3-chloro-4,5-dihydro-5-isoxazoleacetic acid (AT-125; NSC-163501) to γ-glutamyltransferase. *Biochem Biophys Res Commun* 1983;112:564–570.
25. Weiner IM, Wahington JA, Mudge GH. On the mechanism of action of probenecid on renal tubular secretion. *Bull Johns Hopkins Hosp* 1960;106:333–346.
26. Lock EA, Ishmael J. Effect of the organic acid transport inhibitor probenecid on renal cortical uptake and proximal tubular toxicity of hexachloro-1,3-butadiene and its conjugates. *Toxicol Appl Pharmacol* 1985;81:32–42.
27. Elfarra AA, Baggs RB, Anders MW. Structure nephrotoxicity relationships of *S*-(2-chloroethyl)-*DL*-cysteine and analogs. Role for an episulfonium ion. *J Pharmacol Exp Ther* 1985;233: 512–516.
28. Elfarra AA, Jakobson I, Anders MW. Mechanism of *S*-(1,2-dichlorovinyl)-glutathione induced nephrotoxicity. *Biochem Pharmacol* 1986;35:283–288.
29. Monks TJ, Jones TW, Hill BA, Lau SS. Nephrotoxicity of 2-bromo-(cystein-*S*-yl)hydroquinone and 2-bromo-(*N*-acetyl-*L*-cystein-*S*-yl)hydroquinone thioethers. *Toxicol Appl Pharmacol* 1991; 111:279–298.
30. Ullrich KJ, Rumrich G, Gemborys M, Dekant W. Transformation and transport: how does metabolic transformation change the affinity of substrates for the renal contraluminal anion and cation transporters? *Toxicol Lett* 1990:53:19–27.
31. Lau SS, Monks TJ. The *in vivo* disposition of 2-bromo-[^{14}C]-hydroquinone and the effect of γ-glutamyl transpeptidase inhibition. *Toxicol Appl Pharmacol* 1990;103:121–132.
32. Lock EA. The nephrotoxicity of haloalkane and haloalkene glutathione conjugates. In: De Matteis F, Lock EA, eds. *Selectivity and Molecular Mechanisms of Toxicity*. New York: Macmillan, 1987; 59–83.
33. Anders MW, Lash LH, Dekant W, Elfarra AA, Dohn DR. Biosynthesis and biotransformation of glutathione *S*-conjugates to toxic metabolites. *CRC Crit Rev Toxicol* 1988;18:311–341.
34. Lock EA. Studies on the mechanism of nephrotoxicity and nephrocarcinogenicity of halogenated alkenes. *CRC Crit Rev Toxicol* 1988;19:23–42.

35. van Bladeren PJ. Formation of toxic metabolites from drugs and other xenobiotics by glutathione conjugation. *Trends Pharm Sci* 1988;9:295–298.
36. Dekant W, Vamvakas S, Anders MW. Bioactivation of nephrotoxic haloalkenes by glutathione conjugation: formation of toxic and mutagenic intermediates by cysteine conjugate β-lyase. *Drug Metab Rev* 1989;20:43–83.
37. Monks TJ, Lau SS. Sulfur conjugate-mediated toxicities. *Rev Biochem Toxicol* 1989;10:41–90.
38. Monks TJ, Anders MW, Dekant W, Stevens JL, Lau SS, van Bladeren PJ. Contemporary issues in toxicology. Glutathione conjugate mediated toxicities. *Toxicol Appl Pharmacol* 1990;106:1–19.
39. Ozawa N, Guengerich FP. Evidence for formation of an *S*-[2(*N*-guanyl)ethyl] glutathione adduct in glutathione-mediated binding of the carcinogen 1,2-dibromoethane to DNA. *Proc Natl Acad Sci USA* 1983;80:5266–5270.
40. Vadi HV, Schasteen CS, Reed DJ. Interaction of *S*-(2-haloethyl)-mercapturic acid analogs with plasmid DNA. *Toxicol Appl Pharmacol* 1985;80:386–396.
41. Inskeep PB, Koga N, Cmarik JL, Guengerich FP. Covalent binding of 1,2-dihaloethanes to DNA and stability of the major DNA adduct, *S*-[2-(N^7-guanyl)ethyl]-glutathione. *Cancer Res* 1986;46: 2839–2844.
42. Foureman GL, Reed DJ. Formation of *S*-[2-(N^7-guanyl)ethyl] adducts by the postulated *S*-(2-chloroethyl)cysteinyl and *S*-(2-chloroethyl)glutathionyl conjugates of 1,2-dichloroethane. *Biochemistry* 1987;26:2028–2033.
43. Guengerich FP, Peterson LA, Cmarik JL, Koga N, Inskeep PB. Activation of dihaloethanes by glutathione conjugation and formation of DNA adducts. *Environ Health Perspect* 1987;76:15–18.
44. Kim DH, Humphreys WG, Guengerich FP. Characterization of *S*-[2-(N^1-adenyl)ethyl]glutathione as an adduct formed in RNA and DNA from 1,2-dibromoethane. *Chem Res Toxicol* 1990;3:587–594.
45. Kim DH, Guengerich FP. Formation of the DNA adduct *S*-[2-(N^7-guanyl)ethyl] glutathione from ethylene dibromide: effects of modulation of glutathione and glutathione *S*-transferase levels and lack of a role for sulfation. *Carcinogenesis* 1990;11:419–424.
46. Humphreys WG, Kim D-H, Cmarik JL, Shimada T, Guengerich FP. Comparison of DNA alkylating properties and mutagenic responses of a series of *S*-(2-haloethyl)-substituted cysteine and glutathione derivatives. *Biochemistry* 1990;29:10342–10350.
47. Hill DL, Shih TW, Johnston TP, Struck RF. Macromolecular binding and metabolism of the carcinogen 1,2 dibromoethane. *Cancer Res* 1978;38:2438–2442.
48. Rannug U, Sundvall A, Ramel C. The mutagenic effect of 1,2-dichlorethane on *Salmonella typhimurium*. I. Activation through conjugation with glutathione *in vitro*. *Chem Biol Interact* 1978;20: 1–16.
49. Rannug U, Beije B. The mutagenic effect of 1,2-dichloroethane on *Salmonella typhimurium*. II. Activation by the isolated perfused rat liver. *Chem Biol Interact* 1979;24:265–285.
50. van Bladeren PJ, van der Gen A, Breimer DD, Mohn GR. Stereoselective activation of vicinal dihalogen compounds to mutagens by glutathione conjugation. *Biochem Pharmacol* 1979;28: 2521–2524.
51. van Bladeren PJ, Breimer DD, Rotteveel-Smijs GMT, de Jong RAW, Buijs W, van der Gen A, Mohn GR. The role of glutathione conjugation in the mutagenicity of 1,2-dibromoethane. *Biochem Pharmacol* 1980;29:2975–2982.
52. van Bladeren PJ, Breimer DD, Rotteveel-Smijs GMT, De Knijff P, Mohn GR, van Meeteren-Walchi B, Buijs W, van der Gen A. The relation between the structure of vicinal dihalogen compounds and their mutagenic activation via conjugation to glutathione. *Carcinogenesis* 1981;2:499–505.
53. Green T, Odum J. Structure-activity studies of the nephrotoxic and mutagenic action of cysteine conjugates of chloro- and fluoroalkenes. *Chem Biol Interact* 1985;54:15–31.
54. Dekant W, Vamvakas S, Berthold K, Schmidt S, Wild D, Henschler D. Bacterial β-lyase mediated cleavage and mutagenicity of cysteine conjugates derived from the nephrocarcinogenic alkenes trichloroethylene, tetrachloroethylene and hexachlorobutadiene. *Chem Biol Interact* 1986;60:31–45.
55. Vamvakas S, Kordowich FJ, Dekant W, Neudecker T, Henschler D. Mutagenicity of hexachloro-1,3-butadiene and its *S*-conjugates in the Ames test—role of activation by the mercapturic acid pathway in its nephrocarcinogenicity. *Carcinogenesis* 1988;9:907–910.
56. Tate SS. Enzymes of mercapturic acid formation. In: Jakoby WB, ed. *Enzymatic Basis of Detoxication*, vol 2. New York: Academic Press, 1980;95–120.

57. Kozak EM, Tate SS. Glutathione-degrading enzymes of microvillus membranes. *J Biol Chem* 1982;257:6322–6327.
58. Duffel MW, Jakoby WB. Cysteine *S*-conjugate *N*-acetyltransferase from rat kidney microsomes. *Mol Pharmacol* 1982;21:444–448.
59. Rush GF, Smith JH, Newton JF, Hook JB. Chemically induced nephrotoxicity. Role of metabolic activation. *CRC Crit Rev Toxicol* 1984;13:99–160.
60. Tateishi M, Suzuki S, Shimizu H. Cysteine conjugate β-lyase in rat liver. *J Biol Chem* 1978; 253:8854–8859.
61. Tateishi M. Methylthiolated metabolites. *Drug Metab Rev* 1983;14:1207–1234.
62. Stevens J, Jakoby WB. Cysteine conjugate β-lyase. *Mol Pharmacol* 1983;23:761–765.
63. Jakoby WB, Stevens J, Duffel MW, Weisiger RA. The terminal enzymes of mercapturate formation and the thiomethyl shunt. *Rev Biochem Toxicol* 1984;6:97–115.
64. Monks TJ, Highet RJ, Chu PS, Lau SS. Synthesis and nephrotoxicity of 6-bromo-2,5-dihydroxythiophenol. *Mol Pharmacol* 1988;34:15–22.
65. Lau SS, Hill BA, Highet RJ, Monks TJ. Sequential oxidation and glutathione addition to 1,4-benzoquinone: correlation of toxicity with increased glutathione substitution. *Mol Pharmacol* 1988;34:829–836.
66. Monks TJ, Lau SS. Glutathione conjugation, γ-glutamyl transpeptidase and the mercapturic acid pathway as modulators of 2-bromohydroquinone oxidation. *Toxicol Appl Pharmacol* 1990;103: 557–563.
67. Schnellman RG, Monks TJ, Mandel LJ, Lau SS. 2-Bromohydroquinone-induced toxicity to rabbit renal proximal tubules: the role of biotransformation, glutathione and covalent binding. *Toxicol Appl Pharmacol* 1989;99:19–27.
68. Schnellman RG. 2-Bromohydroquinone-induced toxicity to rabbit renal proximal tubules: evidence against oxidative stress. *Toxicol Appl Pharmacol* 1989;99:11–18.
69. Koob M, Kochling A, Weber S, Lau SS, Monks TJ, Dekant W. Cytotoxicity of 2-bromo-(*N*-acetylcystein-*S*-yl)hydroquinone isomers in rat renal tubular epithelial cells. *Toxicol Lett* 1990; 53:143–145.
70. Wefers H, Sies H. Hepatic low-level chemiluminescence during the redox cycling of menadione and the menadione-glutathione conjugate: relation to glutathione and NAD(P)H:quinone reductase (DT-diaphorase) activity. *Arch Biochem Biophys* 1983;224:568–578.
71. Brown PC, Dulik DM, Jones TW. The toxicity of menadione (2-methyl-1,4- naphthoquinone) and two thioether conjugates studied with isolated renal epithelial cells. *Arch Biochem Biophys* 1991; 285:187–196.
72. Lau SS, Jones TW, Highet RJ, Hill BA, Monks TJ. Differences in the localization and extent of the renal proximal tubular necrosis caused by mercapturic acid and glutathione conjugates of menadione and 1,4-naphthoquinone. *Toxicol Appl Pharmacol* 1990;104:334–350.
73. Redegeld FAM, Hofman GA, van de Loo PGF, Koster AS, Noordhoek J. Nephrotoxicity of the glutathione conjugate of menadione (2-methyl-1,4-naphthoquinone) in the isolated perfused rat kidney. Role of metabolism by γ-glutamyltranspeptidase and probenecid-sensitive transport. *J Pharmacol Exp Ther* 1991;256:665–669.
74. Monks TJ, Highet RJ, Lau SS. Oxidative cyclization, 1, 4-benzothiazine formation and dimerization of 2-bromo-3-(glutathion-*S*-yl)hydroquinone. *Mol Pharmacol* 1990;38:121–127.
75. Prota G. Progress in the chemistry of melanins and related metabolites. *Med Res Rev* 1988;8:525–556.
76. Lau SS, Monks TJ. Glutathione conjugation as a mechanism of targeting latent quinones to the kidney. In: Witmer CM, Snyder RR, Jollow DJ, Kalf GF, Kocsis JJ, Sipes IG, eds. *Biological Reactive Intermediates IV. Molecular and cellular effects and human impact*. New York: Plenum, 1991;457–464.
77. Monks TJ, Lau SS. Nephrotoxicity of quinol/quinone-linked *S*-conjugates. *Toxicol Lett* 1990; 53:59–67.
78. Monks TJ, Lo H-H, Kleiner HE, Lau SS. *N*-Acetylation/*N*-deacetylation as determinants of quinol-thioether nephrotoxicity. *Toxicologist* 1991;11:57.
79. Wallin A, Jones TW, Vercesi AE, Cotgreave I, Ormstad K, Orrenius S. Toxicity of *S*-pentachlorobutadienyl-*L*-cysteine studied with isolated rat renal cortical mitochondria. *Arch Biochem Biophys* 1987;258:365–372.
80. Schnellman RG, Cross TJ, Lock EA. Pentachlorobutadienyl-*L*-cysteine uncouples oxidative phosphorylation by dissipating the proton gradient. *Toxicol Appl Pharmacol* 1989;100:498–505.

81. Lash LH, Anders MW. Mechanism of S-(1,2-dichlorovinyl)-*L*-cysteine and *S*-(1,2-dichlorovinyl)-*L*-homocysteine-induced renal mitochondrial toxicity. *Mol Pharmacol* 1987;32:549–556.
82. Schnellman RG, Ewell FPQ, Sgambati M, Mandel LJ. Mitochondrial toxicity of 2-bromohydroquinone in rabbit renal proximal tubules. *Toxicol Appl Pharmacol* 1987;90:420–426.
83. Rivera MI, Monks TJ, Lau SS. Possible cellular target(s) for 2-bromohydroquinone nephrotoxicity. *Toxicologist* 1991;11:257.
84. Lau SS, Jones TW, Sioco R, Hill BA, Pinon RK, Monks TJ. Species differences in renal γ-glutamyl transpeptidase activity do not correlate with susceptibility to 2-bromo-(diglutathion-*S*-yl)hydroquinone mediated nephrotoxicity. *Toxicology* 1990;64:291–311.
85. Tate SS, Khadse V, Wellner D. Renal γ-glutamyl transpeptidases: structural and immunological studies. *Arch Biochem Biophys* 1988;262:397–408.
86. Yamashita K, Totani K, Iwaki Y, Takamisawa I, Tateishi N, Higashi T, Sakamoto Y, Kobata A. Comparative study of the sugar chains of γ-glutamyltranspeptidases purified from human hepatocellular carcinoma and from human liver. *J Biochem* 1989;105:728–735.
87. Rajpert-Demeyts E, Heisterkamp N, Groffen J. Cloning and nucleotide sequence of human γ-glutamyl transpeptidase. *Proc Natl Acad Sci USA* 1988;85:8840–8844.
88. Pawlak A, Lahuna O, Bulle F, Suzuki A, Ferry N, Siegrist S, Chikhi N, Chobert MN, Guellaen G, Laperche Y. γ-Glutamyl transpeptidase: a single copy gene in the rat and a multigene family in the human genome. *J Biol Chem* 1988;263:9913–9916.
89. Reyes E. Rat brain γ-glutamyltranspeptidase: effects of alcohol. *Res Commun Chem Pathol Pharmacol* 1978;21:145–148.
90. Reyes E, Barela TD. Isolation and purification of multiple forms of γ-glutamyl transpeptidase from rat brain. *Neurochem Res* 1980;5:159–170.
91. Antoine B, Visvikis A, Thioudellet C, Rahimi-Pour A, Strazielle N, Wellman M, Siest G. Electrophoretic mobility of γ-glutamyltransferase in rat liver subcellular fractions. Evidence for structure difference from the kidney enzyme. *Biochem J* 1989;262:535–539.
92. Tate SS, Meister A. Interaction of γ-glutamyl transpeptidase with amino acids, dipeptides, and derivatives and analogs of glutathione. *J Biol Chem* 1974;249:7593–7602.
93. Tate SS, Ross ME. Human kidney γ-glutamyl transpeptidase. *J Biol Chem* 1977;252:6042–6045.
94. Bray HG, Franklin TJ, James SP. The formation of mercapturic acids. 3. *N*-Acetylation of *S*-substituted cysteines in the rabbit, rat and guinea pig. *Biochem J* 1959;73:465–473.
95. Buffinton GD, Ollinger K, Brunmark A, Cadenas E. DT-diaphorase-catalysed reduction of 1,4-naphthoquinone derivatives and glutathionyl-quinone conjugates. *Biochem J* 1989;257:561–571.
96. Kari FW. Toxicology and carcinogenesis studies of hydroquinone. *National Toxicology Program; Technical Report Series* 1989;366:1–86.
97. Monks TJ, Hanzlik RP, Cohen GM, Ross D, Graham DG. Contemporary issues in toxicology. Quinone chemistry and toxicity. *Toxicol Appl Pharmacol* 1992;112;2:16.
98. Lau SS, Monks TJ. The contribution of bromobenzene to our current understanding of chemically induced toxicity. *Life Sci* 1988;42:1259–1269.
99. Jaffe M. Ueber die nach einfurung von bromobenzol und chlorobenzol im organismus entstchenden schwelfelthaltigen sauren. *Ber Dtsch Chem Ges* 1879;12:1092–1098.
100. Baumann E, Preusse C. Ueber bromophenylmercaptursaure. *Ber Dtch Chem Ges* 1879;12:806–810.

Toxicology of the Kidney, Second Edition,
edited by Jerry B. Hook and Robin S. Goldstein.
Raven Press, Ltd., New York © 1993.

16

Mechanisms of Metal-Induced Nephrotoxicity

E. A. Conner and B. A. Fowler

Program in Toxicology, University of Maryland, Baltimore, Maryland 21201-1596

The effects of toxic metals on the kidney have been known for many years as a result of occupational or therapeutic exposure to these agents. Studies of the mechanisms underlying these phenomena have been undertaken only in recent years with the advent of cell biology as a scientific discipline and an increased understanding of which cellular organelle systems are most sensitive to a given metal. More recently, molecular factors such as metal-binding proteins, which may markedly alter cellular susceptibility, have received attention due to their capacity to influence dose-response relationships. It should be noted that the kidney is composed of many different cell types and not all cell types are equally sensitive to a given metal. The proximal tubule is the most common component of the nephron to exhibit toxicity from metals but cells in the three distinct anatomical segments vary greatly in their response to a given metal, so that some metals such as cadmium will elicit toxicity in only the first or second segments whereas other metals such as inorganic mercury will selectively damage the third segment. Factors such as metal-metal interactions may also alter expected dose-response relationships in the kidney by changing renal handling characteristics at the level of the target cell, organelle system, or molecular receptor. The need for more sensitive biological indicators of metal-induced nephrotoxicity will also be examined since there is a pressing need for earlier detection of renal damage from these agents.

This chapter will examine the subject areas described above for a number of metals/metalloids and attempt to delineate both the molecular mechanisms of metal-induced nephrotoxicity and molecular factors that regulate these mechanisms, so that the reader may be given a more holistic understanding of this complex subject area. Particular attention will be focused on trying to delineate the biologically active chemical species of a given metal or metalloid following a given route of exposure. The chapter will also delineate needed areas of research, since there is still much to be understood with regard to genetic susceptibility to metal-induced nephrotoxicity and the influence of diet, age, sex, and preexisting renal damage on the toxic process or metal-metal interactions in altering known mechanisms. It is hoped that by taking this approach, this chapter will help the reader develop an overview of the many ways this common class of nephrotoxins may damage this essential organ system. Finally, the chapter will specifically examine the issue of the applicability of mechanistic data derived from animal or cell culture systems to predicting or understanding the response of the human kidney to a given metal. Such a discussion is of increasing importance as the effects and costs of treating chemical-induced renal disease are more fully appreciated.

LEAD

Lead (Pb) is undoubtedly the most ubiquitous nephrotoxic metal in the biosphere and humans are exposed to this agent in food, air, and water. The action of lead on the kidney occurs at several sites including the regulation of blood pressure and the proximal tubule. The relationship(s) that must exist between the accumulation of specific biologically active chemical forms of lead in the kidney and toxicity is currently unknown but clearly essential to understanding mechanisms of lead-induced nephrotoxicity. The following discussion will focus on the lead-induced damage to the kidney proximal tubule with particular emphasis on the known and hypothesized roles of lead-binding proteins in mediating the biochemical effects of lead in various subcellular target organelle systems. The implications of this phenomenon for lead-induced cell injury and clinical outcomes such as chronic renal disease or lead-induced renal adenocarcinoma in animal models will be examined.

Lead-Induced Proximal Tubule Cell Injury

Clinical Manifestations

Clinically, the effects of lead on the renal proximal tubule have been known for many years (1) with manifestations of the Fanconi syndrome, which include decreased tubular reabsorptive capacity for glucose, phosphate, and amino acids. In some reports (1) but not others (2) proteinuria has also been observed. The important component in all these phenomena is that these are substances primarily reabsorbed in the proximal tubule. Histopathological and ultrastructural studies (1,3–10) have demonstrated cellular and mitochondrial swelling, karyomegaly, mitosis, and the formation of pathognomonic lead-containing intranuclear inclusion bodies (1,6,9–12). It appears from these morphological studies that the mitochondrion and nuclear compartments show early manifestations of lead toxicity of this target cell population. These data suggest that since there is strong evidence for intrinsic and essential relationships between organelle structure and biochemical functionality (4,6), these two cellular compartments are likely to play important roles in the mechanisms of lead toxicity to this target cell population.

Renal Handling of Lead

Studies from several laboratories (13–16) have shown that the bioavailable fraction of lead in the circulation is associated with the plasma rather than the red cell component, which contains the largest fraction of lead. It is thus a diffusible fraction of lead that is taken up by the kidney. *In vitro* membrane vesicle transport studies (16) have shown that Pb^{2+} shows extensive membrane binding to the surface coat of the vesicles and no evidence of a membrane transport system. These data suggest that proximal tubule cell uptake of any existing Pb^{2+} in the circulation is due to endocytosis and/or passive diffusion. It is more likely that lead in the circulation is bound to diffusible proteins since Pb^{2+} is such a reactive chemical species. Studies in rodents (17) have shown that lead binds to the rat protein $\alpha_{2\mu}$-globulin, which is synthesized in the liver and transported to the kidney (18). These data suggest that the protein may also act to carry lead from the liver to the kidney in these species and account for the low accumulation of lead in the livers of rodents in comparison with humans or other species. Recently (19), lead-binding proteins similar in size and ion-exchange properties but that did not cross-react with a polyclonal antibody to $\alpha_{2\mu}$- globulin have been isolated from liver and kidneys of humans, suggesting an analogous mechanism for the liver to kidney transport and cellular handling of lead in these two species. The hypothesized central roles of these proteins in mediating lead-induced nephrotoxicity within the renal proximal tubule cells are described below.

Renal Lead-Binding Proteins (PbBP)

Early studies by Moore et al. (20) showed that the pathognomonic lead intranuclear inclusion bodies contained an acidic protein complex with an estimated molecular mass of approximately 28,000 d that was rich in glutamic and aspartic amino acids. This insoluble metal-protein complex contained lead, and also calcium, zinc, and cadmium (18). Due to technical problems associated with recovering the protein from this insoluble matrix, it could not be further characterized. Later studies by Oskarsson et al. (21) focused on examining soluble cytosolic proteins from the kidney using ^{203}Pb and gel column chromatography. These initial studies demonstrated the presence of two forms with estimated molecular masses of 11,500 and 63,000 d. *In vivo* ^{203}Pb injection studies indicated a shift in binding from the lower molecular mass component to the higher molecular mass component with time, suggesting a possible aggregation phenomenon. The 63,000-d component showed tight lead-binding properties even under SDS gel electrophoresis as judged by ^{203}Pb autoradiography. These data suggested formation of a very stable lead-protein complex as perhaps a tetramer of the lower molecular weight PbBP. Studies from other laboratories (22,23) demonstrated the increased presence of an acidic nuclear protein with an approximate molecular mass of 32,000 d associated with intranuclear inclusion bodies. The exact relationships between these molecules are presently not clear, but all appear to be acidic proteins with either similar masses or in comparable ratios to each other, suggesting aggregation phenomena. More recent studies (17) have, in fact, demonstrated that the purified form of the soluble low molecular weight PbBP now known to be $\alpha_{2\mu}$-globulin (17,000 d) does aggregate to form dimers, tetramers, and species of increasingly high molecular weights when metals are bound. The possible significance of this phenomenon to formation of the cytosolic and intranuclear inclusion bodies is discussed below.

PbBP Functionality and Characterization Studies

Utilizing peak fractions from Sephadex column chromatography, Mistry et al. (24,25) demonstrated that the renal PbBP showed an apparent K_d for Pb of approximately 10^{-8} M and that lead bound to this molecule facilitated the cell-free nuclear translocation of lead. Sedimentation studies showed that the low molecular weight peak exhibited an apparent sedimentation coefficient of 2 S, whereas the 63,000-d component showed an apparent sedimentation coefficient of 4.6 S. An additional higher molecular weight peak of 7 to 8 S was also observed. All three peaks showed displaceable binding with cold lead. KCl extraction studies of nuclei used in the cell-free nuclear translocation studies demonstrated that 2-S and 4-S peaks could be recovered from the KCl nuclear extracts, indicating an association of these lead-binding protein peaks with chromatin *in vitro*. The 4-S peak recovered in the KCl extract is undoubtedly the 4.6-S peak that has undergone a structural alteration as a result of nuclear binding. This type of phenomenon is well known for steroid receptors using similar techniques. Metal competition studies (25) conducted on the lead-binding proteins showed that cadmium and zinc were the most effective competitors, whereas calcium did not alter lead binding. Interestingly, zinc actually increased the cell-free translocation of lead, which is similar to the action of zinc on the nuclear translocation of hormone receptors. Overall, the results of these studies are consistent with the hypothesis (17,26) that the lead-binding proteins act in a manner similar to receptors to mediate the well-known effects of lead on renal DNA, RNA, and protein synthesis (5–9). A diagram of the hypothesis is shown in Fig. 1.

The other facet of PbBP functionality that has been examined concerns the ability of these molecules to alter the susceptibility of the lead-sensitive enzyme δ-aminolevulinic acid dehydratase (ALAD) to lead inhibition. Early studies by Fowler et al. (27) showed that this enzyme in rat kidney was highly resistant to lead inhibition following chronic *in vivo* exposure. Subsequent studies (28,29) showed that the renal PbBP was able to prevent Pb inhibition of this highly sensitive enzyme *in vitro* by a mechanism involving both lead chelation and zinc donation, which activates this enzyme. Some of this Zn donation could be due to the Cu, Zn, metallothionein pool (30,31). More recent studies showed that the rat renal PbBP is a cleavage product of the protein $\alpha_{2\mu}$-globulin that is minus nine N-terminal amino acids (17). Our current working hypothesis for the mechanism by which this product may alter

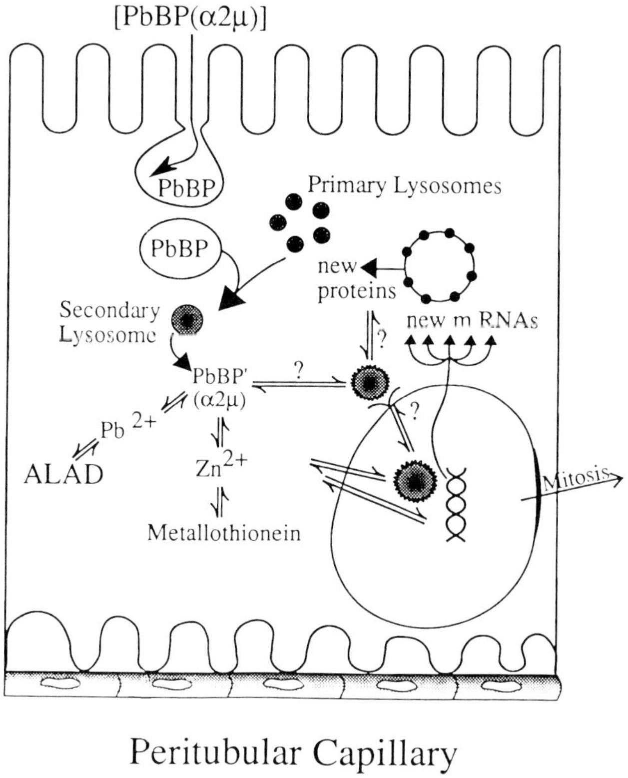

FIG. 1. Renal proximal tubule cell showing known and hypothesized roles for the PbBP (α_2 $_\mu$-globulin cleavage product) in mediating the molecular effects of lead at the molecular level.

renal proximal tubule cell gene expression and regulate Pb inhibition of ALAD is shown in Fig. 1.

More recent preliminary studies (19) have demonstrated the presence of chemically similar but immunologically distinct proteins of similar size and charge properties in both monkey and human kidney and brain and human liver, suggesting analogous proteins in these other species. The importance of these data rests with further testing of the hypothesis described above and in Fig. 1 in these species and the obvious implications such data would have for refining risk assessments in human populations.

Lead-Induced Alterations in Renal Tubule Cell Gene Expression and Carcinogenesis

The ability of chronic high-dose lead exposure to induce renal adenocarcinomas in rodents has been known for many years. The mechanisms underlying this response are less well understood. Studies by Choie and Richter (5–8) demonstrated marked alterations in total DNA, RNA, and protein synthesis in renal proximal tubule cells associated with lead-induced mitosis and formation of the pathognomonic lead intranuclear inclusion bodies. More recent studies (9,32) demonstrated that this phenomenon occurs at lead dosages below those necessary to induce cell death and replacement. Other studies (32,33) utilizing two-dimensional (2-D) gel electrophoresis have demonstrated marked and highly specific alterations in renal gene expression, which show a temporal relationship with the presence of lead intranuclear inclusion bodies. These data suggest that lead at single, low dosages produces changes in renal gene expression that are associated with mitosis under similar conditions. If one or more of these gene products is an oncogene, then a viable hypothesis will be generated for explaining how lead may produce renal carcinogenesis at dosages that do not produce cell death and replacement.

CADMIUM

The nephrotoxicity of cadmium (Cd) in man and experimental animal models has been known for many years (34–38), and there have been a number of extensive reviews (39,40). The primary nephrotoxicity associated with exposure to this element involves the renal proximal tubule development of a characteristic low molecular tubular proteinuria, calciuria, and in some cases glucosuria. The low molecular weight metal-binding protein metallothionein appears to play a central role in the mechanism(s) underlying these phenomena.

Metallothionein

Mammalian metallothionein (MT) is a highly conserved protein with a molecular mass of approximately 6,800 d that is composed of approximately 30% cysteine residues. A number of metals such as cadmium, zinc, copper, mercuric ion, and silver may induce and bind MT. The cysteine residues of this protein act to bind seven metal atoms by forming two metal-binding clusters of four and three metals, respectively, with four cysteines per Cd through a bridging sulfur bond (41). The chemistry and biochemistry of metallothionein has been the subject of intensive research and numerous reviews (42–44), which are outside the scope of the present discussion. Metallothionein synthesized in the liver following exposure to Cd has been shown by numerous researchers (45–51) to be present in the circulation. As a low molecular weight protein, MT is rapidly and efficiently filtered by the glomerulus and reabsorbed by the renal proximal tubule cells, where it is rapidly degraded by the lysosome system with release of Cd^{2+}, which in turn causes the synthesis of renal MT (52–62). Figure 2 shows a representation of this process and the known and hypothesized relationships between this process and tubule cell injury.

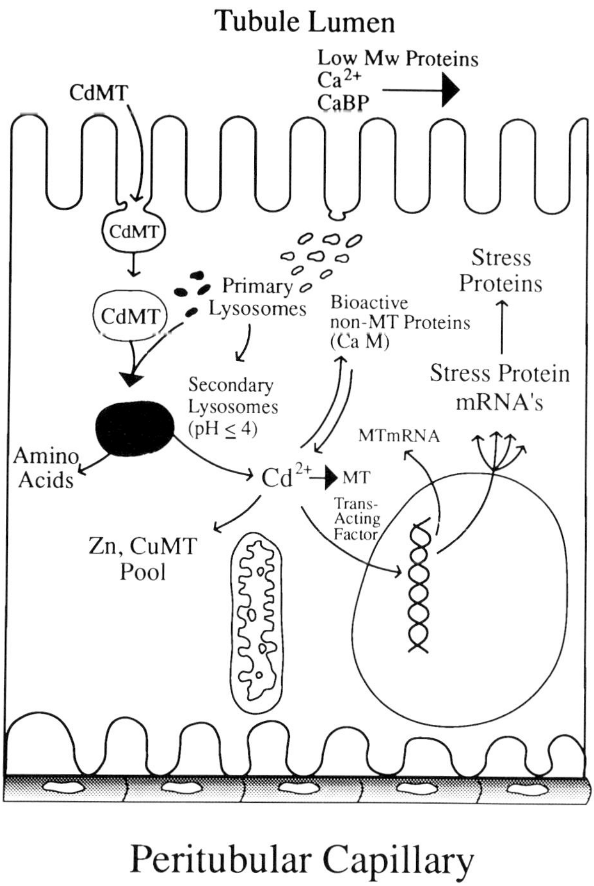

FIG. 2. The roles of metallothionein (MT) in mediating the molecular mechanisms of Cd^{2+} toxicity to renal proximal tubule cells. Reabsorbed MT is degraded by the renal lysosome apparatus with subsequent induction of the renal MT pool. If the capacity of this pool is exceeded due to either elevated chronic exposure or administration of a single high dose of CdMT, then Cd^{2+} is hypothesized to be available to interact with other effector molecules such as calmodulin.

Mechanisms of Cadmium-Induced Cell Injury

As noted above, release of Cd^{2+} from CdMT reabsorbed from the urinary filtrate causes the induction of renal MT, which rebinds the Cd^{2+}, thereby protecting the cell from injury. The ability of Cd^{2+} to produce toxicity appears to be initiated when the binding capacity of the renal MT pool is exceeded as a result of either chronic elevated Cd exposure (39,40) or release/administration of a CdMT bolus to the kidney (53). The ability of Zn^{2+} to induce the renal MT pool has also been shown to markedly influence the nephrotoxicity of subsequent CdMT exposure.

At the ultrastructural level, proximal tubule cells show a characteristic vesiculation and accumulation of small, dense lysosomes (52–54, 56, 58, 59) that contain Cd (52) following parenteral administration of the CdMT complex. These phenomena are associated with development of a tubular proteinuria (53) and calciuria (63–67), which are similar to those found in persons with long-term, elevated exposures (35). The data suggest a perturbation of the process of lysosomal biogenesis by Cd^{2+} with attendant loss of low molecular weight proteins into the urine.

There now appears to be general agreement that it is the non–metallothionein-bound fraction of Cd^{2+} that is biologically active and responsible for producing toxicity via interactions with "effector molecules." The calcium-binding regulatory protein calmodulin is one candidate, since it has been shown (68,69) that Cd^{2+} is highly capable of activating this molecule *in vitro*. Activation of calmodulin could result in the activation of a number of proteases capable of damaging the cytoskeleton. Since the cytoskeleton is regarded as being important for mediating lysosomal biogenesis (70), damage to this structural system could easily explain the disruption of the lysosomal fusion process observed following *in vivo* exposure to CdMT (67).

Alterations of Renal Calcium Metabolism

As noted above, animals administered CdMT also develop a calciuria (63–67) that is similar to that observed in persons following chronic, elevated exposures (35). The mechanisms underlying this phenomenon are presently unknown but may be secondary to the proteinuria since much of the Ca^{2+} in the urine appears to be in a bound form (63) or, alternatively, due to changes in renal membranes, with alterations in Ca^{2+} transport based upon the observation that the major increase in proteinuria occurs after the development of calciuria (64). Of interest is the preliminary set of observations that no measurable changes in renal slice uptake of $^{45}Ca^{2+}$ or intracellular Ca^{2+} occur prior to the vesiculation phenomenon noted above. This means that the cell injury process for these cells, which can lead to cell death and necrosis of proximal tubule cells in the first and second segments (S_1 and S_2), is probably not initiated by alterations in the Ca^{2+} pathway, but that alterations in Ca^{2+} metabolism occur only at a later time point. In any event, the CdMT injection model provides some interesting opportunities for studying both Cd-induced nephrotoxicity and basic mechanisms of cell injury and cell death in the nephron.

MERCURY

The effects of mercurials (Hg) such as inorganic mercury in the form of mercuric chloride (Hg^{2+}) and organic mercury such as methylmercury (CH_3Hg^+) on the renal proximal tubule cell epithelium have been studied for many years. Each chemical form shows some specificity for a different region of the proximal tubule. Hg^{2+} has been utilized for many years to study cell injury in the third (S_3) segment of the proximal tubule (71–75), whereas studies of CH_3Hg^+ and other organomercurials will produce toxicity in both the second (S_2) and third (S_3) segments of the proximal tubule (76,78). There thus appear to be differences in the cell types affected based upon the chemical form of the mercurial administered. Sex differences in susceptibility to CH_3Hg^+-induced nephrotoxicity have also been demonstrated (76,77,79).

The mechanism(s) of mercurial-induced toxicity to the nephron have been extensively studied. A diagram of how mercurials may injure the proximal tubule epithelium is shown in Fig. 3. The mechanism(s) by which Hg^{2+} and CH_3Hg^+ produce toxicity are discussed below on an individual basis.

Inorganic Mercury (Hg^{2+})

The mechanisms by which Hg^{2+} produces damage to the third segment of the renal proximal tubule cell epithelium have been studied for many years (71–75). It

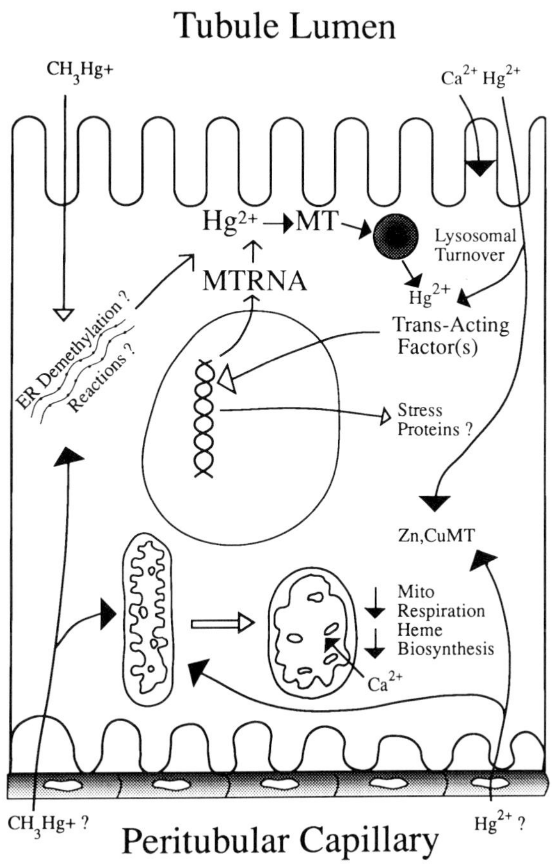

FIG. 3. The known and hypothesized effects of methyl mercury and inorganic mercury on renal proximal tubules cell organelle systems. Note that biologically active chemical species of mercury derived from methyl mercury are currently unknown.

appears that there are several sites of action at both the level of the cell membrane and within the cell (71–75, 80,81). Acute high-dose exposure may produce damage at a number of sites (82–84), whereas more chronic low-dose exposure produces effects that appear to be mediated in part by Hg^{2+} induction of metallothionein in the kidney (85). The mechanisms of damage are thus somewhat different for Hg^{2+} depending upon dose and duration of exposure.

Acute Exposure

As noted above, acute exposure to Hg^{2+} dosages of 2 to 3 mg/kg produces a highly selective necrosis of the S_3 segment of the proximal tubule (71–75). This phenomenon is preceded by damage to the cell membrane (73–74, 80,86), mitochondrial structure and function (80, 86), and loss of cellular control over intracellular Ca^{2+} concentrations (80,86). A complex hypothesis for the sequence of these events has been published and rigorously tested.

Organomercurials

There are a variety of organomercurials that vary in nephrotoxic potential in part as result of their metabolism to inorganic Hg^{2+}. In general, these agents appear to be capable of producing damage to cells in both the S_2 and S_3 segments. The degree of segmental damage appears to rest with how readily the various organomercurials are broken down to yield Hg^{2+}.

Methylmercury is one of the more stable organomercurials that is capable of damaging both the S_2 and S_3 segments of the nephron depending upon the route and duration of exposure (76–78). Sex differences in the susceptibility of rats (76,77) and mice (79) to the nephrotoxicity of this agent have been reported and these may be related to sex differences in the efficiency of demethylation reaction and excretion of Hg^{2+} (87) in renal proximal tubule cells. As a highly lipid soluble chemical, CH_3Hg^+ appears to readily concentrate in renal proximal tubule cells where it may damage the mitochondria and alter the renal lysosome apparatus (88). Mitochondrial damage is associated with the alterations in renal heme biosynthesis and development of an apparent renal porphyrinuria (89). It is interesting to note that, in contrast to Hg^{2+}, CH_3Hg^+ does not induce or bind to metallothionein (90), so that the nephrotoxicity of this agent is probably not markedly influenced by this protein.

Other organomercurials such as ethyl and phenyl mercurials appear to be more rapidly broken down to Hg^{2+} and hence the toxicological manifestations of toxicity for these agents is more like that of Hg^{2+} (91–94).

ARSENIC

The nephrotoxicity of arsenicals (As) has received relatively less attention than that of other toxic elements despite the fact that this element is concentrated by the kidney, reported to cause renal failure (95) in humans, and the urine is the major pathway for elimination of both inorganic and methylated arsenical species from the body. Early studies by Ginsberg (96,97) showed that the kidney actively accumulates arsenate (As^{5+}). Subsequent studies by Vahter and coworkers (98) demonstrated that most species excrete dimethyl arsinic acid (DMA) and methyl arsonic acid (MMA) as the chief urinary metabolites following exposure to inorganic arsenite (As^{3+}) and arsenate (As^{5+}). These methylated species are thought to be primarily formed in the liver (98). The renal tubular epithelium may thus be exposed to all four chemical forms.

The renal mitochondrion appears to be the organelle most greatly damaged by low-dose arsenical exposure. Ultrastructural-biochemical studies by Brown et al. (99) demonstrated that the well-known uncoupling effects of arsenic on mitochondria in other species (100,101) also occurred in rat renal mitochondria and that these biochemical effects were associated with *in situ* mitochondrial swelling. Since these studies were performed following *in vivo* exposure to arsenic, it is likely that the renal tubular cells were exposed to the methylated species. A diagrammatic representation of how exposure of kidney epithelial cells to inorganic arsenicals and methylated species may produce the observed effects is shown in Fig. 4.

INTERACTIONS BETWEEN METALS IN THE KIDNEY

As noted above, concomitant administration of zinc with induction of metallothionein may alter the toxicity of cadmium by providing a molecular binding pool for Cd^{2+} ions, thus preventing their interaction with other effector molecules such as calmodulin. Data from studies by Mistry et al. (24,25) have demonstrated that Cd^{2+} and Zn^{2+} ions are highly effective competitors with Pb^{2+} for binding on $\alpha_{2\mu}$-globulin and that these metals may greatly alter the intranuclear transport of Pb via this mechanism *in vitro*. Such data provide a reasonable mechanistic explanation for data from *in vivo* Pb $\times$ Cd $\times$ As feeding studies (102,103), which showed marked reduction in the formation of lead intranuclear inclusion bodies in rats concomitantly exposed to Pb and Cd but an increase in the excretion of urinary porphyrins in these groups, suggesting that the available lead pool was more available to enzymes in the heme pathway (104). The interaction of Hg with Se in the kidney with formation of HgSe intranuclear inclusions has also been reported (105), with attenuation of Hg-induced tubule cell toxicity as judged by electron microscopy. The overall point of this discussion is that there are published studies that indicate the mechanism(s) of toxicity for a number of metals may be greatly altered by concomitant exposure to other metals that are capable of influencing their intracellu-

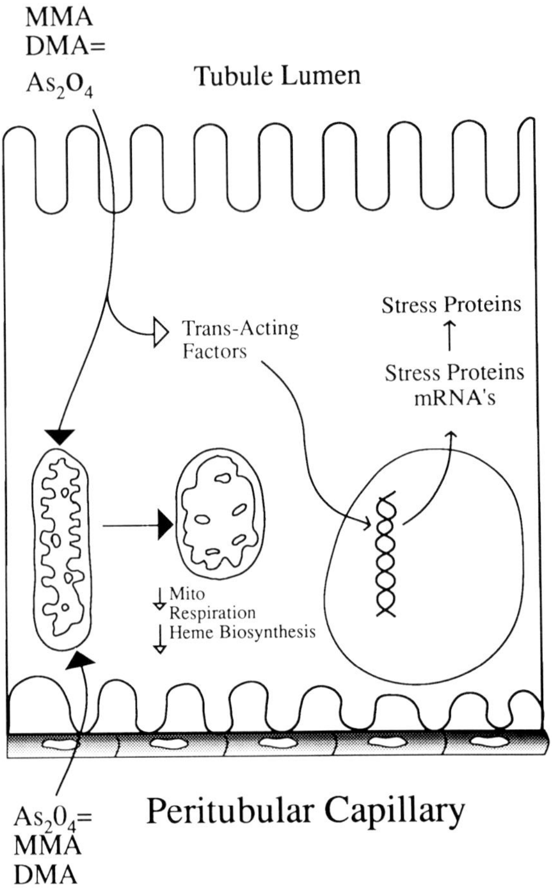

FIG. 4. Effects of inorganic arsenic species, methyl arsonic acid (MMA) and dimethyl arsinic acid (DMA) on proximal tubule cell organelles. High amplitude mitochondrial swelling is a prominent feature *in situ*.

lar molecular binding patterns. Such data should be kept in mind in considering how metals may damage the kidney, since multielement exposures are the rule rather than the exception.

BISMUTH

The main effects of bismuth (Bi) compounds both in man and in animals are exerted in the liver and kidney. High-level exposure causes renal failure associated with degeneration and necrosis of the epithelium of the renal proximal tubules. In children, oral or parenteral administration of bismuth compounds such as triglycolate or thioglycolate causes acute renal failure (106,107). Bismuth nephropathy due to acute and chronic uses of bismuth salts is well recognized. The functional alterations in acute bismuth nephropathy include severe depression of glomerular filtration rate, renal plasma flow, and proximal tubular reabsorption, as indicated by glucosuria, phosphaturia, and aminoaciduria (108). Bismuth inclusions were found in the renal tubular epithelium of 12 out of 14 patients treated parenterally with bismuth compounds (109). A recent case of acute renal failure associated with an overdose of colloidal bismuth subcitrate was reported by Taylor and Klenerman (110). The oral ingestion of colloidal bismuth is thought to be safe since it is less readily absorbed than other bismuth salts.

In rats, the proximal tubules are the most markedly affected site of bismuth toxicity. Early studies by Kolmer et al. (111) showed kidney damage produced by single im injection (0.03 to 1.5 g/kg) of 13 different bismuth compounds. Histological examinations of animals that died and survived had varying degrees of nephritis. Beaver and Burr (112) injected rabbits subcutaneously with bismuth subnitrate (5 g for 3 days). Their results showed degenerative changes and intranuclear and cytoplasmic inclusion in the proximal tubules. These inclusions are pathognomonic for bismuth exposure (113). Hemorrhages in the cortical and cerebral layer of the kidney and lymphohistiocytic infiltrations in rats after 6 months of peroral treatment with potassium-bismuthate and bismuth sulfate were reported by Seljankina et al. (114). Renal concentrations of metallothionein-like proteins and increases in copper have also been reported following subcutaneous injections of bismuth trichloride (115).

CHROMIUM

Both acute and chronic adverse effects of chromium (Cr) are mainly caused by hexavalent compounds. The hexavalent chromium ion (Cr^{+6}) in various animal experiments and occupational health studies has been found to be a potent nephrotoxicant. Acute exposure to Cr^{+6} has been reported to produce acute necrosis of the proximal tubule in humans (116–118). Percutaneous biopsies have also demonstrated large membranous myeloid bodies within these cells that were suggested to be lysosomal in character (117). Histopathological studies of autopsied cases of Cr^{+6} workers showed primary histological changes in the kidney, such as cell degeneration of the renal tubules (119). The effect of Cr^{+6} exposure on glomerular function has also been reported in humans (120–122). In the glomerular tissue a form of lipid degeneration and cell proliferation of the Bowman's capsule occurs (123).

Numerous studies in rats have confirmed the chromium-induced nephrotoxicity observed in humans. Alterations in tubular transport abnormalities, however, are more prominent than alterations in glomerular filtration rate. The first two proximal tubule segments, S_1 and S_2, are the primary cellular targets for Cr^{+6} toxicity (116, 124–129). The earliest ultrastructural lesions involve disruption of the brush border membranes of these cells (124). This structural change has been associated with loss of reabsorptive capacity as measured by glucosuria, tubular proteinuria, and enzymuria (116,124). In addition, a reduction in the specific activity of several brush border marker enzymes in the kidney (128) and decreases in *para*-aminohippurate transport (125,126,129) progressing ultimately to renal failure as measured by increased BUN and serum creatinine (126) has been observed with the above sequence of events.

Prolonged exposure to Cr^{+6} via repeated subcutaneous injections demonstrated ultrastructural and biochemical lesions similar to those reported for acute administration (116). Intraperitoneal injections of Cr^{+6} has also been reported to produce DNA interstrand cross-linking in kidney nuclei (130). It is worth noting that GSH may protect against the acute nephrotoxicity of Cr^{+6}. Standeven and Wetterhahn (131) examined the effect of glutathione (GSH) depletion by L-buthionine sulfoximine (BSO) on Cr^{+6}-induced nephrotoxicity in rats. Their data indicated that a nontoxic dose of Cr^{+6} caused no significant changes in organ GSH levels, although in liver it appeared that Cr^{+6} may have caused an initial decrease of GSH levels followed rapidly by a rebound and an increase. Certain manifestations of Cr^{+6} nephrotoxicity were clearly protentiated by GSH depletion with BSO. The authors concluded that their data support a role for GSH in hepatic and renal metabolism of Cr^{+6}, although GSH appears to protect against the acute toxicity of Cr^{+6} in rats.

PLATINUM

Clinical and animal studies indicate that the administration of anticancer platinum (Pt) derivatives such as cisplatin induce tubular necrosis and degeneration leading to acute renal failure. The functional deficits associated with acute proximal tubular necrosis include enzymuria, proteinuria, altered organic ion transport, and wastage of magnesium. The proximal tubular damage occurs primarily in the pars recta (132–134). Singh (132), using a mouse model, demonstrated both morphological and biochemical changes after 72 hr following a single 10 mg/kg ip dose of cisplatin. The authors concluded that if mitochondrial DNA is damaged then *de novo* synthesis of mitochondrial proteins would not occur and thus degradation of the organelle would result. In addition, Nonclercq et al. (135) encountered histopathological alterations that consisted of progressive cystic tubular degenerations localized in the outer stripe of the outer medulla.

Much evidence has been gathered in recent years suggesting the possible contribution of alterations in heme biosynthesis and degradation to nephrotoxicity of *cis*-platinum (136). The kidney is particularly susceptible to the inhibiting effects of *cis*-platinum. *Cis*-platinum causes a significant decrease in aminolevulinic acid synthetase (ALAS) activity, the rate-limiting enzyme of heme biosynthesis, and an increase in the activity of ferrochelatase, which inserts iron in protoporphyrin-IX. The activity of biliverdin reductase, the enzyme responsible for the conversion of biliverdin to bilirubin in the heme catabolism pathway, is markedly inhibited in response to *cis*-platinum treatment. The mechanisms for *cis*-platinum effects on either heme biosynthesis or catabolism are not clear. Possible events include loss of protein from the kidney or altered turnover of the enzyme and/or inhibition of enzyme production at the transcriptional level (135).

Recent studies have investigated the hypothesis that elevated levels of renal metallothionein (MT) offer protection from the nephrotoxic action of *cis*-platinum (137, 138). Boogaard et al. (139) have shown that pretreatment with MT-inducing metal (Bi^{+3}) reduces lethality of high-dose *cis*-platinum. In addition high levels of GSH in the kidney have been implicated as an effective protector against *cis*-platinum–induced nephrotoxicity (140).

GALLIUM AND INDIUM

Gallium (Ga) and indium (In), major components of the III–V semiconductors, are well known to have toxic effects on the kidney in experimental animals. The mechanisms of toxicity for these metals remain to be investigated. Intratracheal instillation studies with particulate gallium arsenide have shown inhibitory effect on renal ALAD with increased excretion of ALA (141–143). *In vitro* studies demonstrated that ALAD was highly sensitive to gallium in the kidney (141). Recent studies by Aoki et al. (144) demonstrated that 2-D patterns of protein synthesis in proximal tubule epithelial cells were specifically altered by *in vitro* exposure to Ga^{+3}. In addition, a 30K protein was markedly induced and synthesis of several other proteins were stimulated by 30 to 300 μm Ga^{+3} exposure, which did not cause LDH release from the cells. The authors suggest that the induction of 30K protein and stimulation of other proteins in proximal tubules cells may be applicable as early markers of Ga exposure before the onset of cell injury.

A single intravenous injection of indium chloride has been reported to cause extensive necrosis of the renal proximal tubules in both rats and mice (145–147). Woods and Fowler (148) reported a tissue-specific inhibition of ALAD in rat kidney after ip treatment with indium chloride in doses of 10, 20 and 40 mg/kg body weight 16 hr before sacrifice. At the highest dose level, ALAD activity was inhibited to 41% of control levels. Treatment with indium had no significant changes in the renal activities of ALAS, uroporphyrinogen I synthetase (UROS), or ferrochelatase. The inhibited ALAD activity did not result in any changes in the urinary excretion of ALA or porphobilinogen or changes in the renal microsomal content.

REFERENCES

1. Goyer RA, Rhyne BC. Pathological effects of lead. In: Richter GW, Epstein MA, eds. *International review of experimental pathology*. New York: Academic Press, 1973;12:1.
2. Vacca CV, Hines JD, Hall PW. The proteinuria of industrial lead intoxication. *Environ Res* 1986; 41:440–446.

3. Goyer RA. The renal tubule in lead poisoning. I. Mitochondrial swelling and aminoaciduria. *Lab Invest* 1968;19:71–77.
4. Goyer RA, Krall AR. Ultrastructural transformation in mitochondria isolated from kidneys of normal and lead intoxicated rats. *J Cell Biol* 1969;41:393–400.
5. Choie DD, Richter GW. Cell proliferation in rat kidneys after prolonged treatment with lead. *Am J Pathol* 1972;68:359–370.
6. Choie DD, Richter GW, Young LB. Biogenesis of intranuclear lead-protein inclusions in mouse kidney. *Beitr Pathol* 1975;155:197–203.
7. Choie DD, Richter GW. Cell proliferation in mouse kidney induced by lead. I. Synthesis of deoxyribonucleic acid. *Lab Invest* 1974;30:647–657.
8. Choie DD, Richter GW. Cell proliferation in mouse kidney induced by lead II: Synthesis of ribonucleic acid and protein. *Lab Invest* 1974;30:652–656.
9. Hitzfeld B, Planas-Bohne F, Taylor D. The effect of lead on protein and DNA metabolism of normal and lead-adapted rat kidney cells in culture. *Biol Trace Element Res* 1989;21:87–95.
10. Oskarsson A, Fowler BA. Effects of lead inclusion bodies on subcellular distribution of lead in rat kidney: the relationship to mitochondrial function. *Exp Mol Pathol* 1985;43:409–417.
11. Richter GW. Evolution of cytoplasmic fibrillar bodies induced by lead in rat and mouse kidneys. *Am J Pathol* 1976;83:135–149.
12. Murakami M, Kawamura R, Nishi S, Karsunuma H. Early appearance and localization of intranuclear inclusions in the segments of renal proximal tubules of rats, following ingestion of lead. *Br J Exp Pathol* 1983;64:144–155.
13. Vander AJ, Taylor DL, Kalitis K, Mouw DR, Victery W. Renal handling of lead in dogs: clearance studies. *Am J Physiol* 1977;2:F532–F538.
14. Vander AJ, Mouw DR, Cox J, Johnson B. Lead transport by renal slices and its inhibition by tin. *Am J Physiol* 1970;236:F373–F378.
15. Victery W, Vander AJ, Mouw DR. Renal handling of lead in dogs: stop-flow analysis. *Am J Physiol* 1979;237:F408–F414.
16. Victery WW, Miller CR, Fowler BA. Lead accumulation by rat renal brush border membrane vesicles. *J Pharmacol Exp Ther* 1984;231:589–596.
17. Fowler BA, DuVal GE. Effects of lead on the kidney: roles of high affinity lead-binding proteins. *Environ Health Perspect* 1991;91:77–80.
18. Swenberg JA, Short B, Borghoff S, Strasser J, Charboneau M. The comparative pathobiology of $\alpha_{2\mu}$-globulin nephropathy. *Toxicol Appl Pharmacol* 1989;97:35–46.
19. Kahng WM, Conner EA, Fowler BA. Lead-binding proteins (PbBP) in human tissues. *Toxicology* 1992;12:788;1992.
20. Moore JF, Goyer RA, Wilson M. Lead-induced inclusion bodies: solubility, amino acid content and relationship to residual acidic nuclear proteins. *Lab Invest* 1973;29:488–494.
21. Oskarsson A, Squibb KS, Fowler BA. Intracellular binding of lead in the kidney: partial isolation and characterization of postmitochondrial supernatant lead-binding components. *Biochem Biophys Res Commun* 1982;104:290–298.
22. Shelton KR, Egle PM. The proteins of lead-induced intranuclear inclusion bodies. *J Biol Chem* 1982;257:11802–11807.
23. Shelton KR, Todd JM, Egle PM. The inclusion of stress proteins by lead. *J Biol Chem* 1986;261: 1935–1940.
24. Mistry P, Lucier GW, Fowler BA. High affinity lead-binding proteins from rat kidney cytosol: mediate cell-free nuclear translocation of lead. *J Pharmacol Exp Ther* 1985;232:462–469.
25. Mistry P, Mastri C, Fowler BA. Influence of metal ions on renal cytosolic lead-binding proteins and nuclear uptake of lead in the kidney. *Biochem Pharmacol* 1986;35:711–713.
26. Fowler BA. Biological roles of high affinity metal-binding proteins in mediating cell injury. *Comm Toxicol* 1989;3:27–46.
27. Fowler BA, Kimmel CA, Woods JS, McConnel EE, Grant LD. Chronic low level lead toxicity in the rat. III. An integrated toxicological assessment with special reference to the kidney. *Toxicol Appl Pharmacol* 1980;56:59–77.
28. Goering PL, Fowler BA. Regulation of lead inhibition of δ-aminolevulinic acid dehydratase by high affinity renal lead-binding protein. *J Pharmacol Exp Ther* 1984;231:66–71.
29. Goering PL, Fowler BA. Mechanisms of renal lead-binding protein protection against lead-inhibition of Δ-aminolevulinic acid dehydratase. *J Pharmacol Exp Ther* 1985;234:365–371.
30. Goering PL, Fowler BA. Mechanism of kidney metallothionein reversal of lead inhibition of Δ-aminolevulinic acid dehydratase. *Arch Biochem Biophys* 1987;253:48–55.

31. Goering PL, Fowler BA. Metal constitution of metallothionein influences inhibition of Δ-aminolevulinic acid dehydratase (porphobilinogen synthetase) by lead. *Biochem J* 1987;245:339–345.
32. Fowler BA, Mistry P, Victery WW. Ultrastructural morphometric studies of lead inclusion body formation in kidney proximal tubule cells: relationship to altered renal protein synthetic patterns. *Toxicology* 1985;5:53.
33. Mistry P, Mastri C, Fowler BA. Lead-induced alterations of renal gene expression within subcellular compartments. *Toxicology* 1987;7:78.
34. Adams RG, Harrison JF, Scott P. The development of cadmium-induced proteinuria impaired renal function and osteomalacia in alkaline battery workers. *Q J Med* 1969;38:425–436.
35. Kanzantzis G. Renal tubular dysfunction and abnormalities of calcium metabolism in cadmium workers. *Environ Health Perspect* 1979;28:155–159.
36. Lauwerys R, Amery A, Bernard A, Braux P, Pierre Buchet J, Claeys F, DePlaen P, Ducoffre G, Fagard R, Lijnen P, Nick L, Roles H, Rondia D, Saint-Remey A, Sartor F, Staessen J. Health effects of environmental exposure to cadmium: objectives, design and organization of the cadmibel study: a cross-section morbidity study carried out in Belgium from 1985–1989. *Environ Health Perspect* 1990;87:283–289.
37. Buchet JP, Lauwerys R, Roels H, Bernard A, Brauaux P, Claeys F, Ducoffre G, DePlaen P, Staessen J, Amery A, Lijnen P, Thijs L, Rondia D, Sartor F, Saint Remy A, Nick L. Renal effects of cadmium body burden of the general population. *Lancet* 1990;336:699–702.
38. Stassen J, Amery A, Bernard A, Bruauz P, Buchet JP, Claeys F, DePlaen P, Ducoffre G, Fagard R, Lauwerys RR, Lijnen P, Nick L, Saint Remy A, Roels H, Rondia D, Sartor F, Thijs L. Environmental exposure to cadmium influences in calcium metabolism: a population study. (In press).
39. Dunnick J, Fowler BA. Cadmium. In: Seiler HG, Sigel A, eds. *Handbook on the toxicity of inorganic compounds*. New York: Marcel Dekker, 1985;155–174.
40. Kjelstrom T. Renal effects. In: Friberg E, Kjelstrom T, Nordberg GF, eds. *Cadmium and health: a toxicological and epidemiology appraisal*. Boca Raton: CRC Press, 1984;47–86.
41. Kagi JHR, Vasak K, Gilg DEO, Hunziker P, Bernhard WR, Good M. Structure of mammalian metallothionein. *Environ Health Perspect* 1984;54:93–103.
42. Goyer RA, Fowler BA. Metallothionein and cadmium nephrotoxicity conference. *Environ Health Perspect* 1984;54:1–295.
43. Fowler BA, eds. Proceedings of the international conference on the biochemistry of high affinity metal-binding proteins in nonmammalian species: implication for human health. *Environ Health Perspect* 1986;65:3–224.
44. Kagi JHR, Kojima Y, eds. Proceedings of the second international conference on metallothionein and other low molecular weight metal-binding proteins. Basel: Birkhauser Verlag, 1987.
45. Garvey JS, Chang CC. Detection of circulating metallothionein in rats injected with zinc or cadmium. *Science* 1981;241:805.
46. Chang CC, Vander Mallie RJ, Garvey JS. A radioimmunoassay for human metallothionein. *Toxicol Appl Pharmacol* 1980;55:95.
47. Shaikh ZA, Hirayama K. Metallothionein in the extracellular fluids as an index of cadmium toxicity. *Environ Health Perspect* 1979;28:267–271.
48. Sato M, Mehra PK, Bremner I. Measurement of plasma metallothionein-I in the assessment of the zinc status of zinc-deficient and stressed rats. *J Nutr* 1984;114:1683–1689.
49. Vander Mallie RJ, Garvey JS. Radioimmunoassay of metallothioneins. *J Biol Chem* 1979;254: 8416–8421.
50. Bremner I, Mehra PK, Morrison JN, Wood AM. Effects of dietary copper supplementation of rats on the occurrence of metallothionein-I in liver and its secretion into blood, bile, and urine. *Biochem J* 1986;235:735–739.
51. Mehra FK, Bremner I. Development of a radioimmunassay for rat liver metallothionein-I and its application to the analysis of rat plasma and kidneys. *Biochem J* 1983;213:459–465.
52. Squibb KS, Ridlington JW, Carmichael NG, Fowler BA. Early cellular effects of circulating cadmium-thionein on kidney proximal tubules. *Environ Health Perspect* 1979;28:287–296.
53. Squibb KS, Pritchard JB, Fowler BA. Cadmium metallothionein nephropathy: ultrastructural/biochemical alteration and intracellular cadmium binding. *J Pharmacol Exp Ther* 1984;229:311–321.
54. Squibb KS, Fowler BA. Intracellular metabolism and effects in circulating cadmium metallothionein in the kidney following acute treatment. *Environ Health Perspect* 1984;54:31–35.
55. Foulkes EC. Renal transport of cadmium-metallothionein. *Toxicol Appl Pharmacol* 1978;45:505–512.

56. Squibb KS, Pritchard JB, Fowler BA. The renal metabolism and toxicity of metallothionein. In: Foulkes EC, ed. *Biological roles of metallothionein*. New York: Elsevier/North Holland, 1982; 181–192.
57. Webb M, Etienne AT. Studies on the toxicity and metabolism of cadmium thionein. *Biochem Pharmacol* 1977;26:25–30.
58. Fowler BA, Nordberg GF. The renal toxicity of cadmium-metallothionein: morphometric and x-ray microanalytical studies. *Toxicol Appl Pharmacol* 1978;46:609–623.
59. Cherian MG, Goyer RA, Delaquerriere-Richardson L. Cadmium-metallothionein-induced nephrotoxicity. *Toxicol Appl Pharmacol* 1976;38:399–408.
60. Cherian MG, Shaikh ZA. Metabolism of intravenously injected cadmium binding protein. *Biochem Biophys Res Commun* 1975;65:863–869.
61. Shaikh ZA, Smith JC. The biosynthesis of metallothionein in rat liver and kidney after administration of cadmium. *Chem Biol Interact* 1976;15:327–336.
62. Cain K, Holt DE. Studies of cadmium-thionein-induced nephropathy: the course of cadmium-thionein uptake and degradation. *Chem Biol Interact* 1983;43:223–237.
63. Fowler BA, Goering PL, Squibb KS. Mechanism of cadmium-induced metallothionein-induced nephrotoxicity: relationship to altered renal calcium metabolism. In: Kagi JHR, Kojima Y, eds. *Metallothionein*. Basil: Birkhauser Verlag, 1987;66–68.
64. Jin T, Leffler P, Nordberg GF. Cadmium-metallothionein nephrotoxicity in the rat: transient calciuria and proteinuria. *Toxicology* 1987;45:307–317.
65. Leffler P, Jin TY, Nordberg GF. Cadmium-metallothionein-induced kidney dysfunction increases magnesium excretion in the rat. *Toxicol Appl Pharmacol* 1990;103:180–184.
66. Fowler BA, Akkerman M. The role of Ca^{+2} in Cd-induced renal tubular cell injury. In: *Proc. International Conference on cadmium in the human environment: toxicity and carcionogenicity*. Lyon, France: IARC, (in press).
67. Fowler BA, Gandley RE, Akkerman M, Lipsky MM. Proximal tubule cell injury. In: Klassen CD, Suzuki KT, eds. *Proc. U.S. Japan conference on metallothionein in biology and medicine*. CRC Press, Boca Raton, 1991;311–322.
68. Mills JS, Johnson JD. Metal ions as allosteric regulators as calmodulin. *J Biol Chem* 1985;260: 15100–15105.
69. Suzuki Y, Charo S-H, Zysk JR, Cheung WY. Stimulation of calmodulin by calcium ion. *Arch Toxicol* 1985;57:205–211.
70. Wall DA, Maak T. Endocytic uptake, transport, and catabolism of proteins by epithelial cells. *Am J Physiol* 1985;248:C12–C20.
71. Rodin AE, Crowson CN. Mercury nephrotoxicity in the rat. I. Factors influencing the localization of tubular lesions. *Am J Pathol* 1962;41:297–314.
72. Taylor NS. Histochemical studies of nephrotoxicity with sublethal doses of mercury in rats. *Am J Pathol* 1965;46:1–21.
73. Gritzka TL, Trump BF. Renal tubular lesions caused by mercuric chloride: electronic microscopic observations: degeneration of the pars recta. *Am J Pathol* 1968;52:1225.
74. Ganote CE, Reimer KA, Jennings RB. Acute mercuric chloride nephrotoxicity: an electronic microscopic and metabolic study. *Lab Invest* 1975;31:633.
75. Kempson SA, Ellis BG, Price RG. Changes in rat renal cortex, isolated plasma membranes and urinary enzymes following the injection of mercury chloride. *Chem Biol Interact* 1977;18:217.
76. Fowler BA. Ultrastructural evidence for nephropathy induced by longterm exposure to small amounts of methyl mercury. *Science* 1972;175:780–781.
77. Fowler BA. The morphologic effects of dieldrin and methyl mercuric chloride on pars recta segments of the rat kidney proximal tubules. *Am J Pathol* 1972;69:163–174.
78. Klein R, Herman SP, Bullock BC, Talley FA. Early functional and pathological changes in rat kidney during methyl mercury intoxication. *Arch Pathol* 1973;96:83.
79. Yasutake A, Hirayama K, Inouye M. Sex difference in acute renal dysfunction induced by methyl mercury in mice. *Ren Fail* 1990;12:233–240.
80. Trump BF, Berezesky IK, Sato T, Laiho KU, Phelps PC, DeClaris N. Cell calcium, cell injury, and cell death. *Environ Health Perspect* 1984;57:281–287.
81. Trump BF, Berezesky IK, Smith MW, Phelps PC, Elliget KA. The relationship between cellular ion deregulation and acute and chronic toxicity. *Toxicol Appl Pharmacol* 1989;97:6–22.
82. Smith MW, Ambudkar IS, Phelps PC, Regec AL, Trump BF. $HgCl_2$-induced changes in cytosolic Ca^{+2} of cultured rabbits' renal tubular cells. *Biochem Biophys Acta* 1987;931:130–142.

83. Lauwerys R, Buchet JP. Study on the mechanism of lysosome labilization by inorganic mercury in vitro. *Eur J Biochem* 1972;26:535–542.
84. Madsen KM, Christensen EF. Effects of mercury on lysosomal protein digestion in the kidney proximal tubule. *Lab Invest* 1978;38:165.
85. Piotrowski JK, Trojanowska B, Winiewska-Knyol JM, Bolanowska W. Mercury binding in the kidney and liver of rats repeatedly exposed to mercuric chloride: induction of metallothionein by mercury and cadmium. *Toxicol Appl Pharmacol* 1974;27:11.
86. Trump BF, Berezesky IK, Laiho KU, Osornio AR, Mersner WJ, Smith MW. The role of calcium in cell injury. A review. In: Johari OM, ed. *Scan electron microscopy*. 1980;437–462.
87. Fowler BA, Lucier GW, Mushak P. Phenobarbital protection against methyl mercury nephrotoxicity. *Proc Soc Exp Biol Med* 1975;149:75–79.
88. Fowler BA, Brown HW, Lucier GW, Krigman MR. The effect of chronic oral methyl mercury exposure on the lysosome system of rat kidney. Morphometric and biochemical studies. *Lab Invest* 1975;32:313–322.
89. Woods JS, Fowler BA. Renal porphyrinuria during chronic methyl mercury exposure. *J Lab Clin Med* 1977;90:266–272.
90. Chen RW, Ganter HE, Hoekstra WG. Studies on the binding of methylmercury by thionein. *Biochem Biophys Res Commun* 1973;51:383.
91. Ulfvarson U. The effect of the size of the dose on the distribution and excretion of mercury in rats after single intravenous injection of various mercury compounds. *Toxicol Appl Pharmacol* 1969; 15:517–524.
92. Takeda Y, Ukita T. Metabolism of ethylmercuric chloride-^{203}Hg in rats. *Toxicol Appl Pharmacol* 1970;17:181–188.
93. Ulfvarson U. The absorption and distribution of mercury in rats fed organs from rats injected with various mercury compounds. *Toxicol Appl Pharmacol* 1969;15:525–531.
94. Berlin M. Renal uptake, excretion, and retention of mercury II. A study in the rabbit during infusion of methyl- and phenylmercuris compounds. *Arch Environ Health* 1963;6:626–633.
95. Frejaville JP, Bescol J, LeClerc JP, Guillam L, Crabie P, Consco F, Gervais P, Faultier M. Intoxication aigue par les derives arsenicaux; (a propos de 4 observation personnelles); trouble de l'hematose, etude ultramicroscope du foie et du rein. *Ann Med Interne (Paris)* 1972;123:713.
96. Ginsberg JM, Lotspeich WW. Interrelations of arsenate and phosphate transport in the dog kidney. *Am J Physiol* 1963;205:707.
97. Ginsberg JM. Renal mechanism for excretion and transformation of arsenic in the dog. *Am J Physiol* 1965;208:832.
98. Vahter M. Metabolism of arsenic. In: Fowler BA, ed. Biological and environmental effects of arsenic. Amsterdam: Elsevier. 1979;171–198.
99. Brown MM, Rhyne BC, Goyer RA, Fowler BA. The intracellular effects of chronic arsenic administration on renal proximal tubule cells. *J Toxicol Environ Health* 1976;1:507–516.
100. Fluharty AL, Sanadi DR. On the mechanism of oxidative phosphorylation II. Effects of arsenite alone and in combination with 2,3-amercaptopropanol. *J Biol Chem* 1961;236:2772–2778.
101. Squibb KS, Fowler BA. The toxicity of arsenic and its compounds, in biological and environmental effects of arsenic. In: Fowler BA, ed. *Cadmium in the environment*. Amsterdam: Elsevier Science, 1979;chap. 7.
102. Mahaffey KR, Fowler BA. Effects of concurrent administration of dietary lead, cadmium and arsenic in the rat. *Environ Health Perspect* 1977;19:165.
103. Mahaffey KR, Capar SG, Gladen BC, Fowler BA. Concurrent exposure to lead, cadmium, and arsenic: effects of toxicity and tissue metal concentrations in the rat. *J Lab Clin Med* 1981;98:463.
104. Fowler BA, Mahaffey KR. Interaction between lead, cadmium and arsenic in relation to porphyrin excretion patterns. *Environ Health Perspect* 1979;25:87–90.
105. Carmichael NG, Fowler BA. Effects of separate and combined mercuric chloride and sodium selenate administration in rats: histological, ultrastructural and X-ray microanalytical studies of liver and kidney. *J Environ Pathol* 1979;3:399–412.
106. Boyette DP. Bismuth nephrosis with anuria in infant. *J Pediatr* 1946;28:193–197.
107. Urizar R, Vernier RL. Bismuth nephropathy. *JAMA* 1966;198:187–189.
108. Czerwinski AW, Ginn RE. Bismuth nephrotoxicity. *Am J Med* 1964;37:969–975.
109. Beaver DL, Burr RE. Bismuth inclusions in the kidney. *Arch Pathol* 1963;76:89–94.
110. Taylor EG, Klenerman P. Acute renal failure after colloidal bismuth subcitrate overdose. *Lancet* 1990;335:670–671.

111. Kolmer JA, Brown H, Rule AM. Studies in bismuth therapy of syphilis: comparative study of toxicity of therapeutic activity of bismuth compounds commonly employed in treatment of syphilis. *Am J Synph Gonorrhea Vener Dis* 1939;23:7–40.
112. Beaver DL, Burr RE. Electron microscopy of bismuth inclusions. *Am J Pathol* 1963;42:609–617.
113. Fowler BA, Goyer RA. Bismuth localization within nuclear inclusions by x-ray microanalysis: effects of accelerating voltage. *J Histochem Cytochem* 1975;23:722–726.
114. Seljankina KP, Lencenko VG, Petina AA, Petrova NN, El'Nicnik LN. Hygenic standardization of Bismuth of water reservoirs. *Gig Sanit* 1970;35:18–20.
115. Szymanska JA, Zelasowski AJ. Some aspects of bismuth metabolism. *Environ Res* 1979;19:121–126.
116. Franchini I, Mutti A, Cavatorta A, Corradi A, Cosi A, Olivette G, Borghetti A. Nephrotoxicity of chromium. *Contrib Nephrol* 1978;10:98–110.
117. Jao W, Manaligod JR, Gerardo LT, Castillo MM. Myeloid bodies in drug-induced acute tubular necrosis. *J Pathol* 1983;139:33.
118. Langard S, Norseth T. Chromium. In: Fridberg L, Nordberg GG, Vouk VB. *Handbook on the toxicology of metals*. Amsterdam: Elsevier/North Holland, 1979;chap. 22.
119. Linberg E, Vesterberg O. Urinary excretion of proteins in chromeplaters, exchromeplaters and referents. *Scand J Work Environ Health* 1983;9:505–510.
120. Verschoor MA, Bragt PC, Herber RFM, Zeilhuis RL, Zwennis WC. Renal function of chromeplating workers and welders. *Int Arch Occup Environ Health* 1988;60:67–70.
121. Hagberg M, Lindqvist B, Wall S. Exposure to welding fumes and chronic renal diseases, a negative case-referent study. *Int Arch Occup Environ Health* 1986;58:191–195.
122. Lindqvist B. Kidney disease in welders. *IRCS Med Sci Pathol Soc Occup Med* 1983;11:99.
123. Sano T, Ebihara I. Pathological and clinical findings of chromate and chrome plating workers. *J Sci Lab* 1979;55:21–25.
124. Evan AP, Dail WG Jr. The effects of sodium chromate on the proximal tubules of the rat kidney: fine structural damage and lysozymuria. *Lab Invest* 1974;30:704–715.
125. Berndt WO. Renal chromium accumulation and its relationship to chromium induced nephrotoxicity. *J Toxicol Environ Health* 1976;1:449.
126. Kluwe MW. Developed resistance to mercuric chloride nephrotoxicity: failure to protect against other nephrotoxicants. *Toxicol Lett* 1982;12:19.
127. Miyajima H, Hewitt WR, Cote MG, Plaa GL. Relationships between histological and functional indices of acute chemically induced nephrotoxicity. *Fundam Appl Toxicol* 1983;3:543.
128. Kumar A, Rana SVS. Enzymological effects of hexavalent chromium in the rat kidney. *Int J Tissue React* 1984;6:135–139.
129. Baggette JM, Berndt WO. Interaction of potassium dichromate with the nephrotoxins, mercuric chloride and citrinin. *Toxicology* 1984;33:157–169.
130. Tsapakos MJ, Hampton TH, Wetterhahn KE. Chromium (VI)-induced DNA lesions and chromium distribution in rat kidney, liver, and lung. *Cancer Res* 1983;43:56–62.
131. Standeven AM, Wetterhahn KE. Possible role of glutathione in chromium (VI) metabolism and toxicity in rats. *Pharmacol Toxicol* 1991;69:469–476.
132. Singh G. A possible cellular mechanism of cisplatin-induced nephrotoxicity. *Toxicology* 1989;58:71–80.
133. Dobyan DC, Levi J, Jacobs J, Kosek J, Weiner MW. Mechanism of cis-platinum nephrotoxicity: morphologic observations. *J Pharmacol Exp Ther* 1980;213:551.
134. Racusen LC, Solez R. Nephrotoxic tubular and interstitial lesions: morphology and classification. *Toxicol Pathol* 1986;14:45.
135. Nonclercq D, Toubeau G, Tulkens P, Heuson-Stiennon JA, Laurent G. Renal tissue injury and proliferative response after successive treatments with anticancer derivatives and tobramycin. *Virchows Arch [B]* 1990;59:143–158.
136. Maines MD. Effect of cis-platinum on heme, drug, and steroid metabolism pathways: possible involvement in nephrotoxicity and infertility. *Crit Rev Toxicol* 1990;21:1–20.
137. Suzuki AM, Cherian MG. The interactions of cis-diamminedichloroplatinum with metallothionein and glutathione in rat liver and kidney. *Toxicology* 1990;64:113–127.
138. Cacini W, Singh Y. Renal metallothionein and platinum levels in diabetic and nondiabetic rats injected with cisplatin. *Proc Soc Exp Biol Med* 1991;197:285–289.
139. Boogaard P, Slikkerveer A, Nagelkerke JF, Mulder G. The role of metallothionein in the reduction of cis-platin-induced nephrotoxicity by Bi^{+3}-pretreatment in the rat in vivo and in vitro. *Biochem Pharmacol* 1991;41:369–375.

140. Zunino F, Pratesi G, Micheloni A, Cavalletti E, Sala F, Tofanetti O. Protective effect of reduced glutathione against cisplatin-induced renal and systemic toxicity and its influence on the therapeutic activity of the antitumor drug. *Chem Biol Interact* 1989;70:89–101.
141. Goering PL, Fowler BA. Effect of intratracheal gallium arsenide (GaAs) administration of Δ-aminolevulinic acid dehydratase (ALAD) in rats. *Pharmacologist* 1986;28:229.
142. Goering PL, Maronpot RR, Fowler BA. Effect of gallium arsenide administration on Δ-aminolevulinic acid dehydratase in rats: relationship to urinary excretion of aminolevulinic acid. *Toxicol Appl Pharmacol* 1988;92:179–193.
143. Fowler BA, Goering PL. Mechanism of gallium arsenide (GaAs) inhibition of Δ-aminolevulinic acid dehydratase (ALAD). *Pharmacologist* 1986;28:229.
144. Aoki Y, Lipsky MM, Fowler BA. Alteration in protein synthesis in primary cultures of rat kidney proximal tubule epithelial cells by exposure to gallium, indium, and arsenite. *Toxicol Appl Pharmacol* 1990;106:462–468.
145. Downs WL, Scott JK, Steadman LT, Maynard EA. *The toxicity of indium*. University of Rochester Atomic Energy Project Report No. UR558. Rochester, NY: University of Rochester, 1959;57.
146. Castronovo FP. *Factors affecting the toxicity of the element indium*. Doctoral thesis, Johns Hopkins University 1970;73.
147. Castronovo FP, Wagner HN. Factors affecting the toxicity of the element indium. *Br J Exp Pathol* 1971;52:543–559.
148. Woods JS, Fowler BA. Selective inhibition of renal ALA dehydratase by indium: biochemical and ultrastructural studies. *Exp Mol Pathol* 1982;36:306–315.

Toxicology of the Kidney, Second Edition,
edited by Jerry B. Hook and Robin S. Goldstein.
Raven Press, Ltd., New York © 1993.

17

Effects of Selected Fungal Toxins on Renal Function

William O. Berndt

Department of Pharmacology, College of Medicine, University of Nebraska Medical Center, Omaha, Nebraska 68198-6810

The mycotoxins or fungal toxins are secondary products of fungal metabolism produced by a diverse group of fungi. This wide variety of chemicals no doubt are capable of producing a wide range of undesirable effects, including disruption of renal function. The mycotoxicoses produced after exposure to the mycotoxins may reveal themselves as damage to the central nervous system, the liver, the kidney, etc., and these toxicities are known to occur after various routes of exposure, e.g., dermal, oral, etc. An overt fungal infestation is not essential for the production of a mycotoxicosis.

Recently the potential role of naturally occurring chemicals in the production of cancer, and possible other toxic responses, has received considerable notoriety (e.g., 1). How generally involved naturally occurring substances are in the production of a variety of toxicities remains to be determined, but it is quite clear that certain fungal products may be involved. In any event, it is well known that fungal toxins can cause human toxicities and more recently it has become recognized that some can compromise renal function in a variety of species.

Human exposure to fungal products is not a new experience, despite the recent notoriety. The ergotism outbreaks of the Middle Ages are well documented, and there are other suggestions less well documented that even earlier problems existed (2). Modern food storage techniques, where available, have greatly reduced the occurrence of mycotoxicoses in humans, although major problems have persisted with domestic and farm animals. Nonetheless, there have been well-documented human mycotoxicoses in relatively recent times; these were related to aflatoxins. Epidemiological studies in Uganda, Taiwan, Kenya, and elsewhere demonstrated a likely cause-and-effect relationship between certain diseases (e.g., hepatic cancer) and the consumption of foods that were mold-contaminated and/or contained measurable quantities of aflatoxins. A summary of these reports has been given by Hayes (3). Another human disease, endemic Balkan nephropathy, has been suggested to be caused by fungal toxins (e.g., 4), but data confirming a cause-and-effect relationship are less compelling (see below for a more complete discussion).

The diversity of effects produced by mycotoxins is noteworthy. Several mycotoxins are thought to be carcinogenic, e.g., aflatoxins, patulin, and penicillic acid, and an equally chemically diverse group has been shown to produce fetocidal and/or teratogenic effects, e.g., ochratoxin A, rubratoxin B, and T-2 toxin (5,6). In addition, mycotoxin effects have been reported on hepatic function, the cardiovascular system, the skin, the nervous system, and the kidney. The variety of effects produced might well be expected given the wide variety of chemicals involved, although it has not been possible to predict target organ toxicity among the groups of toxins based on chemical structure alone.

Although there are data in the literature to suggest that a number of fungal toxins may have effects on the kidney (7), the major research efforts have been on two substances, citrinin and ochratoxin A. These will be the focus of this chapter.

CHEMISTRY AND OCCURRENCE

Citrinin has been obtained from cultures of several species of *Penicillium*. These molds have been shown to infest various types of grains, and citrinin has been found in samples of wheat, barley, rye, and oats. Although a major concern has been the presence of aflatoxins in Indian ground nuts, citrinin also has been found attributable to infestations with *Penicillium citrinum* and *Aspergillus terreus* (8). Citrinin often occurs in conjunction with ochratoxin A, which is produced by *Aspergillus ochraceus* and other molds. For example, *Penicillium viridicatum* has been reported to produce both ochratoxin A and citrinin, and is known to contaminate cereals and vegetables.

After many years of storage, rice found in warehouses in Japan contained significant quantities of citrinin (9). The presence of citrinin in rice also has been reported from other rice growing areas, including the United States. Similarly, Hokby et al. (10) reported that in Sweden a significant citrinin contamination in stored barley crops had been identified. These barley samples also contained significant quantities of ochratoxin A. In Canada, Van Walbeek (11) reported citrinin as a contaminant in wheat, rye, barley, and oats following a wet harvest in 1968.

Citrinin was first isolated from *P. citrinum* by Hetherington and Raistrick (12). Citrinin is produced readily in the research laboratory utilizing the method of Davis et al. (13) which allows the mold to grow in liquid cultures of 5% sucrose and 2% yeast extract. The structure of citrinin is given in Fig. 1. It has a molecular weight of 250 d, a melting point of 169° to 172°C and UV absorption maxima at 250 and 331 nm. Its virtual insolubility in acidic aqueous solutions makes its isolation from liquid cultures relatively easy. Citrinin has been isolated from various biological fluids including plasma, bile, and urine, and determined quantitatively by high-performance liquid chromatography (14).

Ochratoxin A is one of the most widely occurring mycotoxins. Contaminated

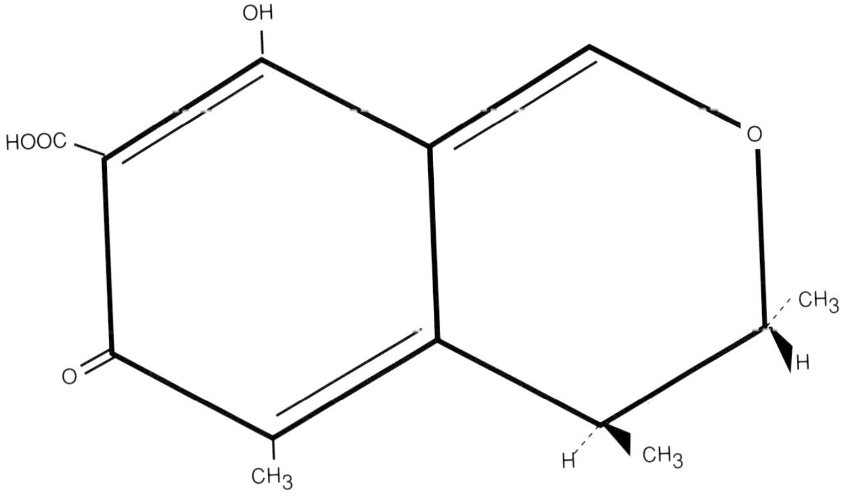

FIG. 1. The chemical structure of citrinin.

food and grain samples have been found in the United States and Canada (15), and in various Eastern European (16) and Latin American countries (17,18). A survey of various foodstuffs in the region where Balkan nephropathy is endemic revealed the presence of ochratoxin A (19,20). The frequency of contamination with ochratoxin A showed a considerable range, but with some frequencies as high as 43%. Petkova-Bocharova and Castegnaro (21) demonstrated a higher presence of ochratoxin A in cereal samples from an area of Bulgaria where the Balkan nephropathy was known to occur than in samples obtained from a control area. Furthermore, ochratoxin A residues in animal tissues may contribute significantly to human contamination (22). For example, pig kidneys have been reported to have significant ochratoxin A concentrations (23), as has blood obtained from slaughter pigs (24). Also chickens fed ochratoxin A experimentally for 150 days had detectable concentrations in muscle and liver (25,26). The possible relationship of ochratoxin A to Balkan nephropathy is discussed below.

In Fig. 2 is the structure of ochratoxin A and some of its congeners. Several of these have been isolated from fungal cultures, e.g., ochratoxin B, and 4-hydroxy ochratoxin A, along with ochratoxin A, have been identified as food and feed contaminants. The biosynthesis of ochratoxin A has been established (27).

CITRININ

Many nonrenal and renal effects of citrinin have been reviewed recently in detail (28).

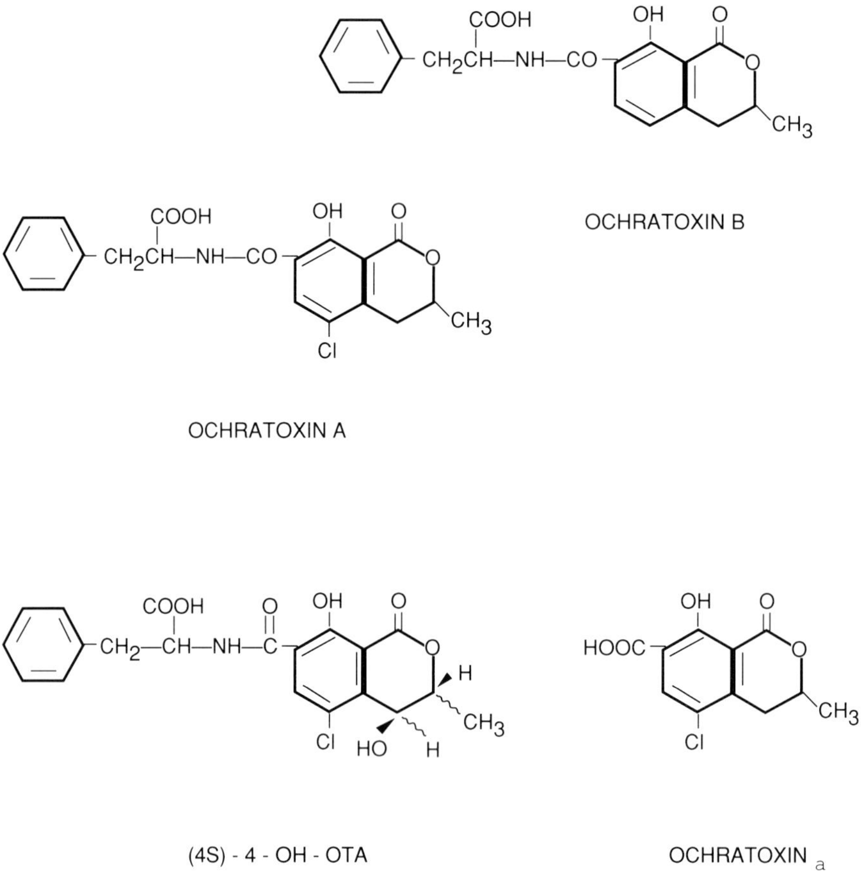

FIG. 2. The chemical structure of ochratoxin A and some of its congeners.

Nonrenal Toxicity

Ambrose and DeEds (29) reported LD_{50} values for citrinin in various animal species. Much of these earlier data have been confirmed by incidental observations in recent studies. Mice exposed to citrinin (30 or 40 mg/kg) on either gestation day 6, 7, 8, or 9 resulted in reduced fetal weight gain and increased fetal lethality. An increased number of maternal deaths also were observed. A relatively high maternal mortality also was found in rats, although citrinin administered subcutaneously (35 mg/kg) on days 3 to 15 of gestation did not alter the number of implants. Fetuses, however, were significantly smaller than those from controls. Enlarged kidneys were found along with internal hydrocephalus and cleft palate (30). The combination of citrinin and ochratoxin A increased the occurrence of gross, soft tissue and skeletal malformations (31). It could not be determined if the response was synergistic or merely additive.

The potential immunotoxicity of citrinin was examined in the mouse (32). Although several effects were observed, the authors concluded that citrinin was not markedly immunotoxic. Hematological changes were produced by citrinin when mice were exposed to the chemical once a week for 6 weeks. For example, a decreased platelet count and hematocrit were observed (33), but as with the immunotoxicity, these effects were not marked.

Several studies have been undertaken to examine the possible carcinogenicity of citrinin. Mice were fed for 70 weeks with diets containing 100 or 200 mg/kg of citrinin and no renal tumors were reported at 40 weeks (34). Sprague-Dawley rats were fed diets containing 0.02% or 0.05% citrinin for 48 weeks and then were killed. Shinohara et al. (35) reported no kidney tumors in those animals. However, when F344 rats were fed 0.1% citrinin in the diet for up to 80 weeks markedly different results were obtained (36). Rats sacrificed at 32 weeks showed an increased incidence of hyperplasia of renal tubular cells, and small adenomas were found in the kidneys of the rats at 40 weeks. By 60 weeks, large tumors were observed grossly in the kidneys of all treated animals. The tumors were "benign" and were classified as clear-cell adenomas.

Relatively minor effects of citrinin on the cardiovascular system and to depress respiration have been reported by Balpin (37) and Chu (38). No mechanistic studies were reported, and neither effect was thought to be significant in situations of citrinin poisoning.

Nephrotoxicity

Perhaps the most important toxicological effect caused by citrinin is its ability to disrupt renal function. This has been reported in both experimental and farm animals, and has been known to occur for many years. Larsen (39) perhaps was the first to associate nephropathy with the feeding of moldy cereal to pigs. This effect has been reproduced experimentally by the feeding of contaminated barley and rye to pigs (40) and by the feeding of purified citrinin (41). Further, except for a few reports (e.g., 42), investigators agree that the effect of citrinin is on the proximal tubule and not on the distal tubule or glomeruli (29,42–45). Some of the differences reported with respect to the tubular site of action of citrinin may relate to species differences. For example, Jordan et al. (46) found in the hamster that both distal and proximal tubules were affected, whereas only the straight segments of the proximal tubule were altered in the mouse (47). In any event, regardless of possible species differences, there is no doubt that citrinin affects the proximal tubule. There is some disagreement, however, about which segment of the proximal tubule is the primary target, i.e., S_1 (45) or S_3 (47).

In the rat, a species studied by several workers (41,48,49), citrinin produced a very characteristic and reproducible response. After the administration of a single dose of citrinin, renal dysfunction persisted for as long as 3 to 4 days (depending on dose) with complete recovery within about 8 days (Table 1). For animals that survive the initial 36 hr, the renal dysfunction is characterized by a nonoliguric ("high

TABLE 1. *Effect of citrinin on renal function in the rat*

Days	Urine Volume	Urine Osmolality	BUN
1	209	53	233
2	282	22	387
3	273	21	480
4	277	22	453
5	227	49	300
6	164	78	187

Data are percent of control collected 24 hr before injection of citrinin (55 mg/kg ip). Adapted from Berndt, ref. 100.

output") renal failure. The urine volume is elevated three to four times normal and the urine osmolality is reduced greatly. In addition, there is marked glucose excretion, and proteinuria, at least late in the toxicity. These events are accompanied by a rise in the blood urea nitrogen (BUN) and creatinine. The animals that die within the first 36 hr after administration of citrinin do so in anuric failure. The overall pattern of response found in the rat is very similar to that reported for the pig (43,50) and in poultry (51).

The increased excretion of glucose in the urine suggests an action of citrinin on the proximal tubule. This supposition is confirmed by various *in vitro* studies that indicate that the renal slice accumulation of *p*-aminohippurate (PAH) and tetraethylammonium (TEA) is compromised by citrinin. This is true both after the addition of citrinin to renal slices and in renal slices prepared from pretreated rats. Although the effect on PAH uptake by slices might be attributed to a competitive effect of citrinin, an organic anion, the effect on TEA accumulation no doubt reflects a more generalized toxicity. Furthermore, studies with isolated membrane vesicles have shown that citrinin can disrupt PAH transport as early as 3 hr after its administration. Also, brush border transport of glucose was similarly inhibited. With *in vitro* studies, only basolateral PAH transport was inhibited (52).

Further evidence for the involvement of proximal tubular cells in citrinin nephrotoxicity comes from studies in which probenecid was administered to rats prior to citrinin. Probenecid blocked the onset of toxicity as measured by slice uptake of PAH and TEA, and mortality (Table 2) (53). Also, citrinin accumulation by the kidney was reduced. In addition, Berndt (54) assessed directly the accumulation of ^{14}C-citrinin by renal cortical slices of the rat and found that this organic anion is accumulated by the same process that is responsible for PAH accumulation and that of other organic anions. Hence, it would appear that the renal accumulation of citrinin by the organic anion transport process is essential for the production of nephrotoxicity and that the likely cellular site of action is the proximal tubule since that is where organic anion transport occurs.

In an effort to understand the mechanism whereby citrinin produces renal damage, several studies have been undertaken (14,55,56). After administration of ^{14}C-citrinin it was found that the label was excreted rapidly in the urine. The radioactivity disappeared from plasma by a double exponential process with as much as 80% to 85% of the administered dose of labeled material found in the urine within 48 hr after the dose was administered. Organ accumulation of the label occurred essentially only in the liver and the kidney. Metabolism of citrinin occurred and high-performance liquid chromatograms of plasma indicated the presence of the parent compound and at least one metabolite. Two metabolites were found in the urine. Dunn et al. (57) identified a urinary metabolite of rats to be dihydrocitrinone. The role of this metabolite, if any, in citrinin-induced nephrotoxicity is not known. Overall, the metabolism of citrinin accounted for only 10% to 20% of the administered dose, with the major amount of label in the urine associated with the parent compound. Unpublished studies (Berndt) with the isolated perfused kidney failed to demonstrate the formation of any metabolites by that organ, which suggests the liver is the primary organ of metabolism. Further, the absence of renal metabolism suggests that formation of a "reactive intermediate" is not likely. On the other hand, renal as well as hepatic glutathione were reduced by 30 min after citrinin administration. The decrease in glutathione amounted to about 30%, somewhat less than reported for other compounds that deplete glutathione as a prelude to target organ toxicity (e.g., acetaminophen). It is also noteworthy that covalently bound ^{14}C was found in renal tissue after the administration of ^{14}C-citrinin. Although hepatic covalent binding did occur, it was at a concentration threefold lower than in kidney, approximately 1.5 ng citrinin equivalents per mg protein and 0.4 ng per mg protein, respectively.

It is difficult to reconcile all of these data with respect to a mechanism of toxicity. The renal slice accumulation studies (53,54) suggest that it is the parent compound that is transported into renal tubular cells as a prerequisite for the production of toxicity. This observation is supported further by the failure of the isolated perfused kidney to generate metabolites of citrinin. However, the ability of citrinin to reduce

TABLE 2. *Effect of probenecid on citrinin-induced reduction of PAH and TEA accumulation by rat renal cortical slices*

Treatment	PAH	PAH with lactate	TEA
Citrinin	36	18	55
Citrinin + probenecid 30	79	50	87
Citrinin + probenecid 60	94	70	88
Citrinin + probenecid 120	125	81	88

Data are given as percent of control. Citrinin was administered in a dose of 55 mg/kg, and probenecid at a dose of 30, 60, or 120 mg/kg. The citrinin was administered 30 min after the probenecid.

PAH, *p*-aminohippurate; TEA, tetraethylammonium.

Adapted from Berndt and Hayes, ref. 53.

renal glutathione (GSH) and to produce a covalently bound compound in kidney tissue suggests that it may be a metabolite rather than the parent compound that produces the nephrotoxic response. Except for the unpublished data with the isolated perfused kidney, all of the data would be consistent with the formation (perhaps in the liver) of an acidic metabolite, the transport of which is blocked by probenecid. Once in the renal tissue, the acidic metabolite produces nephrotoxicity by reacting with some important renal cell component. This reaction would occur once the glutathione conjugation process has been overloaded. A final reconciliation of these differences requires further study. However, the fact that membrane transport processes are affected as early as 3 hr after administration of citrinin complicates this hypothesis (52). How this early effect relates to the overall nephrotoxic response is unclear, since early access into the cell by way of the organic anion transporter appears to be essential for the toxic response. Hence, citrinin must produce a very early intracellular effect, which by 3 hr is reflected in disruption of the transport process responsible for cellular citrinin accumulation.

OCHRATOXIN A

Nonrenal Toxicity

A variety of toxicities have been reported in animals after exposure to ochratoxin A, although many of these have been reported from experimental studies in which relatively high doses were used (61). Liver damage and immunosuppression have been reported (58), although the extent of liver damage is generally considered more variable than the renal damage produced by ochratoxin A. Rahimtula et al. (59) demonstrated that ochratoxin A added to liver or kidney microsomes could enhance lipid peroxidation. The same group (60) has proposed a mechanism whereby ochratoxin A–stimulated lipid peroxidation might occur. The authors acknowledged, however, that it is premature to conclude that enhanced lipid peroxidation is responsible for all of the toxicities observed with ochratoxin A. To date, no organ-specific (e.g., kidney) lipid peroxidative events have been identified *in vivo*.

Certain immunological parameters also are altered by ochratoxin A (58). Haubeck et al. (58) demonstrated a generalized immunosuppression caused by this fungal toxin, and observed that the effects could be prevented by phenylalanine.

Holmberg et al. (62) found ochratoxin A to suppress mitogen-induced blastogenesis of pig blood lymphocytes. Ochratoxin A also suppresses natural killer cell activity in mice by suppressing basal interferon (63). These same workers also showed ochratoxin A to increase the growth of transplantable tumor cells. Possibly this could underlie the carcinogenesis produced by ochratoxin A.

Ochratoxin A is also known to produce teratogenic effects (64). These studies, conducted in rats, demonstrated growth retardation and various soft, tissue anomalies, e.g, microencephaly, stunted limb buds, etc. Mayura et al. (65) also demonstrated that phenylalanine could protect partially against the teratogenic effects of ochratoxin A. Ochratoxin A also affected postimplantation of rat embryos in culture (66). The ability of ochratoxin A to produce teratogenic effects can be enhanced by a reduction in dietary protein intake (67) as well as by a reduction in renal function (68).

Although ochratoxin A did not produce mutagenic effects as demonstrated with short-term tests (69,70), this fungal toxin did induce DNA–single strand breaks in liver, kidney, and spleen of mice. Furthermore, Bendele et al. (71) demonstrated that ochratoxin A was carcinogenic in the (C57BL/6J × C3H) F1 mouse. Both renal adenomas and hepatocellular carcinomas were observed in this strain of mouse. These studies were conducted with the dietary feeding of ochratoxin A at relatively large doses.

Nephrotoxicity

Ochratoxin A has long been studies for its effects on the kidney. For example, Krogh et al. (41,43,50,73), Elling et al. (51), and Berndt and Hayes (72), among others, all have demonstrated that ochratoxin A has adverse effects on renal function in a variety of species. Indeed, this substance was very early identified as a causative agent in porcine nephropathy (74–76). Pigs fed *A. ochraceus* or ochratoxin A–contaminated feed showed renal tubular necrosis, etc., within 1 to 3 weeks of exposure (77). In addition, alterations in gastrointestinal function and changes in liver and lymphoid tissue were seen with high doses of ochratoxin A. In this study and in others with pigs, the alterations in renal function included polyuria, decreased osmolality, proteinuria, glucosuria, and increased excretion of urinary enzymes. Three effects led to an elevation of the blood urea nitrogen and polydipsia. Similar effects were observed in pigs that developed nephropathy after exposure to ochratoxin A through the use of contaminated feed. Morphologically, primary damage was observed on the proximal tubule. In addition, interstitial fibrosis and glomerular atrophy and sclerosis were observed (78).

Elling et al. (51) reported a nephropathy in birds associated with ochratoxin A mycotoxicosis, and the same response was produced in chickens deliberately fed ochratoxin A–contaminated feed (79,80). The effects on renal function were exerted primarily through alterations in the functioning proximal tubule, although glomerular damage also was observed.

In the rat, Berndt and Hayes (72) found that large, single doses of ochratoxin A produced death but without obvious alterations in renal function. Low, single, doses of ochratoxin A failed to alter renal function or animal behavior. However, when small doses were injected repeatedly (daily for 4 to 8 days) alterations in renal function, excessive weight loss, diarrhea, and if continued, death were observed. In contrast to citrinin, ochratoxin A did not produce a dramatic increase in urine volume, although urine osmolality fell significantly. There was also an increase in urinary glucose and ketone excretion, although blood glucose tended to fall rather than rise during the treatment period, i.e., the increased excretion of glucose was not related to large alterations in glucose metabolism.

Ochratoxin A also has significant effects on other proximal tubular functions. For example, utilizing renal slices from animals pretreated with multiple, small doses of ochratoxin A, a reduced PAH and TEA accumulation was observed (72). The primary effect, however, was on the accumulation of the organic anion PAH. Addition of ochratoxin A to healthy renal cortical slices also served to inhibit the transport of organic ions, again with the primary effect being exerted on PAH accumulation. Although these effects may represent a generalized nephrotoxic response, as noted below, the inhibitory effect of ochratoxin A on PAH accumulation in renal slices may be competitive, since ochratoxin A appears to enter proximal tubular cells by the same process.

As with citrinin, several studies have been undertaken with ochratoxin A to assess the role of kinetic factors in the production of nephrotoxicity. These and various biochemical effects of ochratoxin A have been reviewed in detail by Delacruz and Bach (81). Not surprisingly, studies on the distribution of radioactive ochratoxin A after oral administration showed a significant distribution of the compound to the kidney (82). Peak levels were observed within 3 to 12 hr after treatment, after which the concentration of radioactivity declined and subsequently (18 hr) increased in both the liver and intestine. This distribution pattern suggests that ochratoxin A may produce some initial effect on the kidney that is subsequently magnified into the production of the nephrotoxic response.

Rat liver microsomal preparations have been shown to metabolize ochratoxin A into various hydroxylated compounds. Indeed, the 4-hydroxy ochratoxin A has proven to be a major urinary metabolite. Isolated hepatocytes also produce the hydroxylated metabolites (83). None of the metabolism studies, however, has suggested that ochratoxin A need be converted to a reactive intermediate in order to produce its toxic response. As noted above, ochratoxin A does enhance lipid peroxidation (59), but there are not data to indicate that this effect is selective to the kidney, and the role of lipid peroxidation in the production of the nephrotoxic response is unclear.

Several studies have been undertaken to examine biochemical effects of ochratoxin A in an effort to explain the nephrotoxicity. In sufficient concentration, ochratoxin A can block the respiration of isolated liver mitochondria at a site different from that for 2,4-dinitrophenol (84). Whether or not some selective action of ochratoxin A on mitochondrial function occurs in the kidney is not known. In any event, the proximal tubule contains many mitochondria and inhibition of respiration might reduce adenosine triphosphate (ATP) content (see below) and this might underlie the nephrotoxicity.

Endou and colleagues (85,86) have examined the mechanisms by which ochratoxin A enters tubular cells. Studies with isolated tubule suspensions indicated that ochratoxin A added to those suspensions could cause the release of various proximal tubule enzymes. The enzymes released are the same ones that one normally associates with a nephrotoxic response *in vivo*. The treatment of the tubule suspensions

(S_2 and S_3) with probenecid prevented the effect of ochratoxin A. Studies conducted in isolated cell suspensions behaved quite differently. Endou and colleagues (85) have shown that isolated cells from the proximal tubule behave as if they are surrounded by a luminal membrane, i.e., the cellular polarity has been lost. Ochratoxin A did not cause an increase in enzyme release in isolated cells, suggesting that intact cellular polarity is essential for the production of ochratoxin A nephrotoxicity; this may relate to the entrance of the toxin into the cells via the PAH transporter.

These studies demonstrate the requirement for ochratoxin A to enter the cells (presumably by the organic anion transporter), but once inside the cells, what does the fungal toxin do? Jung and Endou (86) have examined cellular ATP content in various nephron segments isolated by dissection. Under *in vitro* conditions, ochratoxin A caused a significant reduction in S_2 tubule ATP at a concentration as low as 10^{-8} M. For the medullary collecting tubule, a concentration of 5×10^{-8} M was required to produce a significant ATP reduction. Jung and Endou examined nine nephron segments and at an ochratoxin A concentration of 5×10^{-5} M. ATP content was reduced significantly only in the S_2 and the S_3 segments. Similarly, mitochondria isolated from renal cortical tissue were responsive to ochratoxin A. Probenecid also protected against the effects of ochratoxin A on ATP content in these experiments as it did for enzyme release from tubule suspension. Jung and Endou suggest that ochratoxin A once inside the cell exerts its toxic effect by disruption of mitochondrial energy metabolism, specifically, ATP production.

Meisner and colleagues (87,89) also have investigated various biochemical events that might explain ochratoxin A nephrotoxicity. These studies resulted in the demonstration, first, that ochratoxin A could inhibit gluconeogenesis in rat renal tissue and second, that a decreased mRNA for coding of phosphoenolpyruvate carboxylase in rat kidney occurred. They have suggested that either through this effect or through some other effect on another critical mRNA might underlie the nephrotoxicity produced by ochratoxin A.

Although a number of studies have been undertaken to examine the biochemical effects that might lead to nephrotoxicity, no absolutely conclusive data have been forthcoming. Undoubtedly several of the effects of ochratoxin A on biochemical parameters have the potential to underlie a nephrotoxic response. However, there seem to be few data to suggest a specificity of this fungal toxin for renal biochemical events over those seen in the liver. For example, although renal tubule ATP content falls after ochratoxin A presumably because of an action on mitochondria, this toxin also affects liver mitochondrial function. Hence, although there may be a number of these biochemical effects that could underlie a nephrotoxic response, details concerning target organ selectivity have not been revealed.

ENDEMIC BALKAN NEPHROPATHY

Because both citrinin and ochratoxin A have been demonstrated to have multiple effects in a wide variety of species, it is not surprising that one or both of these agents might be suggested as causative agents for nephrotoxicity in humans. This sort of extrapolation is not uncommon and, specifically, several workers have suggested that endemic Balkan nephropathy might be the result of intoxication with ochratoxin A, citrinin, or both.

As noted earlier, Barnes (4) suggested, after a process of elimination of other causative agents, that fungal toxins might be involved in the etiology of this disease. Krogh (50) noted the similarities between porcine nephropathy and the human disease. In addition, these workers observed that ochratoxin A was present in various food stuffs and in the blood of various individuals who had this disease. However, Barnes et al. (48) noted that the most frequent mold contamination isolated from the same food samples wherein Krogh et al. (19) noted the presence of ochratoxin A was neither an ochratoxin A nor citrinin producer. Hence, even at the outset of this debate, the circumstances were clouded and little has changed to date.

In an effort to clarify this issue further, many workers examined other effects of ochratoxin A and/or citrinin in an effort to reconcile the experimental and epidemiological findings. Specifically, it has long been recognized that tumors of the urological system occurred in humans suffering from endemic Balkan nephropathy in concert with a disruption of renal function. Recent studies on the tumorigenic potential of ochratoxin A and citrinin were called upon to clarify the issue. Bendele et al. (71) in a 24-month feeding study demonstrated that ochratoxin A was a renal carcinogen in the (C57BL/6J × C3H) F1 mouse. This strain, the B6C3F1 mouse, has been used for many long-term carcinogenesis studies. Interestingly, although ochratoxin A produced renal tumors in males and females of this strain, it was also found to be a hepatic carcinogen in female mice. Hepatic carcinogenesis has not been observed in females suffering from endemic Balkan nephropathy. In addition, Aria and Hibino (36) demonstrated in the F344 male rat that a 73% incidence of renal adenomas occurred after 40 weeks of feeding 0.1% citrinin, whereas no tumors occurred in controls. Hence, although the specific types of tumors produced in animals were not exactly identical to those found in humans, it is true that the two primary mycotoxins thought to be associated with endemic Balkan nephropathy do appear to be tumorigenic. The issue is further complicated by the fact that various tests for *in vitro* mutagenesis were found to be negative for both compounds, although DNA strand breaks were observed with ochratoxin A (90,91).

In a further effort to resolve the discrepancies, several workers have pursued "epidemiological" studies to resolve the matter. As noted above, Krogh et al. (19) were able to demonstrate the presence of ochratoxin A in certain food, and this observation was subsequently confirmed by Pavlovic et al. (20). In both of these studies, several cereals and breads were examined in an area of Yugoslavia where the Balkan nephropathy was known to occur. However, a problem arises when one notes the frequency of occurrence of ochratoxin A as a contaminant. In one study, the frequency was about 9% on average, but with at least one report of an incidence as high as 43%. Although the variability was obviously quite high, it is true that these contaminations were higher in the areas where the disease was prevalent than in control areas. More recently similar studies were undertaken by Petkova-

Bocharova and Castegnaro (21), wherein a variety of cereal samples consumed by humans were analyzed. These studies were conducted in an area of Bulgaria where both the Balkan nephropathy and urinary tract tumors were well documented. In these studies, approximately 17% of the cereal samples analyzed showed the presence of ochratoxin A, whereas only 7% of the samples from a control area were so infected. Where ochratoxin A was found (whether control area or the area where the disease occurred), the concentrations of ochratoxin A in the cereal samples were approximately the same. In 1988, Petkova-Bocharova et al. (92) examined the blood of subjects who lived in the affected and nonaffected areas of Bulgaria. These workers reported that ochratoxin A was found more often in the blood samples from those in the affected area than in blood samples from those in the nonaffected area. Although far from clear-cut, data of this sort have been interpreted to indicate a role for one or more fungal toxins in the production of endemic Balkan nephropathy.

Unfortunately, appropriate experimental studies have not been conducted to resolve this issue. Laboratory experiments in which animals are treated with intermittent doses of one or another fungal toxin at relatively low concentrations should be conducted for a relatively long period of time. Based on the frequency of occurrence of ochratoxin A in human food samples, this approach would mimic the most likely exposure of humans to the fungal toxins. That is to say, it is likely that humans are exposed to the fungal toxins on an irregular, intermittent basis rather than with a fixed dose on a continuous, day-to-day basis. Such an experimental approach might give insights into the likelihood of ochratoxin A as a causative agent in a renal dysfunction similar to endemic Balkan nephropathy.

Although there are data to suggest that fungal toxins may be involved in the production of this human disease, other data suggest the contrary. Hall (93) has summarized much of the earlier data. Nichifor et al. (94) further raised doubt about the causative role of fungal toxins by an examination of the drinking water in affected and nonaffected areas. From this study, several other putative causative agents were revealed. For example, these investigators found that in the endemic areas cadmium, chromium, manganese, and cobalt did exist in the drinking water at higher concentrations than found in the drinking water in nonaffected areas. Radovanovic (95) concluded from an epidemiological investigation that the Balkan nephropathy may be related to the presence of a "slow virus" that contaminates the food and other articles in the households of the affected areas, and is transmitted by rodents. Whatever the causative agent, the studies of Draganescu et al. (96) demonstrated that a blood-borne agent is probably responsible. These workers inoculated guinea pigs with serum samples from patients that had the endemic Balkan nephropathy and were able to produce a morphologically similar disease in the guinea pig. Although the authors argue that this is evidence for the presence of a viral transmission of the disease, any blood-borne agent could be responsible.

Finally, one aspect of this entire issue has not been addressed by any of the workers. The probability is rather high that any individual exposed to one fungal toxin is likely to be exposed to two or more. Furthermore, an individual exposed to fungal toxins, may well be exposed to heavy metals, various viruses, etc. None of the experimental or epidemiological studies has given detailed consideration to the possibility that an interaction of nephrotoxic agents might be involved in the production of the endemic Balkan nephropathy. Studies do exist to suggest that an interaction of fungal toxins may be important in the production of an enhanced mycotoxin response (55,97–99), although this phenomenon has not been studied extensively with respect to effects in the kidney. This is an issue that needs to be resolved before any final decision can be made concerning the etiology of the endemic Balkan nephropathy.

REFERENCES

1. Ames BN, Magaw R, Gold LS. Ranking possible carcinogenic hazards. *Science* 1987;236:271–280.
2. Bagger G. *Ergot and ergotism*. London: Guerney and Jackson, 1931.
3. Hayes AW. Biological activities of mycotoxins. *Mycopathologia* 1979;65:29–41.
4. Barnes JM. Possible nephrotoxic agents. In: Wolstenholme GEW, Knight J, eds. *Ciba Foundation study group*. Massachusetts: Little, Brown, 1967;110.
5. LeBreton E, Frayssinet C, Lafarge C, DeRecondo AM. Alatoxine-Mecanisme dr l'action. *Food Cosmet Toxicol* 1964;2:675–677.
6. Hayes AW. Mycotoxin teratogenicity. In: Rosenberg P, ed. *Toxins: animal, plant, microbial*. New York: Pergamon Press, 1978;739–751.
7. Hayes AW, Williams WL. Acute toxicity of aflatoxin B1 and rubratoxin B in dog. *J Environ Pathol Toxicol* 1977;1:59–70.
8. Subrahmanyam P, Rao AS. Occurrence of aflatoxins and citrinin in groundnuts at harvest in relation to pod condition and kernel moisture content. *Curr Sci* 1974;43:707.
9. Sugimoto T, Miranisawa M, Takano K, Sasamura Y, Tsuguta O. Detection of ochratoxin A, citrinin and sterigmatocystin in stored rice contaminated by a natural occurrence of *Penicillium vindicatum* and *Aspergillus versicolor*. *Shokuhin Eisei Gaku Zasshi* 1977;18:176–181 [Chem Abstr 87:1661689].
10. Hokby F, Hult K, Gatenbeck S, Rutgnist L. Ochratoxin A and citrinin in 1976 crop of barley stored on farms in Sweden. *Acta Agric Scand* 1979;29:174.
11. Van Walbeek W. Fungal toxins in foods. *Can Inst Food Sci Technol J* 1973;6:96–102.
12. Hetherington AC, Raistrick H. *Studies in the biochemistry of micro-organisms*. Part XIV on the production and chemical constitution of a yellow coloring matter, citrinin, produced from glucose by *Penicillium citrinum*. London: Thom Phil Trans Royal Soc, 1931; Ser B. 220–269.
13. Davis ND, Dalby DK, Diener UL, Sansing GA. Medium-scale production of citrinin by *Penicillium citrinum* in a semisynthetic medium. *Appl Microbiol* 1975;29:118–120.
14. Phillips RD, Hayes AW, Berndt WO. High performance liquid chromatographic analysis of the mycotoxin citrinin and its application to biological fluids. *J Chromatogr* 1980;190:419–427.
15. Krogh P, Nesheim A. Ochratoxin A. In: Egan H, Stoloff L, Castegnaro M, Scott P, O'Neill IK, Bartsch H, eds. *Environmental carcinogens: selected methods of analysis*, Vol 5. Lyon: I.A.R.C., *Some mycotoxins* 1982;247–253.
16. Ruprich J, Piscac A, Mala J. Using the radioimmunological assay of the ochratoxin A mycotoxin for the screening control of cereal-type foods and feeds of plant origin. *Vet Med* 1988;33:165–173.
17. Micco C, Grossi M, Miraglia M, Brera C. A study of the contamination by ochratoxin A of green and roasted coffee beans. *Food Addit Contam* 1989;6:333–339.
18. Ysubouchi H, Yamamoto K, Hisada K, Sakabe Y, Udagawa A. Effect of roasting on ochratoxin A level in green coffee beans inoculated with *Aspergillus ochraceus*. *Mycopathologia* 1987;97:111–115.
19. Krogh P, Hald B, Plestina R, Ceovic S. Balkan (endemic) nephropathy and food borne ochratoxin A: preliminary results of a survey of food stuffs. *Acta Pathol Microbiol Scand* 1977;B85:238–245.
20. Pavlovic M, Pestina R, Krogh P. Ochratoxin A contamination of food stuffs in an area with Balkan (endemic) nephropathy. *Acta Pathol Microbiol Scand* 1979;B87:243–246.

21. Petkova-Bocharova T, Castegnaro M. Ochratoxin A contamination of cereals in an area of high incidence of Balkan endemic nephropathy in Bulgaria. *Food Addit Contam* 1985;2:267–270.
22. Kuiper-Goodman T, Scott PM. Risk assessment of the mycotoxin ochratoxin A. *Biomed Environ Sci* 1989;2:179–248.
23. Rousseau DM, Van-Peteghem CH. Spontaneous occurrence of ochratoxin A residues in porcine kidneys in Belgium. *Bull Environ Contam Toxicol* 1989;42:181–186.
24. Marquardt RR, Frohlich AA, Sreemannarayana O, Abramson D, Bernatsky A. Ochratoxin A in blood from slaughter pigs in western Canada. *Can J Vet Res* 1988;52:186–190.
25. Micco C, Miraglia M, Onori R, Ioppolo A, Mantovani A. Long-term administration of low doses of mycotoxins in poultry. 1. Residues of ochratoxin A in broilers and laying hens. *Poult Sci* 1987; 66:47–50.
26. Micco C, Miraglia M, Benelli L, Onori R, Ioppolo A, Mantovani A. Long-term administration of low doses of mycotoxins in poultry. 2. Residues of ochratoxin A and aflatoxins in broilers and laying hens after combined administration of ochratoxin A and aflatoxin B1. *Food Addit Contam* 1988;5:309–314.
27. Vleggaar R, Steyn PS. The biosynthesis of some miscellaneous mycotoxins. In: Steyn PS, ed. *The biosynthesis of mycotoxins*, New York: Academic Press, 1980;395–399.
28. Reddy RV, Berndt WO. Citrinin. In: Sharma RP, Salunkhe DK, eds. *Mycotoxins and phytoalexins*. Caldwell, NJ: CRC Press, Boca Raton, FL, 1991.
29. Ambrose AM, DeEds F. Some toxicological and pharmacological properties of citrinin. *J Pharmacol Exp Ther* 1946;88:173–186.
30. Reddy RV, Mayura K, Hayes AW, Berndt WO. Embryocidal teratogenic and fetotoxic effects of citrinin in rats. *Toxicology* 1982;25:151–160.
31. Mayura K, Berndt WO, Phillips TD. Effects of simultaneous prenatal exposure to ochratoxin A and citrinin in the rat. *J Toxicol Environ Health* 1984;13:553–561.
32. Reddy RV, Taylor MJ, Sharma RP. Evaluation of citrinin toxicity on the immune functions of mice. *J Food Prot* 1988;51:32.
33. Gupta M, Sasmal D, Bandyopadhyay S, Bagchi G, Chatterjee T, Dey S. Hematological changes produced in mice by ochratoxin A and citrinin. *Toxicology* 1983;26:55–62.
34. Kanisawa MC. Synergistic effect of citrinin on hepatorenal carcinogenesis of ochratoxin A in mice. *Dev Food Sci* 1984;7:245.
35. Shinohara Y, Arai M, Hirao K, et al. Combination effect of citrinin and other chemicals on rat kidney tumorigenesis. *Gann* 1976;67:147–155.
36. Arai M, Hibino T. Tumorigenicity of citrinin in male F344 rats. *Cancer Lett* 1983;17:281–287.
37. Balpin O. La citrinie. Nouvelles donnes sar l'action pharmacodynamique de cet. *Antibiotique Therapie* 1959;14:677.
38. Chu WC. Miscellaneous pharmacologic actions of citrinin. *J Lab Clin Med* 1946;31:72–78.
39. Larsen S. On chronic degeneration of the kidneys caused by moldy rye. *Maanedsskr Dyst* 1928;40: 259–284;289–300.
40. Nielsen HE, Hasselager E. Maggent korn til tidlist frauaennede smagnise. *Forsogslab Arbog* 1965; 91.
41. Krogh P, Hasselager E, Friss P. Studies on fungal nephrotoxicity. 2. Isolation of nephrotoxic compounds from *Penicillium viridicatum* westling: citrinin and oxalic acid. *Acta Pathol Microbiol Scand* 1970;B78:401–413.
42. Carlton WW, Sansing G, Szczech GM, Tuite J. Citrinin mycotoxicosis in beagle dogs. *Food Cosmet Toxicol* 1974;12:479–490.
43. Krogh P, Hald B, Pedersen EJ. Occurrence of ochratoxin A and citrinin in cereals associated with mycotoxin porcine nephropathy. *Acta Pathol Microbiol Scand* 1973;B81:689–695.
44. Hamika C, Carlton WW, Hinsman EJ, Tuite J. Citrinin mycotoxicosis in the rabbit: ultrastructural alterations. *Vet Pathol* 1986;23:245–253.
45. Lockard VG, Phillips RD, Hayes AW, Berndt WO, O'Neal RM. Citrinin nephrotoxicity in rats: a light and electron microscopic study. *Exp Mol Pathol* 1980;32:226–240.
46. Jordan WH, Carlton WW, Sansing GA. Citrinin mycotoxicosis in the Syrian hamster. *Food Cosmet Toxicol* 1978;16:355–363.
47. Jordan WH, Carlton WW, Sansing GA. Citrinin mycotoxicosis in the mouse. *Food Cosmet Toxicol* 1977;15:29–34.
48. Barnes JM, Austwide PKC, Carter RL, Flynn FU, Peristianis GC, Aldridge WN. Balkan (endemic) nephropathy and a toxin producing strain of *Penicillium verrucosum*, var. cyclopium: an experimental model in rats. *Lancet* 1977;1:671–675.

49. Berndt WO, Hayes AW. Effects of citrinin on renal tubular transport functions in the rat. *J Environ Pathol Toxicol* 1977;1:93–103.
50. Krogh P. Epidemiology of mycotoxic porcine nephropathy. *Nord Vet Med* 1976;28:452–458.
51. Elling F, Hald B, Jacobsen C, Krogh P. Spontaneous cases of nephropathy in poultry associated with ochratoxin A. *Acta Pathol Microbiol Scand* 1975;3:739–741.
52. Ansari RA, Thakran RS, Berndt WO. The effects of potassium chromate and citrinin on rat renal membrane transport. *Fundam Appl Toxicol* 1991;16:702–709.
53. Berndt WO, Hayes AW. The effect of probenecid on citrinin-induced nephrotoxicity. *Toxicol Appl Pharmacol* 1982;25:118–124.
54. Berndt WO. Transport of citrinin by rat renal cortex. *Arch Toxicol* 1983;54:35–40.
55. Berndt WO, Hayes AW, Phillips RD. Effects of mycotoxins on renal function: mycotoxic nephropathy. In: *Kidney international*, vol 18. New York: Springer-Verlag, 1980;656–664.
56. Phillips RD, Berndt WO, Hayes AW. Distribution and excretion of ^{14}C-citrinin in rats. *Toxicology* 1979;12:285–298.
57. Dunn BB, Stack ME, Park DL, Joshi A, Friedman L, King RL. Isolation and identification of dihydrocitrinone, a urinary metabolite of citrinin in rats. *J Toxicol Environ Health* 1983;12:283–289.
58. Haubeck HD, Lorkoweski G, Kolsh E, Roschenthaler R. Immunosuppression by ochratoxin A and its prevention by phenylalanine. *Appl Environ Microbiol* 1981;41:1040–1042.
59. Rahimtula AD, Bereziat J-C, Bussacchini-Groit V, Bartsch H. Lipid peroxidation as a possible cause of ochratoxin A toxicity. *Biochem Pharmacol* 1988;37:4469–4477.
60. Omar RF, Hasinoff BB, Mejilla F, Rahimtula AD. Mechanism of ochratoxin A stimulated lipid peroxidation. *Biochem Pharmacol* 1990;40:1183–1191.
61. Harwig J. Ochratoxin A and related metabolites. In: Purchase IFH, ed. *Mycotoxins*. Amsterdam: Elsevier, 1974;345–368.
62. Holmberg T, Thuvander A, Hult K. Ochratoxin A as a suppressor of mitogen-induced blastogenesis of porcine blood lymphocytes. *Acta Vet Scand* 1988;29:219–223.
63. Lea T, Steien K, Stormer FC. Mechanism of ochratoxin A-induced immunosuppression. *Mycopathologia* 1989;107:153–159.
64. Mayura K, Hayes AW, Berndt WO. Teratogenic effects of ochratoxin A in rats. *Toxicology* 1982; 25:176–185.
65. Mayura K, Parker R, Berndt WO, Phillips TD. Ochratoxin A induced teratogenicity in rats: partial protection with phenylalanine. *Appl Environ Microbiol* 1985;48:1186–1188.
66. Mayura K, Edwards JF, Maull EA, Phillips TD. The effects of ochratoxin A on postimplantation rat embryos in culture. *Arch Environ Contam Toxicol* 1989;18:411–415.
67. Mayura K, Hayes AW, Berndt WO. Effects of dietary protein on teratogenecity of ochratoxin A in rats. *Toxicology* 1983;27:147–157.
68. Mayura K, Stein A, Berndt WO, Phillips TD. Teratogenic effects of ochratoxin A in rats with impaired renal function. *Toxicology* 1984;32:277–286.
69. Umeda TM, Tsutsu T, Saito M. Mutagenicity and inducibility of single-strand breaks and chromosome aberrations by various mycotoxins. *Gann* 1977;58:619–625.
70. Wehner FC, Thiel PG, van Rensburg SJ, Demasius IPC. Mutagenicity to *Salmonella typhimurium* of some *Aspergillus* and *Penicillium* mycotoxins. *Mutat Res* 1978;58:193–203.
71. Bendele AM, Carlton WW, Krough P, Lillehoj EB. Ochratoxin A carcinogenesis in the (C57BL/6J × C3H) F1 Mouse. *J Natl Cancer Inst* 1985;75:733–739.
72. Berndt WO, Hayes AW. *In vivo* and *in vitro* changes in renal function caused by ochratoxin A in the rat. *Toxicology* 1979;12:5–17.
73. Krogh P, Azelsen NE, Elling F, et al. Experimental porcine nephropathy. Changes of renal function and structure induced by ochratoxin A-contaminated feed. *Acta Pathol Microbiol Scand Suppl* 1974;246:1–21.
74. Krogh P, Elling F, Friis C, et al. Porcine nephropathy induced by long-term ingestion of ochratoxin A. *A Vet Pathol* 1979;16:466–475.
75. Elling F, Moller T. Mycotoxic nephropathy in pigs. *Bull WHO* 1973;49:411–418.
76. Rutgvist I, Bjurklund NE, Hult K, Hukby E, Carlsson B. Ochratoxin A as the cause of spontaneous nephropathy in fattening pigs. *Appl Environ Microbiol* 1978;36:920–925.
77. Szczech GM, Carlton WW, Tuite J, Caldwell R. Ochratoxin A toxicosis in swine. *Vet Pathol* 1973;10:347–364.
78. Elling F, Nielsen JP, Lillehoj EB, Thomassen MS, Stormer FC. Ochratoxin A-induced porcine

nephropathy: enzyme and ultrastructure changes after short-term exposure. *Toxicon* 1985;23:247–254.

79. Krogh P, Elling F, Hald B, et al. Experimental avian nephropathy: changes of renal function and structure induced by ochratoxin A-contaminated feed. *Acta Pathol Microbiol Scand* 1976;A84: 429–434.
80. Svendsen C, Skadhauge E. Renal functions in hens fed graded dietary levels of ochratoxin A. *Acta Pharmacol Toxicol* 1976;38:186–194.
81. Delacruz L, Bach PH. The role of ochratoxin A metabolism and biochemistry in animal and human nephrotoxicity. *J Biopharmaceut Sci* 1990;1:278–304.
82. Lillehoj EB, Kwolek WF, Elling F, Krogh P. Tissue distribution of radioactivity from ochratoxin A-^{14}C in rats. *Mycopathologia* 1979;68:175–177.
83. Hansen CE, Dueland S, Drevon CA, Stormer FC. Metabolism of ochratoxin A by primary cultures of rat hepatocytes. *Appl Environ Microbiol* 1982;43:1267–1271.
84. Moore JH, Truelove B. Ochratoxin A: inhibition of mitochondrial respiration. *Science* 1970;168: 1102–1103.
85. Endou H, Obara T, Ueno Y. Use of isolated nephron segments and isolated renal cells for the evaluation of nephrotoxicity. In: Bach PH, Lock EA, eds. *Renal heterogenicity and target cell toxicity*. New York: John Wiley, 1984;535–538.
86. Jung KY, Endou H. Nephrotoxicity assessment by measuring cellular ATP content. II. Intranephron site of ochratoxin A nephrotoxicity. *Toxicol Appl Pharmacol* 1989;100:383–390.
87. Meisner H, Selanik S. Inhibition of renal gluconeogenesis in rats by ochratoxin. *Biochem J* 1979;180:681–684.
88. Meisner H, Meisner P. Ochratoxin A, an *in vivo* inhibition of renal phosphoenolpyruvate carboxykinase. *Arch Biochem Biophys* 1981;208:146–153.
89. Meisner H, Cimbala MA, Hanson RW. Decrease of renal phosphoenolpyruvate carboxykinase RNA and poly(A) RNA level by ochratoxin A. *Arch Biochem Biophys* 1983;223:264–270.
90. Creppy EE, Kane A, Dirheimer G, Lafarge-Frayssinet C, Mousset S, Frayssinet C. Genotoxicity of ochratoxin A in mice: DNA single-strand break evaluation in spleen, liver and kidney. *Toxicol Lett* 1985;28:29–35.
91. Kane A, Creppy EE, Roth A, Roschenthaler R, Dirheimer G. Distribution of [^{3}H]-label from low doses of radioactive ochratoxin A ingested by rats, and evidence for DNA single-strand breaks caused in liver and kidneys. *Arch Toxicol* 1986;58:219–244.
92. Petkova-Bocharova T, Chernozemsky IN, Castegnaro M. Ochratoxin A in human blood in relation to Balkan endemic nephropathy and urinary system tumors in Bulgaria. *Food Addit Contam* 1988; 5:299–301.
93. Hall PW III. Endemic Balkan nephropathy. In: Porter G, ed. *Nephrotoxic mechanisms and environmental toxins*. New York: Plenum Publishing, 1982;227–240.
94. Nichifor E, Balea M, Rusu G, et al. Studies on the familial character of endemic Balkan nephropathy. Possible role of the toxic hydric factor in the determination of "familial agglomerations" in endemic Balkan nephropathy. *Med Interne* 1985;23:229–237.
95. Radovanovic Z. Epidemiological evidence on Balkan nephropathy as a viral disease. *Med Hypotheses* 1987;22:171–175.
96. Draganescu N, Antipa C, Girjabu E, Melencu M. Endemic Balkan nephropathy, a slow virus disease? *Virologie* 1983;34:3–6.
97. Huff WE, Doerr JA. Synergism between aflatoxin and ochratoxin A in broiler chickens. *Poult Sci* 1981;60:550–555.
98. Rati ER, Basappa SC, Murthy V, Sreenivasa, Ramesh HP, Ramesh BS, Singh GB. The synergistic effect of aflatoxin B1 and ochratoxin A in rats. *J Food Sci Technol* 1981;18:176–179.
99. Huff WE, Kubena LF, Harvey RB, Doerr JA. Mycotoxin interactions in poultry and swine. *J Anim Sci* 1988;66:2351–2355.
100. Berndt WO. The nephrotoxicity of mycotoxins and botanicals. In: Bach PH, Bonner FW, Bridges JW, Lock EA, eds. *Nephrotoxicity, assessment and pathogenesis*. New York: John Wiley, 1982; 378–395.

Toxicology of the Kidney, Second Edition,
edited by Jerry B. Hook and Robin S. Goldstein.
Raven Press, Ltd., New York © 1993.

18

Male Rat–Specific Light Hydrocarbon Nephropathy

Lois D. Lehman-McKeeman

Human and Environmental Safety Division, Miami Valley Laboratories, Procter and Gamble Company, Cincinnati, Ohio 45239-8707

Light hydrocarbon nephropathy is a chemically induced toxicological syndrome that occurs exclusively in adult male rats. Currently, a diverse group of more than 20 chemicals has been reported to cause this unusual nephrotoxicity (Table 1). The acute histopathological hallmark of the toxicity is marked accumulation of protein (hyaline) droplets within the renal cortical proximal tubule cells, and consequently, the syndrome has also been referred to as hyaline droplet nephropathy. It is now well established that α_{2u}-globulin, a protein synthesized exclusively by adult male rats, is the only protein involved in the development of this chemically induced renal protein overload. It is also established that chemicals (or their metabolites) that produce this syndrome must first bind to α_{2u}-globulin to initiate biochemical changes leading to renal lysosomal protein overload. Chronic exposure to the chemicals producing this syndrome causes renal injury and compensatory renal cell proliferation, and results in a low, but significant incidence of renal tubular tumors, again limited to male rats. Whereas a significant research effort has been directed toward understanding the mechanisms by which hyaline droplet nephropathy occurs, the issue of male rat–specific renal carcinogens has received considerable attention from regulatory agencies. This chapter reviews the histopathological characteristics of the nephropathy, the biochemical mechanisms underlying its development, and the current thinking on the relevance of this unusual male rat–specific nephrotoxicity and nephrocarcinogenicity to human health.

α_{2u}-GLOBULIN

Because light hydrocarbon nephropathy begins as a renal tubular cell protein overload, initial studies to determine how chemicals could produce such an overload focused on identifying what protein(s) was(were) accumulating following chemical exposure. The separation power of two-dimensional gel electrophoresis

TABLE 1. *Chemicals reported to cause the male rat–specific hyaline droplet nephropathy*

Chemical	References
Decahydronapthalene (decalin)	1
Naphthas	2,3
2,4,4-Trimethylpentane	4
Tetralin	5
60 solvent, 70 solvent	3
C_{10}–C_{12} Isoparaffinic solvent	6
Stoddard solvent	3
Napthenic aromatic solvent	3
Diisobutyl ketone	7
Methylisobutyl ketone	8
Isopropylcyclohexane	9
BW540C, BW58C	10
Levamisole	10
3,5,5-Trimethylhexanoyl-oxybenzene sulfonate	11
Tridecyl acetate	12
Lindane	13
Chemicals also shown to be male rat–specific renal carcinogens	
d-Limonene	14,15
Unleaded gasoline	3,16
1,4-Dichlorobenzene	17,18
Isophorone	19
Perchloroethylene	20,21
Pentachloroethane	20,22
Jet fuels (JP-5, JP-4, JP-10, RJ-5)	23
Dimethylmethylphosphonate	24

Adapted from Flamm and Lehman-McKeeman, ref. 25.

was used to answer this pivotal question, and as indicated in Fig. 1, showed that only one protein had accumulated following chemical treatment. Subsequently, this protein was identified as α_{2u}-globulin (26).

The discovery of the involvement of α_{2u}-globulin in this lesion immediately put some perspective around the male rat specificity of light hydrocarbon nephropathy. α_{2u}-globulin, synthesized exclusively by adult male rats, is the most abundant protein in male rat urine (Table 2) (27). It is estimated that more than 15 mg of α_{2u}-globulin is excreted daily by adult male rats, accounting for 35% to 40% of the total urinary protein fraction (27,28). Despite its abundance in urine and its accumulation in the kidney, α_{2u}-globulin is not synthesized in renal parenchyma. Rather, the protein is synthesized almost exclusively in the liver, where it is rapidly secreted into the circulation. The molecular weight of α_{2u}-globulin is approximately 18,500 d (27), allowing it to be freely filtered across the glomerulus. Thus, the protein that accumulates in the kidney is that which has been filtered and reabsorbed into the organ.

In the liver, α_{2u}-globulin is encoded by a multigene family clustered on chromosome 5 (29,30). The expression of the α_{2u}-globulin gene family is regulated by a complex interaction of testosterone, glucocorticoids, insulin, growth hormone, and

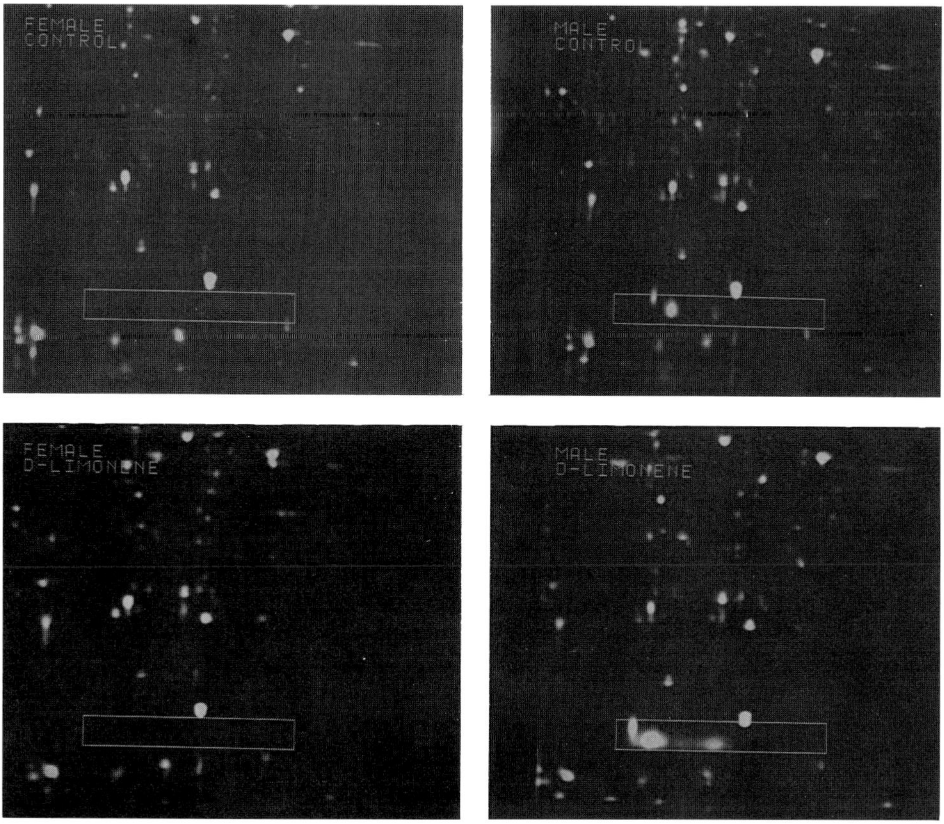

FIG. 1. Two-dimensional gel electrophoretic profiles of rat kidney proteins showing the presence of α_{2u}-globulin exclusively in male rat kidneys. α_{2u}-Globulin is outlined on the gels. In male rats treated with d-limonene (200 mg/kg) there is a marked accumulation of α_{2u}-globulin within 24 hr of receiving a single oral dosage. (Reproduced from Webb et al., ref. 14, with permission.)

TABLE 2. *Characteristics of α_{2u}-globulin*

Major urinary protein excreted by adult male rats
Molecular weight of approximately 18,500
Hormonal regulation of hepatic gene expression (testosterone, growth hormone, thyroid hormone, glucocorticoids, insulin)
Estrogen inhibits hepatic gene expression
Function is not known
Not synthesized by any other species

thyroid hormone (31–36). In a hormonally intact rat, the protein is considered to be fully induced (31). Furthermore, given its regulation by male sex hormones, α_{2u}-globulin is not synthesized until male rats reach puberty (37).

On the other hand, estrogen is a very effective repressor of α_{2u}-globulin synthesis (33,38). Consequently, although female rats have the entire complement of hepatic α_{2u}-globulin genes, no α_{2u}-globulin is synthesized in female rat liver. Female rats synthesize a small amount of α_{2u}-globulin in extrahepatic tissues and excrete a virtually nondetectable quantity in urine (39). The extrahepatic sites of α_{2u}-globulin synthesis include the salivary, lachrymal, preputial, meibomian, and perianal glands (41–42). This extrahepatic protein is electrophoretically distinct from the major urinary protein in male rats. The hormonal regulation of α_{2u}-globulin synthesis in each of these tissues is unique, and most notably, synthesis is not sex-specific in the lachrymal, salivary, and preputial glands (40,41).

The renal handling of α_{2u}-globulin is one of its most unusual features. Unlike most other proteins, α_{2u}-globulin is very poorly reabsorbed by the kidney, with only 60% of the filtered load being reabsorbed (43,44). This is in contrast to proteins such as albumin or lysozyme where renal reabsorption approaches 100% (45,46). It is estimated that male rats synthesize a total of 50 mg of α_{2u}-globulin daily (27,43,44). Thus, the 15 to 20 mg of this protein that is excreted daily, representing that which is filtered but not reabsorbed, accounts for nearly 40% of the total amount synthesized per day.

Although male rats dedicate significant energy to the synthesis of α_{2u}-globulin, the function of this abundant protein remains unknown. Recent work with structurally similar proteins has suggested that the tertiary structure of α_{2u}-globulin features a hydrophobic pocket that may serve to bind endogenous ligands (47–49). In this regard, the specific localization of α_{2u}-globulin and its mRNA in pheromone-producing sebaceous glands (preputial, meibomian, and perianal glands) may be suggestive of a pheromone-carrying function for the protein (42). The transport of a pheromone might also explain why so much of this protein is wasted into the urine. To date, however, no endogenous ligand for α_{2u}-globulin has been identified. Other functions ascribed to α_{2u}-globulin include potential roles as a renal fatty-acid binding protein (50) or as an important physiological modulator in spermatogenesis (51).

HISTOPATHOLOGICAL CHARACTERIZATION OF LIGHT HYDROCARBON NEPHROPATHY

The abundance of α_{2u}-globulin in the glomerular filtrate accounts for sex-related differences in the ultrastructural features of rat proximal convoluted tubules. The most notable distinction is the larger size and abundance of phagolysosomes (hyaline droplets) in the P_2 segment of the proximal tubule in male rats (52,53). Light microscopically, hyaline droplets can be visualized with Mallory-Heidenhain staining (26), as shown in Fig. 2. Other stains, including Lee's methylene blue basic

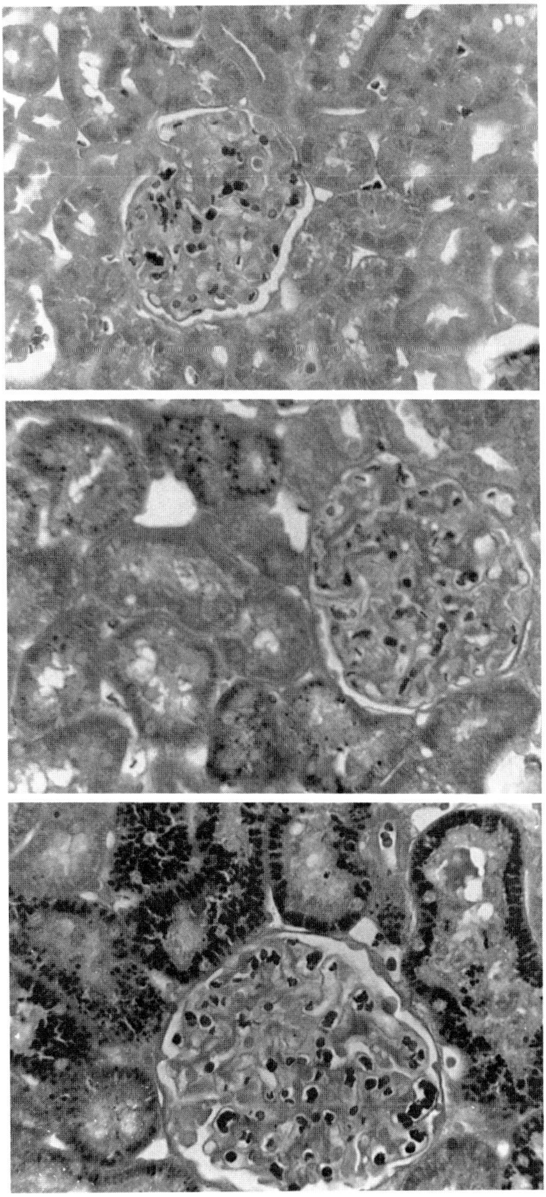

FIG. 2. Histopathological characterization of the spontaneous and exacerbated formation of hyaline droplets in male rat kidneys (×320). When stained with Mallory-Heidenhain stain, female rats do not show these droplets (*top panel*), whereas the spontaneous formation of the droplets in male rat kidneys (*middle panel*) is obvious. A single oral dosage of d-limonene (150 mg/kg) produced a dramatic increase in the number of and size of the hyaline droplets 24 hr after dosing (*bottom panel*).

fuchsin, have also been used to evaluate the droplets (4). As depicted in Fig. 2, the acute, pathognomonic feature of light hydrocarbon nephropathy is exacerbated accumulation and size of hyaline droplets in male rat kidneys. At the ultrastructural level, it has been shown that the droplets represent lysosomes that are so engorged with protein that, in fixed tissue, they appear polyangular and contain crystalloid material (54,55). Whereas exacerbated hyaline droplet accumulation is evident within 24 hr following a single exposure to any of the chemicals listed in Table 1, repeated exposure (3 to 4 weeks) produces progressive renal injury characterized by renal proximal tubular cell degeneration and necrosis. These dead cells are sloughed into the lumen of the nephron and contribute to the formation of granular casts at the corticomedullary junction. Finally, papillary mineralization is noted and there is an accelerated onset of cortical changes typical of chronic progressive nephrosis which is commonly seen in aging male rats (4,26). It must be emphasized that these renal changes are not seen in female rats, nor has renal toxicity been observed in other species including mice (15,18,19,21,22,24) and dogs (56).

No studies have been conducted to specifically follow the histopathological progression from accelerated chronic progressive nephrosis to renal tubular tumor formation. With the onset of cell death, there is a compensatory increase in renal cell proliferation (4,57), and for several chemicals this cell proliferation, detected as renal tubular cell hyperplasia, appears to be sustained throughout a 2-year exposure regimen (15). Therefore, it is generally considered that the renal tumors ultimately seen following chronic chemical treatment, represent a histopathological continuum that begins as hyaline droplet exacerbation and progresses to hyperplasia and tumorigenesis.

BIOCHEMICAL MECHANISMS OF LIGHT HYDROCARBON NEPHROPATHY

Research conducted in several laboratories has indicated that the essential prerequisite for the development of light hydrocarbon nephropathy is an interaction between the chemical (or metabolites) and α_{2u}-globulin (11,58–60). To characterize this binding, equilibrium dialysis of kidney cytosol has been performed. As presented in Fig. 3, when cytosol from d-limonene–treated rats was dialyzed against neutral Tris buffer, approximately 40% of the d-limonene equivalents in male rat kidney remained bound to renal proteins. In contrast, virtually no binding was seen in female rat kidney. Sequential dialysis against an SDS-containing buffer eliminated the protein binding in the male rat kidney cytosol, thereby indicating that the interaction with protein was reversible in nature. Additional analyses in which α_{2u}-globulin is resolved from all other renal proteins has shown that the xenobiotic-protein interaction is indeed specific for α_{2u}-globulin (11,59). Finally, *in vitro* equilibrium saturation binding studies have indicated that the dissociation constant of the xenobiotic-α_{2u}-globulin interaction is approximately 10^{-7} M (61).

Whereas the biochemical experiments described above have been conducted for

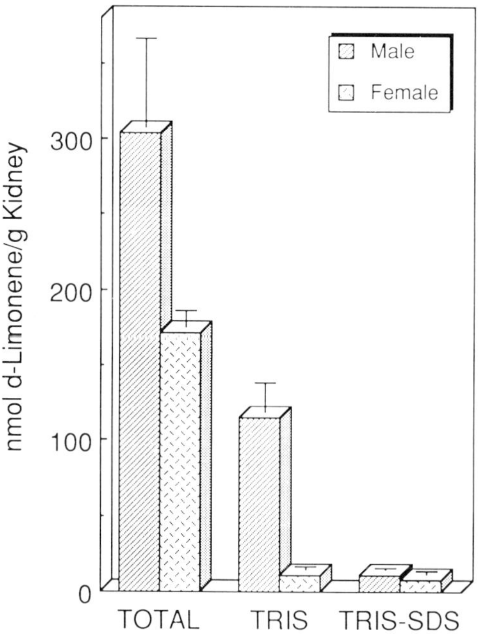

FIG. 3. Equilibrium dialysis of rat kidney cytosol from d-limonene–treated male and female rats. The total d-limonene concentration in the male rat kidney was significantly higher than in the female rat kidney. Cytosols were dialyzed for 24 hr against the respective buffer. Results (mean ± SE of four rats) are expressed as the amount of d-limonene–derived radioactivity retained in the dialysis bag at the end of the 24-hr period. (Adapted from Lehman-McKeeman et al., ref. 59)

only five of the chemicals listed in Table 1, the results have consistently shown that approximately 20% to 40% of the chemical present in male rat kidney is reversibly bound to α_{2u}-globulin. Moreover, it appears that this binding contributes to the selective retention of the compound in the male rat kidney. For example, as noted in Fig. 3, the total d-limonene equivalents in male rat kidney was approximately two times higher than the concentration in female rat kidney. For some chemicals, the sex-dependent retention of chemical in male rat kidney is as much as ten times higher than the female rat (11).

For d-limonene, 2,4,4-trimethylpentane (TMP), 1,4-dichlorobenzene, isophorone, and 3,5,5-trimethylhexanoyloxybenzene sulfonate (THBS) experiments have also been conducted to identify the moieties that are bound to α_{2u}-globulin. These experiments have demonstrated that the chemicals that bind to α_{2u}-globulin are structurally diverse (Fig. 4), as they include d-limonene and *cis*-d-limonene-1,2-oxide (59), 2,4,4-trimethyl-2-pentanol (58), 1,4-dichlorobenzene and 2,5-dichlorophenol (60), isophorone (62), and the γ-lactone of 3,5,5-trimethylhexanoic acid (11), for d-limonene, TMP, 1,4-dichlorobenzene, isophorone, and THBS, respectively. It is particularly interesting to note that d-limonene-1,2-oxide, an epoxide intermediate, will bind reversibly to α_{2u}-globulin. It must also be noted, however, that in all cases, the amount of xenobiotic that binds to α_{2u}-globulin is actually quite small relative to the dosage administered to the rat. For example, with d-limonene, the epoxide bound to α_{2u}-globulin represents less than 0.04% of the dosed chemical (59).

Although it is quite clear that α_{2u}-globulin binds these chemicals, the nature of the protein binding site and the orientation of the chemical in that binding site are not known. Given that d-limonene-1,2-oxide binds reversibly to α_{2u}-globulin, it has been assumed that the epoxide moiety does not participate directly in the binding, thereby suggesting that the binding occurs on the more hydrophobic portion of the molecule (59). Likewise, the chemicals shown in Fig. 4 have distinct hydrophobic domains, and it is likely that the hydrophobicity of the chemical is important for binding (61).

It is also not known where in the body the interaction between the xenobiotic and α_{2u}-globulin takes place. However, because the xenobiotic-protein complex appears to be localized to the renal lysosomal compartment, it is reasonable to assume that the complex does not form in the kidney, but rather, the complex may form in the liver or in the circulation. Based on this assumption, following glomerular filtration, the chemical-protein complex would enter the tubular cell by endocytosis, the endosome would fuse with a primary lysosome, and the complex would remain in the lysosome until degraded.

The principal biological consequence of the binding of xenobiotics to α_{2u}-globulin is a reduction in the rate of the lysosomal degradation of the protein (Table 3). In *in vitro* experiments, with renal cortical lysosomes from untreated male rats as the enzyme source, the binding of d-limonene-1,2-oxide, 2,5-dichlorophenol, and isophorone to α_{2u}-globulin decreased the *in vitro* degradation of the protein by renal lysosomal cathepsins by approximately 30% (63). This change in lysosomal degradation of proteins such as albumin is not affected by the presence of any one of these chemicals (63). Moreover, there is no generalized reduction in lysosomal cathepsin activity in association with the nephropathy as evidenced by the fact that no other protein accumulates in the kidney. Additionally, lysosomal cathepsin activity actually increases following exposure to unleaded gasoline (64), whereas d-limonene treatment has no effect on lysosomal cathepsin levels (65).

The renal half-life of native α_{2u}-globulin is reported to be 5 to 6 hr (63,66). When a xenobiotic is bound to α_{2u}-globulin, its renal half-life increases to about 10 hr (63). Therefore, the exacerbated accumulation of α_{2u}-globulin–containing hyaline droplets results from the xenobiotic-induced reduction in lysosomal degradation of the protein.

Given the biochemical mechanism underlying the development of hyaline droplet nephropathy, the male rat specificity of this toxicity is attributed to the fact that only male rats synthesize large quantities of α_{2u}-globulin. No nephrotoxicity is seen in female rats where α_{2u}-globulin is synthesized in very small quantities. If, however, female rats are injected with α_{2u}-globulin prior to treatment with a hyaline droplet–inducing agent, α_{2u}-globulin will accumulate and the ensuing nephropathy will be

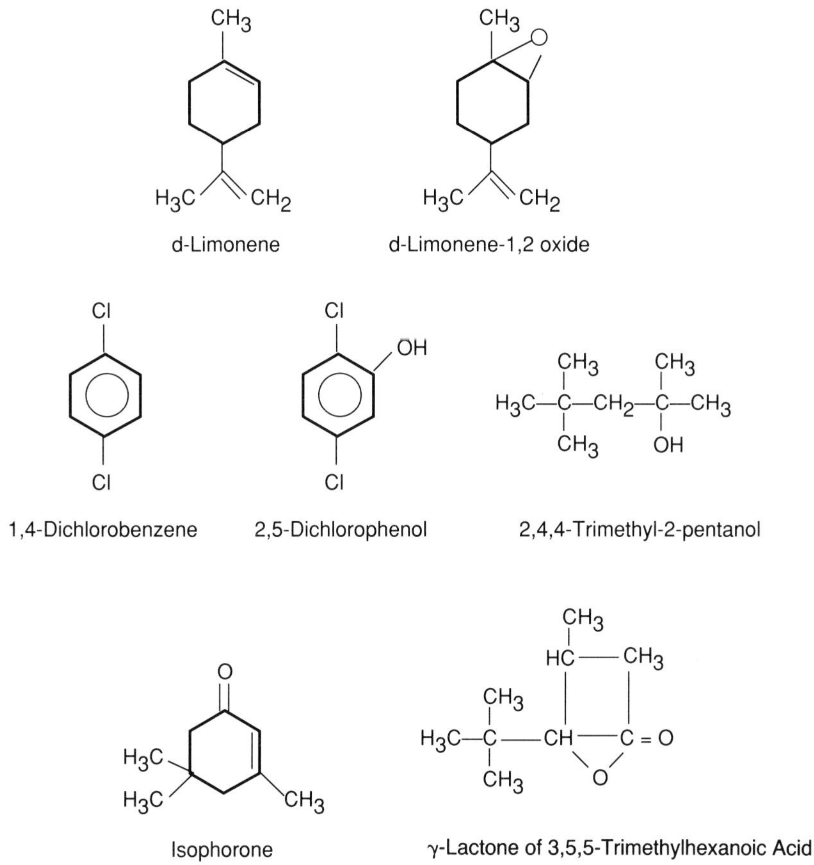

FIG. 4. The five chemicals (or chemical metabolites) that have been identified to bind to α_{2u}-globulin.

TABLE 3. *Lysosomal degradation of [^{14}C] α_{2u}-globulin–xenobiotic conjugates*

Conjugate	% Degraded
Control	29.4 ± 2.6
d-Limonene-1,2-oxide	20.6 ± 1.0
Isophorone	22.4 ± 1.5
2,5-Dichlorophenol	19.6 ± 0.8

Adapted from Lehman-McKeeman et al., ref. 63.

observed (67). In addition, the acute nephropathy cannot be produced in 2-year-old male rats (68) because the levels of α_{2u}-globulin decline dramatically in senescent rats (69–71). Furthermore, it has recently been demonstrated that the NIH black rat, an unusual strain in which adult males do not synthesize α_{2u}-globulin because of a gene-specific regulatory defect (72), does not show spontaneous hyaline droplet accumulation or chemically induced hyaline droplet nephropathy (13,67).

Whereas the biochemical mechanisms underlying the development of the acute changes seen in light hydrocarbon nephropathy have been well characterized, the cellular and biochemical sequelae that lead to the subchronic changes seen in male rat kidneys are poorly understood. It has been suggested by several investigators that lysosomal overload featuring engorged, enlarged, polyangular lysosomes results in lysosomal rupture and cell death (61,73). However, there are currently no data to support this hypothesis. In fact, it has been shown that cells containing these enlarged lysosomes appear otherwise perfectly normal (55). Furthermore, whereas exacerbated hyaline droplet nephropathy is observed in entire cross sections of tubules (as shown in Fig. 2), the cytotoxicity seen histopathologically is confined to single cell necrosis (4). Clearly, more research in this area is required to define how this protein overload can lead to cell death.

LIGHT HYDROCARBON NEPHROPATHY AND NEPHROCARCINOGENICITY

Renal tubular tumors are generally regarded as uncommon lesions in rats, occurring spontaneously at incidences of 0.35% and 0.17% for male and female Fischer 344 rats, respectively (74). To date, only eight of the chemicals listed in Table 1 have been tested in 2-year bioassays. Each of these chemicals has produced renal tubular tumors exclusively in male rats. Collectively, the overall incidence of renal cell tumors (not adjusted for mortality) does not exceed 25%. Therefore, the chemicals in this class can be distinguished from classical renal carcinogens such as dimethylnitrosamine or other substituted nitrosamines where the renal tumor incidence approaches 100% (75). Moreover, the tumors associated with hyaline droplet nephropathy appear to have a long latency period, as they are typically not seen until after at least 18 months of continued dosing. Finally, the male rat–specific renal carcinogens, unlike classic renal carcinogens, are not highly mutagenic as a class. In general, hyaline droplet–inducing agents are not mutagenic in *Salmonella* (with or without metabolic activation) or mouse lymphoma cells, and are not clastogenic in Chinese hamster ovary (CHO) cells (15,18,19,21,22,24).

The identification of a potentially reactive epoxide intermediate of d-limonene that binds to α_{2u}-globulin might raise some concern that this epoxide is directly involved in the carcinogenicity of d-limonene. However, this epoxide is an unusually stable one. Moreover, d-limonene-1,2-oxide has also tested negative for mutagenicity in several strains of *Salmonella* (76–78); it did not induce sister chromatid exchange in V79 cells, and it caused no unscheduled DNA synthesis in rat hepatocytes (79).

The overall lack of genotoxicity for chemicals causing male rat–specific renal tumors supports the concept that nongenotoxic mechanisms are integrally involved in the carcinogenic response. In this regard, it has been suggested that increased renal cell proliferation may be responsible for the low incidence of renal tumors seen with exposure to these chemicals. Specifically, it has been argued that persistent elevations in renal cell proliferation may facilitate fixation of spontaneously altered DNA or may serve to promote spontaneously initiated cells (57,61,73).

To test this hypothesis, studies to evaluate renal cell proliferation resulting from subchronic or chronic hyaline droplet nephropathy have been conducted. Data showing increased cell proliferation in male rat kidneys, but not in female rat kidneys, are consistent with the cell proliferation hypothesis (4,57,80). Furthermore, an initiation-promotion study conducted with ethyl-hydroxy-ethylnitrosamine (EHEN) as the initiator and unleaded gasoline as the promoter, showed a significant linear trend in the incidence of renal cell tumors in male rats treated with increasing dosages of unleaded gasoline for 24 weeks (80).

There are, however, inconsistencies in the cell proliferation concept that must be resolved before it can be totally accepted. For example, in the initiation-promotion study discussed above, there was an increased renal tumor incidence in rats treated with unleaded gasoline for 24 weeks, but this increase was not observed in rats treated for 59 weeks (80). Moreover, renal cell proliferation rates, determined with up to 1 year of treatment, remain higher than control values but decline over time (57,73). It has been argued that the decline in cell proliferation correlated with the age-dependent decline in α_{2u}-globulin synthesis. However, as presented by Short et al. (57), the amount of α_{2u}-globulin in kidney (evaluated immunohistochemically) remained constant from 3 to 48 weeks of treatment, whereas cell proliferation declined by as much as 50% over the same time interval. The inconsistencies in the cell proliferation data suggest that, whereas cell proliferation may play a pivotal role in the nephrocarcinogenicity of hyaline droplet–inducing agents, other (as yet unidentified) factors might also be involved in the carcinogenic response.

HUMAN RELEVANCE OF LIGHT HYDROCARBON NEPHROPATHY

Given that α_{2u}-globulin is essential to the development of this male rat–specific nephrotoxicity, and that the protein is synthesized exclusively by adult male rats, it seems reasonable to conclude that light hydrocarbon nephropathy is unique to the male rat. However, there is a group of proteins that is similar to α_{2u}-globulin in both primary sequence homology and tertiary structure, and that is synthesized by many species, including humans. The proteins, classified as an α_{2u}-globulin superfamily (81), are listed in Table 4. As mentioned earlier, many of the proteins in this superfamily serve to bind and transport endogenous ligands (47,48). For several of these proteins, the three-dimensional structure has been deduced from x-ray crystallographic studies (91,96–98). The results of this work have revealed that all these proteins have a very unusual structure featuring a β-barrel core (a hydrophobic pocket) into which ligands are bound (49,99). For proteins like odorant-binding

TABLE 4. *Members of the $\alpha_{2\mu}$-globulin superfamily*

Protein	Species	Ligand	References
α_{2u}-Globulin	Rat	Unknown	42
Mouse urinary protein	Mouse	Unidentified	82
Retinol-binding protein	Mammals	Retinol	83
α_1-Acid glycoprotein	Mammals	Drugs, steroids	84,85
Odorant-binding protein	Mammals	Odorants	86
Apolipoprotein D	Human	Cholesterol	87
Protein HC	Human	Unidentified	88
Pregnancy-associated endometrial α_2-globulin	Human	Unknown	89
Protein 1	Human	Unknown	90
β-Lactoglobulin	Cow	Retinol, alkanes	91,92
Androgen-dependent secretory protein	Rat	Unknown	93
Aphrodisin	Hamster	Unknown	94
Purpurin	Chicken	Retinol, heparin	95
Insecticyanin	Insects	Biliverdin IX	96,97

protein (47), α_1-acid glycoprotein (84,85), and retinol-binding protein (100), a variety of ligands have been identified. In contrast, although it is clear that α_{2u}-globulin will bind a variety of exogenously administered chemicals, no endogenous ligand has been identified for this protein.

The superfamily protein that is most similar to α_{2u}-globulin is mouse urinary protein (MUP). This protein, which shares approximately a 90% sequence homology with α_{2u}-globulin, is essentially the mouse equivalent of α_{2u}-globulin (82, 101). MUP is the major urinary protein excreted by mice (102–104), as adult male mice excrete nearly 15 mg of MUP daily (105). Like α_{2u}-globulin, its synthesis is hormonally regulated (106), but unlike α_{2u}-globulin, female mice synthesize and excrete MUP, albeit at levels that are five to ten times lower than those observed for male mice (102,105). If the presence of a member of this protein superfamily represents a risk factor for other species to develop a protein overload nephropathy, mice should represent the species most likely to develop this unusual toxicity. However, studies conducted in mice indicate that no renal changes are observed following exposure to hyaline droplet inducing agents. In fact, for d-limonene (105) and THBS (11), the complete lack of any *in vivo* interaction between these chemicals and MUP has been demonstrated. These results suggest that similarity in protein structure is not a sufficient criterion by which to evaluate species predilection to develop light hydrocarbon nephropathy.

The presence of endogenous ligands for structurally similar proteins may play a very important role in preventing other proteins from causing this toxicity. For example, the dissociation constants of the endogenous ligand-protein complexes are similar to that for α_{2u}-globulin–xenobiotic conjugates, in the 10^{-7} M range (91, 107). Given this affinity, an exogenously administered hyaline droplet inducer would have to be present in very high concentrations in order to displace the endogenous ligand from the protein. However, as noted earlier, the hyaline droplet–inducing moieties tend to be very minor metabolites (59). In this regard, a putative ligand for MUP has been isolated (Lehman-McKeeman and Rodriguez, unpublished observation). Although the identity of it has yet to be established, it seems likely that this ligand also blocks binding of hyaline droplet–inducing agents to MUP.

Finally, it should be noted that, with the resolving power of two-dimensional gel electrophoresis, the potential for proteins in the α_{2u}-globulin superfamily to contribute to hyaline droplet nephropathy has been evaluated. Specifically, several of these proteins (like retinol-binding protein and α_1-acid glycoprotein) are present in both male and female rats. However, these structurally similar proteins do not accumulate in kidneys of either male or female rats, again suggesting that this toxicity is specific for male rats because of unique properties of α_{2u}-globulin.

CONCLUSION

Over the past 10 years, hyaline droplet nephropathy has emerged as an important xenobiotic-induced nephrotoxicity that has received considerable attention in the toxicology community. As more and more research is done in this area, it is obvious that this toxicity is not limited to light hydrocarbons. Rather a diverse (and ever-increasing) group of chemicals can produce this toxicity. This issue, however, is also extremely significant in regulatory arenas, where there has been considerable discussion regarding how to evaluate the human risk associated with this class of chemicals (25). The biochemical mechanisms underlying the development of this male rat–specific nephrotoxicity are well defined, and criteria describing the critical events progressing from hyaline droplet to tumor can be established (Table 5). Therefore, this issue presents the opportunity to incorporate mechanistic data into the risk assessment process. Although there are some data gaps as noted throughout this chapter, the fact remains that, without α_{2u}-globulin, there is no risk of protein overload nephrotoxicity. Thus, it is reasonable to conclude that this toxicity is unique to male rats because of the unusual properties of α_{2u}-globulin and consequently, this toxicity is unlikely to occur in other species including humans.

TABLE 5. *Criteria describing xenobiotic-induced hyaline droplet nephropathy and male rat–specific renal carcinogenicity*

Exacerbated hyaline droplet accumulation in renal proximal tubule epithelial cells of male rats
Hyaline droplets contain α_{2u}-globulin
The xenobiotic binds reversibly to α_{2u}-globulin in kidney
The xenobiotic or its metabolites are not genotoxic
Increased renal cell proliferation and hyperplasia
Renal tubular tumors are seen exclusively in male rats

Adapted from Flamm and Lehman-McKeeman, ref. 25.

ACKNOWLEDGMENTS

The author gratefully acknowledges the outstanding technical support provided by Mr. Douglas Caudill, Ms. Judy Young, Ms. Cindy Eddy, and Ms. Monica Fey in completing experiments referred to in this chapter. I am also indebted to Drs. Pedro "Pete" Rodriguez and George Daston for both their friendship and their critical evaluation of the research efforts ongoing in my laboratory.

REFERENCES

1. Kanerva RL, McCracken MS, Alden CL, Stone LC. Morphogenesis of decalin-induced renal alterations in the male rat. *Food Chem Toxicol* 1987;25:53–61.
2. Halder CA, Warne TM, Hatoum NS. Renal toxicity of gasoline and related petroleum naphthas in male rats. In: Mehlman MR, Hemstreet CP, Thorpe JJ, Weaver NK, eds. *Renal effects of petroleum hydrocarbons. Advances in modern environmental toxicology*, vol VII. Princeton, NJ: Princeton Science Publishers, 1984;73–88.
3. Phillips RD, Cockrell BY. Effect of certain light hydrocarbons on kidney function and structure in male rats. In: Mehlman MA, Hemstreet CP, Thorpe JJ, Weaver NK, eds. *Renal effects of petroleum hydrocarbons. Advances in modern environmental toxicology*, vol VII. Princeton, NJ: Princeton Science Publishers, 1984;89–105.
4. Short BG, Burnett VL, Cox MG, Bus JS, Swenberg JA. Site-specific renal cytotoxicity and cell proliferation in male rats exposed to petroleum hydrocarbons. *Lab Invest* 1987;57:564–577.
5. Servé MP, Llewelyn BM, Yu KO, McDonald GM, Olson CT, Hobson DW. Metabolism and nephrotoxicity of tetralin in male Fischer 344 rats. *J Toxicol Environ Health* 1989;26:267–275.
6. Viau C, Bernard A, Gueret F, Maldague P, Gengoux P, Lauwerys R. Isoparaffinic solvent-induced nephrotoxicity in the rat. *Toxicology* 1986;38:227–240.
7. Dodd DE, Losco PE, Troup CM, Pritts IM, Tyler TR. Hyalin droplet nephrosis in male Fischer 344 rats following inhalation of diisobutyl ketone. *Toxicol Ind Health* 1987;3:443–457.
8. Phillips RD, Moran EJ, Dodd DE, Fowler EH, Kary CD, O'Donoghue J. A 14-week vapor inhalation toxicity study of methyl isobutyl ketone. *Fundam Appl Toxicol* 1987;9:380–388.
9. Henningsen GM, Salomon RA, Yu KO, Lopez I, Roberts J, Servé MP. Metabolism of nephrotoxic isopropylcyclohexane in male Fischer 344 rats. *J Toxicol Environ Hlth* 1988;24:19–25.
10. Read NG, Astbury PJ, Morgan RJI, Parsons DN, Port CJ. Induction and exacerbation of hyaline droplet formation in the proximal tubular cells of the kidneys from male rats receiving a variety of pharmacological agents. *Toxicology* 1988;52:81–101.
11. Lehman-McKeeman LD, Rodriguez PA, Caudill D, Fey ML, Eddy CL, Asquith TN. Hyaline droplet nephropathy resulting from exposure to 3,5,5-trimethylhexanoyloxybenzene sulfonate. *Toxicol Appl Pharmacol* 1991;107:429–438.
12. Daugherty WC, Smith JH, Hinz JP, Biles RW. Subchronic toxicity evaluation of tridecyl acetate in rats. *Fundam Appl Toxicol* 1990;14:104–112.
13. Dietrich DR, Swenberg JA. Lindane induces nephropathy and renal accumulation of α_{2u}-globulin in male but not in female Fischer 344 rats or male NBR rats. *Toxicol Lett* 1990;53:179–181.
14. Webb DR, Ridder GM, Alden CL. Acute and subchronic nephrotoxicity of d-limonene in Fischer 344 rats. *Food Chem Toxicol* 1989;27:639–649.
15. National Toxicology Program. Toxicology and carcinogenesis studies of d-limonene in F344/N rats and B6C3F1 Mice (gavage studies). *NTP Technical Report 347*. Washington, DC: U.S. Dept. Health & Human Services, Public Health Service, NIH, 1990.
16. Kitchen DN. Neoplastic renal effects of unleaded gasoline in Fischer 344 rats. In: Mehlman MA, Hemstreet CP, Thorpe JJ, Weaver NK, eds. *Renal effects of petroleum hydrocarbons. Advances in modern environmental toxicology*, vol VII. Princeton, NJ: Princeton Scientific Publishers, 1984; 65–71.
17. Bomhard E, Luckhaus G, Voight WH, Loeser E. Induction of light hydrocarbon nephropathy by p-dichlorobenzene. *Arch Toxicol* 1988;61:433–449.
18. National Toxicology Program. Toxicology and carcinogenesis studies of 1,4-dichlorobenzene in

F344/N rats and B6C3F1 mice. *NTP Technical Report 319*. Washington, DC: U.S. Dept. Health & Human Services, Public Health Service, NIH, 1987.

19. National Toxicology Program. Toxicology and carcinogenesis studies of isophorone in F344/N rats and B6C3F1 mice (gavage study). *NTP Technical Report No. 291*. Research Triangle Park, NC: National Toxicology Program, 1986.
20. Goldsworthy TL, Lyght O, Burnett VL, Popp JA. Potential role of α_{2u}-globulin, protein droplet accumulation, and cell replication in the renal carcinogenicity of rats exposed to trichloroethylene, perchloroethylene and pentachloroethane. *Toxicol Appl Pharmacol* 1988;96:367–379.
21. National Toxicology Program. Carcinogenesis bioassay of tetrachloroethylene (perchloroethylene) in F-344/N rats and B6C3F1 mice (inhalation study). *NTP Technical Report 311*. Washington, DC: U.S. Dept. Health & Human Services, Public Health Service, NIH, 1986.
22. National Toxicology Program. Carcinogenesis bioassay of pentachloroethane in F-344/N rats and B6C3F1 mice (gavage study). *NTP Technical Report 232*. Washington, DC: U.S. Dept. Health & Human Services, Public Health Service, NIH, 1983.
23. Bruner RH. Pathologic findings in laboratory animals exposed to hydrocarbon fuels of military interest. In: Mehlman MA, Hemstreet III CP, Thorpe JJ, Weaver NK, eds. *Renal effects of petroleum hydrocarbons. Advances in modern environmental toxicology*, vol VII. Princeton, NJ: Princeton Scientific Publishers, 1984;133–140.
24. National Toxicology Program. Carcinogenesis studies of dimethylmethylphosphonate in F-344/N rats and B6C3F1 mice (gavage study). *NTP Technical Report 323*. Washington, DC: U.S. Dept. Health & Human Services, Public Health Service, NIH, 1987.
25. Flamm WG, Lehman-McKeeman LD. The human relevance of the renal tumor-inducing potential of d-limonene in male rats. Implications for risk assessment. *Reg Toxicol Pharmacol* 1991;13: 70–86.
26. Alden CL, Kanerva RL, Ridder G, Stone LC. The pathogenesis of the nephrotoxicity of volatile hydrocarbons in the male rat. In: Mehlman MA, Hemstreet III CP, Thorpe JJ, Weaver NK, eds. *Renal effects of petroleum hydrocarbons. Advances in modern environmental toxicology*, vol VII. Princeton, NJ: Princeton Scientific Publishers 1984;107–120.
27. Roy AK, Neuhaus OW, Harmison HR. Preparation and characterization of a sex-dependent rat urinary protein. *Biochim Biophys Acta* 1966;127:72–81.
28. Lehman-McKeeman LD, Caudill D. Quantitation of α_{2u}-globulin and albumin by reverse-phase high performance liquid chromatography. *J Pharmacol Methods* 1991;26:239–247.
29. Kurtz DT. Rat α_{2u}-globulin is encoded by a multigene family. *J Mol Appl Gen* 1981;1:29–38.
30. Roy AK, Neuhaus OW. Proof of the hepatic synthesis of a sex-dependent protein in the rat. *Biochim Biophys Acta* 1966;127:82–87.
31. Kurtz DT, Feigelson P. Multihormonal control of the messenger RNA for the hepatic protein α_{2u}-globulin. In: Litwack G, ed. *Biochemical action of hormones*, vol V. New York: Academic Press, 1978.
32. Kurtz DT, Sippel AE, Feigelson P. Effect of thyroid hormones on the level of the hepatic mRNA for α_{2u}-globulin. *Biochemistry* 1976;15:1031–1036.
33. Kurtz DT, Sippel AE, Ansah-Yiadom R, Feigelson P. Effects of sex hormones on the level of messenger RNA for the rat hepatic protein α_{2u}-globulin. *J Biol Chem* 1976;251:3594–3598.
34. Kurtz DT, Chan KM, Fiegelson P. Translational control of hepatic α_{2u}-globulin synthesis by growth hormone. *Cell* 1978;15:743–750.
35. Roy AK, Chatterjee B, Prasad MSK, Unakar N. Role of insulin in the regulation of the hepatic messenger RNA for α_{2u}-globulin in diabetic rats. *J Biol Chem* 1980;255:11614–11618.
36. Kurtz DT, Chan KM, Fiegelson P. Glucocorticoid induction of hepatic α_{2u}-globulin synthesis and messenger RNA level in castrated male rats in vivo. *J Biol Chem* 1978;253:7886–7890.
37. Roy AK. Androgenic induction of α_{2u}-globulin in rats: androgen insensitivity in prepubital animals. *Endocrinology* 1973;92:957–960.
38. Roy AK, McMinn DM, Biswas NM. Estrogenic inhibition of the hepatic synthesis of α_{2u}-globulin in the rat. *Endocrinology* 1975;97:1501–1508.
39. Vandoren G, Mertens B, Heyns W, Van Baelen H, Rombauts W, Verhoeven G. Different forms of α_{2u}-globulin in male and female rat urine. *Eur J Biochem* 1983;134:175–181.
40. MacInnes JI, Nozik ES, Kurtz DT. Tissue-specific expression of the rat alpha α_{2u}-globulin gene family. *Mol Cell Biol* 1986;6:3563–3567.
41. Murty CVR, Sarkar FH, Mancini MA, Roy AK. Sex-independent synthesis of α_{2u}-globulin and its messenger riboneucleic acid in the rat preputial gland: biochemical and immunocytochemical analyses. *Endocrinology* 1987;121:1000–1005.

42. Mancini MA, Majumdar D, Chatterjee B, Roy AK. α_{2u}-globulin in modified sebaceous glands with pheromonal functions: localization of the protein and its mRNA in preputial, meibomian and perianal glands. *J Histochem Cytochem* 1989;37:149–157.
43. Neuhaus O, Flory W, Biswas N, Hollerman CE. Urinary excretion of α_{2u}-globulin by adult male rats following treatment with nephrotoxic agents. *Nephron* 1981;28:133–140.
44. Caudill D, Asquith TN, Lehman-McKeeman LD. Biochemical differences between α_{2u}-globulin (α_{2u}) and mouse urinary protein (MUP): explanation of murine resistance to develop hyaline droplet nephropathy (HDN). *Toxicologist* 1991;11:137(abstract).
45. Neuhaus OW. Renal reabsorption of low molecular weight proteins in adult male rats: α_{2u}-globulin. *Proc Soc Exp Biol Med* 1986;182:531–539.
46. Maack T, Johnson V, Kau ST, Figueiredo J, Sigulem D. Renal filtration, transport and metabolism of low-molecular-weight proteins: a review. *Kidney Int* 1979;16:251–270.
47. Snyder SH, Sklar PB, Pevsner J. Molecular mechanisms of olfaction. *J Biol Chem* 1988;263: 13971–13974.
48. Pevsner J, Reed RR, Feinstein PG, Snyder SH. Molecular cloning of odorant-binding protein: member of a ligand carrier family. *Science* 1988;241:336–339.
49. Godovac-Zimmerman J. The structural motif of β-lactoglobulin and retinol-binding protein: a basic framework for binding and transport of small hydrophobic molecules? *Trends Biochem Sci* 1988; 13:64–66.
50. Kimura H, Odani S, Suzuki JI, Arakawa M, Ono T. Kidney fatty acid-binding protein: identification as α_{2u}-globulin. *FEBS Lett* 1989;246:101–104.
51. Roy AK, Byrd JG, Biswas NM, Chowdhury AK. Protection of spermatogenesis by α_{2u}-globulin in rats treated with oestrogen. *Nature* 1976;260:719–721.
52. Maunsbach AB. Electron microscopic observations of cytoplasmic bodies with cystalline patterns in rat kidney proximal tubule cells. *J Ultrastruct Res* 1966;14:167–196.
53. Kretchmer N, Bernstein J. The dynamic morphology of the nephron: morphogenesis of the "protein droplet." *Kidney Int* 1974;5:96–105.
54. Stone LC, Kanerva RL, Burns JM, Alden CL. Decalin-induced nephrotoxicity: light and electron microscopic examination of the effects of oral dosing on the development of kidney lesions in the rat. *Food Chem Toxic* 1987;25:43–52.
55. Garg BD, Olson MJ, Li LC, Roy AK. Phagolysosomal alterations induced by unleaded gasoline in epithelial cells of the proximal convoluted tubules of male rats: effect of dose and treatment duration. *J Toxicol Environ Health* 1989;26:101–118.
56. Webb DR, Kanerva RL, Hysell DK, Alden CL, Lehman-McKeeman LD. Assessment of the subchronic oral toxicity of d-limonene in dogs. *Food Chem Toxicol* 1990;28:669–675.
57. Short BG, Burnett VL, Swenberg JA. Elevated proliferation of proximal tubule cells and localization of accumulated α_{2u}-globulin in F344 rats during chronic exposure to unleaded gasoline or 2,2,4-trimethylpentane. *Toxicol Appl Pharmacol* 1989;101:414–431.
58. Lock EA, Charbonneau M, Strasser J, Swenberg JA, Bus JS. 2,2,4-Trimethylpentane-induced nephrotoxicity. II. The reversible binding of a TMP metabolite to a renal protein fraction containing α_{2u}-globulin. *Toxicol Appl Pharmacol* 1987;91:182–192.
59. Lehman-McKeeman LD, Rodriguez PA, Takigiku R, Caudill D, Fey ML. d-Limonene-induced male-rat-specific nephrotoxicity: evaluation of the association between d-limonene and α_{2u}-globulin. *Toxicol Appl Pharmacol* 1989;99:250–259.
60. Charbonneau M, Strasser J, Lock EA, Turner MJ, Swenberg JA. Involvement of reversible binding to α_{2u}-globulin in 1,4-dichlorobenzene-induced nephrotoxicity. *Toxicol Appl Pharmacol* 1989; 99:122–132.
61. Borghoff SJ, Short BG, Swenberg JA. Biochemical mechanisms and pathobiology of α_{2u}-globulin nephropathy. *Annu Rev Pharmacol Toxicol* 1990;30:349–367.
62. Strasser J, Charbonneau M, Borghoff SJ, Turner MJ, Swenberg JA. Renal protein droplet formation in male Fischer 344 rats after isophorone (IPH) treatment. *Toxicologist* 1988;8:136(abstract).
63. Lehman-McKeeman LD, Rivera-Torres MI, Caudill D. Lysosomal degradation of α_{2u}-globulin and α_{2u}-globulin-xenobiotic conjugates. *Toxicol Appl Pharmacol* 1990;103:539–548.
64. Olson MJ, Mancini MA, Garg BD, Roy AK. Leupeptin-mediated alteration of renal phagolysosomes: similarity to hyaline droplet nephropathy of male rats exposed to unleaded gasoline. *Toxicol Lett* 1988;41:245–254.
65. Caudill D, Lehman-McKeeman LD. Effect of d-limonene-induced hyaline droplet exacerbation on lysosomal proteolytic function and urinary protein excretion. *Toxicologist* 1990;10:267(abstract).

66. Ekstrom RC. *Characterization and metabolism of α_{2u}-globulin-a male sex-dependent protein of the rat*. Ph.D. Thesis, U. Wisconsin, 1983.
67. Ridder GM, VonBargen EC, Alden CL, Parker RD. Increased hyaline droplet formation in male rats exposed to decalin is dependent on the presence of α_{2u}-globulin. *Fundam Appl Toxicol* 1990; 15:732–743.
68. Murty CVR, Olson MJ, Garg BD, Roy AK. Hydrocarbon-induced hyaline droplet nephropathy in male rats during senescence. *Toxicol Appl Pharmacol* 1988;96:380–392.
69. Roy AK, Nath TS, Motwani NM, Catterjee B. Age-dependent regulation of the polymorphic forms of α_{2u}-globulin. *J Biol Chem* 1983;258:10123–10127.
70. Chatterjee B, Fernandes G, Yu BP, Song C, Kim JM, Demyan W, Roy AK. Calorie restriction delays age-dependent loss in androgen responsiveness of the rat liver. *FASEB J* 1989;3:169–173.
71. Sarkar FH, Sarkar PK, Hunter S, Poulik MD, Roy AK. Cytoplasmic androgen binding protein of rat liver: molecular characterization after photoaffinity labeling and function correlation with age-dependent synthesis of α_{2u}-globulin. *Biochemistry* 1987;26:3965–3970.
72. Chatterjee B, Demyan WF, Song CS, Garg BD, Roy AK. Loss of androgenic induction of α_{2u}-globulin gene family in the liver of NIH black rats. *J Endocrinol* 1989;125:1385–1388.
73. Swenberg JA, Short B, Borghoff S, Strasser J, Charbonneau M. The comparative pathobiology of α_{2u}-globulin nephropathy. *Toxicol Appl Pharmacol* 1989;97:35–46.
74. Solleveld HA, Haseman JK, McConnell EE. Natural history of body weight gain, survival and neoplasia in the F344 rats. *J Natl Cancer Inst* 1984;72:929–940.
75. Hard GC. High frequency, single-dose model of renal adenoma/carcinoma induction using dimethylnitrosamine in CrL:(W)BR rats. *Carcinogenesis* 1984;5:1047–1050.
76. Watabe T, Hiratsuka A, Isobe M, Ozawa N. Metabolism of d-limonene by hepatic microsomes to non-mutagenic epoxides toward *Salmonella typhimurium*. *Biochem Pharmacol* 1980;29:1068–1071.
77. Watabe T, Hiratsuka A, Ozawa N, Isobe M. A comparative study on the metabolism of d-limonene and 4-vinylcyclohex-1-ene by hepatic microsomes. *Xenobiotica* 1981;11:333–344.
78. Basler A, von der Hude W, Seelbach A. Genotoxicity of epoxides. Investigations with the SOS Chromotest and the salmonella/mammalian microsome test. *Mutagenesis* 1989;4:313–314(abstract).
79. von der Hude W, Basler A, Mateblowski R, Obe G. Genotoxicity of epoxides. II. In vitro investigations with the sister-chromatid exchange (SCE) test and the unscheduled DNA synthesis (UDS) test. *Mutagenesis* 1979;4:323–324(abstract).
80. Short BG, Steinhagen WH, Swenberg JA. Promoting effects of unleaded gasoline and 2,4,4-trimethylpentane on the development of atypical cell foci and renal tubular cell tumors in rats exposed to N-ethyl-N-hydroxyethylnitrosamine. *Cancer Res* 1989;49:6369–6378.
81. Brooks DE. The major androgen-regulated secretory proteins of the rat epididymus bear sequence homology with members of the α_{2u}-globulin superfamily. *Biochem Int* 1987;14:235–240.
82. Shaw PH, Held WA, Hastie ND. The gene family for major urinary proteins: expression in several secretory tissues of the mouse. *Cell* 1983;32:755–761.
83. Blaner WS. Retinol-binding protein: the serum transport protein for vitamin A. *Endocr Rev* 1989; 19L:308–316.
84. Ganguly M, Carnigham RH, Westphal U. Steroid-protein interactions. XIV. Interaction between human α_1-acid glycoprotein and progesterone. *Biochemistry* 1967;6:2803–2814.
85. Urien S, Albengres E, Zini R, Tillement JP. Evidence for binding of certain acidic drugs to α_1-acid glycoprotein. *Biochem Pharmacol* 1982;31:3687–3689.
86. Pevsner J, Trifiletti RR, Strittmatter SM, Snyder SH. Isolation and characterization of an olfactory receptor protein for odorant pyrazines. *Proc Natl Acad Sci USA* 1985;82:3050–3054.
87. Drayna DT, McLean JW, Wion KL, Trent JM, Drablein HA, Lawn RM. Human apolipoprotein D gene: gene sequence, chromosome localization, and homology to α_{2u}-globulin superfamily. *DNA* 1987;6:199–204.
88. Otin CL, Grubb AO, Mendez E. The complete amino acid sequence of human complex-forming glycoprotein heterogeneous in charge (Protein HC) from one individual. *Arch Biochem Biophys* 1984;228:544–554.
89. Julkunen M, Seppala M, Janne OA. Complete amino acid sequence of human placental protein 14: a progesterone-regulated uterine protein homologous to β-lactoglobulins. *Proc Natl Acad Sci USA* 1988;85:8845–8849.

90. Bernard AM, Lauwerys RR, Noel A, Vandeleene B, Lambert A. Urine protein 1: a sex-dependent marker of tubular or glomerular dysfunction. *Clin Chem* 1989;35:2141–2142(abstract).
91. Papiz MZ, Sawyer L, Eliopoulos EE, North ACT, et al. The structure of β-lactoglobulin and its similarity to plasma retinol-binding protein. *Nature* 1986;324:383–385.
92. Wishnia A, Pinder TW. Hydrophobic interactions in proteins. The alkane binding site of β-lactoglobulins A and B. *Biochemistry* 1966;5:1535–1542.
93. Brooks DE, Means AR, Wright EJ, Singh SP, Tiver KK. Molecular cloning of the cDNA for two major androgen-dependent secretory proteins of 18.5 kilodaltons synthesized by the rat epididymus. *J Biol Chem* 1986;26:4956–4961.
94. Henzel WJ, Rodriguez H, Singer AG, Stults IT, Macrides F, Agosta WC, Niall H. The primary structure of aphrodisin. *J Biol Chem* 1988;263:16682–16687.
95. Berman P, Gray P, Chen E, et al. Sequence analysis, cellular localization and expression of a neuroretina adhesion and cell survival molecule. *Cell* 1987;51:135–142.
96. Holden HM, Rypniewski WR, Law JH, Rayment I. The molecular structure of insecticyanin from the tobacco hornworm. *Manduca sexta L* at 2.6 A resolution. *EMBO J* 1987;6:1565–1570.
97. Huber R, Schneider M, Epp O, Mayr I, Messerschmidt A, Pflugrath J. Crystallization, crystal structure analysis and preliminary molecular model of the bilin-binding protein from the insect *Pieris brassicae*. *J Mol Biol* 1987;195:423–434.
98. Newcomer ME, Jones TA, Aqvist J, Sundelin J, Eriksson U, Rask L, Peterson PA. The three-dimensional structure of retinol-binding protein. *EMBO J* 1984;3:1451–1454.
99. Cowan SA, Newcomer ME, Jones TA. Crystallographic refinement of human serum retinol binding protein at 2A resolution. *Proteins* 1990;8:44–61.
100. Hase J, Kobashi K, Nakai N, Onosaka S. Binding of retinol-binding protein obtained from human urine with vitamin A derivatives and terpenoids. *J Biochem* 1976;79:373–380.
101. Hastie ND, Held WA, Toole JJ. Multiple genes coding for the androgen-regulated major urinary proteins of the mouse. *Cell* 1979;17:449–457.
102. Finlayson JS, Potter M, Runner CR. Electrophoretic variation and sex dimorphism of the major urinary protein complex in inbred mice: a new genetic marker. *J Natl Cancer Inst* 1963;31:91–107.
103. Rumke PH, Thung PJ. Immunological studies on the sex-dependent prealbumin in mouse urine and its occurrence in the serum. *Acta Endocrinol* 1965;47:156–164.
104. Finlayson JS, Asofsky R, Potter M, Runner CC. Major urinary protein complex of normal mice: origin. *Science* 1965;149:981–982.
105. Lehman-McKeeman LD, Caudill D, Takigiku R, Schneider RE, Young JA. Comparative disposition of d-limonene in rats and mice: relevance to male rat specific nephrotoxicity. *Toxicol Lett* 1990;53:193–195.
106. Knopf JL, Gallagher JF, Held WA. Differential, multihormonal regulation of the mouse major urinary protein gene family in the liver. *Mol Cell Biol* 1983;3:2232–2240.
107. Cogan U, Kopelman M, Mokady S, Shinitzky M. Binding affinities of retinol and related compounds to retinol binding proteins. *Eur J Biochem* 1976;65:71–78.

Toxicology of the Kidney, Second Edition,
edited by Jerry B. Hook and Robin S. Goldstein.
Raven Press, Ltd., New York © 1993.

19

Renal Carcinogenesis

Daniel R. Dietrich and *James A. Swenberg

*Institute of Toxicology, Swiss Federal Institute of Technology and University of Zurich, CH-8603 Schwerzenbach, Switzerland; and *Departments of Environmental Sciences and Engineering and Pathology, University of North Carolina, Chapel Hill, North Carolina 27599-7095*

Renal carcinogenesis is a broad, complex area of research that encompasses the work of scientists from many fields including biology, chemistry, and medicine, and focuses on understanding the mechanisms involved in the genesis of renal tumors in a multitude of animal species, including man. The most broadly practiced approach to studying the induction of tumors, for evaluating the carcinogenic potential of a chemical, and for predicting possible risk of cancer for man, is the animal carcinogenicity bioassay. Such an approach is only of value if the mechanisms of tumor formation in the surrogate species are similar to the mechanisms in man. Nearly all renal tumor types observed in man (1,2) have been experimentally induced in rodents by various chemical carcinogens, hormones, viruses, and radiation (reviewed by Hamilton [3], Hiasa and Ito [4], Bannasch and Zerban [5], Dietrich and Swenberg [6]). Although the kidneys of experimental animals can respond to carcinogenic stimuli with the development of a number of different morphological types of renal tumors, e.g., nephroblastoma (NB), renal mesenchymal tumor (RMT), renal cell tumor (RCT), and renal transitional cell tumor (RTCT), renal cell tumors constitute the vast majority of the induced tumors (7). This pattern of tumor development is similar to that observed in humans, where over 90% of the diagnosed renal tumors are of epithelial origin, i.e., renal cell tumor (8,9).

A number of compounds from diverse chemical classes have induced renal tumors in different species of experimental animals. The types of chemicals capable of inducing renal tumors include procarcinogens, which require metabolism to exert their carcinogenic potential, direct-acting alkylating agents, direct-acting nonalkylating agents, and metals.

In this chapter, we will discuss spontaneous, chemically induced, and hereditary renal tumors in experimental animals and humans. The discussion will focus on the pathogenesis of renal tumors, the presence of preneoplastic lesions and their importance as precursors for tumor formation, the types of etiologic agents, and their mechanisms of action. Emphasis is placed on tumors in experimental animals rather than on those in humans.

CLASSIFICATION OF RENAL TUMORS

Nephroblastomas

Morphology of Preneoplastic and Neoplastic Lesions

True nephroblastomas, like renal mesenchymal tumors (discussed below), are neoplasms of young animals (10,11) and have been observed in rat, mouse, multimammate mouse (*Praomys natalensis*), rabbit, opossum, swine, cow, horse, sheep, goat, cat, dog, nonhuman primates, chicken, fish, and amphibia (10–18). Histologically, NBs are quite distinguishable from renal mesenchymal tumors. As summarized in Table 1, rat NBs have a distinct pseudocapsule and do not contain mesenchymal components such as striated muscle, hyperplastic smooth muscle, cartilage, and osteoid. Rodent NBs consist of homogeneous populations of highly basophilic, epitheloid blastemal cells with the potential for organoid differentiation into epithelial structures such as tubular and glomeruloid profiles (Figs.1 and 2), but not into secondary mesenchyme (4,7,19). This potential for epithelial organoid differentiation is a rather consistent feature shown by nephroblastomas across phyletic boundaries, with the exception of humans.

TABLE 1. *Summary of discriminating features between nephroblastoma and renal mesenchymal tumor in rats*

	Nephroblastoma	Renal mesenchymal tumor
General form	Circumscribed, clear demarcation, pseudocapsule	Irregular outline, infiltration of tumor cells, no capsule
General histology	Homogeneous tumor cells	Heterogeneous tumor cells
Tumor components	Blastema/epithelium	Secondary mesenchyme
Mesenchyme	Normal connective tissue consistent with supportive, vascular stroma	Neoplastic spindle cells, smooth muscle, embryonic, mesenchyme, vascular tissue, striated muscle, cartilage, osteoid (collagen, reticulin)
Epithelial structures	Blastema with primitive tubules, ducts, glomeruloid bodies as products of neoplastic differentiation	Mature tubules, glomeruli, cysts, urothelium, as entrapped remnants of preexisting parenchyma
Fate of engulfed existing epithelium	Disappears beyond tumor periphery	Frequently survives within tumor mass
Origin	Cortex	Outer stripe—outer zone of medulla
Tissue origin	Metanephrogenic blastema?	Intertubular connective tissue

Modified from Hard, ref. 7.

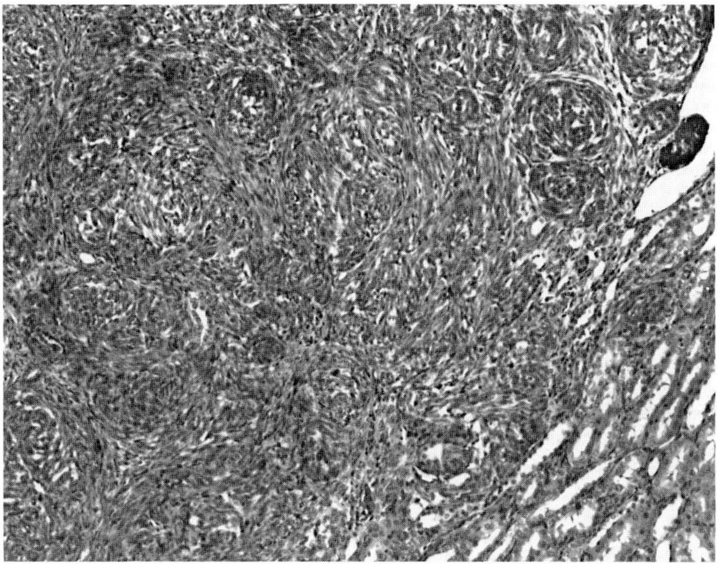

FIG. 1. Spontaneous nephroblastoma in a female F344 rat treated with tetrachlorophtalic anhydrate 94 mg/kg/day for 90 days. Note the absence of preexisting renal tubules or mesenchymal structures within the tumor tissue. (H&E $\times$ 90.)

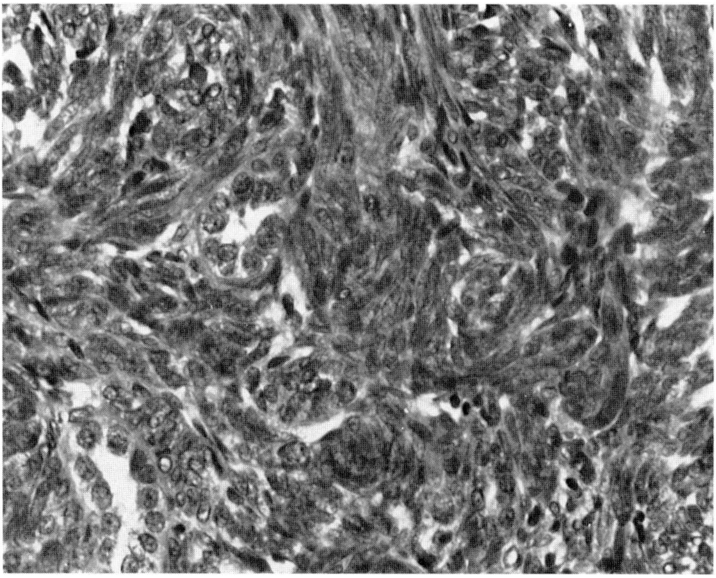

FIG. 2. High-power field of the nephroblastoma depicted in Fig. 1. The predominant cells are highly basophilic, epitheloid blastemal cells partially undergoing organoid differentiation into tubular epithelium. (H&E $\times$ 360.)

In man, Wilms' tumor has the bipotential of differentiating into neoplastic secondary mesenchyme as well as into blastema and epithelium (20); thus, a range of histological varieties are reported for this one tumor type. Congenital malformations of nonrenal organs (21) and preneoplastic lesions, e.g., nodular renal blastema or nephroblastomosis (22), as observed in humans with Wilms' tumor, have never been described in conjunction with NB of animals. In contrast to NB observed in animals, the etiology of Wilms' tumor is fairly well known, in that the genesis of Wilms' tumor has been associated with the absence of one or more genes on the short arm of chromosome 11 (23,24).

Incidence of Spontaneous Nephroblastomas

Nephroblastomas are rare tumors. Although no NBs are reported for wild rats (0/100,000), laboratory rats seem to have a higher predisposition to the spontaneous formation of NBs (10). Indeed, the inbred Nb-Hooded rat, WAB/Not rat, and F344 male rat have higher incidences of NB, 40/100,000, 39/24,000, and 1/2,320, respectively, than the 9/100,000 observed in laboratory rats in general (10,15, 17,25). Rabbits also have a slightly higher incidence (66/100,000) of NB than is found in other domestic animals, e.g., swine (4/100,000), cattle (1/1,3000,000), and chicken (9/100,000) (11,14,26). A similar incidence (1/10,000) is reported for the occurrence of Wilms' tumor in children (24).

Induction of NB in Animals

Chemical Induction

Nephroblastomas were chemically induced in rabbits (27–29), opossum (30), mice (31), rats (31–38), dogs, non-human primates (10), and fish (39). They were predominantly induced by treating either the offspring transplacentally or postnatally with 1,2-dimethylhydrazine, 1-methylhydrazine, DMBA, *N*-ethylnitrosourea (ENU), MNU, dimethylnitrosamine (DMN) or nickel compounds.

Hormonal Induction

Renal tumors, classified as renal cell tumors and NB (40,41), have been induced in the Syrian golden hamster (*Mesocricetus auratus*) with estrogen derivatives such as diethylstilbestrol (DES). However, given the observation that these renal tumors are derived from residual metanephric blastema located in the intertubular stroma, the correct classification should be nephroblastoma (41).

Viral Induction

Chickens infected with the leukosis virus strains BAI A (avian myeloblastosis virus [AMV]) and MC29 developed nephroblastomas (42–44). Infection by AMV induced tumors with epithelial and nephroblastemal characteristics having the bipotential of differentiating into neoplastic secondary mesenchyme as well as into blastema and epithelium, a characteristic also noted for the human Wilms' tumor (see Table 4). In contrast, MC29 virus induced only epithelial growths representing principally aberrant and malformed glomerular and tubular structures, similar to NB described in rats (45).

Renal Mesenchymal Tumors

Morphology of Preneoplastic and Neoplastic Lesions

Renal mesenchymal tumors (RMTs) have been the subject of much confusion with respect to diagnosis and classification, the literature revealing no less than 13 synonyms for this complex neoplasm (19). Most commonly, RMT are mistaken for embryonal kidney tumors and are misclassified as nephroblastomas (NBs) or Wilms' tumors. It is thus very difficult to verify whether some of the renal tumors described in the literature are RMT or actually NB. RMTs have been diagnosed in mice, guinea pigs, rabbits, rats, sheep, cats, dogs, and in the ring-tailed lemur (*Lemur catta*), a nonhuman primate (10–12,16,19,46–49).

Histopathologically, RMT is a very heterogeneous connective tissue neoplasm consisting of a range of mesenchymal cell types (Figs. 3 and 4, Table 1) that reflect their origin from a multipotential stem cell (7,19). This heterogeneity led Riopelle and Jasmin (37) to distinguish three putatively different subgroups. However, subgrouping RMT may lead more to confusion than to clarity, as each neoplasm consists not only of one predominant cell type, but varies from area to area within an individual tumor (4).

A sequential study of the pathogenesis of RMT revealed the existence of preneoplastic lesions as early as 3 to 5 days after treatment of the rats with DMN (50). Interstitial lesions, such as small aggregations of cells undergoing mitosis, developed in the immediate vicinity of the glomerular hilus. This stage was followed by a mononuclear inflammatory reaction, with focal aggregations of plasma cells, the appearance of tumor cell aggregations, and finally microscopic tumors. Hard and Butler (50–52) reported that not all hypercellular foci develop into tumor cell aggregations, but that small residual lesions resembling fibrous scars can be found 12 weeks after DMN treatment, indicating that some of the hypercellular foci may regress to scar tissue. From the data presented by Hard and Butler (50), it is not possible to determine what percentage of the original number of hypercellular foci actually progress to RMT. It is interesting though to note that the incidence of

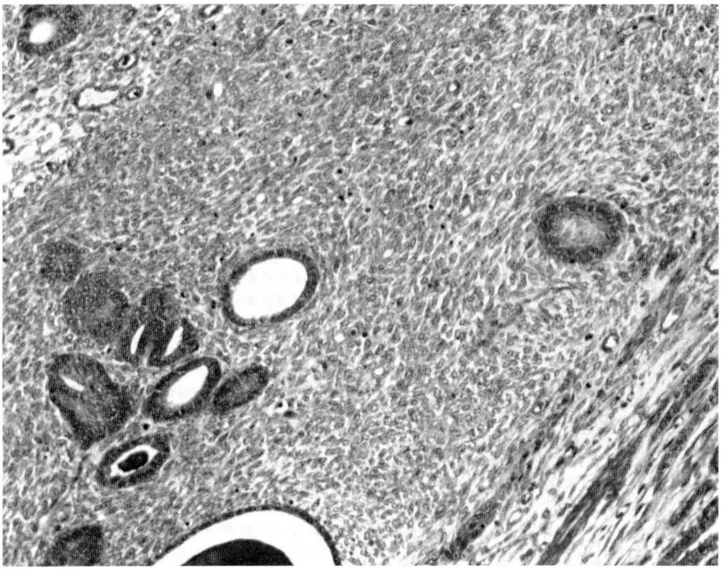

FIG. 3. Mesenchymal tumor. Cellular area with residual renal tubules that are flattened and atrophic, or hyperplastic. (H&E × 135.) (Reproduced from Hard, ref. 301, with permission.)

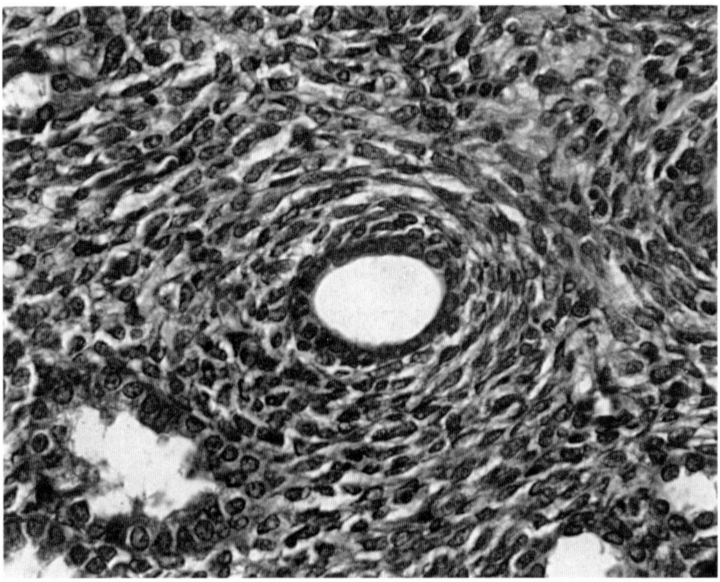

FIG. 4. Mesenchymal tumor. The predominant cell form is spindle shaped and often aligned in layers around preexisting renal tubules. (H&E × 270.) (From Hard and Butler, ref. 50, with permission.)

interstitial lesions (percentage of animals with interstitial lesions), counted 3 days after treatment, corresponds to the incidence of RMT appraised 25 weeks after treatment, suggesting that the incidence of preneoplastic interstitial lesions early in the experiment could give a fairly close prediction of the incidence of RMT at the end of the experiment (Table 2). However, this very suggestion was questioned by Driver and coworkers (53), who, although observing a similar dose-response relationship for preneoplastic lesions, did not find that the incidence of preneoplastic lesions was directly proportional to the tumor incidence at the end of the experiments. They suggested that the mechanisms that operate to remove the majority of the early proliferative foci determine the shape of the dose-response curve for the tumors, and that these are independent of the initial alkylation levels in rats treated with a single dose of DMN.

As indicated earlier, RMT observed in animals are clearly distinguished from the human Wilms' tumor. However, within the overall spectrum of Wilms' tumors, one variant has been described with mesenchymal characteristics clearly distinguishable in its morphology and clinical behavior from the classical Wilms' tumors described above (54–59). In addition to the RMT variant of Wilms' tumors, there have been reports of RMT in humans in conjunction with tuberous sclerosis (60). However, in contrast to Wilms' tumors, the etiology of this disease is unknown.

Incidence of Spontaneous RMT

Renal mesenchymal tumors are rare tumors; however, they are more frequent than NBs. Gilbert and Gillman (61) found 3/641 and 1/701 RMTs in untreated male and female Wistar rats, respectively. Slightly lower numbers, 4/2,320 and 0/2,370 RMTs were observed in 2-year-old untreated male and female F344 rats, respectively. However, at termination of the natural life span, the incidences of RMT increased to 1/529 and 2/529 for male and female F344 rats, respectively (25). A study by Goodman and coworkers (62) indicated that Osborne-Mendel rats seemed more susceptible to the formation of spontaneous RMT (male 19/975, female 25/970). No RMTs were found in 251 19-month-old male and female Swiss mice (18), whereas Slye and coworkers (63) reported seven sarcomas in 33,000 autopsied mice. In a 12-month survey of cattle, sheep, and pigs slaughtered in Great Britain

TABLE 2. *Doses of dimethylnitrosamine (DMN) and incidences (percent of affected animals) of preneoplastic interstitial lesions (3 days beyond treatment) and of renal mesenchymal tumors (25 weeks after treatment)*

DMN mg/kg	Interstitial lesions (%)	Mesenchymal tumors (%)
60	100	100
50	83	90
30	30	24
0	0	0

Compiled from data published by Hard and Butler, ref. 50.

only one RMT was found in 1,300,000 cattle and one RMT in 3,700,000 pigs, whereas no RMTs were found in 4,500,000 sheep, emphasizing the rarity of this tumor (26). Similarly no RMTs were observed during 450 autopsies performed in a United States colony of rhesus monkeys (*Macaca mulatta*) (64).

Induction of RMT in Animals

Chemical Induction

Next to renal epithelial cell tumors (see below), RMTs are the most common renal neoplasm of rats and mice induced by chemical agents. Dimethylnitrosamine (DMN) has been the most extensively employed chemical for studying RMT. A single dose of DMN administered to protein-deprived, immature Wistar rats resulted in virtually a 100% incidence of RMT (50,65). RMTs were generally induced at high incidences in DMN-treated rats of very young age (66), whereas no RMTs were found in 5-month-old DMN-treated rats (66,67), thus emphasizing the importance of age with respect to the induction of this tumor. Other chemicals that induce this tumor in relatively high incidence include cycasin (68,69), ethyl methanesulfonate (70), 1,2-dimethylhydrazine (31,71), streptozotocin (72), *N*-methylnitrosourea (73,74), and transplacentally administered *N*-ethylnitrosourea (33). Lower incidences of RMT are achieved by treating 2-month-old F344 rats with nickel compounds (38).

Viral Induction

Sarcomas predominantly containing collagen and elastic fibers have been induced by treating newborn Wistar rats with a single injection of SE-polyomavirus 1530 (75,76). SE-polyomavirus-induced RMTs (see Table 4) were also reported for mice, hamsters, and rabbits (75).

Renal Cell Tumors

Morphology of Preneoplastic and Neoplastic Lesions

Renal cell tumors (RCT), also known as renal epithelial tumors due to their epigenesis in renal tubule epithelial cells, are the most frequent of renal tumors and have been reported in rats, mice, hamsters, guinea pigs, rabbits, cats, dogs, horses, sheep, cows, pigs, squirrels, nonhuman primates, birds, fish, reptiles, amphibians (12,16,26,47,49,77–79), and humans (1). Of the renal tumors found in humans, approximately 90% are RCTs (9). Nearly all renal cell tumor types observed in man (1,2) have also been found as spontaneous or experimentally induced tumors in animals (3–6). With the exception of the hereditary RCT in the shepherd dog (80) and rats, carrying a specific gene mutation first described by Eker (81), the etiology of RCT in animals is unknown. In contrast, both spontaneous and hereditary human RCT seem to share one common feature in their etiology, namely the loss of a putative tumor suppressor gene, via deletion or translocation, located on the short arm of the human chromosome 3 (82,83).

Sequential observations on the appearance of neoplastic lesions in rats and mice treated with ENU, *N*-ethyl-*N*-hydroxyethylnitrosamine (EHEN), FBPA, and DMN, as well as stop-assays carried out with *N*-nitrosomorpholine (NNM)-treated rats, led to the discovery of early lesions that shared morphological characteristics with RCT and the identification of at least five different cell types, i.e., clear, basophilic, eosinophilic, chromophobic, and oncocytic cells in RCT (84–94). These findings and the similarity of the types of lesions and tumors observed in rodents to tumor types observed in humans, led to renewed investigation and eventually to a tentative new classification of human renal cell tumors (2,95–97). The in-depth discussion of these cell types and the corresponding RCT would certainly exceed the scope and the intentions of this chapter; therefore, the reader is referred to the reviews by Bannasch and coworkers (99), Bannasch and Zerban (5), and Dietrich and Swenberg (6) for more comprehensive information on this matter. Recent studies on the importance of preneoplastic lesions as predictive tools in renal carcinogenesis, resulted in a new simplified nomenclature for preneoplastic lesions of RCT (6). All cell types mentioned above have been observed in these preneoplastic and neoplastic lesions (Figs. 5 to 10), the morphological criteria of which are listed in Table 3. In a subsequent study, Dietrich and Swenberg (100) showed that using the new nomenclature for preneoplastic and neoplastic lesions of RCT simplified the evaluation of carcinogenesis studies and, in conjunction with mechanistic data, may improve the interpretation of animal studies with regard to human risk assessment.

Incidence of Spontaneous RCT

As with the previous tumors, most data on the spontaneous incidence of RCT are reported for laboratory mice and rats. Shinohara and Frith (101) reported 13 RCTs in 3,495 female BALB/C mice, whereas Horn and Stewart (48) observed a spontaneous RCT frequency of only 0.02% in various strains of mice. Prejean and coworkers (18), on the other hand, reported one RCT in 101 male Swiss-Webster mice. In F344 rats sacrificed after 2 years 0.34% (8/2,320) and 0.17% (4/2,370) of the male and female rats, respectively, had RCT (25). In a lifetime study, Goodman and coworkers (62,102) observed incidences of 0.16% and 0.05% in male and female F344 rats as well as 0.3% and 0.0% in male and female Osborne-Mendel rats. In contrast to the data by Goodman and coworkers, Solleveld and coworkers (25) found that the spontaneous incidences of RCT in F344 rats held for their entire life span to be higher, 3/529 (0.57%) and 5/529 (0.95%) for males and females, respectively. Slightly higher incidences of spontaneous RCT were reported in Syrian golden hamsters, namely 0.55% in males and 0.50% in females (103). In do-

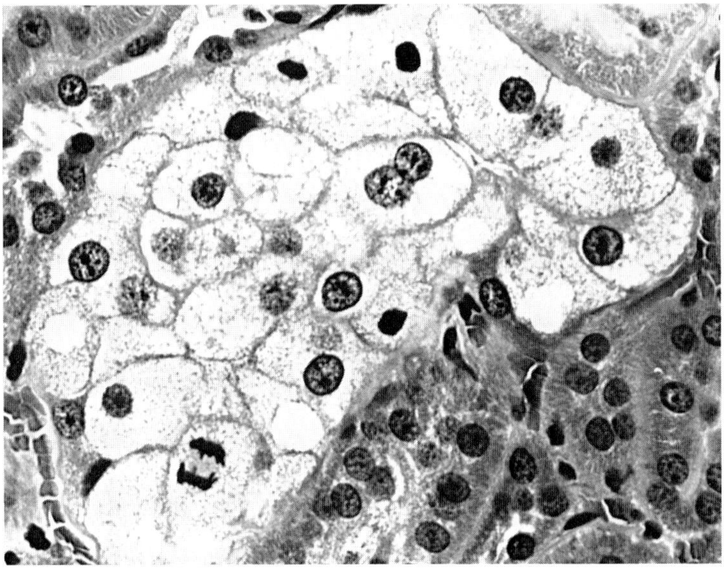

FIG. 5. Atypical tubule containing clear cells observed in the renal cortex of a male F344 rat initiated with EHEN and then promoted with d-limonene as described by Dietrich and Swenberg (100). (H&E × 540.)

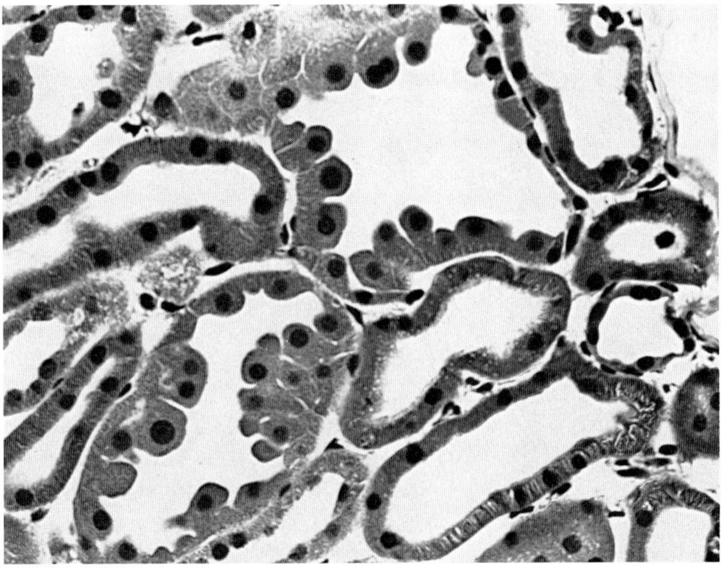

FIG. 6. Atypical tubule containing oncocytic cells observed in the renal cortex of a male NBR rat initiated with EHEN and then gavaged with corn oil as described by Dietrich and Swenberg (100). (H&E × 90.)

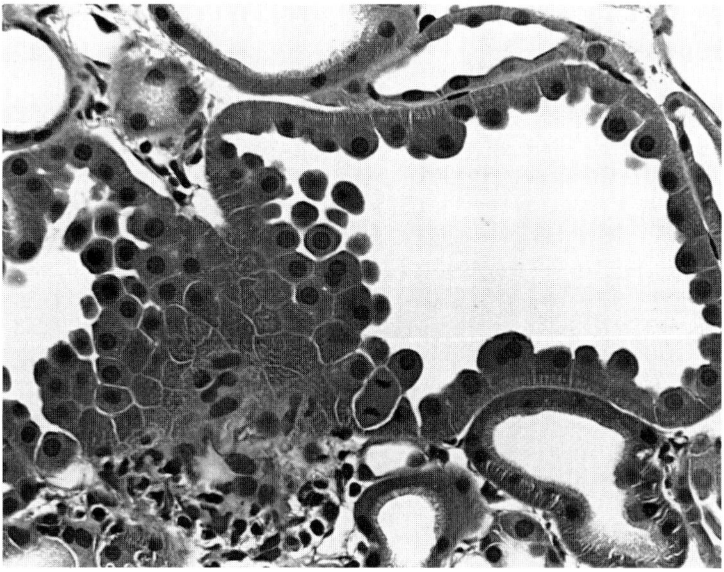

FIG. 7. Atypical hyperplasia containing oncocytic cells observed in the renal cortex of a male NBR rat treated water and then promoted with d-limonene as described by Dietrich and Swenberg (100). (H&E × 360.)

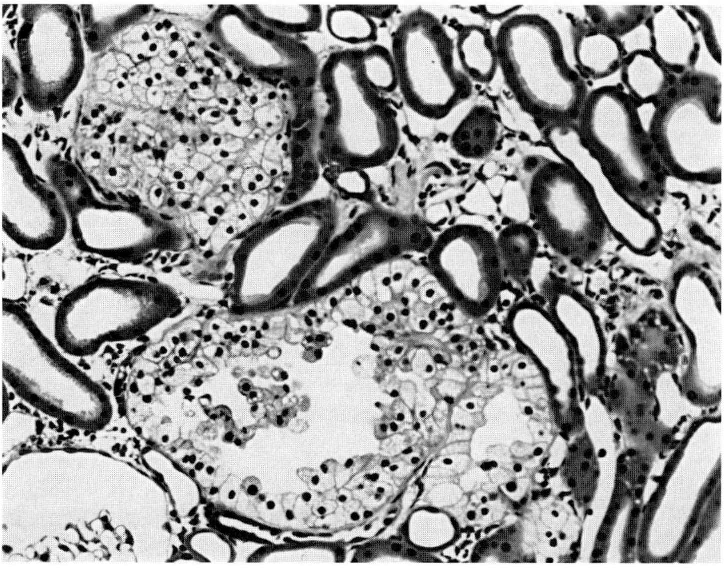

FIG. 8. Atypical hyperplasia containing clear cells observed in the renal cortex of a male F344 rat initiated with EHEN and then promoted with d-limonene as described by Dietrich and Swenberg (100). (H&E × 180.)

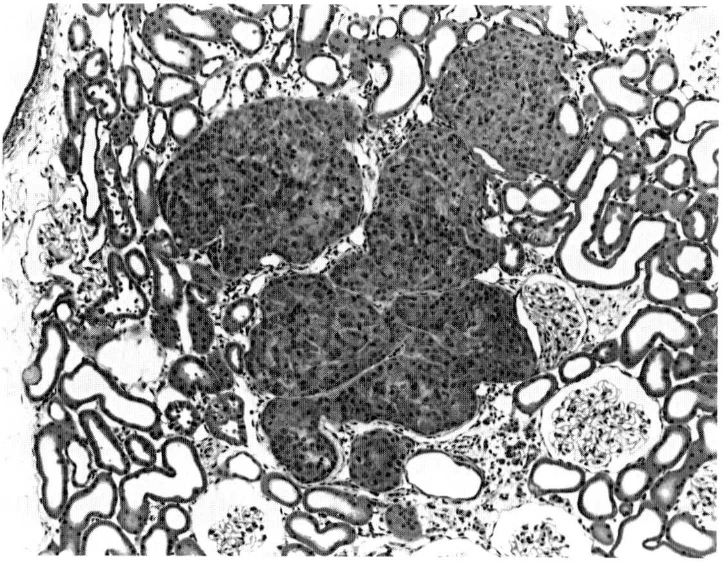

FIG. 9. Basophilic renal cell adenoma observed in the renal cortex of a male F344 rat initiated with EHEN and then gavaged with corn oil as described by Dietrich and Swenberg (100). (H&E × 90.)

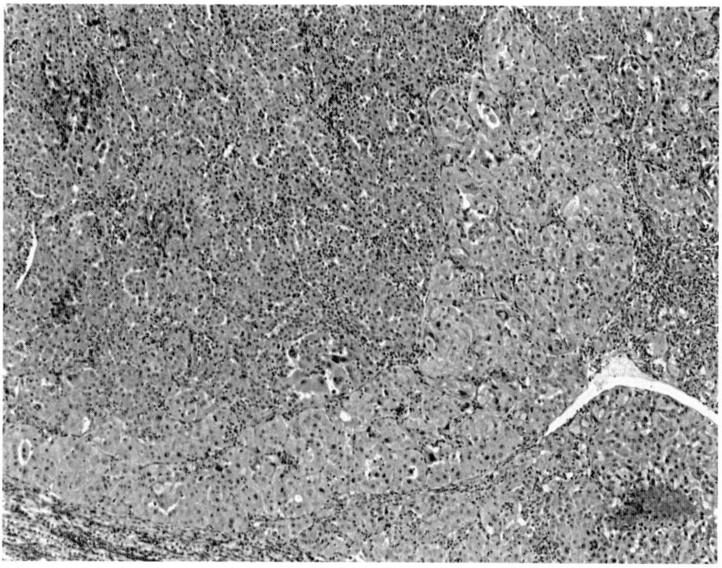

FIG. 10. Renal cell carcinoma containing acidophilic, basophilic, and oncocytic cells observed in the renal cortex of a male F344 rat treated with 210 μg ochratoxin A kg/day for 2 years. (H&E × 17.) (From Dietrich and Swenberg, ref. 6, with permission.).

TABLE 3. *Morphological criteria of preneoplastic and neoplastic lesions observed in the formation of RCT*

Lesion	Size	Morphological criteria
Atypical tubules (AT)	<2 adjacent tubules	Contain atypical cells. Mitotic figures are possible but rare. The lumen is dilated or obstructed with atypical cells or cellular debris.
Atypical hyperplasia (AH)	<10 adjacent tubules	Homogeneous or heterogeneous aggregation of atypical cells. Single or multilayered with or without central necrosis and mitotic figures.
Adenoma	>10 adjacent tubules	Homogeneous or heterogeneous aggregation of atypical cells. Mitotic figures and necrotic foci. Encapsulated, noninvasive but surrounding tissue shows signs of compression. Three types of adenomas: solid, cystic, cystopapillary.
Carcinoma	Varying size	Not clearly delineated, compresses and invades surrounding parenchyma. Mitotic figures and focal necrosis are frequent. Tends to metastasize to other organs. Cell types are atypical and pleomorphic but not necessarily highly prolific. Solid, tubular, or papillary growth structure.

Compiled from data published by Dietrich and Swenberg, ref. 6.

mestic animals, Sandison and Anderson (26) found spontaneous RCT in 0.0007% of cattle, 0.001% of sheep, and 0.00003% of pigs slaughtered during a 12-month survey. Human RCTs occur at a rate of approximately 6.5 and 3.7 per 100,000 in males and females per year (1,9); however, these numbers also include RCT thought to be induced by etiologic agents such as tobacco (20) as well as RCT having a hereditary or familial epigenesis.

Induction of RCT in Animals

Chemical Induction

In order to study the genesis of RCT, rats have been treated with a multitude of agents including inorganic reagents, nitrosamines, solvents, metals, mycotoxins, and irradiation (4,5), all of which are listed in Table 4 and will be discussed in Etiological Agents, below. Similarly, the induction of RCT in mice has been achieved by injecting mice with a single dose of ENU or streptozotocin (35,84) or repeated ip injections of Fe-NTA (104).

Hormonal Induction

Mice developed RCT after being treated with stilbestrol for 4 to 8 weeks and then being kept for their life span (105). However, the incidence of RCT after this treat-

TABLE 4. *Summary table of agents reported to induce preneoplastic and neoplastic lesions in the kidneys of experimental animals*

Agent class	Agent	Abbrev.	Species	Tumor	References
Nitroso compounds and other alkylating agents	Dimethylnitrosamine	DMN	Rat	NB	135
				RMT	7,36,37,50–53, 66,190
				RCT	19,28,36,66,85, 86,90,190, 263–265
	Niethylnitrosamine	DEN	Rat	RMT	121,266,267
				RCT	137,267–268
	N-butyl-*N*-hydroxybutylnitrosamine	BBN	Rat	RMT	36
				RTCT	36,136,269
	N-ethyl-*N*-hydroxyethylnitrosamine	EHEN	Rat	RCT	89,90,134,136, 143,189,191, 235,236, 270–276
	N-ethylnitrosourea	ENU	Rat	NB	33
				RMT	33
				RCT	33
			Mouse	RCT	84
			Rabbit	NB	27–29
				RCT	27
			Opossum	NB	30
	N-methylnitrosourea	MNU	Rat	NB	33
				RMT	33,73,277
				RCT	33,277
			Mouse	RMT	74
				RCT	74,277
	N-methyl-*N*-nitro-*N*-nitrosoguanidine	MNNG	Fish	NB	39
	Di-isopropanolnitrosamine	DIPN	Rat	RTCT	120
	N-nitrosomorpholine	NNM	Rat	RCT	5,90–94,141, 142,268,278
	Ethyl methanesulphonate	EMS	Rat	RMT	70,150
				RCT	70,150
			Mouse	RCT	150
	1,2-Dimethylhydrazine	1,2-DMH	Rat	RMT	71
	1,1-Dimethylhydrazine	1,1-DMH	Mouse	RCT	149
	Methylazoxymethanol	MAM	Rat	NB	68
				RMT	68
				RCT	68
	Cycasin	-	Rat	NB	144,145
				RMT	69,144,145,279
				RCT	69,144,145, 280,281
				RTCT	144,145
			Mouse	RCT	146
			Hamster	RCT	147
	Streptozotocin	-	Rat	NB	72,282
				RMT	72
				RCT	72,282,284

TABLE 4. *Continued.*

Agent class	Agent	Abbrev.	Species	Tumor	References
			Mouse	RCT	35
Arylamines and amides	2-Acetylamino-fluorene	2-AAF	Mouse	RCT	101
	N-(4′-fluoro-4-biphenyl) acetamide	FBPA	Rat	RCT	87,88,151,152
Nitrofurans	2-[4-(5-Nitro-2-furyl)-2-thiazolyl] hydrazide	FNT	Rat	RMT	156
				RCT	156
				RTCT	156
	N-[4-(5-nitro-2-furyl)-2-thiazolyl] formamide	FANFT	Rat	RTCT	119,157–159
Volatile hydrocarbons and $\alpha_{2\mu}$-globulin nephropathy–inducing agents	Unleaded gasoline	UG	Rat	RCT	285,286
	1,4-Dichlorobenzene	1,4-DCB	Rat	RCT	287
	Hexachloroethane	HCE	Rat	RCT	288
	Pentachloroethane	PCE	Rat	RCT	289
	Perchloroethylene	-	Rat	RCT	290
	Isophorone	IP	Rat	RCT	291
	Dimethyl methyl phosphonate	DMMP	Rat	RCT	122,292
				RTCT	122,292
	d-Limonene	dL	Rat	RCT	100,293
Antibiotics and analgesics	Niridazole	-	Rat	RMT	167,168
				RCT	167,168
	Daunomycin	-	Rat	RCT	169
	Acetaminophen	-	Rat	RTCT	294
	Phenacetin	-	Rat	RCT	116
				RTCT	116–118,291
	Antipyrine	-	Rat	RTCT	294
	Paracetamol	-	Rat	RTCT	116
	Phenazone	-	Rat	RTCT	116
	Caffeine	-	Rat	NB	116
Metal compounds	Lead acetate	PbA	Rat	RCT	137,170,295, 296
	Nickel acetate	NiA	Rat	RCT	123
	Nickel compounds	Ni(X)	Rat	NB	38
				RMT	38
				RCT	38
	Ferric nitriloacetate	Fe-NTA	Mouse	RCT	104
Hormones	Estrogen	-	Hamster	NB	41
				RCT	41,107,175–177,179
	Stilbestrol-cholesterol	-	Mouse	RCT	105
Mycotoxins	Citrinin	-	Rat	RCT	297
	Ochratoxin A	OA	Rat	RCT	131
			Mouse	RCT	183
	Aflatoxin B_1	-	Rat	RCT	185,298
Viruses	Avian myeloblastosis virus	BAIA	Chicken	NB	42–45
				RMT	45
		MC29	Chicken	NB	45
	SE-Polyomavirus	-	Rat	RMT	76

TABLE 4. *Continued.*

Agent class	Agent	Abbrev.	Species	Tumor	References
	Lucke's virus	-	Frog	RCT	78
Radiation	Gamma rays	-	Rat	RCT	47,187
				RTCT	187
			Mouse	RCT	47
Tumor promoters	Sodium barbital	NaBB	Rat	RCT	121,123,124, 192,266
				RTCT	121,123,192
	β-Cylodextrin	β-C	Rat	RCT	4
	N-(3,5-dichloro-phenyl) suc-cinimide	NDPS	Rat	RCT	189,190
				RTCT	189
	Folic acid	FA	Rat	RCT	189
	DL-Serine	-	Rat	RCT	191
	Di-(2-ethylhexyl)-phthalate	DEHP	Rat	RCT	188
Other agents	Nitrilotriacetate	NTA	Rat	RCT	195–197,233, 236,237
				RTCT	197,234
	Potassium bro-mate	$KBrO_3$	Rat	RCT	275,299,300
			Mouse	RCT	203
			Hamster	RCT	203
	7,12-Dimethyl-benz[a]-anthra-cene	DMBA	Rat	NB	32
	Chloroform		Rat	RCT	193,194
			Mouse	RCT	193
	Tris(2,3-dibromo-propyl) phos-phate	TBP	Rat	RCT	198,199
			Mouse	RCT	198,199
	Dichloroacetylene	DCA	Rat	RCT	201
			Mouse	RCT	201
	Urethane	-	Rat	NB	202
				RMT	202
				RCT	202
				RTCT	202
	C.I. Acid Orange 3	-	Rat	RTCT	200

ment was very low (2%). On the other hand, bilateral renal tumors can be induced by estrogens and estrogen-derivatives in both intact and castrated male Syrian hamsters with an incidence approaching 100% (106). The induction of renal tumors termed RCT in the Syrian golden hamster treated with estrogen or estrogen derivatives, as reported by Bloom and coworkers (107), was questioned, especially as the lesions described by these authors did not seem to have evolved from epithelial cells. Indeed, the classification of estrogen-induced renal neoplasm has been the subject of considerable controversy. The tumors have been classified as either adenocarcinoma (108), nephroblastoma (41), or renal mesenchymal tumor (109). The most recent study shows that renal cells, involved in the formation of estrogen-induced neoplasms, harbor both epithelial and mesenchymal characteristics; however, they morphologically bear resemblance to developing embryonic kidney cells, which seem to be committed to an epithelial differentiation (110).

Viral Induction

RCT incidences of 70.8% and 29.9% in male and female leopard frogs (*Rana pipiens*) have been reported by Lucke (78). These RCTs (Table 4) induced by a herpes type virus, named Lucke virus, develop predominantly from renal proximal tubule epithelial cells (3), and frequently metastasize to the lung and the liver (78).

Renal Transitional Cell Tumors

Morphology of Preneoplastic and Neoplastic Lesions

Renal transitional cell tumors (RTCTs) have been reported in rats (111), cats, dogs, cows, pigs, horses (12,16,112), nonhuman primates (49), and humans (113). In many reviews and scientific articles, RTCTs have not been treated as an entity by themselves, but rather as variants of renal epithelial tumors or treated in conjunction with bladder tumors, due to their site of origin, the transitional cell epithelium of the renal pelvis.

In general four lesions are distinguished: transitional cell hyperplasia, atypical hyperplasia, transitional cell carcinoma, and squamous cell carcinoma (111,114).

Transitional cell hyperplasia is considered to be a nonneoplastic lesion of the renal pelvis (Figs. 11 and 12). It can consist of focal or multifocal nodular growths that protrude into the pelvis. These projections more often occur at the junction of the papilla and pelvis and are several cell layers thick. Transitional cell hyperplasia is characterized by an increased number of urothelial cells in the fornices of the papilla or pelvis that appear indistinguishable from normal cells covering the pelvis.

Atypical hyperplasia is characterized by the presence of cellular pleomorphism, nuclear abnormalities, alteration of cytologic polarity with respect to basement membranes, and increased mitotic activity. Being generally larger than transitional cell hyperplasia, but lacking poor demarcation and invasive growth, this lesion represents a precursor of transitional cell carcinoma.

Transitional cell carcinoma has a poorly demarcated lobular growth pattern, shows varying cellular atypia, tends to fill the pelvis and invade the adjacent renal structures, and metastasizes readily (Figs. 13 and 14). Mitotic figures may be frequent. Typically this tumor is associated with a prominent inflammatory reaction and areas of necrosis and hemorrhage are present in the larger lesions.

Squamous cell carcinoma consists entirely of neoplastic squamous epithelium, often contains abundant keratin, can elicit an extensive scirrhous response, and may metastasize. Squamous cell carcinomas are thought to arise from transitional cell epithelium that has undergone squamous metaplasia.

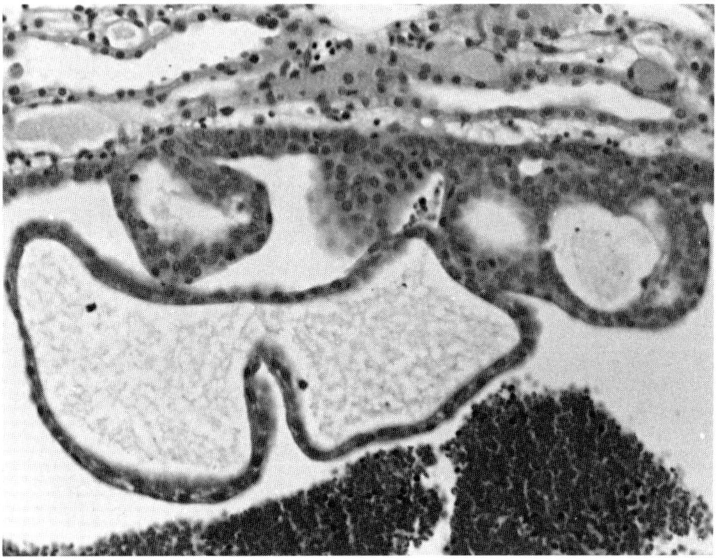

FIG. 11. Transitional cell hyperplasia in the pelvis of a male F344 rat treated with 210 μg/kg/day of ochratoxin A for 2 years (131). Note the absence of cellular atypia. (H&E × 180.)

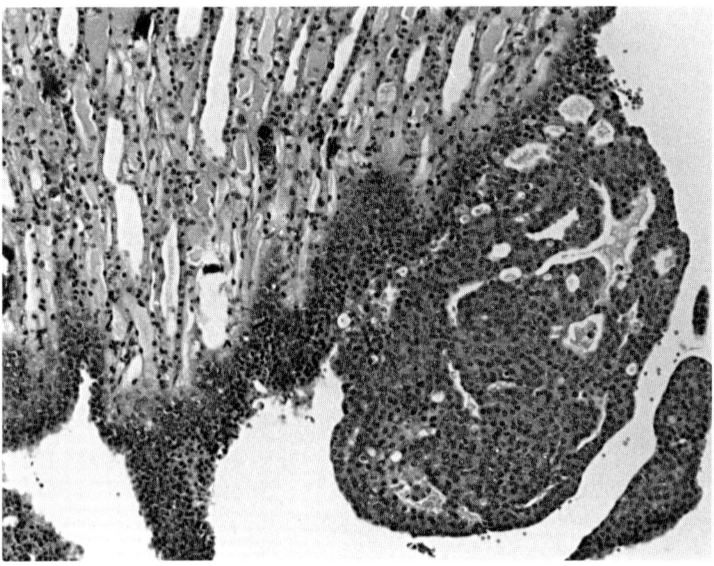

FIG. 12. Transitional cell hyperplasia in the pelvis of a male F344 rat treated with 500 mg/kg/day of dimethyl methylphosphonate for 2 years (292). Note the absence of cellular atypia. (H&E × 119.)

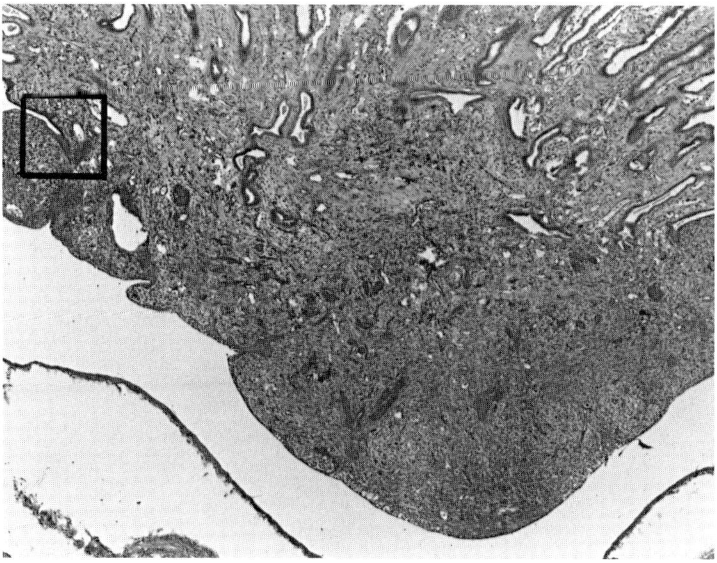

FIG. 13. Transitional cell carcinoma in the pelvis of a female F344 rat treated with 750 mg/kg/day of C.I. acid orange 3 for 2 years (200). Note the invasive characteristic of the lesion. (H&E × 36.)

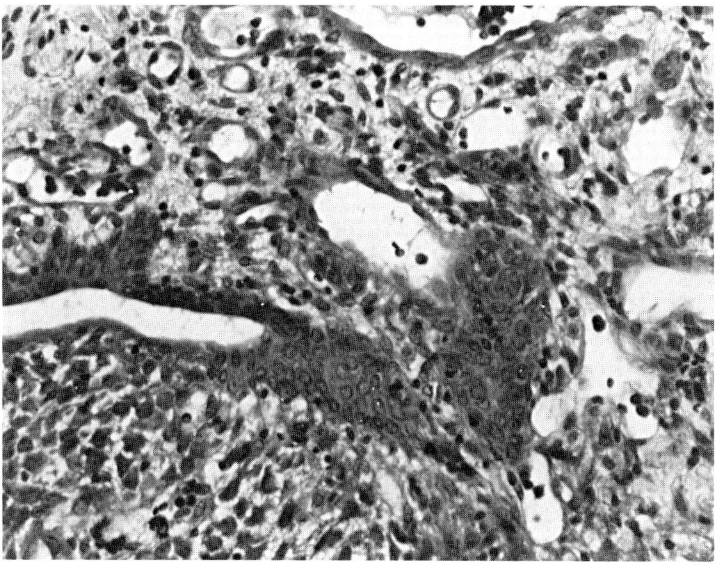

FIG. 14. High-power field of the encased area of the transitional cell carcinoma depicted in Fig. 13. Note the cellular heterogeneity and atypia as well as the invasive growth pattern. (H&E × 288.)

Incidence of Spontaneous RTCT

Perusal of the available literature revealed little information regarding the incidence of spontaneous RTCT. Solleveld and coworkers (25) observed an incidence of 0.04% for transitional cell carcinomas in control male and female F344 rats kept for 2 years. They also reported three papillomas (atypical hyperplasias) in 2,320 autopsied male F344 rats, whereas none were found in 2,370 female F344 rats. Goodman and coworkers (102) noted similar incidences of carcinomas in F344 rats, 0.6% and 0.11% in male and female rats, respectively. No papillomas were reported. On the other hand, 975 male and 970 female Osborne-Mendel rats kept for their lifespan, did not have any transitional cell carcinomas, whereas one papilloma was reported in a female rat. In humans the background incidence of RTCT has been estimated to be between 1 in 183,000 and 1 in 156,000 in Sweden (115).

Induction of RTCT

Chemical Induction

In a series of experiments RTCTs were induced in rats following treatment with nongenotoxic analgesics such as phenacetin, paracetamol (acetaminophen), caffeine, and phenazone (116–118). Genotoxic compounds, especially di-isopropanolnitrosamine (DIPN), MNU, and N-[4-(5-nitro-2-furyl)-2-thiazolyl]formamide (FANFT) have been associated in particular with the development of pelvic tumors (119,120). Renal transitional cell tumors in rats have also been reported in conjunction with barbital sodium (NaBB) and dimethyl methylphosphonate treatment (121–124).

In humans, the significant increase in incidence of RTCT has been associated with the abuse of analgesics, although not definitively demonstrated (113,125–127). Analgesic abuse has been very common in Switzerland, Sweden, and Australia. The estimated incidence of new cases of analgesic-associated pelvic tumors has risen from 240 (1963 to 1966) to 2,900 (1972 to 1977) per 100,000 inhabitants per year in Basel, Switzerland (115).

Bacterial Induction

A low number of RTCTs has been induced in female Sprague-Dawley rats following a single injection of a 0.5 ml suspension of *Escherichia coli* (06k13H1) into the bladder of the animals (119).

Mycotoxic Induction

High incidences of pelvic tumors have been reported in association with Balkan endemic nephropathy (BEN). In the Vratza district of Bulgaria, a region endemic for this nephropathy, Chernozemsky and coworkers (128) found hyperendemic villages with age-adjusted incidences of BEN and RTCT of 0.51% and 0.10% in females, and 0.32% and 0.09% in males, respectively. Analysis of the food staples in these areas revealed the presence of appreciable concentrations of ochratoxin A, a mycotoxin shown primarily to induce renal cell tumors in rats and mice (6,129–131). Although there is considerable evidence linking the presence of ochratoxin A in food staples with the development of mycotoxic porcine nephropathy (132) and BEN (130), the role of ochratoxin A in the formation of RTCT has yet to be elucidated.

ETIOLOGIC AGENTS

Since a large number and variety of agents have been shown to induce renal tumors, it would exceed the scope of this chapter to discuss them all individually. However, it is possible to group a great many of these agents under general agent classes, and thus general agent classes will be discussed. In addition, all etiologic agents are listed separately under their agent class, the abbreviation used in this chapter, the types of renal tumors that were induced, and in which species it was observed along with the corresponding literature reference (Table 4). Some of these agent classes have been treated in previous chapters of this book *in extentio*, thus only the most important aspects of these agents will be discussed and the reader will be referred to the respective chapter(s) for further reading.

Nitroso Compounds and Other Alkylating Agents

Nitrosamines and other nitroso derivatives have been shown to be highly reactive DNA-alkylating agents as well as potent renal carcinogens in experimental animals (4,7,36,133). Extensive studies of the carcinogenicity of dimethylnitrosamine (DMN) not only demonstrated that the incidence of tumors induced with DMN is largely dependent on its rate of metabolism, which can be modulated by the protein content of the diet (65), but also that specific nitrosamines induce only certain types of renal tumors (7,134). Renal cell tumors and RMTs have been induced following treatment with DMN, but neither NBs nor RTCTs have been reported (Table 4). The only NB in conjunction with DMN treatment was observed by Thomas and Schmaehl (135); however, the lack of a pathological description of this tumor prevents confirmation of it as NB, rather than RMT. On the other hand, *N*-butyl-*N*-(4-hydroxybutyl)nitrosamine (BHBN) predominantly induced RMT and RTCT in rats, whereas few RCT and no NB have been reported (36,136). In contrast to DMN and BHBN, *N*-ethylnitrosourea (ENU) given transplacentally to rabbits and rats primarily induced NB and only a few RCTs in the kidneys of the offspring (27–29). Single postnatal injections of ENU in mice induced RCT, but no NB, RMT, or RTCT (84). In addition, reports of histogenesis with other carcinogenic nitrosamines indicate that the origin of the preneoplastic and neoplastic lesions within the renal epithelial segment varies with the chemical. For instance, diethylnitrosamine (DEN) induces tumors of the P_2 and cortical P_3 segments (137), whereas DMN-induced tumors are believed to arise from the P_1 segment of the proximal convoluted tubule (85). Furthermore, *N*-nitrosomorpholine (NNM)-induced tumors were shown to originate from proximal convoluted tubules as well as from the intercalated cells of the collecting duct (91–93,138–142), whereas *N*-ethyl-*N*-hydroxyethylnitrosamine (EHEN)-induced tumors are believed to arise exclusively from the proximal convoluted tubules (90,143).

Cycasin, a component of the nut of *Cycas circinalis* L., is one of the best studied aliphatic carcinogens having DNA-alkylating capabilities (69,144,145). Cycasin induces not only all four types of kidney tumors, but also tumors in the lung, gall bladder, liver, and the intestine, which were reported in exposed rats, mice, and hamsters (144–148). Cycasin-related compounds such as methylazoxymethanol (MAM), 1,2-dimethylhydrazine, and 1,1-dimethylhydrazine have also been demonstrated to be kidney carcinogens in rats and mice (31,71,149). Other kidney tumor-inducing alkylating compounds not related to cycasin include streptozotocin and ethyl methanesulfonate (EMS) (35,70,72,133,150).

Arylamines and Amides

With respect to renal carcinogenesis, one of the most extensively studied compounds in this class is *N*-(4′-fluoro-4-biphenylyl)acetamide (FBPA). In all studies conducted with FBPA the development of RCT was reported (87,88,151,152). Several different stages of RCT development were observed (87,151) and it was suggested that these preneoplastic and neoplastic lesions originate in the proximal tubules, specifically in the P_3 segment of the cortical proximal tubule (88). The carcinogenicity of compounds such as FBPA or 2-acetylaminofluorene (2-AAF) is dependent on metabolic conversion to reactive metabolites via *N*-hydroxy derivatives (10).

Nitrofurans

Nitrofurans are potent carcinogens that induce tumors in a variety of organs, including the kidney, of mice and rats (153–155). The two best studied nitrofurans are 2-[4-(5-nitro-2-furyl)-2-thiazolyl]hydrazide (FNT) and *N*-[4-(5-nitro-2-furyl)-2-thiazolyl]formamide (FANFT). Although FNT induces RMT, RCT, and RTCT in the rat (156), only RTCT is reported following treatment of rats with FANFT (119, 157–159). Considering that the renal pelvis and bladder have a very similar morphology, it is not surprising that nitrofurans in general and specifically FANFT are potent bladder carcinogens (119,157–160).

Volatile Hydrocarbons and $\alpha_{2\mu}$-Globulin Nephropathy–Inducing Agents

A number of compounds including volatile hydrocarbons have been shown to induce renal tumors in male rats (Table 4). Characteristic to all these compounds is that the majority of them are nongenotoxic and that nephropathy and tumors are induced only in male rats but not in female rats or in either sex of mice, guinea pigs, dogs, or nonhuman primates (162–164). Indeed, studies with some of these compounds showed that the induction of renal neoplasia is preceded by a characteristic nephropathy, with the most consistent component being the accumulation of hyaline droplets containing the male rat–specific urinary protein $\alpha_{2\mu}$-globulin (165,166), single cell necrosis, and sustained increases in cell proliferation (100). The mechanisms by which these compounds exert their nephrotoxic and carcinogenic potentials are well understood and are discussed in the chapter by Lehman-McKeeman and in the section Mechanisms Involved in the Genesis of Renal Neoplasia, below.

Antibiotics and Analgesics

The antibiotic daunomycin, as well as the antischistosomal drug niridazol, induce renal tumors in rats and mice (167–169). More detailed information on the nephrotoxic potentials of antibiotics is given in the chapter by Tune. Analgesics such as phenacetin, acetaminophen, and phenazone have been closely associated with increased incidences of pelvic tumors in patients with confirmed abuse of analgesics (113,115,125–127). In experimental animals, the nongenotoxic phenacetin was shown to induce a low, but significantly increased incidence of renal pelvic and bladder tumors in treated rats (116). A more detailed discussion of the nephrotoxicity of analgesics is found in the chapter by Duggin.

Metal Compounds

Several metal compounds have been shown to be nephrotoxic and to induce renal neoplasia. The nephrotoxicity of metals, with emphasis on heavy metals, is discussed in the chapter by Conner and Fowler. The induction of renal neoplasia by metals was most intensively studied with lead acetate and nickel compounds (38,123,137,170). Although lead is not mutagenic in most test systems (171), it is a potent mitogen in the rat and mouse kidney (172,173) and decreases the fidelity of deoxyribonucleic acid (DNA) repair polymerases (174). Nickel acetate (NiA), on the other hand, has been observed to form increased concentrations of 8-hydroxy-2′-deoxyguanosine in DNA extracted from kidneys of exposed rats (123). It must be stated, however, that the link between 8-hydroxy-2′-deoxyguanosine and renal tumor formation has yet to be established.

Hormones

Estrogens including a variety of synthetic derivatives have been used to induce renal neoplasms in Syrian golden hamsters and in mice (3,40,47,105,175). The hamster model has been used to study the role of hormones in the neoplastic process (107,176–178). Estrogen-induced neoplasia in hamsters could be blocked by administration of antiestrogens, vitamin C (176,179), androgen, progesterone, or ethinyl estradiol (106). Further insight into the carcinogenic process of estrogen in Syrian golden hamsters was obtained by studying the effects of estrogen on cultured Syrian hamster proximal tubular cells. A proliferative response of these cells was observed after estrogen treatment in Syrian hamster proximal tubular cells but not in cultured cells of the same type isolated from either rat or guinea pig (180). Most recently, Liehr and coworkers (181) presented data that indicate that estrogen treatment of male Syrian hamsters resulted in the formation of estrogen metabolites that bind covalently to kidney DNA. Because of their target organ specificity, these adducts formed by endogenous electrophiles have been postulated to play an etiological role in tumor induction by estrogens.

Mycotoxins

One of the most potent renal carcinogens known today is ochratoxin A (OA), a mycotoxin produced by fungal strains within the genera *Aspergillus* and *Penicillium* (182). Ochratoxin A induced RCT in high incidences in rats and mice (131,183) and many of these tumors were metastatic carcinomas. It has to be pointed out that ochratoxin A is one of the most potent carcinogens among all of the nongenotoxic and many of the genotoxic carcinogens ever tested by the National Toxicology Program, in that it induces high incidences of RCT of a clearly malignant nature. Ochratoxin A has also been investigated for its role in Balkan endemic nephropathy and the high incidences of renal pelvic tumors observed in conjunction with this nephropathy (128–130). However, recent findings also point to a mycotoxin from *Penicillium aurantiogriseum* as the active agent in the Balkan endemic nephropathy (184). Thus, it appears that ochratoxin A may not be the only mycotoxin involved in the genesis of BEN-associated renal pelvic tumors (Dr. Gordon Hard, personal communication).

Other mycotoxins that induce renal tumors are citrinin and aflatoxin B_1, the former a product of the fungus *Penicillium viridicatum* (132) and the latter of *Aspergillus flavus* (185). More detailed information to the nephrotoxic potentials of mycotoxins are presented in chapter 17.

Radiation

Reports on the effects of radiation on neoplasia of the kidney are limited to rats and mice (47). Gamma rays were shown to specifically induce early changes in renal epithelial cells (186); thus, it is no surprise that only RCT and RTCT are reported in rats and mice following whole body irradiation (47,187).

Tumor Promoters

Various agents have been shown to increase the renal tumor incidence in experimental animals when given after a complete carcinogen such as a nitrosamine

(188–190). One characteristic inherent to these agents is their nephrotoxicity (4, 191). Increased cell proliferation rates can be a sequel to sustained nephrotoxicity, as was shown for sodium barbital (192). Increased cell proliferation could enhance fixation and clonal expansion of spontaneous and induced mutations, thus explaining the promoting potential of these agents (6,100). Clonal expansion of spontaneous mutations to veritable preneoplastic and neoplastic lesions would also explain the increased incidences of RCT and RTCT in rats following chronic administration of sodium barbital (NaBB) at high concentrations (121,123,124).

Other Agents

A wide variety of different agents can also induce renal neoplasia in experimental animals, including the polycyclic aromatic hydrocarbon, 7,12-dimethylbenzanthracene (DMBA); the halogenated hydrocarbon, chloroform (193,194); the cationic chelator, nitrilotriacetic acid (NTA) (195–197); the flame retardant, tris(2, 3-dibromopropyl) phosphate (198,199); the dye, C.I. acid orange 3 (200); the by-product of chlorinated aliphatic hydrocarbon synthesis, dichloroacetylene (201); the alcohol decomposition product, urethane (202); and the food additive, potassium bromate (203).

MECHANISMS INVOLVED IN THE GENESIS OF RENAL NEOPLASIA

Much research has been conducted in recent years to understand better the mechanisms involved in the induction of neoplasia. These efforts led to the discovery of many critical events in the pathogenesis of neoplasia (204) and to the understanding of the mechanisms involved in the tissue-specific carcinogenesis of yet a small number of compounds, such as the induction of skin papillomas by DMBA, mammary carcinomas induced in pregnant rats with NMU, or thymic lymphomas also induced with NMU (205). Despite these advances, the mechanisms responsible for the induction of cancer are not known for the majority of carcinogenic compounds.

Carcinogenesis is known to be a multistep process that involves two or more genetic events and requires cell proliferation (206–210). The genetic events can result from point mutations, chromosomal rearrangements, insertions or deletions of genes, and gene amplification. Cell proliferation is required to convert DNA damage to point mutations and for clonal expansion of initiated cells. Such clonal expansion increases the probability of additional genetic events occurring in initiated populations, leading to progression (211). In contrast to the liver, where an abundance of data has accumulated regarding the mechanisms of a variety of compounds involved in the genesis of liver tumors, there is a paucity of data pertaining to mechanisms in renal tumor formation. However, there are a few excellent examples of mechanisms in renal carcinogenesis including the effects of genotoxic and nongenotoxic chemicals, as well as hereditary factors, which will be reviewed in the following paragraphs.

Mechanism of Genotoxic Chemicals

A majority of renal carcinogens studied appear to act via a genotoxic/mutagenic mechanism, i.e., the chemicals or their metabolites interact with DNA. In general, a chemical carcinogen and/or its metabolite covalently binds to one of the bases in the DNA of a target cell. The chemical-DNA adduct can be translated into a heritable alteration (mutation) during DNA replication. This process leads to the formation of altered cells believed to be precursors for tumor formation.

One of the best studied mechanisms involving genotoxic chemicals is the induction of renal mesenchymal tumors by DMN. A single median lethal dose of DMN given to rats will induce RCT and RMT in about 20% of surviving animals (212), whereas it takes several doses of DMN to induce similar tumor incidences in the liver (213). The incidence of kidney tumors can be increased to 100% by temporary modification of dietary conditions (214). Swann and McLean (65) demonstrated that rats fed a diet deficient in protein become resistant to the acute toxic effects of DMN, permitting administration of a larger amount in a single dose. This resistance appeared to be the result of lower metabolism of DMN by liver and kidney of exposed rats. However, whereas the metabolism of the liver was reduced to 26% of normal by the protein-free diet, the DMN metabolism of the kidney was reduced to only 56% of normal (212). This selective inhibition of metabolism in the liver greatly increased the proportion of the dose metabolized in the kidney and thus increased the alkylation of kidney DNA. Indeed, the amount of alkylation of kidney DNA of rats fed protein-free diet was reported to be 1.7 times greater than the amount measured in the kidneys of rats on a normal diet. Furthermore, of the two major DNA adducts formed, 7-methylguanine and O^6-methylguanine, the potentially mutagenic O^6-methylguanine (215) was shown to be much longer lived in kidney than in liver DNA (216), thus possibly explaining the higher susceptibility of the kidney toward tumor induction. Nicoll and coworkers (216) also demonstrated that O^6-methylguanine was much longer lived in kidney DNA following a large dose of DMN that after a small dose (216), indicating that the enzyme system responsible for the removal of O^6-methylguanine, O^6-alkylguanine–DNA transferase, is saturable and is present in varying amounts in different organs (217–219).

Following the discovery that the dose-response curve for the methylation of kidney DNA by DMN is linear (53), one would expect that the dose-response curve for DMN-induced RMT would also be linearly related to dose. However, several studies showed that the dose-response curve for DMN-induced RMT is nonlinear, having a sigmoidal shape (53,212). No RMT developed after a single intraperitoneal injection with 2 mg DMN/kg (53). On the other hand, early lesions of RMT (50–52) were shown to follow a linear dose-response, were discovered even at doses that did not induce RMT, and the number of early lesions observed was found to be directly proportional to the amount of DNA methylation (53). No threshold was found for either methylation of kidney DNA or the formation of early lesions. Although these early lesions are present as early as 2 weeks after the administration of DMN and seem to represent precursors of RMT, not all early lesions develop into RMT (50–53). Apparently some of these early lesions regress, as was shown to be the case for precursors of RCT (6). It appears that both the regression of early lesions and the initial amount of DNA alkylation determine the shape of the final tumor dose-response curve.

Mechanisms of Nongenotoxic Chemicals

Nongenotoxic carcinogens obviously do not induce DNA damage themselves. However, nongenotoxic carcinogens can induce enhanced cell proliferation (220) and thus contribute to enhanced fixation of spontaneous mutations, leading to increased numbers of initiated cells, clonal expansion of such initiated cell populations, and the formation of tumors. Spontaneous mutations are assumed to stem from spontaneous genetic events such as depurination and deamination of DNA, formation of covalent DNA adducts by normal, active cellular metabolites, DNA damage by oxygen free-radicals produced in cellular metabolism, and errors in DNA replication (221). This assumption is corroborated by the observation that control animals of certain stocks and strains of laboratory rodents develop an appreciable incidence of preneoplastic lesions and spontaneous tumors (100,222). These incidences vary greatly from tissue to tissue, strain to strain, sex to sex, and species to species (6,222). A common feature of many nongenotoxic chemicals tested at high doses in carcinogenesis bioassays is the concurrent induction of cytotoxicity and/or hyperplasia in the same tissues of exposed rodents that develop neoplasia.

$\alpha_{2\mu}$-*Globulin Nephropathy–Inducing Agents*

One of the best studied chemically induced renal diseases resulting in renal tumors and believed to occur through a nongenotoxic mechanism is $\alpha_{2\mu}$-globulin nephropathy. This renal disease was shown to occur only in male rats. It does not occur in female rats or in either sex of any other rodent species, dogs, or nonhuman primates (162,163). It also does not occur in male NBR rats, a rat strain that does not synthesize this protein (166,223). Nongenotoxic chemicals and/or their metabolites that cause this syndrome, e.g., PS-6 unleaded gasoline, d-limonene, 1,4-dichlorobenzene, trimethylpentane, or isophorone, are not cytotoxic by themselves, but bind reversibly to $\alpha_{2\mu}$-globulin, leading to an accumulation of the chemical-protein complex in the lysosomes, cell necrosis, and compensatory cell proliferation.

$\alpha_{2\mu}$-Globulin is synthesized by the male rat liver, except in NBR rats (224), beginning at the onset of puberty and is excreted in great amounts via the urine (225,226). Approximately half of the $\alpha_{2\mu}$-globulin is reabsorbed by the proximal tubules of the renal cortex and enzymatically hydrolyzed to amino acids and peptides via lysosomal digestion (227). Possibly due to the relatively high resistance of $\alpha_{2\mu}$-globulin toward catabolism (228,229), this protein has a natural tendency to accumulate in the lysosomes of the P_2 segment of the proximal tubules (165,220).

Hyaline droplets observed in hematoxylin-eosin–stained tissue sections of control male rats often represent lysosomal accumulations of $\alpha_{2\mu}$-globulin. This site-specific accumulation of $\alpha_{2\mu}$-globulin can elicit slightly higher cell turnover of the affected cells in the P_2 segment of control male versus female rats (230).

The reversible binding of chemical and/or their metabolites to $\alpha_{2\mu}$-globulin, however, is thought to alter the protein, making it even less digestible (164,229). This results in an exacerbated accumulation of altered genesis in the lysosomes and in increased cell necrosis within the P_2 segment, which is thought to be due to a combination of lysosomal dysfunction, release of digestive enzymes into the cytoplasm, and decreased plasma membrane availability (231). Male rats treated with PS-6 unleaded gasoline or trimethylpentane were shown to compensate for the enhanced loss of proximal tubule cells by increasing the rate of cell proliferation in the P_2 segment. This sustained increase in cell proliferation exhibited a dose-response similar to that of renal tumor induction observed in male rats treated with unleaded gasoline in a 2-year bioassay (220,232). In an ensuing 65-week initiation-promotion study, using male and female F344 rats, with EHEN as the initiator and unleaded gasoline or trimethylpentane as the promoter, Short and coworkers (134) observed significant dose-related increases in the incidence of preneoplastic lesions such as atypical hyperplasia of basophilic, eosinophilic, and clear cell types in the male rat initiation-promotion, initiation-control, and promotion-control groups. In addition, a significant linear trend in the incidence of RCT was reported in male rats treated with unleaded gasoline. In female rats, on the other hand, neither the incidence of atypical cell foci nor RCT was elevated following promotion with unleaded gasoline or trimethylpentane (231). Increased P_2-cell proliferation rates and incidences of preneoplastic lesions and RCT were also reported from an initiation-promotion study using male F344 and the $\alpha_{2\mu}$-globulin–deficient male NBR rats, with EHEN as the initiator and d-limonene as the promoter (100). However, these increased P_2-cell proliferation rates and incidences of preneoplastic lesions and RCT only occurred in F344 rats, but not in NBR rats treated with EHEN and d-limonene or d-limonene alone. This indicates that the presence of $\alpha_{2\mu}$-globulin is mandatory for the formation of male rat kidney tumors by d-limonene. In addition, these experiments suggest that sustained increases in cell proliferation rates are causally related to the formation of preneoplastic and neoplastic lesions. The presence of low incidences and numbers of preneoplastic lesions in control groups of both rat strains corroborate the assumption that tumors induced by nongenotoxic chemicals stem from spontaneous mutations that progress to preneoplastic and neoplastic lesions.

Nitrilotriacetate

Chronic exposure to high concentrations of nitrilotriacetate (NTA) have been shown to induce sustained cytotoxicity, preneoplastic lesions, and RCT in either sex of rat and mouse (104,233). The earliest lesions observed are cells with cytoplasmic vacuolization, followed by sloughing and necrosis or proliferation of these cells, and the formation of hyperplastic foci of the eosinophilic, basophilic, or clear cell type (234–237). These latter lesions are thought to be precursors for the eosinophilic, basophilic, and clear cell adenomas and adenocarcinomas found in rats and mice chronically exposed to NTA (195,196). NTA, which is not metabolized in the mammalian system, is assumed to induce a redistribution of systemic zinc, leading to an increased resorption of zinc in the proximal tubules of the kidney. This site-specific increase in tissue zinc has been demonstrated to be a necessary condition for both the initiation and progression of the NTA-associated renal tubular toxicity that precedes and accompanies neoplasia at this site (233,238,239).

Renal Tumor Promoters

A number of nongenotoxic compounds have been shown to enhance tumor formation when administered to experimental animals after treatment with an alkylating agent as the initiator (Table 4). The mechanism of action has not been elucidated for any of these compounds; however, some effects appearing pertinent to renal tumor formation will be discussed. Some compounds such as NaBB, NDPS, FA, DL-serine, and β-C have been shown to be highly nephrotoxic (189,191,192). NaBB was reported to induce low incidences of RCT and RTCT when given at high concentrations (121,124,192). The nephrotoxicity of the aforementioned compounds was generally localized within the cortical epithelium and always associated with an enhanced regenerative response. In the cases of NaBB and NDPS, an increased rate of cell proliferation and/or the presence of increased numbers of preneoplastic lesions were observed (189,192). Although the mechanism of cytotoxicity for these compounds is unknown, it seems reasonable to assume that the increased rate of cell proliferation enhanced the possibility of mutations leading to the formation and progression of preneoplastic lesions to veritable tumors.

Hereditary Mechanisms

Renal tumors occur in humans and animals not only as a result of spontaneous formation or following exposure to carcinogenic agents, but also as a consequence of an inherited predisposition to cancer formation (240). *Human renal tumors* such as Wilms' tumor, von Hippel–Lindau disease, and familial renal cell carcinoma exist in the spontaneous as well as in the hereditary form. The hereditary form of Wilms' tumor, found in 1% of all Wilms' tumor cases (241), involves the formation of tumors in both kidneys of an affected patient and stands in contrast to the generally unilateral formation of renal tumors in spontaneous Wilms' tumor cases. Although deletions on the short arm of chromosome 11 can be detected in the spontaneous as well as the hereditary form of Wilms' tumor (241,242), the genetic alteration distinctly characteristic for the hereditary form has not been identified to date (243,244). However, the question arises as to whether the spontaneous form of Wilms' tumor really possesses a genetic alteration distinctly different from the hereditary form, or whether this genetic alteration is the same, with one being formed spontaneously, the other inherited. Indeed, recent advances in cytogenetic analysis of individuals with Wilms' tumor, have resulted in the isolation and cloning of a gene on human chromosome 11 (band 13) assumed to be responsible for the formation of Wilms' tumor (245,246).

Von Hippel–Lindau (VHL) disease is an autosomal dominant inherited disorder characterized by a predisposition to develop a variety of tumors, most frequently hemangioblastomas of the central nervous system and retina, renal cell carcinoma, pheochromocytoma and renal, pancreatic, and epididymal cysts (247). Renal cell carcinomas constitute a particularly frequent cause of death in this disorder, occurring as bilateral and multifocal tumors, and presenting at an earlier stage than spontaneous, nonhereditary cases of this tumor type (248). The inherited mutation (VHL gene) responsible for this disease has been mapped to the short arm of chromosome 3 (3p25) and appears to be linked to the locus encoding the human homologue of the *raf*-1 oncogene (248–250). However, crossovers with the VHL locus suggest that the defect responsible for the VHL phenotype is not a mutation in the *raf*-1 oncogene itself, but a mutation leading to the inactivation of a putative "tumor suppressor gene" (248,250).

Renal cell carcinoma may appear spontaneously or in the inherited form. The hereditary form is characterized by bilateral formation of renal cell carcinoma. An example of cytogenic alterations associated with the hereditary form of this disease is a constitutional cytogenetic defect, i.e., a balanced reciprocal translocation between chromosomes 3 and 8 (82,83,251,252). All family members presenting renal cell carcinoma had karyotypes with this translocation, whereas nonaffected family members had normal karyotypes (251). In other families with hereditary renal cell carcinoma, balanced translocations were described that occurred between chromosomes 3 and 6, or 3 and 11 (83,253). All these hereditary cases are thus associated with changes on chromosome 3, and in all of them the chromosome 3 breakpoint was located on the short arm (83). In some cases of the spontaneous form of renal cell carcinoma, loss of heterozygosity in alleles on the short arm of chromosome 3 have also been observed (254,255), indicating that the same putative tumor suppressor gene may be involved in both the spontaneous and hereditary form of this disease.

Deletion of DNA sequences on chromosome 3p may be associated with the initiation of renal cell carcinoma and is consistent with the cytogenetic alterations observed in tumor DNA (254) and with the hypothesis that inactivation of a tumor suppressor gene on 3p may be important in tumorigenesis as was suggested to be the case in von Hippel–Lindau disease (82,248,250). However, cases of familial renal cell carcinoma have been reported where no deletions or aberrations of chromosome 3 were observed (253). This observation allows two possible interpretations: (a) that there are a multitude of mechanisms by which tumors may be induced, or (b) that this observation is a result of an inactivation of the same suppressor gene by point mutations or deletions unobservable at the level of cytogenetics.

In animals, only two hereditary forms are known: multifocal renal cell tumors of the shepherd dog (79,80) and bilateral renal cell tumors of the rat carrying the Eker mutation (81,256,257). Very little is known to date on the etiology of hereditary renal tumors of the shepherd dog. The only indication for a hereditary mechanism is the simultaneous formation of tumors in both kidneys in 90% of affected dogs (80). In rats carrying the Eker mutation, a single gene mutation predisposes to renal cell carcinoma with an autosomal dominant pattern of inheritance (81,256,257); 100% of the heterozygous animals, which inherit one copy of the mutation, develop renal cell tumors. Homozygosity for the mutation is lethal, whereas animals that inherit two normal copies of the gene remain normal with respect to tumor formation (81). Funaki and coworkers (258) cytogenetically analyzed cell lines derived from the hereditary Eker rat renal cell carcinomas and reported loss and/or deletion of chromosome 5 and 6 in all seven cell lines examined, as well as alterations in chromosomes 5 and 6 primary tumor cells. In addition, expression of epithelial growth factor (EGF) receptor transcripts and overexpression of transforming growth factor–α(TGFα) by the cell lines was observed. Increased expression of TGFα was also detected in renal cell tumor tissue, indicating that altered expression of this growth factor occurred during tumor formation and progression (259). These results compare well with observations made for human renal cell carcinoma, where both primary tumors and tumor-derived cell lines have consistently been reported to overexpress TGFα (260–262). Loss and/or deletion of chromosome(s) are reported in human renal cell carcinoma as well as in Eker rat tumors, suggesting that loss of a tumor suppressor gene(s), as implicated in human renal cell carcinoma, may be involved in tumor development of the hereditary Eker rat renal tumors. Additional understanding of von Hippel–Lindau disease, as well as the role of tumor suppressor genes in renal cell tumors, may be sought by using this Eker rat model, especially as the renal cell tumors observed in rats are comparable in histology and biochemistry to the renal cell tumors observed in humans (2,5). Furthermore, Eker rats also develop hemangioblastomas, similar to those reported in von Hippel–Lindau disease (personal communication by Dr. J. Everitt).

CONCLUSIONS

In reviewing the literature it became apparent that the pathology (nomenclature, histology, biochemistry) of renal tumors in animals and humans is very similar. However, this review also shows the paucity of data pertaining to mechanisms of renal tumor induction and progression. The most recent developments with emphasis on a more generalized nomenclature in the pathology of renal tumors, including preneoplastic lesions, should facilitate interpretation and comparison of data, and thus should eventually lead to a better insight into the mechanisms involved in renal carcinogenesis.

ACKNOWLEDGMENTS

We are indebted to Drs. C. Walker and J. Everitt for helpful comments regarding hereditary tumors, the Eker rat model, and for reviewing this chapter. We also would like to thank Dr. G. Hard for allowing us to use some of his photographs as well as for the comments pertaining to the nomenclature and pathology of renal lesions. Furthermore, the efforts by the personnel of the NTP Archives in locating lesions for photography are gratefully acknowledged. Finally we would like to thank C. Dietrich for preparing the photographs and for typing parts of this manuscript.

REFERENCES

1. Mostofi FK. Tumors of the renal parenchyma. In: Churg J, Spargo BH, Mostofi FK, Abell MR, eds. *Kidney disease: present status*, vol 1. Baltimore: Williams & Wilkins, 1979;356–412.
2. Thoenes W, Stoerkel St, Rumperl HJ. Histopathology and classification of renal cell tumors (adenomas, oncocytomas and carcinomas). *Pathol Res Pract* 1986;181:125–143.
3. Hamilton JM. Renal carcinogenesis. *Adv Cancer Res* 1975;22:1–56.
4. Hiasa Y, Ito N. Experimental induction of renal tumors. *CRC Crit Rev Toxicol* 1987;17(4):279–343.
5. Bannasch P, Zerban H. Animal models and renal carcinogenesis. In: Eble JN, ed. *Contemporary issues of surgical pathology*, New York: Churchill Livingstone, 1990;1–34.
6. Dietrich DR, Swenberg JA. Preneoplastic lesions in rodent kidney induced spontaneously or by genotoxic agents: predictive nature and comparison to lesions induced by genotoxic carcinogens. *Mutat Res* 1991;248:239–260.
7. Hard GC. Experimental models for the sequential analysis of chemically induced renal carcinogenesis. *Toxicol Pathol* 1986;1:112–122.
8. Bennington JL, Kradjian RM. *Renal carcinoma*. Philadelphia: Saunders, 1967.
9. Lipsky MM, Trump BF. Chemically induced renal epithelial neoplasia in experimental animals. *Int Rev Exp Pathol* 1988;30:357–383.
10. Hard GC. Comparative oncology. I. Nephroblastoma in laboratory mammals. In: Pochedly C, Baum ES, eds. *Wilms' tumor, clinical and biological manifestations*. New York: Elsevier, 1984;147–167.
11. Hard GC. Comparative oncology. II. Nephroblastoma in domesticated and wild animals. In: Pochedly C, Baum ES, eds. *Wilms' tumor, clinical and biological manifestations*. New York: Elsevier, 1984;169–189.
12. Baskin GB, De Paoli A. Primary renal neoplasms of the dog. *Vet Pathol* 1977;14:591–605.
13. Bennett BT, Beluhan FZ, Welsh TJ. Malignant nephroblastoma in *Macaca fascicularis*. *Lab Animal Sci* 1982;32(4):403–404.
14. Green HSN. The occurrence and transplantation of embryonal nephromas in the rabbit. *Cancer Res* 1943;3:434–440.
15. Hard GC, Noble R. Occurrence, transplantation, and histologic characteristics of nephroblastoma in the Nb Hooded rat. *Invest Urol* 1981;18(5):371–376.
16. Jubb KVF, Kennedy PC, Palmer N. *Pathology of domestic animals*, 3rd ed. San Diego: Academic Press, 1985.
17. Middle JG, Robinson G, Embleton MJ. Naturally arising tumors of the inbred WAB/Not rat strain. I. Classification, age and sex distribution, and transplantation behavior. *J Natl Cancer Inst* 1981; 67(3):629–636.
18. Prejean JD, Peckham JC, Casey AE, Griswold DP, Weisburger EK, Weisburger JH. Spontaneous tumors in Sprague-Dawley rats and Swiss mice. *Cancer Res* 1973;33:2768–2773.
19. Hard GC. Mesenchymal tumour, kidney, rat. In: Jones TC, Mohr U, Hunt RD, eds. *Monographs on pathology of laboratory animals, urinary system*. Berlin, Heidelberg, New York: Springer-Verlag, 1986;61–71.
20. Bennington JL, Beckwith JR. *Atlas of tumor pathology: tumors of the kidney, renal pelvis and ureter*. American Forces Institute of Pathology, Bethesda, MD: 1975.
21. Miller RW, Fraumeni JF, Manning MD. Association of Wilms' tumor with aniridia, hemihypertrophy and other congenital malformations. *N Engl J Med* 1964;270(18):922–927.
22. Bove KE, McAdams AJ. The nephroblastomatosis complex and its relationship to Wilms' tumor: a clinicopathologic treatise. *Perspect Pediatr Pathol* 1976;3:185–223.

23. Riccardi VM, Sujansky E, Smith AC, Francke U. Chromosomal imbalance in the Aniridia-Wilms' tumor association: 11p interstitial deletion. *Pediatrics* 1978;61(4):604–610.
24. Lewis R. Wilms' tumor: The genetic plot thickens. *J NIH Res* 1990;2:72–77.
25. Solleveld HA, Haseman JK, McConnell EE. Natural history of body weight gain, survival, and neoplasia in the F344 rat. *J Natl Cancer Inst* 1984;72(4):929–940.
26. Sandison AT, Anderson LJ. Tumors of the kidney in cattle, sheep, and pigs. *Cancer Res* 1968; 21:727–742.
27. Fox RR, Diwan BA, Meier H. Transplacental induction of primary renal tumors in rabbits treated with 1-ethyl-1-nitrosourea. *J Natl Cancer Inst* 1975;54(6):1439–1448.
28. Hard GC, Fox RR. Electron-microscopic analysis of nephroblastomas induced transplacentally in the IIIVO/J rabbit by a single dose of N-ethylnitrosourea. *Am J Pathol* 1984;117(2):239–251.
29. Hard GC, Fox RR. Histologic characterization of renal tumors (nephroblastomas) induced transplacentally in IIIVO/J and WH/J rabbits by N-ethylnitrosourea. *Am J Pathol* 1983;113(1):8–18.
30. Jurgelski W, Hudson P, Falk HL. Tissue differentiation and susceptibility to embryonal tumour induction by ethylnitrosourea in the opossum. *Natl Cancer Inst Monogr* 1979;51:123–158.
31. Hawks A, Hicks RM, Holsman JW, Magee PN. Morphological and biochemical effects of 1,2-dimethylhydrazine and 1-methylhydrazine in rats and mice. *Br J Cancer* 1974;30:429–439.
32. Jasmin G, Riopelle JL. Nephroblastomas induced in ovariectomized rats by dimethylbenzanthracene. *Cancer Res* 1970;30:321–326.
33. Turusov VA, Alexandrov VA, Timoshenko IV. Nephroblastoma and renal mesenchymal tumour induced in rats by N-nitrosoethyl- and N-nitrosomethylurea. *Neoplasma* 1980;27:229–235.
34. Hara H, Miyao M, Moriki T, Kutsukake F, Yamane T. Histological and ultrastructural studies of nephroblastoma in rats induced transplacentally by ethylnitrosourea. *Acta Pathol Jpn* 1982;32: 385–398.
35. Hard GC. Identification of a high-frequency model for renal carcinoma by the induction of renal tumours in the mouse with a single dose of streptozotocin. *Cancer Res* 1985;45:703–708.
36. Ito N, Hiasa Y, Kamamoto Y, Makiura S, Sugihara S, Marugami M, Okajima E. Histopathological analysis of kidney tumors in rats induced by chemical carcinogens. *GANN* 1971;62:435–444.
37. Riopelle JL, Jasmin G. Nature, classification, and nomenclature of kidney tumours induced in the rat by dimethylnitrosamine. *J Natl Cancer Inst* 1969;42:643–662.
38. Sunderman FW, McCully KS, Hopfer SM. Association between erythrocytosis and renal cancers in rats following intrarenal injection of nickel compounds. *Carcinogenesis* 1984;5(11):1511–1517.
39. Hendricks JD, Scanlan RA, Williams JL, Sinnhuber RO, Grieco MP. Carcinogenicity of N-methyl-N′-nitro-N-nitroguanidine to the livers and kidneys of rainbow trout (*Salmo gairdneri*) exposed as embryos. *J Natl Cancer Inst* 1980;64(6):1511–1519.
40. Kirkman H. Autonomous derivatives of estrogen-induced renal carcinomas and spontaneous renal tumors in the Syrian hamster. *Cancer Res* 1974;34:2728–2744.
41. Llombart-Bosch A, Peydro A. Morphological, histochemical and ultrastructural observations of diethylstilboestrol-induced kidney tumors in the Syrian golden hamster. *Eur J Cancer* 1975;11: 403–412.
42. Ishiguro H, Beard D, Sommer JR, Heine U, de The G, Beard JW. Multiplicity of cell response to the BAI strain A (myeloblastosis) avian tumor virus. I. Nephroblastoma (Wilms' tumor): gross and microscopic pathology. *J Natl Cancer Inst* 1962;29:1–39.
43. Heine U, de The G, Ishiguro H, Sommer JR, Beard D, Beard JW. Multiplicity of cell response to the BAI strain A (myeloblastosis) avian tumor virus. II. Nephroblastoma (Wilms' tumor): ultrastructure. *J Natl Cancer Inst* 1962;29:41–105.
44. Ogura H, Gelderblom H, Bauer H. Isolation of avian nephroblastoma virus from avian myeloblastosis virus by the infections DNA technique. *Intervirology* 1974;4:69–76.
45. Beard JW, Chabot JF, Beard D, Heine U, Houts GE. Renal neoplastic response to leukosis virus strains BAI A (avian myeloblastosis virus) and MC29. *Cancer Res* 1976;36:339–353.
46. Fitts RH. Bilateral feline embryonal sarcoma. *J Am Vet Med Assoc* 1960;136(12):616.
47. Guerin M, Chouroulinkov I, Riviere MR. Experimental kidney tumors. In: Rouiller C, Mueller AF, eds. *The kidney, morphology, biochemistry, physiology*, vol 2. New York: Academic Press, 1969;199–268.
48. Horn HA, Stewart HL. A review of some spontaneous tumours in noninbred mice. *J Natl Cancer Inst* 1952;13:591–603.
49. Jones SR, Casey HW. Primary renal tumours in nonhuman primates. *Vet Pathol* 1981;18(6):89–104.

50. Hard GC, Butler W. Cellular analysis of renal neoplasia: light microscope study of the development of interstitial lesions induced in the rat kidney by a single carcinogenic dose of dimethylnitrosamine. *Cancer Res* 1970;30:2806–2815.
51. Hard GC, Butler WH. Ultrastructural study of the development of interstitial lesions leading to mesenchymal neoplasia induced in the rat renal cortex by dimethylnitrosamine. *Cancer Res* 1971;31:337–347.
52. Hard GC, Butler W. Ultrastructural analysis of renal mesenchymal tumor induced in the rat by dimethylnitrosamine. *Cancer Res* 1971;31:348–365.
53. Driver HE, White INH, Butler WH. Dose response relationships in chemical carcinogenesis: renal mesenchymal tumours induced in the rat by a single dose of dimethylnitrosamine. *Br J Exp Pathol* 1987;68:133–143.
54. Beckwith JB, Palmer NF. Histopathology and prognosis of Wilms' tumor. *Cancer Res* 1978; 41:1937–1948.
55. Bolande RP, Brough AJ, Izant RJ. Congenital mesoblastic nephroma of infancy. *Pediatrics* 1967;40(2):272–278.
56. Marsden HB, Lawler W. Bone metastasizing renal tumour of childhood. *Virchows Arch [A]* 1980;387:341–351.
57. Marsden HB, Lawler W, Kumar PM. Bone metastasizing renal tumor of childhood. *Cancer Res* 1978;42:1922–1928.
58. Morgan E, Kidd JM. Undifferentiated sarcoma of the kidney. *Cancer Res* 1978;42:1916–1921.
59. Penchansky L, Gallo G. Rhabdomyosarcoma of the kidney in children. *Cancer Res* 1979;44:285–292.
60. Golji H. Tuberous selerosis and renal neoplasms. *J Urol* 1961;85(6):919–923.
61. Gilbert C, Gillman J. Spontaneous neoplasms in the albino rat. *S Afr J Med Sci* 1958;23:257–272.
62. Goodman G, Ward JM, Squire RA, et al. Neoplastic and nonneoplastic lesions in aging Osborne-Mendel rats. *Toxicol Appl Pharmacol* 1980;55:433–447.
63. Slye M, Holmes HF, Wells HG. Primary spontaneous tumors in the kidney and adrenal of mice. *Cancer Res* 1921;6:305–336.
64. Kent SP, Pickering JE. Neoplasms in monkeys (*Macaca mulatta*): spontaneous and irradiaton induced. *Cancer Res* 1958;11(1):138–147.
65. Swann P, McLean A. Cellular injury and carcinogenesis: the effect of a protein-free high-carbohydrate diet on the metabolism of dimethylnitrosamine in the rat. *J Biochem* 1971;124:283–288.
66. Hard GC. Effect of age at treatment on incidence and type of renal neoplasm induced in the rat by a single dose of dimethylnitrosamine. *Cancer Res* 1979;39:4965–4970.
67. Murphy GP, Mirand EA, Johnston GS, Schmidt JD, Scott WW. Renal tumors induced by single dose of dimethylnitrosamine: morphologic, functional, enzymatic and hormonal characterizations. *Invest Urol* 1966;4:39–56.
68. Laqueur GL, Matsumoto H. Neoplasms in female Fischer rats following intraperitoneal injection of methylazoxymethanol. *J Natl Cancer Inst* 1966;37:217–232.
69. Laqueur GL, Mickelsen O, Whiting MG, Kurland LT. Carcinogenic properties of nuts from *Cycas circinalis L.* indigenous to Guam. *J Natl Cancer Inst* 1963;31:919–951.
70. Swann PF, Magee PM. Induction of rat kidney tumours by ethyl methanesulfonate and nervous tissue tumours by methyl methanesulfonate and ethyl methanesulfonate. *Nature* 1969;223:947–949.
71. Sunter JP, Senior PV. Induction of renal tumours in rats by the administration of 1,2-dimethylhydrazine. *J Pathol* 1983;140:69–76.
72. Horton L, Fox C, Corrin B, Soenksen PH. Streptozotocin-induced renal tumours in rats. *Br J Cancer* 1977;36:692–699.
73. Leaver DD, Swann PF, Magee PN. The induction of tumours in the rat by a single oral dose of N-nitrosomethylurea. *Br J Cancer* 1969;23:177–187.
74. Terracini B, Testa MC, Cabral JR, Rossi L. The roles of age at treatment and dose in carcinogenesis in C3Hf/Dp mice with a single administration of N-nitroso-N-methylurea. *Br J Cancer* 1976; 33:427–439.
75. Desselberger U, Georgii A, Zobl H, Ostertag H. On the oncogenic activity of polyomavirus in the rat. *Zentralbl Bakteriol Mikrobial Hyg [A]* 1972;219:28–38.
76. Georgii A, Thiele J, Reale E. Die Feinstruktur eines Polyomavirus-induzierten Sarkoms der Rattenniere waehrend seines Wachstums. *Z Krebsforschung* 1973;80:255–264.
77. Haschek WM, King JM, Tennant BC. Primary renal cell carcinomas in two horses. *J Am Vet Med Assoc* 1981;179(10):992–994.

78. Lucke B. Kidney carcinoma in the Leopard frog: a virus tumor. *Ann NY Acad Sci* 1952;54:1093–1109.
79. Yang YH. The multicentric renal adenocarcinomas in situ of a dog. *Pathol Microbiol* 1966; 29:181–185.
80. Lium B, Moe L. Hereditary multifocal renal cystadenocarcinomas and nodular dermatofibrosis in the German shepherd dog: macroscopic and histopathologic changes. *Vet Pathol* 1985;22:447–455.
81. Eker R, Mossige J, Johannessen JV, Aars H. Hereditary renal adenomas and adenocarcinomas in rats. *Diagn Histopathol* 1981;4:99–110.
82. Li FP. Cancer families: human models of susceptibility to neoplasia—the Richard and Hinda Rosenthal Foundation Award Lecture. *Cancer Res* 1988;48:5381–5386.
83. Daniel LN, Linehan WM. Genetics of renal cell carcinoma. *Semin Urol* 1989;4:258–263.
84. Lombard LS, Rice JM, Vesselinovitch SD. Renal tumours in mice: light microscopic observations of epithelial tumours induced by ethylnitrosourea. *J Natl Cancer Inst* 1974;53:1677–1685.
85. Hard GC, Butler WH. Ultrastructural aspects of renal adenocarcinoma induced in the rat by dimethylnitrosamine. *Cancer Res* 1971;31:366–372.
86. Hard GC, Butler WH. Morphogenesis of epithelial neoplasms induced in the rat kidney by dimethylnitrosamine. *Cancer Res* 1971;31:1496–1505.
87. Dees JH, Heatfield BM, Reuber MD, Trump BJ. Adenocarcinoma of the kidney. III. Histogenesis of renal adenocarcinomas induced in rats by N-(4′-fluoro-4-biphenylyl)acetamide. *J Natl Cancer Inst* 1980;64:1537–1545.
88. Dees JH, Heatfield BM, Trump BJ. Adenocarcinoma of the kidney. IV. Electron microscopic study of the development of renal adenocarcinomas induced in rats by N-(4′-fluoro-4-biphenylyl)acetamide. *J Natl Cancer Inst* 1980;64:1547–1562.
89. Tsuda H, Sakata T, Tamano S, Okumura M, Ito N. Sequential observations on the appearance of neoplastic lesions in the liver and kidney after treatment with N-ethyl-N-hydroxyethylnitrosamine followed by partial hepatectomy and unilateral nephrectomy. *Carcinogenesis* 1983;4:523–528.
90. Tsuda H, Hacker HJ, Katayama H, Masui T, Ito N, Bannasch P. Correlative histochemical studies on preneoplastic and neoplastic lesions in the kidney of rats treated with nitrosamines. *Virchows Arch [B]* 1986;51:385–404.
91. Bannasch P, Schacht U, Storch E. Morphogenese und Mikromorphologie epithelialer Nierentumoren bei Nitrosomorpholin-vergifteten Ratten. I. Induktion und Histologie der Tumoren. *Z Krebsforsch* 1974;81:311–331.
92. Bannasch P, Krech R, Zerban H. Morphogenese und Mikromorphologie epithelialer Nierentumoren bei Nitrosomorpholin-vergifteten Ratten. II. Tubulaere Glykogenose und die Genese von klar- und acidophilzelligen Tumoren. *Z Krebsforsch* 1978;92:63–86.
93. Bannasch P, Krech R, Zerban H. Morphogenese und Mikromorphologie epithelialer Nierentumoren bei Nitrosomorpholin-vergifteten Ratten. III. Onkocytentubuli und Onkocytome. *Z Krebsforsch* 1978;92:87–104.
94. Bannasch P, Krech R, Zerban H. Morphogenese und Mikromorphologie epithelialer Nierentumoren bei Nitrosomorpholin-vergifteten Ratten. IV. Tubulaere Laesionen und basophile Tumoren. *J Cancer Res Clin Oncol* 1980;98:243–265.
95. Thoenes W, Stoerkel S, Rumpelt HJ. Human chromophobe cell renal carcinoma. *Virchows Arch [B]* 1985;48:204–217.
96. Thoenes W, Stoerkel S, Rumpelt HJ, Moll R, Baum HP, Werner S. Chromophobe cell renal carcinoma and its variants—a report on 32 cases. *J Pathol* 1988;155:277–287.
97. Stoerkel S, Pannen B, Thoenes W, Steart PV, Wagner S, Drenckhahn D. Intercalated cells as a probable source for the development of renal oncocytomas. *Virchows Arch [B]* 1988;56:185–189.
98. Stoerkel S, Steart PV, Drenckhahn D, Thoenes W. The human chromophobe cell renal carcinoma: its probable relation to intercalated cells of the collecting duct. *Virchows Arch [B]* 1988;56:237–245.
99. Bannasch P, Nogueira E, Zerban H. Zytologie und Zytogenese experimenteller epithelialer Nierentumoren. *Verh Dtsch Ges Pathol* 1989;73:301–313.
100. Dietrich DR, Swenberg JA. The presence of alpha$_{2\mu}$-globulin is necessary for d-limonene promotion of male rat kidney tumors. *Cancer Res* 1991;51:3512–3521.
101. Shinohara Y, Frith CH. Morphologic characteristics of benign and malignant renal cell tumours in control and 2-acetylaminofluorene-treated BALB/c female mice. *Am J Pathol* 1980;100:455–468.
102. Goodman DG, Ward JM, Squire RA, Chu KC, Linhart MS. Neoplastic and nonneoplastic lesions in aging F344 rats. *Toxicol Appl Pharmacol* 1979;48:237–248.

103. Fortner J. Spontaneous tumors, including gastrointestinal neoplasms, and malignant melanomas in the Syrian hamster. *Cancer Res* 1957;10:1153–1156.
104. Li JL, Okada S, Hamazaki S, Ebina Y, Midorikawa O. Subacute nephrotoxicity and induction of renal cell carcinoma in mice treated with ferric nitrilotriacetate. *Cancer Res* 1987;47:1867–1869.
105. Richardson FL. Incidence of mammary and pituitary tumours in hybrid mice treated with stilbestrol for varying periods. *J Natl Cancer Inst* 1957;18:813–829.
106. Li JJ, Li SA. Estrogen carcinogenesis in hamster tissues: a critical review. *Endocr Rev* 1990; 11(4):524–531.
107. Bloom HJG, Dukes CE, Mitchley BCV. Hormone dependent tumours of the kidney. I. The oestrogen induced renal tumour of the Syrian hamster. Hormone treatment and possible relationship to carcinoma of the kidney in man. *Br J Cancer* 1963;17:611–645.
108. Horning ES, Whittick JW. The histogenesis of stilbestrol-induced renal tumours in the male golden hamster. *Br J Cancer* 1954;8(2):451–457.
109. Hacker HJ, Bannasch P, Liehr JG. Histochemical analysis of the development of estradiol-induced kidney tumors in male Syrian hamsters. *Cancer Res* 1988;48:971–976.
110. Gonzalez A, Oberley TD, Li JJ. Morphological and immunohistochemical studies of the estrogen-induced Syrian hamster renal tumor: probable cell of origin. *Cancer Res* 1989;49:1020–1028.
111. Montgomery CA, Seely JC. Kidney. In: Boorman GA, Eustis SL, Elwell MR, Montgomery CA, Mackenzie WF, eds. *Pathology of the Fischer rat*. San Diego: Academic Press, 1990;127–153.
112. Wimberly HC, Lewis RM. Transitional cell carcinoma in the domestic cat. *Vet Pathol* 1979; 16:223–228.
113. Bach PH, Gregg NJ. Experimentally induced renal papillary necrosis and upper urothelial carcinoma. *Int Rev Exp Pathol* 1988;30:1–54.
114. Hard GC, Alden CL, Stula EF, Trump BF. Proliferative lesions of the kidney in rats. Society of Toxicologic Pathologists. *Standard System of Nomenclature and Diagnostic Pathology* 1993;in press.
115. Bach PH, Bridges JW. Chemically induced renal papillary necrosis and upper urothelial carcinoma. *CRC Crit Rev Toxicol* 1985;15(3):217–329.
116. Johansson SL. Carcinogenicity of analgesics: long-term treatment of Sprague-Dawley rats with phenacetin, phenazone, caffeine, and paracetamol (acetaminophen). *Int J Cancer* 1981;27:521–529.
117. Johansson SL, Angervall L. Urothelial hyperplasia of the renal papillae in female Sprague-Dawley rats induced by long-term feeding of phenacetin. *Acta Pathol Microbiol Scand Sect A* 1976; 84:353–354.
118. Johansson SL, Angervall L. Urothelial changes of the renal papillae in Sprague-Dawley rats induced by long-term feeding of phenacetin. *Acta Pathol Microbiol Scand Sect A* 1976;84:375–383.
119. Johansson SL, Anderstroem C, von Schultz L, Larson P. Enhancement of N-[4-(5-Nitro-2-furyl)-2-thiazolyl]formamide-induced carcinogenesis by urinary tract infection in rats. *Cancer Res* 1987;47:559–562.
120. Reznik G, Mohr U. Induction of renal pelvic tumours in Sprague-Dawley rats by di-isopropanolnitrosamine. Cancer Lett 1976;2:87–92.
121. Diwan BA, Nims RW, Ward JM, Hu H, Lubet RA, Rice JM. Tumor promoting activities of ethylphenylacetylurea and diethylacetylurea, the ring hydrolysis products of barbiturate tumor promoters phenobarbital and barbital, in rat liver and kidney initiated by N-nitrosodiethylamine. *Carcinogenesis* 1989;10(1):189–194.
122. Dunnick JK, Eustis SL, Haseman JK. Development of kidney tumors in the male F344/N rat after treatment with dimethyl methylphosphonate. *Fundam Appl Toxicol* 1988;11:91–99.
123. Kasprzak KS, Diwan BA, Konishi N, Misra M, Rice JM. Initiation by nickel acetate and promotion by sodium barbital of renal cortical epithelial tumors in male F344 rats. *Carcinogenesis* 1990,11(4):647–652.
124. Konishi N, Diwan BA, Ward JM. Amelioration of sodium barbital-induced nephropathy and regenerative tubular hyperplasia after a single injection of streptozotocin does not abolish the renal tumor promoting effect of barbital sodium in male F344/NCr rats. *Carcinogenesis* 1990; 11(12):2149–2156.
125. McCredie M, Ford JM, Taylor JS, Stewart JH. Analgesics and cancer of renal pelvis in New South Wales. *Cancer Res* 1982;49:2617–2625.
126. McCredie M, Stewart JH, Mahony JF. Is phenacetin responsible for analgesic nephropathy in New South Wales? *Clin Nephrol* 1982;17(3):134–140.

127. McCredie M, Stewart JH, Ford JM, MacLennan RA. Phenacetin-containing analgesics and cancer of the bladder or renal pelvis in women. *Br J Urol* 1983;55:220–224.
128. Chernozemsky IN, Stoyanov IS, Petkova-Bocharova TK, et al. Geographic correlation between the occurrence of endemic nephropathy and urinary tract tumours in Vratza district, Bulgaria. *Int J Cancer* 1977;19:1–11.
129. Petkova-Bocharova T, Castegnaro M. Ochratoxin A contamination of cereals in an area of high incidence of Balkan endemic nephropathy in Bulgaria. *Food Addit Contam* 1985;2(4):267–270.
130. Castegnaro M, Bartsch H, Cherozemsky I. Endemic nephropathy and urinary tract tumors in the Balkans. *Cancer Res* 1987;47:3608–3609.
131. National Toxicology Program. Toxicology and carcinogenesis studies of ochratoxin A in F344/N rats. *Tech Rep No 358* 1989.
132. Krogh P, Hald B, Pedersen EJ. Occurrence of ochratoxin A and citrinin in cereals associated with mycotoxic porcine nephropathy. *Acta Pathol Microbiol Scand Sect B* 1973;81:689–695
133. International Agency for Research on Cancer. *IARC monographs on the evaluation of the carcinogenic risk of chemicals to humans*, vol 17 Lyon: 1978.
134. Short BG, Steinhagen WH, Swenberg JA. Promoting effects of unleaded gasoline and 2,2,3-trimethylpentane on the development of atypical cell foci and renal tubular cell tumors in rats exposed to N-ethyl-N-hydroxyethylnitrosamine. *Cancer Res* 1989;49:6369–6378.
135. Thomas C, Schmaehl D. Zur Morphologie der Nierentumoren bei der Ratte. *Z Krebsforsch* 1964;66:125–137.
136. Fukushima S, Hirose M, Hagiwara A, Hasegawa R, Ito N. Inhibitory effect of 4,4′-diaminodiphenylmethane on liver, kidney and bladder carcinogenesis in rats ingesting N-ethyl-N-hydroxyethylnitrosamine or N-butyl-N-(4-hydroxybutyl)nitrosamine. *Carcinogenesis* 1981;2(10):1033–1037.
137. Nogueira E. Rat renal carcinogenesis after chronic simultaneous exposure to lead acetate and N-nitrosodiethylamine. *Virchows Arch [B]* 1987;53:365–374.
138. Krech R, Zerban H, Bannasch P. Mitochondrial anomalies in renal oncocytes induced in rat by N-nitrosomorpholine. *Eur J Cell Biol* 1981;25:331–339.
139. Mayer D, Weber E, Kadenbach B, Bannasch P. Immunocytochemical demonstration of cytochrome c oxidase as a marker for renal oncocytes and oncocytomas. *Toxicol Pathol* 1989;17:46–49.
140. Nogueira E, Bannasch P. Histogenese von onkocytaeren und klarzelligen Nierentumoren der Ratte. *Verh Dtsch Ges Pathol* 1987;71:562.
141. Nogueira E, Bannasch P. Cellular origin of rat renal oncocytoma. *Lab Invest* 1988;59:337–343.
142. Nogueira E, Klimek F, Weber E, Bannasch P. Collecting duct origin of rat renal clear cell tumours. *Virchows Arch [B]* 1989;57:275–283.
143. Ohmori T, Hiasa Y, Murata Y, Williams GM. Gamma glutamyl transpeptidase activity in carcinogen-induced epithelial lesions of rat kidney. *GANN* 1982;73:543–548.
144. Hirono I, Laqueur GL, Spatz M. Tumor induction in Fischer and Osborne-Mendel rats by a single administration of cycasin. *J Natl Cancer Inst* 1968;40:1003–1010.
145. Hirono I, Laqueur GL, Spatz M. Transplantability of cycasin-induced tumors in rats, with emphasis on nephroblastomas. *J Natl Cancer Inst* 1968;40:1011–1025.
146. Hirono I, Shibuya C, Fushimi K. Tumor induction in C57BL/6 mice by a single administration of cycasin. *Cancer Res* 1969;29:1658–1662.
147. Hirono I, Hayashi K, Mori H, Miwa T. Carcinogenic effects of cycasin in Syrian golden hamsters and the transplantability of induced tumors. *Cancer Res* 1971;31:283–287.
148. Hirono I. Carcinogenicity and neurotoxicity of cycasin with special reference to species differences. *Fed Proc* 1972;31(5):1493–1499.
149. Toth B. 1,1-Dimethylhydrazine (unsymmetrical) carcinogenesis in mice: light microscopic and ultrastructural studies on neoplastic blood vessels. *J Natl Cancer Inst* 1973;50:181–194.
150. Montesano R, Mohr U, Magee PN, Hilfrich J, Haas H. Additive effect in the induction of kidney tumours in rats treated with dimethylnitrosamine and ethylmethanesulphonate. *Br J Cancer* 1974;29:50–58.
151. Dees JH, Reuber MD, Trump BF. Adenocarcinoma of the kidney. I. Ultrastructure of renal adenocarcinomas induced in rats by N-(4′-fluoro-4-biphenylyl)acetamide. *J Natl Cancer Inst* 1976;57:779–794.
152. Tanner DC, Lipsky MM. Effect of lead acetate on N-(4′-fluoro-4-biphenyl)acetamide induced renal carcinogenesis in the rat. *Carcinogenesis* 1984;5(9):1109–1113.

153. Price JM, Morris JE, Lalich JJ. Evaluation of the carcinogenic activity of 5-nitro-furan derivatives in the rat. *Fed Proc* 1966;25:419.
154. Stein RJ, Yost D, Petroliunas F, et al. Carcinogenic activity of nitrofurans. A histologic evaluation. *Fed Proc* 1966;25:291.
155. Cohen SM, Ertuerk E, Bryan GT. Carcinogenicity of formic acid 2-[4-(5-nitro-2-furyl)-2-thiazolyl]-hydrazide in Swiss mice. *Cancer Res* 1970;30:906–912.
156. Ertuerk E, Cohen SM, Bryan GT. Induction, histogenesis, and isotransplantability of renal tumors induced by formic acid 2-[4-(5-nitro-2-furyl)-2-thiazolyl]hydrazide in rats. *Cancer Res* 1970; 30:2098–2106.
157. Ertuerk E, Price JM, Morris JE, et al. The production of carcinoma of the urinary bladder in rats by feeding N-[4-(5-nitro-2-furyl)-2-thiazolyl]formamide. *Cancer Res* 1967;27:1998–2002.
158. Ertuerk E, Cohen SM, Price JM, et al. Pathogenesis, histology, and transplantability of urinary bladder carcinomas induced in albino rats by oral administration of N-[4-(5-nitro-2-furyl)-2-thiazolyl]formamide. *Cancer Res* 1969;29:2219–2228.
159. Anderstroem C, Johansson SL, von Schultz L. The influence of phenacetin or mechanical perforation on the development of renal pelvic and urinary bladder tumors in FANFT-induced urinary tract carcinogenesis. *Acta Pathol Microbiol Immunol Scand Sect A* 1983;91:373–380.
160. Cohen MS, Murasaki G, Fukuschima S, Greenfield RE. Effect of regenerative hyperplasia on the urinary bladder: carcinogenicity of sodium saccharin and N-[4-(5-Nitro-2-furyl)-2-thiazolyl] formamide. *Cancer Res* 1982;42:65–71.
161. Jacobs JA, Arai M, Cohen SM, Friedell GH. A long-term study of reversible and progressive urinary bladder cancer lesions in rats fed N-[4-(5-nitro-2-furyl)-2-thiazolyl]formamide. *Cancer Res* 1977;37:2817–2821.
162. Alden CL. A review of unique male rat hydrocarbon nephropathy. *Toxicol Pathol* 1986;14(1):109–111.
163. Swenberg JA, Short BG, Borghoff SJ, Strasser J, Charbonneau M. The comparative pathobiology of alpha2-microglobulin nephropathy. *Toxicol Appl Pharmacol* 1989;97:35–46.
164. Borghoff SJ, Short BG, Swenberg JA. Biochemical mechanisms and pathobiology of alpha2-microglobulin nephropathy. *Annu Rev Pharmacol Toxicol* 1990;30:349–367.
165. Burnett VL, Short BG, Swenberg JA. Localization of alpha2-microglobulin within protein droplets of male rat kidney: immunohistochemistry using perfusion-fixed, GMA-embedded tissue sections. *J Histochem Cytochem* 1989;37:813–818.
166. Dietrich DR, Swenberg JA. NCI-Black-Reiter (NBR) male rats fail to develop renal disease following exposure to agents that induce α-2μ-globulin ($\alpha_{2\mu}$) nephropathy. *Fundam Appl Toxicol* 1991;16:749–762.
167. Bulay O, Clayson DB, Shubik P. Carcinogenic effects of niridazole in rats. *Cancer Lett* 1978; 4:305–310.
168. Bulay O, Patil K, Wilson R, Shubik P. Kidney tumors induced in rats by the antischistosomal drug niridazole. *Cancer Res* 1979;39:4996–5002.
169. Sternberg SS, Philips FS, Cronin AP. Renal tumors and other lesions in rats following a single intravenous injection of daunomycin. *Cancer Res* 1972;32:1029–1036.
170. Mao P, Molnar JJ. The fine structure and histochemistry of lead-induced renal tumours in rats. *Am J Pathol* 1967;50:571–603.
171. Rossman TG. Effect of metals on mutagenesis and DNA repair. *Environ Health Perspect* 1981; 40:189–195.
172. Choie DD, Richter GW. Cell proliferation in kidney induced by lead. I. Synthesis of deoxyribonucleic acid. *Lab Invest* 1974;30(5):647–651.
173. Choie DD, Richter GW. Cell proliferation in mouse kidney induced by lead. II. Synthesis of ribonucleic acid and protein. *Lab Invest* 1974;30(5):652–656.
174. Gerber GB, Leonard AM, Jacquet P. Toxicity, mutagenicity and teratogenicity of lead. *Mutat Res* 1980;76:15–141.
175. Liehr JG, Ballatore AM, McLachlan JA, Sirbasku DA. Mechanism of diethylstilbestrol carcinogenicity as studied with the fluorinated analogue E-3′,3″,5′,5″-tetrafluorodiethylstilbestrol. *Cancer Res* 1983;43:2678–2682.
176. Li JJ, Cuthbertson TL, Li SA. Inhibition of estrogen tumorigenesis in the Syrian golden hamster kidney by antiestrogens. *J Natl Cancer Inst* 1980;64:795–800.
177. Li JJ, Li SA. Estrogen-induced tumorigenesis in hamsters: roles for hormonal and carcinogenic activities. *Arch Toxicol* 1984;55:110–118.

178. Lin YC, Loring JM, Villee CA. Permissive role of the pituitary in the induction and growth of estrogen-dependent renal tumors. *Cancer Res* 1982;42:1015–1019.
179. Liehr JG, Wheeler WJ. Inhibition of estrogen-induced renal carcinoma in Syrian hamsters by vitamin C. *Cancer Res* 1983;43:4638–4642.
180. Oberley TD, Lauchner LJ, Pugh TD, et al. Specific estrogen-induced cell proliferation of cultured Syrian hamster renal proximal tubular cells in serum-free chemically defined media. *Proc Natl Acad Sci USA* 1989;86:2107–2111.
181. Liehr JG, Gladek A, Macatee T, Randerath E, Randerath K. DNA adduct formation in liver and kidney of male Syrian hamsters treated with estrogen and/or α-naphthoflavone. *Carcinogenesis* 1991;1263:385–389.
182. Marquardt RR, Frohlich A, Abramson D. Ochratoxin A: an important western Canadian storage mycotoxin. *Can J Physiol Pharmacol* 1990;68:991–999.
183. Bendele AM, Carlton WW, Krogh P, Lilehoj EB. Ochratoxin A carcinogenesis in the (C57BL/6J × C3H)F_1 mouse. *J Natl Cancer Inst* 1985;75:733–742.
184. Yeulet SE. *Penicillium nephrotoxin and associated metabolites in the etiology of Balkan endemic nephropathy (BEN)*. Ph.D-thesis, University of London, UK; 1986.
185. Epstein SM, Bartus B, Farber E. Renal epithelial neoplasms induced in male Wistar rats by oral aflatoxin B_1. *Cancer Res* 1969;29:1045–1050.
186. Leak LV, Rosen VJ. Early ultrastructural alterations in proximal tubular cells after unilateral nephrectomy and X-irradiation. *J Ultrastruct Res* 1966;15:326–348.
187. Rosen VJ, Castanera TJ, Kimeldorf DJ, Jones DC. Renal neoplasms in the irradiated and nonirradiated Sprague-Dawley rat. *Renal Neoplasm* 1961;38(3):359–369.
188. Kurokawa Y, Takamura N, Matushima Y, Imayawa T, Hayashi Y. Promoting effect of peroxisome proliferators in two-stage rat renal tumorigenesis. *Cancer Lett* 1988;43:145–149.
189. Shirai T, Ohshima M, Masuda A, Tamano S, Ito N. Promotion of 2-(ethylnitrosamino)ethanol-induced renal carcinogenesis in rat by nephrotoxic compounds: positive responses with folic acid, basic lead acetate, and N-(3,5-dichlorophenyl)succinimide but not with 2,3-di-bromo-1-propanol phosphate. *J Natl Cancer Inst* 1984;72:477–482.
190. Shinohara Y, Arai M, Hirao K, Sugihara S, Nakanishi K, Tsumoda H, Ito N. Combination effect of citrinin and other chemicals on rat kidney tumourigenesis. *GANN* 1976;67:147–155.
191. Hiasa Y, Enoki N, Kitahori Y, Konishi N, Shimoyama T. DL-serine: promoting activity on renal tumourigenesis by N-ethyl-N-hydroxyethylnitrosamine in rats. *J Natl Cancer Inst* 1984;73:297–299.
192. Hagiwara A, Diwan BA, Ward JM. Barbital sodium, a tumor promoter for kidney tubules, urinary bladder, and liver of the F344 rat, induces persistent increases in levels of DNA synthesis in renal tubules but not in urinary bladder epithelium or hepatocytes. *Fundam Appl Toxicol* 1989;13:332–340.
193. Weisburger EK. Carcinogenicity studies on halogenated hydrocarbons. *Environ Health Perspect* 1977;21:7–16.
194. Jorgenson TA, Meierhenry EF, Rushbrook CJ, Bull RJ, Robinson M. Carcinogenicity of chloroform in drinking water to male Osborne-Mendel rats and female B6C3F1 mice. *Fundam Appl Toxicol* 1985;5:760–769.
195. Alden CL, Kanerva RL. The pathogenesis of renal cortical tumours in rats fed 2% trisodium nitrilotriacetate monohydrate. *Food Chem Toxic* 1982;20:441–490.
196. Alden Cl, Kanerva RL. Reversibility of renal cortical lesions induced in rats by high doses of nitrilotriacetate monohydrate. *Food Chem Toxic* 1982;20:935–937.
197. Myers MC, Kanerva RL, Alden CL, Anderson RL. Reversibility of nephrotoxicity induced in rats by nitrilotriacetate in subchronic feeding studies. *Food Chem Toxic* 1982;20:925–934.
198. Reznik G, Ward JM, Hardisty JF, Russfield A. Renal carcinogenic and nephrotoxic effects of the flame retardant tris(2,3-dibromopropyl)phosphate in F344 rats and (C57BL/6N × C3H/HcN)F_1 mice. *J Natl Cancer Inst* 1979;63:205–212.
199. Reznik G, Reznik-Schueller HM, Rice JM, Hague BF. Pathogenesis of toxic and neoplastic renal lesions induced by the flame retardant tris(2,3-dibromopropyl)phosphate in F344 rats, and development of colonic adenomas after prolonged oral administration. *Lab Invest* 1981;44(1):74–83.
200. National Toxicology Program. Toxicology and carcinogenesis of C.I. acid orange 3 in F344 rats and B6C3F1 mice. *Technical Report No 335* 1988.
201. Reichert D, Spengler U, Romen W, Henschler D. Carcinogenicity of dichloroacetylene: an inhalation study. *Carcinogenesis* 1984;5(11):1411–1420.

202. Vesselinovitch SD, Mihailovitch N. The development of neurogenic neoplasms, embryonal kidney tumors, Harderian gland adenomas, Anitschkow cell sarcomas of the heart, and other neoplasms in urethane treated newborne rats. *Cancer Res* 1968;28:888–897.
203. Kurokawa Y, Maekawa A, Takahashi M, Hayashi Y. Toxicity and carcinogenicity of potassium bromate—a new renal carcinogen. *Environ Health Perspect* 1990;87:309–335.
204. Swenberg JA, Fedtke N, Fennell TR, Walker VE. Relationships between carcinogen exposure, DNA adducts and carcinogenesis. In: Clayson DB, Munro IC, Shubik P, Swenberg JA eds. *Progress in predictive toxicology*. Amsterdam: Elsevier, 1990;161–184.
205. Balmain A, Brown K. Oncogene activation in chemical carcinogenesis. *Adv Cancer Res* 1988; 51:147–182.
206. Pitot HC, Goldsworthy T, Moran S. The natural history of carcinogenesis: implications of experimental carcinogenesis in the genesis of human cancer. *J Supramol Struct Cell Biochem* 1981; 17:133–146.
207. Barrett JC, Wiseman RW. Cellular and molecular mechanisms of multistep carcinogenesis; relevance to carcinogen risk assessment. *Environ Health Perspect* 1987;76:65–70.
208. Farber E, Sarma DRS. Hepatocarcinogenesis: a dynamic cellular perspective. *Lab Invest* 1987; 56:4–22.
209. Knudson AG. A two-mutation model for human cancer. In: Klein G ed. *Advances in viral oncology*, vol. 7. New York: Raven Press, 1987;1–17.
210. Cerutti PA. Commentary: response modification creates promotability in multistage carcinogenesis. *Carcinogenesis* 1988;9(4):519–526.
211. Swenberg JA, Richardson FC, Boucheron JA, Deal FH, Belinsky SA, Charbonneau M, Short BG. High- to low-dose extrapolation: critical determinants involved in the dose response of carcinogenic substances. *Environ Health Perspect* 1987;76:57–63.
212. Swann PF, Kaufman DG, Magee PN, Mace R. Induction of kidney tumours by a single dose of dimethylnitrosamine: dose response and influence of diet and benzo(a)pyrene pretreatment. *Br J Cancer* 1980;41:285–294.
213. Peto R, Gray R, Brantom P, Grasso P. Nitrosamine carcinogenesis in 5120 rodents: chronic administration of sixteen different concentrations of NDEA, NDMA, NPXR and NPIP in water of 4440 inbred rats with parallel studies in NDEA alone of the effect of age at starting (3, 6, or 20 weeks) and of species (rats, mice or hamsters). *IARC Sci Publ* 1984;57:627–665.
214. Swann PF, McLean AEM. The effect of diet on toxic and carcinogenic action of dimethylnitrosamine. *Biochem J* 1968;107:14–15.
215. Swann PF. Why do O^6-alkylguanine and O^4-alkylthymine miscode? The relationship between the structure of DNA containing O^6-alkylguanine and O^4-alkylthymine and the mutagenic properties of these bases. *Mutat Res* 1990;233:81–94.
216. Nicoll JW, Swann PF, Pegg AE. Effect of dimethylnitrosamine on persistence of methylated guanines in rat liver and kidney DNA. *Nature* 1975;254:261–262.
217. Goth R, Rajewsky MF. Persistence of O^6-ethylguanine in rat-brain DNA: correlation with nervous system specific carcinogenesis by ethylnitrosourea. *Proc Natl Acad Sci USA* 1974;71(3):639–643.
218. Kleihues P, Margison GP. Brief communication: carcinogenicity of N-methyl-N-nitrosourea: possible role of excision repair of O^6-methylguanine from DNA. *J Natl Cancer Inst* 1974;53:1839–1841.
219. Pegg AE. Properties of mammalian O^6-alkylguanine-DNA transferases. *Mutat Res* 1990;233:165–175.
220. Short BG, Burnett VL, Cox MG, Bus JS, Swenberg JA. Site-specific renal cytotoxicity and cell proliferation in male rats exposed to petroleum hydrocarbons. *Lab Invest* 1987;57:564–577.
221. Loeb LA. Endogenous carcinogenesis: molecular oncology into the twenty-first century—presidential address. *Cancer Res* 1989;49:5489–5496.
222. Swenberg JA, Short BG. Influence of cytotoxicity on the induction of tumors. In: Butterworth BE, Slaga TJ eds. *Nongenotoxic mechanisms of carcinogenesis*. Cold Spring Harbor, NY: Banbury Report, 1987;25:151–161.
223. Ridder GM, van Bargen EC, Alden CL, Parker RD. Increased hyaline droplet formation in male rats exposed to decalin is dependent on the presence of $\alpha_{2\mu}$-globulin. *Fundam Appl Toxicol* 1990;15:732–743.
224. Chatterjee B, Demyan WF, Song CS, Garg BD, Roy AK. Loss of androgenic induction of $\alpha_{2\mu}$-globulin gene family in the liver of NIH-Black rats. *Endocrinology* 1989;125:1385–1388.
225. Roy AK, Neuhaus OW, Harmison CR. Preparation and characterization of a sex-dependent rat urinary protein. *Biochim Biophys Acta* 1966;127:72–81.

226. Neuhaus OW, Leserth DS. Dietary control of the renal reabsorption and excretion of $\alpha_{2\mu}$-globulin. *Kidney Int* 1979;16:409–415.
227. Maack T, Park CH, Camargo MJF. Renal filtration, transport, and metabolism of proteins. In; Seldin PW, Giebisch G eds. *The kidney: physiology and pathophysiology*. New York: Raven Press 1985;1773–1803.
228. Charbonneau MJ, Strasser J, Borghoff SJ, Swenberg JA. In vitro hydrolysis of [$_{14}$C]-alpha2-microglobulin isolated from male rat kidney. *Toxicologist* 1988;8:537.
229. Lehman-McKeeman LD, Rivera-Torres MI, Caudill D. Lysosomal degradation of alpha2-microglobulin and alpha2-microglobulin-xenobiotic conjugates. *Toxicol Appl Pharmacol* 1990;103:539–548.
230. Short BG. *Unleaded gasoline renal carcinogenesis in rats*. Ph.D-thesis, University of North Carolina, 1988.
231. Short BG, Burnett VL, Swenberg JA. Elevated proliferation of proximal tubule cells and localization of accumulated $\alpha_{2\mu}$-globulin in F344 rats during chronic exposure to unleaded gasoline or 2,2,4-trimethylpentane. *Toxicol Appl Pharmacol* 1989;101.414–431.
232. Short BG, Burnett VL, Swenberg JA. Histopathology and cell proliferation induced by 2,2,4-trimethylpentane in the male rat kidney. *Toxicol Pathol* 1986;14:194–203.
233. Anderson RL, Alden CL, Merski JA. The effects of nitrilotriacetate on cation disposition and urinary tract toxicity. *Food Chem Toxicol* 1982;20:105–122.
234. Alden CL, Kanerva RL, Anderson RL, Adkins AG. Short-term effects of dietary nitrilotriacetic acid in the male Charles River rat kidney. *Vet Pathol* 1981;18:549–559.
235. Hiasa Y, Kitahori Y, Konishi N, Enoki N, Shimoyama T, Miyashiro A. Trisodium nitrilotriacetate monohydrate: promoting effects on the development of renal tubular cell tumors in rats treated with N-ethyl-N-hydroxyethylnitrosamine. *J Natl Cancer Inst* 1984;72:483–489.
236. Hiasa Y, Kitahori Y, Konishi N, Shimoyama T. Dose-related effect of trisodium nitrilotriacetate monohydrate on renal tumorigenesis initiated with N-ethyl-N-hydroxyethylnitrosamine in rats. *Carcinogenesis* 1985;6:907–910.
237. Miyashiro A. Promoting effect of trisodium nitrilotriacetate monohydrate on the development of tumors in kidneys and urinary bladders of rats treated with N-ethyl-N-hydroxyethylnitrosamine or N-butyl-N-(4-hydroxybutyl)nitrosamine. *J Nara Med Ass* 1984;35:550–565.
238. LeBoef RA, Kerckaert GA, Aardema MJ, Poiley JA, Raineri R. Enhanced morphological and neoplastic transformation of Syrian hamster embryo cells cultured at pH 6.70. In: Mendelsohn ML, Albertini RJ, eds. *Mutation and the environment, part D: carcinogenesis*, vol 340. New York: John Wiley, 1990;219–228.
239. LeBoef RA, Thompson ED, Kerckaert GA, Reeder BA, Putman DL, Morris MJ. Genotoxicity of zinc chelates of nitrilotriacetic acid (NTA) and EDTA. *Environ Mol Mutagen* 1990;15:117.
240. Knudson AG. Hereditary cancer, oncogenes and antioncogenes. *Cancer Res* 1985;45:1437–1443.
241. Huff V, Compton DA, Chao L, Strong LC, Geiser CF, Saunders GF. Lack of linkage of familial Wilms' tumour to chromosomal band 11p13. *Nature* 1988;336:377–378.
242. Grundy P, Koufos A, Morgan K, Li FP, Meadows AT, Cavanee WK. Familial predisposition to Wilms' tumour does not map to the short arm of chromosome 11. *Nature* 1988;336:374–376.
243. Jeanpierre C, Antignac C, Beroud C, Lavedan C, Henry I, Saunders G, Williams B, Glaser T, Junien C. Constitutional and somatic deletions of two different regions of maternal chromosome 11 in Wilms' tumor. *Genomics* 1990;7:434–438.
244. Compton DA, Weil MM, Bonetta L, et al. Definition of the limits of the Wilms' tumor locus on human chromosome 11p13. *Genomics* 1990;6:309–315.
245. Call KM, Glaser T, Ito CY, et al. Isolation and characterization of a zinc finger polypeptide gene at the human chromosome 11 Wilms' tumor locus. *Cell* 1990;60:509–520.
246. Gessler M, Poustka A, Cavanee W, Neve RL, Orkin SH, Bruns GAP. Homozygous deletion in Wilms tumours of a zinc-finger gene identified by chromosome jumping. *Nature* 1990;343:774–778.
247. Maher ER, Yates JRW, Ferguson-Smith MA. Statistical analysis of the two stage mutation model in von Hippel-Lindau disease, and in sporadic cerebellar haemangioblastoma and renal cell carcinoma. *J Med Genet* 1990;27:311–314.
248. Seizinger BR, Rouleau GA, Ozelius LJ, et al. Von Hippel-Lindau disease maps to the region of chromosome 3 associated with renal cell carcinoma. *Nature* 1988;332:268–269.
249. King CR, Schimke RN, Arthur T, Davoren B, Collins D. Proximal 3p deletion in renal cell carcinoma cells from a patient with von Hippel-Lindau disease. *Cancer Genet Cytogenet* 1987;27:345–348.

250. Maher ER, Yates JRW, Harries R, Benjamin C, Harris R, Moore AT, Ferguson-Smith MA. Clinical features and natural history of von Hippel-Lindau disease. *Q J Med* 1990;77(283):1151–1163.
251. Cohen AJ, Li FP, Berg S, Marchetto DJ, Tsai S, Jacobs SC, Brown RS. Hereditary renal cell carcinoma associated with a chromosomal translocation. *N Engl J Med* 1979;301:592–595.
252. Outzen HC, Maguire HC. The etiology of renal cell carcinoma. *Semin Oncol* 1983;10(4):378–384.
253. Levinson AK, Johnson DE, Strong LC, Pathak S, Huff V, Saunders GF. Familial renal cell carcinoma: hereditary or coincidental? *J Urol* 1990;144:849–851.
254. Zbar B, Brauch H, Talmadge C, Linehan M. Loss of alleles of loci on the short arm of chromosome 3 in renal cell carcinoma. *Nature* 1987;327:721–724.
255. Walter TA, Berger CS, Sandberg AA. The cytogenetics of renal tumors: where do we stand, where do we go? *Cancer Genet Cytogenet* 1989;43:15–34.
256. Eker R. Familial renal adenomas in Wistar rats. *Acta Pathol Microbiol Scand* 1954;34:554–562.
257. Eker R, Mossige J. A dominant gene for renal adenomas in the rat. *Nature* 1961;189:858–859.
258. Funaki K, Knudson AG, Freed JJ, Everitt J, Walker C. Hereditary renal cell carcinoma in the rat associated with nonrandom loss of chromosomes 5 and 6. *Proc Am Assoc Cancer Res* 1991;32: 305.
259. Walker C, Everitt J, Freed JJ, Knudson AG, Whiteley LO. Altered expression of transforming growth factor-α in rat hereditary renal cell carcinoma. *Cancer Res* 1991;51(11):2973–2978.
260. Mydlo JH, Michaeli J, Cordon-Cardo C, Goldenberg AS, Heston WDW, Fair WR. Expression of transforming growth factor α and epidermal growth factor receptor messenger RNA in neoplastic and nonneoplastic human kidney tissue. *Cancer Res* 1989;49:3407–3411.
261. Gomella LG, Sargent ER, Wade TP, Anglard P, Linehan WM, Kasid A. Expression of transforming growth factor α in normal human adult kidney and enhanced expression of transforming growth factors α and β_1 in renal cell carcinoma. *Cancer Res* 1989;49:6972–6975.
262. Petrides PE, Bock S, Bovens S, Hofmann R, Jakse G. Modulation of pro-epidermal growth factor, pro-transforming growth factor α and epidermal growth factor receptor gene expression in human renal cell carcinomas. *Cancer Res* 1990;50:3934–3939.
263. Jasmin G, Cha J. Renal adenomas induced in rats by dimethylnitrosamine. An electron microscopic study. *Arch Pathol* 1969;87:267–278.
264. Jasmin G, Riopelle J. Renal adenomas induced by dimethylnitrosamine. Enzyme histochemistry in the rat. *Arch Pathol* 1968;85:298–305.
265. McGiven A, Ireton H. Renal epithelial dysplasia and neoplasia in rats given dimethylnitrosamine. *J Pathol* 1972;108:187–190.
266. Diwan BA, Rice JM, Ohschima M, Ward JM, Dove LF. Comparative tumor-promoting activities of phenobarbital, amobarbital, barbital sodium, and barbituric acid on livers and other organs of male F344/NCr rats following initiation with N-nitrosodiethylamine. *J Natl Cancer Inst* 1985; 74(2):509–516.
267. Mohr U, Hilfrich J. Brief communication: effect of a single dose of N-diethylnitrosamine on the rat kidney. *J Natl Cancer Inst* 1972;49:1729–1731.
268. Druckrey H, Steinhoff D, Preussmann R, Ivankovic S. Erzeugung von Krebs durch eine einmaliage Dosis von Methylnitroso-Harnstoff und verschiedenen Dialkylnitrosaminen an Ratten. *Z Krebsforsch* 1964;66:1–10.
269. Nakanishi K, Fukushima S, Shibata M, Shirai T, Ogiso T, Ito N. Effect of phenacetin and caffeine on the urinary bladder of rats treated with N-butyl-N-(4-hydroxybutyl)nitrosamine. *GANN* 1978; 69:395–400.
270. Hiasa Y, Ohshima M, Iwata C, Tanikake T. Histopathological studies on renal tubular cell tumors in rats treated with N-ethyl-N-hydroxyethylnitrosamine. *GANN* 1979;70:817–820.
271. Hiasa Y, Enoki N, Kitahori Y, Konishi N, Shimoyama T. DL-Serine: promoting activity on renal tumorigenesis by N-ethyl-N-hydroxyethylnitrosamine in rats. *J Natl Cancer Inst* 1984;73(1):297–299.
272. Hiasa Y, Ohshima M, Kitahori Y, Fujita T, Yuasa T, Miyashiro A. Basic lead acetate: promoting effect on the development of renal tubular cell tumors in rats treated with N-ethyl-N-hydroxyethylnitrosamine. *J Natl Cancer Inst* 1983;70(4):761–765.
273. Kurata Y, Tsuda H, Sakata T, Yamashita T, Ito N. Reciprocal modifying effects of isomeric forms of aminophenol on induction of neoplastic lesions in rat liver and kidney initiated by N-ethyl-N-hydroxyethylnitrosamine. *Carcinogenesis* 1987;8(9):1281–1285.
274. Hirose M, Shirai T, Tsuda H, Fukushima S, Ogiso T, Ito N. Effect of phenobarbital, polychlorinated biphenyl and sodium saccharin on hepatic and renal carcinogenesis in unilaterally nephrec-

tomized rats given N-ethyl-N-hydroxyethylnitrosamine orally. *Carcinogenesis* 1981;2(12):1299–1302.
275. Kurokawa Y, Takahashi M, Kokubo T, Ohno Y, Hayashi Y. Enhancement by potassium bromate of renal tumorigenesis initiated by N-ethyl-N-hydroxyethylnitrosamine in F-344 rats. *GANN* 1983;74:607–610.
276. Ohshima M. N-ethyl-N-hydroxyethylnitrosamine studies on the development of renal cell tumors in rats by N-ethyl-N-hydroxyethylnitrosamine. *J Nara Med Ass* 1980;31:361–378.
277. Terracini B, Testa MC. Carcinogenicity of a single administration of N-nitrosomethylurea: a comparison between new-born and 5-week-old mice and rats. *Br J Cancer Res* 1970;24:588–598.
278. Bannasch P, Mayer D, Krech R. Neoplastische und praeneoplastische Veraenderungen bei Ratten nach einmaliger oraler Applikation von N-Nitrosomorpholin. *J Cancer Res Clin Oncol* 1979;94: 233–248.
279. Uchida E, Hirono I. Effect of phenobarbital on the development of neoplastic lesions in the liver of cycasin-treated rats. *J Cancer Res Clin Oncol* 1981;100:231–238.
280. Williams PD, Murphy GP. Dose related effects of cycasin induced renal and hepatic tumors. *Res Commun Chem Pathol Pharmacol* 1971;264:627–632.
281. Gusek W, Mestwerdt W. Cycasin-induzierte Nierentumoren bei der Wistarratte unter besonderer Beruecksichtigung der Adenome. *Beitr Pathol Anat* 1969;139:199–218.
282. Bleasel AF, Yong LCJ. Streptozotocin induced diabetic nephropathy and renal tumors in the rat. *Experientia* 1982;38:129–130.
283. Rakieten N, Gordon BS. Metastatic renal adenocarcinoma produced by streptozotocin. *Cancer Chemother Rep* 1975;59(5):891–892.
284. Mauer SM, Lee CS, Najarian JS, Brown DM. Induction of malignant kidney tumors in rats with streptozotocin. *Cancer Res* 1974;34:158–160.
285. Kitchen DN. Neoplastic renal effects of unleaded gasoline in Fischer 344 rats. In: Mehlman MA, eds. *Renal effects of petroleum hydrocarbons*. Princeton, NJ: Princeton Sci, 1984;65–71.
286. MacFarland HN, Ulrich CE, Hodsworth CE, Kitchen DN, Halliwell WH, Blum SC. A chronic inhalation study with unleaded gasoline vapor. *J Am Coll Toxicol* 1984;3(4):231–248.
287. National Toxicology Program. Carcinogenesis studies of 1,4-dichlorobenzene in F-344/N rats and B6C3F1 mice. *Tech Rep No 319*, 1987.
288. National Toxicology Program. Toxicology and carcinogenesis studies of hexachloroethane in F-344/N rats. *Tech Rep No 361*, 1989.
289. National Toxicology Program. Carcinogenesis bioassay of pentachloroethane in F-344/N rats and B6C3F1 mice. *Tech Rep No 232*,1983.
290. National Toxicology Program. Carcinogenesis bioassay of tetrachloroethylene (perchloroethylene) in F-344/N rats and B6C3F1 mice. *Tech Rep No 311*, 1986.
291. National Toxicology Program. Carcinogenesis studies of isophorone in F-344/N rats and B6C3F1 mice. *Tech Rep No 291*, 1986.
292. National Toxicology Program. Carcinogenesis studies of dimethylmethylphosphonate in F-344/N rats and B6C3F1 mice. *Tech Rep No 323*, 1987.
293. National Toxicology Program. Carcinogenesis studies of d-limonene in F-344/N rats and B6C3F1 mice. *Tech Rep No 347*, 1990.
294. Johansson SL, Radio SJ, Saidi J, Sakata T. The effects of acetaminophen, antipyrine and phenacetin on rat urothelial cell proliferation. *Carcinogenesis* 1989;10(1):105–111.
295. Hinton DE, Lipsky MM, Heatfield BM, Trump BF. Opposite effects of lead on chemical carcinogenesis in kidney and liver of rats. *Bull Environ Contam Toxicol* 1979;23:464–469.
296. Koller LD, Kerkuliet NI, Exon JH. Neoplasia induced in male rats fed lead acetate, ethylurea, and sodium nitrite. *Toxicol Pathol* 1985;13(1):50–57.
297. Arai M, Hibino T. Tumorigenicity of citrinin in male F344 rats. *Cancer Lett* 1983;17:281–287.
298. Merkow LP, Epstein S, Slifkin M, Pardo M. The ultrastructure of renal neoplasms induced by aflatoxin B_1. *Cancer Res* 1973;33:1608–1614.
299. Kurokawa Y, Matushima Y, Takamura N, Imazawa T, Hayashi Y. Relationship between the curation of treatment and the incidence of renal cell tumors in male F344 rats administered potassium bromate. *J Cancer Res (GANN)* 1987;78:358–364.
300. Kurokawa Y, Hayashi Y, Maekawa A, Takahashi M, Kokubo T. Induction of renal cell tumors in F-344 rats by oral administration of potassium bromate, a food additive. *GANN* 1982;73:335–338.
301. Hard GC. Tumours of the kidney, renal pelvis and ureter. In: Turusov VS, ed. *Pathology of tumors in laboratory animals—tumours of the rat*, vol 1, part 2. Lyon: IARC, 1976;73.

Subject Index

S